PSYCHIATRIC SECRETS

Second Edition

JAMES L. JACOBSON, MD
Associate Professor
Department of Psychiatry
University of Vermont Medical School
Burlington, Vermont

ALAN M. JACOBSON, MD
Professor
Department of Psychiatry
Harvard Medical School
Senior Vice President
Strategic Initiatives
Joslin Diabetes Center
Boston, Massachusetts

HANLEY & BELFUS, INC. / Philadelphia

Publisher: HANLEY & BELFUS, INC.
                  Medical Publishers
                  210 South 13th Street
                  Philadelphia, PA 19107
                  (215) 546-7293; 800-962-1892
                  FAX (215) 790-9330
                  Web site: http://www.hanleyandbelfus.com

Note *to the reader*: Although the information in this book has been carefully reviewed for correctness of dosage and indications, neither the authors nor the editor nor the publisher can accept any legal responsibility for any errors or omissions that may be made. Neither the publisher nor the editor makes any warranty, expressed or implied, with respect to the material contained herein. Before prescribing any drug, the reader must review the manufacturer's current product information (package inserts) for accepted indications, absolute dosage recommendations, and other information pertinent to the safe and effective use of the product described.

Library of Congress Cataloging-in-Publication Data

Psychiatric secrets / written [i.e. edited] by James L. Jacobson, Alan M. Jacobson.—2nd ed.
        p. ; cm. — (The Secrets Series®)
     Includes bibliographical references and index.
     ISBN 1-56053-418-4 (alk. paper)
        1. Psychiatry—Examinations, questions, etc.   I. Jacobson, James L., 1951–
II. Jacobson, Alan (Alan M.)   III. Series.
     [DNLM: 1. Mental Disorders—diagnosis—Examination Questions.   2. Mental
Disorders—therapy—Examination Questions.   WM 18.2 P9727 2000]
RC457.P76 2001
616.89'0076—dc21

                                                                    00-037043

PSYCHIATRIC SECRETS, 2nd ed.   ISBN 1-56053-418-4

Last digit is the print number: 9   8   7   6   5   4   3   2   1

CONTENTS

Contents

XII. ETHICAL AND LEGAL ISSUES IN PSYCHIATRY

CONTRIBUTORS

C. Alan Anderson, MD
Assistant Professor of Neurology and Emergency Medicine, University of Colorado School of Medicine, Denver; Attending Physician, Denver Veterans Affairs Medical Center, Denver, Colorado

Elissa Mary Ball, MD
Senior Instructor, Department of Psychiatry, University of Colorado Health Sciences Center, Denver; Staff Psychiatrist, Colorado Mental Health Institute, Pueblo, Colorado

Loisa Bennetto, PhD
Assistant Professor, Department of Clinical and Social Sciences in Psychology, University of Rochester, Rochester, New York

Mark A. Blais, PsyD
Assistant Professor, Department of Psychiatry, Harvard Medical School; Associate Chief of Psychology, Massachusetts General Hospital, Boston, Massachusetts

Kerry Lewis Bloomingdale, MD
Instructor, Department of Psychiatry, Harvard Medical School, Boston; Physician, Beth Israel Deaconess Hospital, Boston, Massachusetts

Archie Brodsky, BA
Research Associate, Department of Psychiatry, Harvard Medical School, Boston; Program in Psychiatry and the Law, Massachusetts Mental Health Center, Boston, Massachusetts

Andrew W. Brotman, MD
Clinical Professor and Vice Dean, Department of Psychiatry, New York University School of Medicine, New York, New York

Harold J. Bursztajn, MD
Associate Professor, Department of Psychiatry, Harvard Medical School, Boston; Co-Director, Program in Psychiatry and the Law, Massachusetts Mental Health Center, Boston, Massachusetts

Lester Butt, PhD
Director, Department of Psychology, Craig Hospital, Englewood, Colorado

Randall D. Buzan, MD
Assistant Professor, Director of Outpatient Services, Department of Psychiatry, University of Colorado, Denver, Colorado

Carl Clark, MD
Assistant Clinical Professor, Department of Psychiatry, University of Colorado, Denver, Colorado

S. Tziporah Cohen, MD
Clinical Fellow in Psychiatry, Harvard Medical School, Boston; Fellow in Psychosocial Oncology, Dana Farber Cancer Institute, Boston, Massachusetts

C. Munro Cullum, PhD
Associate Professor, Departments of Psychiatry and Neurology, University of Texas Southwestern Medical Center, Dallas, Texas

Robert D. Davies, MD
Assistant Professor, Department of Psychiatry; Director, Anxiety and Mood Disorders Clinic, University of Colorado Health Sciences Center, Denver, Colorado

William W. Dodson, MD
Assistant Professor, Department of Psychiatry, University of Colorado Health Sciences Center, Denver, Colorado

Jane L. Erb, MD
Instructor, Department of Psychiatry, Harvard Medical School, Boston; Director of Psychopharmacology, Brigham and Women's Hospital, Boston, Massachusetts

Gordon K. Farley, MD
Professor Emeritus of Psychiatry, University of Colorado School of Medicine, Denver, Colorado

Christopher M. Filley, MD
Professor of Neurology and Psychiatry, University of Colorado School of Medicine, Denver; Attending Physician, Denver Veterans Affairs Medical Center, Denver, Colorado

Judith E. Fox, PhD
Assistant Clinical Professor, Department of Psychiatry, University of Colorado Health Sciences Center; Assistant Professor of Psychology, University of Denver, Graduate School of Professional Psychology, Denver, Colorado

Michael H. Gendel, MD
Associate Clinical Professor of Psychiatry, University of Colorado Health Sciences Center; Medical Director, Colorado Physicians' Health Program, Denver, Colorado

Alexis A. Giese, MD
Associate Professor, Department of Psychiatry, University of Colorado Health Sciences Center, Denver, Colorado

Benjamin P. Green, MD
Assistant Clinical Professor of Psychiatry, University of Colorado School of Medicine; Private Practice (psychiatry), Denver, Colorado

Doris C. Gundersen, MD
Assistant Professor, Department of Psychiatry, University of Colorado Health Sciences Center, Denver, Colorado

Frederick B. Hebert, MD, FAACAP, FAPA
Associate Professor, Department of Psychiatry, University of Colorado Health Sciences Center, Denver; Former Associate Director, Psychiatric Services, Denver General Hospital, Denver, Colorado

Robert M. House, MD
Associate Professor, Department of Psychiatry, University of Colorado Health Sciences Center, Denver; Director, Consult/Liaison Psychiatry, Colorado Psychiatric Hospital, Denver, Colorado

Alan M. Jacobson, MD
Professor, Department of Psychiatry, Harvard Medical School, Boston; Senior Vice President, Strategic Health Initiatives, Joslin Diabetes Center, Boston, Massachusetts

James L. Jacobson, MD
Clinical Assistant Professor, Department of Psychiatry, University of Colorado School of Medicine, Denver, Colorado; August 2000—Associate Professor, Department of Psychiatry, University of Vermont College of Medicine, Burlington, Vermont

Robert N. Jamison, PhD
Associate Professor, Departments of Anesthesia and Psychiatry, Harvard Medical School, Boston, Massachusetts

Michael A. Jenike, MD
Professor of Psychiatry, Harvard Medical School, Boston; Associate Chief of Psychiatry Research, Massachusetts General Hospital, Boston, Massachusetts

Michael W. Kahn, MD
Instructor, Department of Psychiatry, Harvard Medical School, Boston, Massachusetts

Jane A. Kennedy, DO
Associate Clinical Professor, Department of Psychiatry, University of Colorado School of Medicine, Denver, Colorado

Steven Kick, MD, MSPH
Associate Professor of Medicine and Psychiatry, University of Colorado Health Sciences Center, Denver, Colorado

Mary Lou Klem, PhD
Assistant Professor, Department of Psychiatry, University of Pittsburgh School of Medicine, Pittsburgh, Pennsylvania

John J. Kluck, MD
Assistant Professor, Department of Psychiatry, University of Colorado Health Sciences Center, Denver, Colorado

Joyce Seiko Kobayashi, MD
Associate Professor, Department of Psychiatry, University of Colorado Health Sciences Center, Denver, Colorado

Lyle Laird, PharmD, BCPP

Andrew B. Littman, MD
Instructor, Department of Psychiatry, Harvard Medical School; Director, Behavioral Medicine Division, Preventive Cardiology, Massachusetts General Hospital, Boston, Massachusetts

Theo C. Manschreck, MD, MPH
Clinical Professor, Consolidated Department of Psychiatry, Harvard Medical School, Fall River; Senior Psychiatrist, Massachusetts General Hospital, Boston, Massachusetts

Harold P. Martin, MD
Associate Professor, Department of Psychiatry, University of Colorado School of Medicine, Denver, Colorado

Mary Jane Massie, MD
Attending Psychiatrist, Memorial Sloan-Kettering Cancer Center, New York; Professor of Clinical Psychiatry, Weill Medical College of Cornell University, New York, New York

Robin April McCann, PhD
Division Chief Psychologist, Institute for Forensic Psychology, Colorado Mental Health Institute, Pueblo, Colorado

John A. Menninger, MD
Assistant Clinical Professor, Department of Psychiatry, University of Colorado Health Sciences Center, Denver, Colorado

Jeffrey L. Metzner, MD
Clinical Professor, Department of Psychiatry, University of Colorado Health Sciences Center, Denver, Colorado

Herbert T. Nagamoto, MD
Associate Professor, Department of Psychiatry, University of Colorado Health Sciences Center, Denver; Staff Physician, Denver Veterans Administration Medical Center, Denver, Colorado

Kim Nagel, MD
Assistant Clinical Professor, Department of Psychiatry, University of Colorado School of Medicine, Denver, Colorado

Deirdre Ann Opp, RPh, BCPP
Instructor, Clinical Pharmacy Practice, University of Colorado School of Pharmacy, Denver, Colorado

Richard L. O'Sullivan, MD
Assistant Professor, Harvard Medical School, Boston; Assistant in Psychiatry, Massachusetts General Hospital, Boston, Massachusetts

William H. Polonsky, PhD
Assistant Clinical Professor, Department of Psychiatry, University of California/San Diego, La Jolla, California

Michael Kenneth Popkin, MD
Professor, Departments of Psychiatry and Medicine, University of Minnesota Medical School, Minneapolis, Minnesota

William H. Redd, MD
Professor, Mt. Sinai School of Medicine, New York; Associate Director, Ruttenberg Cancer Center, Mt. Sinai/New York University Medical School, New York, New York

Martin Reite, MD
Professor, Department of Psychiatry, University of Colorado Health Sciences Center, Denver; Chief, Psychiatry Service, Veterans Affairs Medical Center, Denver, Colorado

Roberta M. Richardson, MD
Assistant Clinical Professor, Department of Psychiatry, University of Colorado Health Sciences Center, Denver, Colorado

Paula DeGraffenreid Riggs, MD
Assistant Professor, Department of Psychiatry, Division of Substance Dependence, University of Colorado School of Medicine, Denver, Colorado

Margaret Roath, MSW, LCSW
Associate Professor, Department of Psychiatry, University of Colorado Health Sciences Center, Denver, Colorado

Sally J. Rogers, PhD
Professor, Department of Psychiatry, University of Colorado Health Sciences Center, Denver, Colorado

Andrew J. Roth, MD
Assistant Professor, Department of Psychiatry, Weill Medical College, Cornell University, New York; Assistant Attending Psychiatrist, Memorial Sloan-Kettering Cancer Center, New York, New York

Jacqueline A. Samson, PhD
Assistant Professor, Department of Psychiatry, Harvard Medical School, Boston; Associate Psychologist, McLean Hospital, Belmont, Massachusetts

Christopher Douglas Schneck, MD
Assistant Professor, Department of Psychiatry; Medical Director, Inpatient Services, University of Colorado Health Sciences Center, Denver, Colorado

Ronald Schouten, MD, JD
Assistant Professor, Department of Psychiatry, Harvard Medical School, Boston, Massachusetts

Stephen R. Shuchter, MD
Professor, Department of Psychiatry, University of California, San Diego, California

Thomas D. Stewart, MD
Associate Clinical Professor, Department of Psychiatry, Yale University; Chairman, Department of Psychiatry, Hospital of St. Raphael, New Haven, Connecticut

Marshall R. Thomas, MD
Associate Professor, Department of Psychiatry, University of Colorado Health Sciences Center, Denver, Colorado

Hubert H. Thomason, Jr, MD
Assistant Clinical Professor, Department of Psychiatry, University of Colorado Health Sciences Center, Denver, Colorado

Laetitia L. Thompson, PhD
Associate Professor, Departments of Psychiatry and Neurology, University of Colorado School of Medicine, Denver, Colorado

Russell G. Vasile, MD
Associate Professor, Department of Psychiatry, Harvard Medical School; Staff Psychiatrist, Beth Israel Deaconess Medical Center, Boston, Massachusetts

Robert Waldinger, MD
Assistant Professor of Psychiatry, Harvard Medical School, Boston; Researcher at Judge Baker Children's Center, Boston, Massachusetts

Myron F. Weiner, MD
Professor, Department of Psychiatry, University of Texas Southwestern Medical Center, Dallas, Texas

Garry Welch, PhD
Investigator and Assistant Professor, Department of Behavioral and Mental Health Research, Joslin Diabetes Center and Harvard Medical School, Boston, Massachusetts

Elizabeth A. Whitmore, PhD
Assistant Professor, Department of Psychiatry, Division of Substance Dependence, University of Colorado School of Medicine, Denver, Colorado

Rena R. Wing, PhD
Professor, Department of Psychiatry and Human Behavior, Brown University School of Medicine, Providence, Rhode Island

Leslie Winter, MD
Resident, Department of Psychiatry, University of Colorado Health Sciences Center, Denver, Colorado

Lawson R. Wulsin, MD
Associate Professor, Departments of Primary Care Psychiatry and Family Medicine, University of Cincinnati College of Medicine, Franciscan Family Practice Center, Cincinnati, Ohio

Claire Zilber, MD
Assistant Professor, Departments of Psychiatry and Internal Medicine, University of Colorado Health Sciences Center, Denver, Colorado

Sidney Zisook, MD
Professor, Department of Psychiatry, University of California, San Diego, California

John Zrebiec, MSW
Lecturer, Department of Psychiatry, Harvard Medical School; Senior Clinical Social Worker, Joslin Diabetes Center, Boston, Massachusetts

Dedication

To our parents
whose support and encouragement
has meant so much to us
throughout our lives

PREFACE TO FIRST EDITION

Psychiatric Secrets presents an up-to-date approach to the assessment and treatment of psychiatric disorders in children, adults, and the elderly. It uses a question and answer format to address key principles in clinical practice in keeping with the concept of *The Secrets Series*®. The questions raise central issues and provide the organizational structure for each chapter. This process of question and answer yields a dialogue through which the expert clinicians who authored each chapter can provide their best "pearls of wisdom" often gained from years of experience as researchers, educators, and practicing clinicians.

Psychiatric Secrets is divided into twelve sections that address in systematic fashion the steps in the treatment process. The book has a heavy emphasis on diagnosis, for it is the belief of the editors that careful, thoughtful diagnosis is the "springboard" to treatment. The first two sections outline a general approach to gathering and presenting clinical information. The next three sections on major psychiatric syndromes and clinical problems focus primarily on issues related to diagnosis, including careful descriptions of common clinical characteristics, etiology, course of illness, and, when appropriate, basic features of treatment. The section devoted to therapeutic approaches presents introductions to both psychotherapeutic and biologic treatments, and includes indications, contraindications, and side effects of interventions. The final section provides integrating information related to common problems and settings, such as child psychiatry, assessment and treatment of suicidal and violent patients, and consultation-liaison psychiatry, as well as ethical and legal aspects of psychiatry.

This text is intended to reinforce concepts for the mental health professional, yet is geared primarily for the medical student, house officer, and general practitioner. The chapters are designed to be read independently, and thus there is occasional overlap of information. Each author was given complete freedom to utilize his or her expertise in expressing views about assessment or treatment. Thus, *Psychiatric Secrets* presents both basic information as well as the approach of experienced practitioners to specific topics.

We are grateful to the authors for contributing their knowledge, time, and talent. In addition, we would like to thank Linda Belfus and Polly E. Parsons, who encouraged us to undertake this project, and the many unsung heroes who typed, re-typed, re-re-typed, critiqued, proofread, and helped us move the book to completion. Without all of their efforts, this book would not have happened.

James L. Jacobson, M.D.
Alan M. Jacobson, M.D.

PREFACE TO SECOND EDITION

Psychiatric Secrets presents an up-to-date approach to the assessment and treatment of psychiatric disorders in children, adults, and the elderly. It uses a question and answer format to address key principles in clinical practice in keeping with the concept of *The Secrets Series*®. The questions raise central issues and provide the organizational structure for each chapter. This process of question and answer yields a dialogue through which the expert clinicians who authored each chapter can provide their best "pearls of wisdom," gained from years of experience as researchers, educators, and practicing clinicians.

This second edition of *Psychiatric Secrets* follows the same general outline and format as the first edition. It is divided into twelve sections that address in systematic fashion the steps in the treatment process. The book heavily emphasizes diagnosis, for it is the belief of the Editors that careful, thoughtful diagnosis is the "springboard" to treatment. The first two sections outline a general approach to gathering and presenting clinical information. The next three sections on major psychiatric syndromes and clinical problems focus primarily on issues related to diagnosis. These sections include careful descriptions of common clinical care characteristics, etiology, course of illness, and basic features of treatment. The section devoted to therapeutic approaches presents introductions to both psychotherapeutic and biologic treatments, and includes indications, contraindications, and side effects of interventions. The final sections provide integrating information related to common problems and settings as well as developmental stages of life. The sections include topics such as child psychiatry, assessment and treatment of suicidal and violent patients, and consultation-liaison psychiatry, as well as ethical and legal aspects of psychiatry.

While the format of the second edition remains largely unchanged, the material in each of the chapters has been updated to take advantage of developments in psychiatry. In particular, those chapters devoted to psychopharmacology have been revised to reflect the rapid advances in treatment. Because of the increasing complexity of the pharmacology of psychiatric disorders, we have added one new chapter that addresses the complex drug interactions now involved in treating patients, especially those with both psychiatric and medical problems.

This text is intended to reinforce concepts for the mental health professional, yet is geared primarily for the medical student, house officer, and general practitioner. The chapters are designed to be read independently; consequently, there is occasional overlap of information. Each author was given complete freedom to utilize his or her expertise in expressing views about assessment and treatment. Thus, *Psychiatric Secrets, 2nd edition* presents both basic information as well as the approach of experienced practitioners to specific topics.

We are grateful to the authors for contributing their knowledge, time, and talent. In addition we would like to thank Linda Belfus and Polly E. Parsons, who encouraged us to undertake the project in the beginning, and Madeleine Jacobson, for her unflagging support through each of our two editions. Moreover, Jacqueline Mahon has played a critical role as our editor for the second edition, and Nora Hallinan has "bird-dogged" this project from beginning to end. Without all of these efforts, this book would not have happened.

Finally, this book has been a special pleasure for the co-editors because it has allowed us to mix the fun and pleasure of our work with that of our brotherly love. It is not an exaggeration to say that the last several years have been a true labor of love.

James L. Jacobson, M.D.
Alan M. Jacobson, M.D.

I. Approach to Clinical Interviewing and Diagnosis

1. THE INITIAL PSYCHIATRIC INTERVIEW

Robert Waldinger, M.D., and Alan M. Jacobson, M.D.

1. What are the primary aims of the first psychiatric interview?

To make an initial differential diagnosis and to formulate a treatment plan. These goals are achieved by:

- Gathering information

Chief complaint	History of current and past suicidal and
History of presenting problem(s)	homicidal ideation
Precipitating factors	Current and past history of victimization
Symptoms	(e.g., domestic violence, child abuse)
Affective	History of psychiatric problems, including
Cognitive	treatment and response
Physical	Social and developmental history
Substance use and abuse	Family psychiatric and social history
Changes in role and social	Mental history
functioning	Medical history

- Arriving at an empathic understanding of how the patient feels. This understanding is a critical base for establishing rapport with the patient. When the clinician listens carefully and then communicates an appreciation of the patient's worries and concerns, the patient gains a sense of being understood. This sense of being understood is the bedrock of all subsequent treatment, and allows the clinician to initiate a relationship in which an alliance for treatment can be established.

2. That's a lot to focus on in the first meeting. What about *helping* the patient?

The initial diagnosis and treatment plan may be rudimentary. Indeed, when patients present in a crisis, the history may be confused, incomplete, or narrowly focused. As a result, some interventions are started even when basic information about history, family relationships, and ongoing stressors is being gathered. It is critical to remember that emotional difficulties often are isolating. The experience of sharing one's problem with a concerned listener can be enormously relieving in and of itself. Thus, the initial interview is the start of treatment even before a formal treatment plan has been established.

3. How should the initial interview be organized?

There is no single ideal, but it is useful to think of the initial interview as having three components:

Establish initial rapport with the patient, and ask about the presenting complaint or problems, i.e., what has brought the patient to the first meeting. Some patients tell their stories without much guidance from the interviewer, whereas others require explicit instructions in the form of specific questions to help them organize their thoughts. During this phase of the first interview, the patient should be allowed to follow his or her own thought patterns as much as possible.

Elicit specific information, including a history of the presenting problems, pertinent medical information, family background, social history, and specific symptom and behavioral patterns. Formally test mental status (see Chapter 2).

Ask if the patient has any questions or unmentioned concerns. Initial recommendations are then made to the patient for further evaluation and/or beginning treatment.

Although the three parts of the interview can be considered separately, they often weave together, e.g., mental status observations can be made from the moment the clinician meets the patient. Pertinent medical and family history may be brought up in the course of presenting other concerns, and patients may pose important questions about treatment recommendations as they present their initial history.

4. Is the initial assessment different for complex situations?

The initial psychiatric assessment may require more than one session for complex situations—for example, when evaluating children or families, or when assessing a patient's suitability for a particular therapeutic approach, such as brief psychotherapy. The initial assessment also may require information gathering from other sources: parents, children, spouse, best friend, teacher, police officers, and/or other healthcare providers. These contacts may be incorporated into the first visit, or may occur later. The first step in making such arrangements is to explain the reason for them to the patient and to obtain explicit, written permission for the contact.

5. How should a referral source be approached?

It is almost always appropriate to call the referral source to gather information and to explain the initial diagnostic impressions and treatment plans. Exceptions may occur when the referral comes from other patients, friends, or other nonprofessionals, whom the patient wishes to exclude from treatment.

6. Are there any variations on these guidelines for an initial assessment?

Specific theoretical orientations may dictate important variations in the initial assessment. For example, a behavioral therapist guides discussion to specific analyses of current problems and spends little time on early childhood experiences. The psychopharmacologic evaluation emphasizes specific symptom patterns, responses to prior medication treatment, and family history of psychiatric illness. The approach presented in this chapter is a broadly applicable set of principles that can be used in evaluating most patients.

7. How is information gathered from an interview?

The interviewer must discover as much as possible about how the patient thinks and feels. During the clinical interview, information is gathered from what the patient tells the interviewer; critically important clues also come from how the history unfolds. Thus, both the content of the interview (i.e., **what the patient says**) and the process of the interview (i.e., **how the patient says it**) offer important routes to understanding the patient's problems. Consider the order of information, the degree of comfort in talking about it, the emotions associated with the discussion, the patient's reactions to questions and initial comments, the coherence of the presentation, and the timing of the information. The full elaboration of such information may take one or several sessions over the course of days, weeks, or months, but in the first interview hints of deeper concerns may be suggested.

For example, a 35-year-old woman presented with worries about her son's recurrent asthma and associated difficulties in school. She talked freely about her worries and sought advice on how to help her son. When asked about her husband's thoughts, she became momentarily quiet. She then said that he shared her concern and switched the discussion back to her son. Her hesitancy hinted at other problems, which were left unaddressed in the initial session. Indeed, she began the next session by asking, "Can I talk about something else besides my son?" After being reassured, she described her husband's chronic anger at their son for his "weakness." His anger and her own feelings in response became an important focus of subsequent treatment.

8. How should the interview be started?

The here and now is the place to begin all interviews. Any one of a number of simple questions can be used: "What brings you to see me today? Can you tell me what has been troubling you? How is it that you decided to make this appointment?" For anxious patients, structure is useful: early inquiry about age, marital status, and living situation may give them time to become comfortable before embarking on a description of their problems. If the anxiety is evident, a simple comment about the anxiety may help patients to talk about their worries.

9. Is a highly structured format important?

No. Patients must be given some opportunity to organize their information in the way that they feel most comfortable. The interviewer who prematurely subjects the patient to a stream of specific questions limits information about the patient's own thinking process, does not learn how the patient handles silences or sadness, and closes off the patient's opportunities to hint at or introduce new topics. Furthermore, the task of formulating one specific question after another may intrude on the clinician's ability to listen and to understand the patient.

This does not mean that specific questions should be avoided. Often, patients provide elaborate answers to specific questions such as "When were you married?" Their responses may open new avenues to the inquiry. The key is to avoid a rapid-fire approach and to allow patients to elaborate their thoughts.

10. How should questions be asked?

Questions should be phrased in a way that invites patients to talk. Open-ended questions that do not indicate an answer tend to allow people to elaborate more than specific or leading questions. In general, leading questions (e.g., "Did you feel sad when your girlfriend moved out?") can be conversation stoppers, because they may give the impression that the interviewer expects the patient to have certain feelings. Nonleading questions ("How did you feel when your girlfriend moved out?") are as direct and more effective.

11. What is an effective way to deal with patient hesitancy?

When patients need help in elaborating, a simple statement and/or request may elicit more information: "Tell me more about that." Repeating or reflecting what patients say also encourages them to open up (e.g., "You were talking about your girlfriend."). Sometimes comments that specifically reflect the clinician's understanding of the patient's feelings about events may help the patient to elaborate. This approach provides confirmation for both the interviewer and the patient that they are on the same wavelength. When the interviewer correctly responds to their feelings, patients frequently confirm the response by further discussion. The patient whose girlfriend left may feel understood and freer to discuss the loss after a comment such as "You seem discouraged about your girlfriend moving out."

12. Give an example of how comprehensive information-gathering can pinpoint a problem.

An elderly man was referred for increasing despondency. In the initial interview, he first described financial difficulties and then brought up the recent development of medical problems, culminating with the diagnosis of prostatic carcinoma. As be began talking about the cancer and his wish to give up, he fell silent. At this point in the interview, the clinician expressed his recognition that the patient seemed to feel overwhelmed by the build-up of financial and, most of all, medical reversals. The patient nodded quietly and then elaborated his particular concerns about how his wife would get on after he died. He did not feel that his children would be helpful to her. It was not yet clear whether his pessimism reflected a depressive overreaction to the diagnosis of cancer or an accurate appraisal of the prognosis. Further assessment of his symptoms and mental state and a brief discussion with his wife later in the meeting revealed that the prognosis was quite good. The treatment then focused on his depressive reactions to the diagnosis.

13. How are questions best worded?

The interviewer should use language that is not technical and not overly intellectual. When possible, the patient's own words should be used. This is particularly important in dealing with intimate matters such as sexual concerns. People describe their sexual experience in language that is quite varied. If a patient says that he or she is gay, use that exact term rather than an apparently equivalent term such as

homosexual. People use some words and not others because of the specific connotations that different words carry for them; at first, such distinctions may not be apparent to the interviewer.

14. What about patients who are unable to communicate coherently?

The interviewer must remain aware at all times of what is going on during the interview. If the
patient is hallucinating or intensely upset, failure to acknowledge the upset or the disconcerting experience may elevate the patient's anxiety. Discussing the patient's current upset helps to alleviate
tension and tells the patient that the clinician is listening. If the patient's story rambles or is confusing, acknowledge the difficulty of understanding the patient and evaluate the possible reasons (e.g,
psychosis with loosened associations vs. anxiety about coming to the visit).

When general questions (e.g., "Tell me something about your background.") are ineffective, it
may be necessary to ask specific questions about parents, schooling, and dates of events. Realize,
however, that it can be tempting to ask endless questions to alleviate your own anxiety rather than
the patient's.

15. Summarize key points to remember about the initial interview.

Allowing the patient freedom to tell his or her own story must be balanced by attending to the
patient's ability to focus on relevant topics. Some people require guidance from the interviewer to
avoid getting lost in tangential themes. Others may need consistent structure because they have trouble ordering their thoughts, perhaps due to a high degree of anxiety. An empathic comment about the
patient's anxiety may reduce it and thus lead to clearer communication.

Some Interviewing Guidelines

- Let the first part of the initial interview follow the patient's train of thought.
- Provide structure to help patients who have trouble ordering their thoughts or to finish obtaining
  specific data.
- Phrase questions to invite the patient to talk (e.g., open-ended, nonleading questions).
- Use the patient's words.
- Be alert to early signs of loss of behavioral control (e.g., standing up to pace).
- Identify the patient's strengths as well as problem areas.
- Avoid jargon and technical language.
- Avoid questions that begin with "why."
- Avoid premature reassurance.
- Do not allow patients to act inappropriately (e.g., break or throw an object).
- Set limits on any threatening behavior, and summon help if necessary.

16. What specific pitfalls should be avoided during the initial interview?

Avoid jargon or technical terms, unless clearly explained and necessary. Patients may use
jargon, for example, "I was feeling paranoid." If patients use a technical word, ask about their meaning for the term. You may be quite surprised by the patient's understanding. For example, patients
may use "paranoid" to suggest fear of social disapproval or pessimism about the future. Also, be
careful about assigning a diagnostic label to the patient's problems during the interview. The patient
may be frightened and confused by the label.

In general, **avoid asking questions that begin with "why."** Patients may not know why they
have certain experiences or feelings, and can feel uncomfortable, even stupid, if they believe their
answers aren't "good." Asking why also implies that you expect the patient to provide quick explanations. Patients discover more about the roots of their problems as they reflect on their lives during
the interview and in subsequent sessions. When tempted to ask why, rephrase the question so that it
elicits a more detailed response. Alternatives include "What happened?" "How did that come
about?" or "What thoughts do you have about that?"

Avoid premature reassurance. When patients are upset, as they often are during first interviews, the interviewer may be tempted to allay the patient's fear by saying "Everything will be fine"

or "There is nothing really seriously wrong here." However, reassurance is genuine only when the clinician (1) has explored the precise nature and extent of the patient's problems and (2) is certain of what he or she is telling the patient. Premature reassurance can heighten the patient's anxiety by giving the impression that the clinician has jumped to a conclusion without a thorough evaluation or is just saying what the patient wants to hear. It also leaves patients alone with their fears about what is really wrong. Furthermore, premature reassurance tends to close off discussion rather than encourage further exploration of the problem. It may be more reassuring to ask what the patient is concerned about. The process (i.e., the nature of the interaction) comforts the patient more than any single thing the interviewer may say.

Set limits on behavior. Because of their psychiatric problems, some patients may lose control in the session. Although the approach described here emphasizes letting the patient direct much of the verbal discussion, at times limits must be set on inappropriate behavior. Patients who are aroused and want to take off their clothes or threaten to throw an object need to be controlled. This goal is most often accomplished by commenting on the increasing arousal, discussing it, inquiring about sources of upset, and letting patients know the limits of acceptable behavior. On rare occasions outside help may be necessary (e.g., security guards in an emergency department), especially if the behavior is escalating, and if the interviewer senses danger. The interview should be stopped until the patient's behavior can be managed so that it is safe to proceed.

17. What is commonly forgotten in evaluating patients?

The new patient initiates contact with the clinician because of problems and worries; these are the legitimate first topics of the interview. It also is helpful to gain an understanding of the patient's strengths, which are the foundation on which treatment will build. Strengths include ways in which the patient has coped successfully with past and current distress, accomplishments, sources of inner value, friendships, work accomplishments, and family support. Strengths also include hobbies and interests that patients use to battle their worries. Questions such as "What are you proud of?" or "What do you like about yourself?" may reveal such information.

Often the information comes out as an afterthought in the course of conversation. For example, one patient took great pride in his volunteer work through the church. He mentioned it only in passing as he discussed his activities of the week before the meeting. Yet this volunteer work was his only current source of personal value. He turned to it when he became upset about his lack of success in his career.

18. What is the role of humor in the interview?

Patients may use humor to deflect the conversation from anxiety-provoking or troubling topics. At times, it may be useful to allow such deviations to help patients maintain emotional equilibrium. However, probe further if the humor seems to lead to a radical change in focus from a topic that seemed important and/or emotionally relevant. Humor also can direct the interviewer toward new areas for investigation. A light joke by the patient (e.g., about sex) may be the first step in introducing a topic that later takes on importance.

On the part of the interviewer, humor may be protective and defensive. Just as the patient can feel anxious or uncomfortable, so can the interviewer. Be careful, because humor can backfire. It may be misunderstood as ridicule. It also can allow both patient and interviewer to avoid important topics. Sometimes humor is a wonderful way to show the human qualities of the interviewer and thus build a therapeutic alliance. Nonetheless, keep in mind the problematic aspects of humor, especially when you and your patient don't know each other well.

19. How is suicidal intent assessed?

Because of the frequency of depressive disorders and their association with suicide, it always is necessary to address the possibility of suicidal intent in a first interview. Asking about suicide will not provoke the act. If the subject does not arise spontaneously, several questions can be used to draw out the patient's thoughts on suicide (listed in the order that they may be used for beginning a discussion):

- How badly have you been feeling?
- Have you thought of hurting yourself?
- Have you wanted to die?
- Have you thought of killing yourself?
- Have you tried?
- How, when, and what led up to your attempt?
- If you have not tried, what led you to hold back?
- Do you feel safe to go home?
- What arrangements can be made to increase your safety and to decrease your risk of acting on suicidal feelings?

Such discussion may need to be extended until it is clear whether the patient may safely leave or needs hospital admission (see Chapters 75 and 76).

20. What is the best way to bring a first evaluation interview to a close?

One way is to ask the patient if he or she has any specific questions or concerns that have not been addressed. After addressing such issues, briefly summarize important impressions and diagnostic conclusions and then suggest the course of action. Be as clear as possible about the formulation of the problem, diagnosis, and next steps. This is the time to mention the need for any tests, including laboratory examinations and further psychological assessments, and to obtain permission for meeting or talking with important others who may provide needed information or should be included in the treatment plan.

Both clinician and patient should recognize that the plan is tentative and may include alternatives that need further discussion. If medication is recommended, the clinician should describe the specific benefits and expected time course as well as inform the patient about potential side effects, adverse effects, and alternative treatments. Often patients want to think over suggestions, get more information about medications, or talk with family members. In most instances, the clinical situation is not so emergent that clear action must be taken in the first interview. However, be clear in presenting recommendations, even if they are tentative and primarily oriented to further diagnostic assessment.

At this point it is tempting to provide false reassurance, such as "I know everything is going to be okay." It is perfectly legitimate—and indeed better—to allow for uncertainty when uncertainty exists. Patients can tolerate uncertainty, if they see that the clinician has a plan to elucidate the problem further and to arrive at a sound plan for treatment.

BIBLIOGRAPHY

1. Edgerton JE, Campbell RJ III (eds): American Psychiatry Glossary. 7th ed. Washington, DC, American Psychiatric Press, 1994.
2. MacKinnon R, Yudofsky S: The Psychiatric Evaluation in Clinical Practice. Philadelphia, J.B. Lippincott, 1986.
3. Morrison J: The First Interview. New York, Guilford Press, 1993.
4. Orthmer E, Orthmer SC: The Clinical Interview Using DSM IV. Washington, DC, American Psychiatric Association Press, 1994.
5. Sullivan HS: The Psychiatric Interview. New York, Norton, 1954.
6. Waldinger R: Psychiatry for Medical Students, 3rd ed. Washington, DC, American Psychiatric Press, 1996.

2. THE MENTAL STATUS EXAMINATION

Robert M. House, M.D.

1. What is the mental status examination?

The mental status examination (MSE) is a component of all medical exams and may be viewed as the psychological equivalent of the physical exam. It is especially important in neurologic and psychiatric evaluations. The purpose is to evaluate, quantitatively and qualitatively, a range of mental functions and behaviors at a specific point in time. The MSE provides important information for diagnosis and for assessment of the disorder's course and response to treatment. Observations noted throughout the interview become part of the MSE, which begins when the clinician first meets the patient. Information is gathered about the patient's behaviors, thinking, and mood.

At an appropriate point in the evaluation the formal MSE is undertaken to compile specific data about the patient's cognitive functioning. Earlier informal observations about mental state are woven together with the results of specific testing. For example, the interviewer will have considerable information about attention span, memory, and organization of thought from the process of the interview. Specific questions during the formal exam clarify more precisely the degree of attention or memory dysfunction.

Case. A 55-year-old man presented with recent complaints of sadness and fear of being alone. He also expressed thoughts about death. As he presented his concerns, he rambled to unrelated topics and seemed to lose track of the interviewer's questions. During the formal inquiry he was able to recall only 1 of 3 objects he was asked to memorize and made several mistakes in serial subtractions of 7 from 100. Specific questioning about suicidal wishes and actions revealed that he had overdosed with aspirin 1 month earlier and still experienced suicidal thoughts and wishes to die. The cognitive tests were compatible with mild dementia, and the differential diagnosis included major depression. Further work-up and treatment supported this diagnosis. Cognitive functioning improved with antidepressants.

2. Is the MSE a separate part of the patient evaluation?

No. The MSE must be interpreted along with the presenting history, physical exam, and laboratory and radiologic studies. Separate interpretation makes you vulnerable to erroneous conclusions. Collateral information from families and friends is also invaluable to confirm or supply missing data.

Case. A 27-year-old man presented to the psychiatric emergency department with somewhat grandiose behavior, pressured speech, irritability, and psychomotor agitation. The initial diagnostic impression was bipolar disorder, manic or drug-induced mania. The patient denied drug abuse. However, questioning his wife uncovered a history of substance abuse, and laboratory evaluation revealed the presence of amphetamine metabolites. The correct diagnosis was amphetamine-induced mood disorder.

3. What key factors should be considered along with the MSE?

To assess properly the patient's mental status, it is important to have some understanding of the patient's social, cultural, and educational background. What may be abnormal for someone with more intellectual ability may be normal for someone with less intellectual ability. Patients for whom English is a second language may have difficulty understanding various components of the MSE, such as the proverbs. Age may be a factor. In general, patients over the age of 60 years tend to do less well on the cognitive elements of the MSE. Often this is related to less education rather than to aging alone.

4. What are the major components of the MSE?

Components vary somewhat from author to author. However, most detailed MSEs include information about appearance, motor activity, speech, affect, thought content, thought process, perception, intellect, and insight.

Major Components of the Mental Status Examination

Appearance	Age, sex, race, body build, posture, eye contact, dress, grooming, manner, attentiveness to examiner, distinguishing features, prominent physical abnormalities, emotional facial expression, alertness
Motor	Retardation, agitation, abnormal movements, gait, catatonia
Speech	Rate, rhythm, volume, amount, articulation, spontaneity
Affect	Stability, range, appropriateness, intensity, affect, mood
Thought content	Suicidal ideation, death wishes, homicidal ideation, depressive cognitions, obsessions, ruminations, phobias, ideas of reference, paranoid ideation, magical ideation, delusions, overvalued ideas
Thought process	Associations, coherence, logic, stream, clang associations, perseveration, neologism, blocking, attention
Perception	Hallucinations, illusions, depersonalization, derealization, déjà vu, jamais vu
Intellect	Global impression: average, above average, below average
Insight	Awareness of illness

Adapted from Zimmerman M: Interviewing Guide for Evaluating DSM-IV Psychiatric Disorders and the Mental Status Examination. Philadelphia, Psychiatric Press Products, 1994, pp 121–122.

5. What is the first step in the MSE?

A determination of consciousness must be the first step in MSE. Basic brain function determines the patient's ability to relate to the surroundings and cooperate with the interviewer. Disturbance of this basic function affects higher level mental processes that make up the major portions of the exam. The Glasgow Coma Scale was developed by Teasdale and Jennett in 1974 to assess impaired consciousness. It is based on eye opening and motor and verbal responses to stimuli. The scale ranges from 3 (deep coma) to 14 (full-alert wakefulness).

Glasgow Coma Scale

CATEGORY	SCORE
Eyes open (E)	
Spontaneously	4
To speech	3
To pain	2
None	1
Best motor response (M)	
Obeys command	5
Localizes pain	4
Flexion to pain	3
Extension to pain	2
None	1
Best verbal response (V)	
Oriented	5
Confused	4
Inappropriate words	3
Incomprehensible sounds	2
None	1
Summed coma scale = E + M + V	

6. Are there short forms of the MSE?

Several shortened forms of the MSE have been developed as screening instruments. All are composed of a combination of measures to detect cognitive impairments more accurately. Although helpful, such exams must be combined with clinical history. The diagnosis of dementia and delirium also requires the demonstration of a decline in cognitive functioning from a higher baseline. All screening exams have difficulty in identifying patients with mild cognitive impairment and patients with focal neurologic lesions, such as subdural hematomas or meningiomas. The key point is that *MSEs should not be used as the sole criteria for diagnosing delirium or dementia.*

7. What are some of the more common screening exams?

The Mini-Mental State Examination (MMSE) is probably the best known. The MMSE tests orientation, immediate and short-term memory, concentration, arithmetic ability, language, and praxis. It takes about 10 minutes to administer. The Cognitive Capacity Screening Examination (CCSE) tests orientation, serial subtraction, memory, and similarities. It is less sensitive to delirium or dementia in the elderly. The Neurobehavioral Cognitive Status Examination (NCSE) is especially good for medically ill patients; it focuses on consciousness, orientation, attention, language, construction, memory, calculations, and reasoning. It tends to be more sensitive in detecting impairment because it is more detailed.

Mini-Mental State Examination

MAXIMAL SCORE	SCORE	
		Orientation
5	( )	What is the (year) (season) (date) (day) (month)?
5	( )	Where are we: (state) (country) (town) (hospital) (floor)?
		Registration
3	( )	Name 3 objects: take 1 second to say each. Then ask patient to repeat them. Give 1 point for each correct answer.
		Attention and Calculation
5	( )	Serials 7s from 100. 1 point for each correct answer. Stop after 5 answers. Alternatively, spell "world" backward.
		Recall
3	( )	Ask for the 3 objects named above. 1 point for each correct answer.
		Language
9	( )	Ask patient to name a pencil and watch. (2 points)
		Repeat the following: "No ifs, ands, or buts." (2 points)
		Follow a 3-stage command: "Take a paper in your right hand, fold it in half, and put it on the table." (3 points)
		Read and obey the following:
		Close your eyes (1 point)
		Write a sentence (1 point)
		Copy a drawing of intersecting pentagons (1 point)

Adapted from Folstein MF, Folstein SE, McHugh PR: Mini-Mental State: A practical method for grading the cognitive states of patients for the clinician. J Psychiatr Res 12:189–198, 1975.

Additional questions can be used to extend and expand the components of a screening exam:

Attention can be tested by counting by 2s to 20. This task is easier and can be used for patients with poor arithmetic skills.

Calculation abilities can be tested by asking the patient to add simple combinations of two-digit numbers. The task can be graded in difficulty.

Immediate recall can be assessed by asking patients to repeat number sequences up to seven forward and four in reverse order. Start with shorter sequences.

Memory can be assessed by asking about news events, sports, television shows, or recent meals.

Long-term memory can be assessed by using past events confirmed by family members and also by repeating names of historical figures, such as presidents of the U.S.

Language ability can be assessed by asking patients to explain similarities and differences between common objects (e.g., tree-bush, car-plane, air-water).

Thinking processes can be assessed by asking patients to explain common proverbs with which they are familiar.

8. Can the MSE help to detect organic brain disease?

Emotional and behavioral change is frequently the first presentation of organic brain disease, especially in patients with frontal and temporal tumors, hydrocephalus, or cortical atrophy. Brain tumors, subdural hematomas, small infarcts, and cerebral atrophy may be undetected on routine neurologic exam, whereas the cognitive effects of such lesions may be apparent on mental status examination. For patients with known brain lesions, a thorough MSE documents cognitive or emotional changes.

9. Does a normal MSE or MMSE score mean competence?

No. Competence relates to patients' ability to make reasonable decisions for themselves and others. Such decisions include ability to provide food and shelter, to manage money, and to participate in activities such as deciding a course of medical care. Patients who score well on an MSE may have deficits in understanding or completing common tasks of daily living. Among a population with a probable diagnosis of Alzheimer's disease, 50% of patients scoring between 26 and 30 on the MMSE had difficulty with basic tasks such as coping with small sums of money or finding their way around familiar streets. The MSE is only one component needed to assess competency. Medical condition, current ability for self-care, and corroborating information from family or friends must be taken in consideration. A more detailed discussion of competency and its evaluation is provided in Chapter 83.

Probability of Alzheimer's Disease Among Patients with Specific Problems of Daily Living

SPECIFIC ABILITY	MMSE RANGE (%)*			
	0–10	11–20	21–25	26–30
Cope with small sums of money	98	78	53	50
Perform household tasks	97	87	63	56
Recall recent events	97	92	89	91
Remember short lists of items	95	89	83	84
Find way around familiar streets	92	72	59	53
Recognize surroundings	82	44	30	19
Dress self	82	38	15	16
Find way about indoors	68	40	20	16
Tendency to dwell in the past	50	57	48	34
Feed self	44	05	02	06
Bowel and bladder continence	41	14	17	12

* Values are percentages of probable Alzheimer's disease among patients with MMSE scores falling in each range and difficulty performing the indicated activities.

Adapted from Mungas D: In-office mental status testing: A practical guide. Geriatrics 46:54–66, 1991, with permission.

10. Does an abnormal MSE or MMSE score mean incompetence?

Not necessarily. Many patients with cognitive limitations develop alternative means of coping with their deficits that allows them to live fairly independent and satisfying lives. As with patients with a normal MSE or MMSE score, **collateral history** helps to determine whether the patient is able to provide for basic needs.

11. What are the major limitations of MSE screening questionnaires?

Although structured, screening questionnaires are still subject to interpretive bias and depend on the skill and experience of the interviewer. All screening questionnaires have a fairly significant false-negative rate, especially in patients with focal lesions of the right hemisphere. Age (especially > 60 years), education (< 9th grade), cultural experience, and low socioeconomic standing limit the usefulness of MSE screening questionnaires. Unlike a detailed mental status exam, screening questionnaires are less to sensitive to subtle cognitive impairment.

12. What are executive functions?

Complex cognitive abilities mediated primarily by the frontal lobes, dorsolateral prefrontal cortex, head of the caudate nucleus, and medial thalamus are referred to as executive functions. Disorders in these areas can be assessed by evaluating the patient's ability to self-regulate and plan. For example, can the patient inhibit impulsive responses to a stimulus and deliberate before acting? Failure to do so suggests a frontal lobe disorder. Perseveration of motor activity is another example of frontal lobe dysfunction: ask the patient to perform an alternating task such as palm up–palm down, and later insert a third task (e.g., palm up–palm down–fist). The impaired patient may be able to repeat only two components of the assigned task. Focal lesions or degenerative disorders, such as Huntington's chorea, that affect these structures may lead to disorders of executive function.

13. Is the MSE important to perform in patients who appear cognitively intact?

Yes. The exam can be abbreviated, but testing of cognitive functions provides a useful baseline. Patients may deteriorate during follow-up. The initial exam provides a point for comparison. Furthermore, mental status observations are a key tool for psychiatrists. Honing observational skills through informal assessment and formal exams helps to alert the clinician to subtle aspects of affect, speech, and behavior, especially as they change during the course of meetings. Subtle fluctuations are important sources of information throughout treatment. Learning to detect subtleties is a critical component of learning to become a skilled psychiatric clinician.

GLOSSARY

Aphasia: inability to communicate by speech, writing, or symbols.

Apraxia: inability to complete purposeful movements.

Catatonia: form of schizophrenia marked by periods of rigidity, excitement, and stupor.

Clang association: speech in which words are repeated based on similarity of sound, without regard to meaning.

Déjà vu: sense that one is seeing or experiencing something that has been seen before.

Delusion: a false belief that is not shared by others.

Dysarthria: difficulty in speech production.

Echolalia: imitative repetition of speech of another person

Flight of ideas: rapid shifting from one topic to another, often with a common theme.

Loosening of association: disturbance of associations that render speech vague and unfocused.

Neologism: creation of new words; often a mixture of other words.

Perseveration: excessive continuation of a response or action, usually verbal.

Thought insertion: a delusion that thoughts are placed in one's mind by an outside source.

BIBLIOGRAPHY

1. Beresford T, Holt R, Hall R, et al: Cognitive screening at the bedside: Usefulness of a structured examination. Psychosomatics 26:319–326, 1985.
2. Crum RM, Anthony JC, Bassett SS, et al: Population-based norms for the MMSE by age and educational level. JAMA 269:2386–2391, 1993.
3. Cummings JL: The mental status examination. Hosp Pract 28:56–68, 1993.
4. Folstein MF, Folstein SE, McHugh PR: "Mini-Mental State": A practical method for grading the cognitive state of patients for the clinician. J Psychiatr Res 12:189–198, 1975.

5. Kiernan RJ, Mueller J, Langston JW, et al: The neurobehavioral cognitive status examination: A brief but differentiated approach to cognitive assessment. Ann Intern Med 107:481–485, 1987.
6. Nelson A, Fogel B, Faust D: Bedside cognitive screening instruments: A critical assessment. J Nerv Ment Disease 174:73–83, 1986.
7. Strub RL, Black FW: The Mental Status Examination in Neurology, 2nd ed. Philadelphia, F.A. Davis, 1985.
8. Teasdale G, Jennett B: Assessment of coma and impaired consciousness: A practical scale. Lancet 2:81–84, 1974.
9. Zauberts TS, Viederman M, Fins JJ: Ethical, legal, and psychiatric issues in capacity, competency, and informed consent: An annotated bibliography. Gen Hosp Psychiatry 18:155–172, 1996.
10. Zimmerman M: Interview Guide for Evaluating DSM-IV Psychiatric Disorders and the Mental Status Examination. Philadelphia, Psychiatric Press Products, 1994.

3. ORGANIZATION AND PRESENTATION OF PSYCHIATRIC INFORMATION

Michael W. Kahn, M.D.

1. Which principles guide the organization and presentation of clinical data?

After you have done the initial interview(s), performed the mental status exam, and gathered the results of various tests, you are left with the task of organizing and presenting the data coherently. This task often is daunting. Keep in mind that your primary goal is to be able to tell a concise yet sufficiently detailed story about the patient's current state so that (1) you have at least a few working hypotheses about the patient's problems, and (2) a person hearing (or reading) about the patient has enough information to arrive at his or her own hypotheses. The success of any effort toward organization and presentation of information is founded on **the clearest presentation of the most relevant facts.**

2. Where do I start?

The psychiatric presentation differs little from the standard way of presenting a medical patient, and often is organized in the following order:

a. Chief complaint
b. History of present illness
c. Past psychiatric history
d. Past medical history
e. Psychosocial history
f. Family psychiatric history
g. Physical exam
h. Mental status exam
i. Assessment and plan

3. How do the write-ups for a patient with schizophrenia and a patient with diabetes differ?

In theory, nothing is different; in practice, however, psychiatrists tend to work more effectively when they have even a rudimentary grasp of who the patient is *as a person*, and not just as the vehicle for an array of signs and symptoms. Of course, this could be said to be true for *all* physicians, not just psychiatrists. However, because psychiatrists deal with disturbances in patients' behaviors, thoughts, moods, and feelings, a vivid and lifelike description of the patient's history can be especially helpful in diagnosis and treatment.

4. What does assessing the patient "as a person" mean in practice?

Compare these two hypothetical histories of present illness:

> Mr. Jones is a 54-year-old married white man who was in his usual state of health until 3 weeks prior to admission, when he lost his job. He then noted subacute onset of early-morning awakening, weight loss, fatigue, decreased concentration, and depressed mood. His wife, noticing that he had suicidal ideation, brought him to the hospital.

> Mr. Jones is a 54-year-old married white man who derived much of his sense of self-esteem and accomplishment from his job as an accountant, which he held for over 30 years. Three weeks ago, when he was laid off (due to cutbacks in the firm where he worked), he felt that "The rug was pulled out from under me." He had always made his job the center of his life, and was left with nothing to do at home. His wife was overwhelmed as well. He says that he began to feel that "Nothing made sense any more . . . I felt all washed up," and gradually lost his appetite as well as his interest in and energy for the few hobbies he had. He developed insomnia with early-morning awakening, and after a while began to tell his wife that "I'm no use to anyone anymore." When he asked his wife if she'd miss him "if he were gone," she brought him to the hospital.

Although both histories give a clear picture of someone developing an episode of major depression, the second one conveys a more detailed and useful assessment of the patient as a person, as well as of the circumstances leading up to the hospital admission. It presents at least the beginning of an understanding of the patient's personality and home life. The use of direct quotations greatly contributes to the sense of vividness and immediacy, and begins to help the listener empathize with the patient's suffering. When reading or hearing such a presentation, important questions readily come to mind: Had Mr. Jones seen the cutbacks coming but failed to plan for them? Why was the job the center of his life? Why couldn't his wife have been more of a support? Why does he frame his anguish in terms of his not being any "use" to anyone?—and so forth.

The essential point is to make the history of present illness as **vivid and richly detailed** as possible, making use of direct patient quotations when applicable and useful, and minimizing use of standard "boiler-plate" jargon about symptoms and behavior.

5. What sort of boiler-plate jargon should be avoided?
The kind that describes symptoms in concise but impoverished ways that lack important complexity. For example, rather than saying:

> "The patient demonstrated intense affect when faced with his illness."

Consider saying instead:

> "The patient became tearful and sad when discussing the isolation caused by his psychotic thinking."

Rather than saying:

> "The patient exhibited agitated and threatening behavior in her relationship."

Consider saying:

> "The patient shouted angrily and shook her fist at her boyfriend."

Once again, the more successful you are at depicting a clear, detailed, and evocative history, the greater the chances will be of reaching a more accurate assessment that leads directly to a rational treatment plan. Avoid clinical clichés!

6. How should the past psychiatric history be incorporated?
This part of the presentation should document not only what prior treatment the patient has received, but also the *circumstances* and *outcome* of such treatment. Outlining *untreated* episodes of illness also can be helpful, as can describing the initial onset of symptoms.

Hospitalizations: Note precipitating factors, length of stay, success/failure of different treatments used, working diagnoses.

Somatic treatments: Note dosage of medication, duration, usefulness, and side effects. If appropriate, mention whether electroconvulsive therapy has been used.

Therapy: Note session length, frequency, duration, focus (e.g., supportive, exploratory, behavioral, cognitive), and usefulness.

Suicidality/homicidality: Note stressors, prior attempts (in detail), and treatment measures that proved effective. Classifying prior attempts in terms of relative risk and rescue potential can be particularly helpful. For example: the patient who lightly lacerated a wrist in full view of a family member would be considered a low-risk/high-rescue attempt; taking an overdose of acetaminophen behind a locked bathroom door would be high-risk/low-rescue.

Remember: eliminate vagueness! Saying "The patient failed a lithium trial" is less helpful than saying "A two-month trial of lithium at therapeutic plasma levels resulted in intolerable tremor and polyuria." Direct patient quotations can be quite useful, as well.

7. Is taking a past medical history in a psychiatric setting different than in a nonpsychiatric setting?

Not substantially. Clearly, any illness with possible psychiatric complications (e.g., Parkinson's disease, multiple sclerosis, stroke, Lyme disease, hyopthyroidism) should be explored in some detail. Given the protean psychiatric manifestations of several different types of seizures, the presence or absence of a seizure disorder is especially important to determine. Mood disorders, hallucinations, delusions, and unusual character traits may be sequelae of a seizure focus, usually in the temporolimbic area. Because these symptoms may represent ictal manifestations of a *nonconvulsive* seizure, a patient's seizures may have gone undiagnosed. Therefore, inquire about any history of head trauma, particularly if it led to loss of consciousness.

8. Describe some key points of the psychosocial history.

Given the importance of early relationships to personality development and coping skills, a few essential facts about the patient's upbringing can shed light on his or her current functioning. A brief outline of the structure of the patient's **family** is essential, and should include the place of the patient in the birth order, whether or not the parents were ever married or remain married, and whether either parent is deceased. Patients often fail to spontaneously mention losses of other family members; therefore, ask whether any siblings or grandparents were lost to the patient either recently or in childhood.

Physical and sexual abuse—two obviously sensitive subjects—should be mentioned tactfully but candidly if they are clinically relevant. Clearly, taking a history of abuse must be done with care, with special attention to the patient's clinical condition and whether or not discussion of such events could be traumatizing or intrusive.

Information about the patient's **work history** and **relationships** is invaluable for an accurate assessment of personality functioning. How does the patient respond to the responsibility of a job? How does he or she deal with interpersonal conflict and intimacy? Similarly, even a brief history of how the patient performed in **school** can convey a sense of early social relationships as well as any possible learning difficulties that may have gone undetected.

Substance abuse often is presented in this section. The same overall suggestions for detail and richness apply, e.g.: "The patient typically drinks alone, on weekends only, consuming 'anything I can get my hands on' until he passes out. He has never had seizures or DTs, and does not like Alcoholics Anonymous because 'it's hard to be around so many strangers.'" This description is so much more evocative than "Patient is alcohol-dependent."

The patient's **religion** and whether it is important also should be mentioned, especially if the patient is struggling with suicidal impulses.

Finally, any **military** and **legal** elements are important and should not be neglected.

9. What about the family psychiatric history?

A careful exploration of the family's history of mental illness frequently offers helpful data. Not uncommonly, patients remember that a family member was psychiatrically ill but don't know the diagnosis. Certain facts can be revealing: The patient's mother was "nervous a lot" and was hospitalized five times for "shock treatments." The patient's uncle was "always hyper," "drank too much," and was arrested three times for passing bad checks.

Not surprisingly, such details often are more revealing than the "diagnosis" remembered by the patient.

10. What are the pitfalls in presenting the mental status exam?

This is where boiler-plate jargon can easily get out of hand (see Question 5). "Patient has auditory hallucinations" can be true, if the examiner was careful, or quite false, if the exam was cursory. Be specific! If a patient mentions hearing voices, you need to ask: How many voices? Are they there all the time? Do they comment on the patient? Are they perceived as coming from inside or outside the head? Do they tell the patient to do anything? Are they threatening or comforting? *Don't just mention the symptom—describe it.* Describe the patient's appearance, interpersonal style, and mannerisms or idiosyncrasies. This principle applies to all portions of the mental status exam, including cognitive testing.

11. How is everything pulled together in the formulation (or assessment) section?

Remarkably little consensus exists about what it means to formulate a case. A common belief is that formulation involves an esoteric and sophisticated explanation of the patient's difficulties that displays the examiner's ability to extrapolate more from details of the case than meets the eye. Rather, perhaps the essence of formulation is that it arranges facts in such a way as to suggest a differential diagnosis and a treatment plan. A focus on *basic* psychiatric knowledge, common sense, and a willingness to think in terms of *hypotheses* rather than *conclusions* usually lead to a clarifying and useful formulation.

12. Give some examples of successful formulations.

One main function of the formulation is to summarize known pertinent clinical facts, emphasizing the *stressors* and *sequence of events* that led to the patient seeking help. Features essential to any formulation are:

- An indication of baseline functioning (no prior psychosis)
- A description of a likely stressor (the loss of the job)
- A response to that stressor (humiliation, followed by cocaine use)
- A summary of the salient symptomatic phenomenology (e.g., grandiosity, irritability)
- A differential diagnosis

The following is a simple but useful formulation:

> In summary, Ms. Smith is a 19-year-old woman with the new onset of a psychotic disorder that has developed over the past 3 weeks. The symptoms appeared to begin fairly abruptly after she was fired from her job and began using cocaine daily to avoid her feelings of shame and disappointment. Her grandiosity, irritability, sleeplessness, and pressured speech all suggest the diagnosis of bipolar disorder, manic phase; however, given the amount of cocaine that she has been using, it is worth considering the possibility of a substance-induced mood disorder with manic features, secondary to cocaine.

The hypothesis that the patient used cocaine to avoid the pain of her loss is clearly based more on common sense and empathy rather than on any formula concerning human behavior. Here is a more complex formulation (referring to the patient in Question 4):

> In summary, Mr. Jones is a man without prior psychiatric history whose self-esteem is closely tied to his ability to be an effective worker and to provide for his family. The loss of his job is a tremendous blow to his self-image and quickly has led to his feeling worthless, guilty, and hopeless. He has developed all the signs of a major depressive episode. His suicidal state may be the outcome of his hopelessness and his inward-turned rage about the layoff.

13. The previous formulation indicates that the patient is turning his rage onto himself. Explain.

That is a hypothesis based on psychodynamic theory, which holds that human behavior is, to a large extent, governed by hidden (or, more specifically, *unconscious*) meanings and forces within the mind. Psychodynamic principles can be useful tools for probing and unraveling patients' difficulties; these principles are most helpful when used to generate *hypotheses*, which then require further data to be confirmed or refuted. In this case, for example, further discussions with this patient while he was recovering clinically might reveal the rage (perhaps directed against a harsh and over-demanding father) masked by the acute symptoms. Exploration and venting of the rage might lead to further improvement and reduced vulnerability to future depression.

14. Are there other hypotheses that can be used as tools in case formulation?

Three other sets of hypotheses, which are well-summarized by Lazare, are the *sociocultural*, the *behavioral*, and the *biologic/syndromal*. Although a complete description of each of these is beyond the scope of this chapter, some familiarity with each can greatly enhance a clinician's skill in reaching an accurate and thorough formulation. The biologic/syndromal approach underlies the classification system contained in the Diagnostic and Statistical Manual (DSM-IV) of the American Psychiatric Association, which is the prevailing diagnostic system within American psychiatry.

15. What if the formulation is wrong?

Revise it. The value of a formulation is that it provides a starting point for an informed understanding and discussion of the case. It is less important to be "right" than to be flexible. Think of the initial formulation as leading to a **working diagnosis** that will guide the initial work-up and treatment and may be modified as you become more familiar with the patient. In summary:

- Emphasize clinical detail.
- Avoid clinical clichés and boiler-plate jargon.
- Quote the patient where applicable.
- Describe symptoms rather than label them.
- Use the formulation to summarize the facts, generate hypotheses, and arrive at a working diagnosis.

APPENDIX: A SAMPLE WRITE-UP

Chief complaint: "I think I can go home; I'm feeling fine."

History of present illness: Mr. Williams is a 36-year-old, single, white man well-known to our system who carries the diagnosis of bipolar affective disorder. He was doing well living in his own apartment and working as a salesman, and was coming to see his therapist weekly for psychotherapy and lithium. About 2 weeks ago, his girlfriend of 3 years broke up with him; he began to drink daily (6 to 10 beers) and failed to show up for his appointments. The therapist estimates he should have run out of lithium 1 week before. On the night of admission Mr. Williams arrived at his girlfriend's house intoxicated; he was verbally threatening, and tried to break down her door. The police were called and he was taken to the emergency room at a city hospital. There his blood alcohol level was initially .256 and he was placed in restraints overnight. When sober, he continued to be pressured, hyperalert, and grandiose, and showed markedly impaired insight and judgment, with plans to "charge two tickets on the Concorde to take my girlfriend to Paris" despite the fact that he has no money left in the bank. He was sent to this hospital on a temporary commitment paper because of severely impaired judgment and the inability to care for himself.

Past psychiatric history: First hospitalization was at age 22 for 4 weeks for typical manic symptoms. Responded well to lithium 1200 mg q.d. and complied with followup treatment.

Second hospitalization was at age 26 for severe depression that seemed to begin after stopping lithium "to see if I needed it any more." He overdosed on aspirin but immediately called his doctor and then an ambulance; there were no medical sequelae. Depression responded well to fluoxetine, although he had some hypomania; dose of fluoxetine stabilized at 10 mg q.d. Lithium level was 1.0 mEq/L on 1200 mg q.d.

Third hospitalization was for mania at age 34, again after stopping medication because "It was making me sleepy." Quickly improved when lithium was restarted.

He has never had electroconvulsive therapy or received valproic acid or carbamazepine. Had a significant acute dystonic reaction to haloperidol during first admission.

Weekly psychotherapy sessions have focused on helping the patient accept his illness and improve self-esteem. Only suicide attempt was the aspirin overdose mentioned above.

Past medical history: No known allergies or significant medical problems. Lost consciousness for "about 10 seconds" after a childhood accident. No resulting headaches, behavior changes, or seizures. Twice-yearly creatinine levels have been stable. No evidence exists of impaired renal function due to lithium. Thyroid function has been normal.

Psychosocial history: He is the oldest of two sons born to a still-married retired couple. Younger brother is healthy and works as an engineer. Mother and father are in good health.

Patient did well in school and "always had friends." Received a degree in history from a state college and has worked as an appliance salesman. He has never married but has had several long-term relationships. He was arrested for driving recklessly during a manic episode but otherwise has had no legal problems. He was never in the military. He is Protestant and does not attend church.

When manic he tends to drink to excess, but otherwise drinks socially. As a teenager, he experimented with marijuana.

Family psychiatric history: Father has had problems with depression and is on desipramine, but has never been hospitalized. Maternal grandmother had clear-cut bipolar illness, and was hospitalized over 20 times for both depression and mania until she began taking lithium in 1972; since then she has had two hospitalizations and is doing well.

Mental status exam: On admission he was a gaunt, dishevelled young man who was pacing around the room throughout the interview and was very difficult to interrupt. He showed clear pressured speech and flight of ideas: "I wanted to take the Concorde but they wouldn't let me . . . you seem to be a brilliant doctor . . . Maybe I'll just move to Hollywood . . . " etc. He was irritable when asked questions. Claims he hears "God's voice every morning when I wake up" but otherwise denies auditory or visual hallucinations. Mood is described as "terrific," but affect is irritable and elated. He has no homicidal or suicidal thoughts: "Why should I hurt anyone?"

He is hyper-alert and oriented in all three spheres. He refused cognitive testing: "I hate remembering those three things and doing those sevens." When asked about proverbs he said "A rolling stone is a rolling stone is Mick Jagger." Analogies were deferred. Judgment and insight were both obviously severely compromised.

Formulation: This is the fourth hospitalization in 14 years for this 36-year-old man with what appears to be clear-cut bipolar disorder, with a history of both mania and depression following discontinuation of lithium. This present episode seems to have been precipitated by his sense of helplessness after a girlfriend left him. He ran out of medicine and began drinking heavily; his anger at the girlfriend came out while he was manic and intoxicated. Because he has never had mania or depression while actually taking lithium, it would make sense to start this medication again. Because of a history of dystonia with high-potency neuroleptics, thorazine is prescribed to control the acute manic symptoms.

Diagnoses: Axis I: Bipolar I disorder, most recent episode manic, 296.44
        Axis II: No diagnosis
        Axis III: No diagnosis
        Axis IV: Loss of important relationship
        Axis V: Global assessment of functioning = 20 (see Chapter 4)
Plan: Lithium 600 mg b.i.d.
        Thorazine 100 mg t.i.d.
        Daily meetings as tolerated by patient to monitor side effects and develop alliance.

BIBLIOGRAPHY

1. Clinical hypothesis testing. In Lazare A (ed): Outpatient Psychology. Baltimore, Williams & Wilkins, 1989.
2. McWiliams N: Psychoanalytic Case Formulation. New York, Guilford Press, 1999.

4. INTRODUCTION TO DSM-IV

Michael W. Kahn, M.D.

1. What is the conceptual orientation of DSM-IV?

The Diagnostic and Statistical Manuals (DSM) are handbooks developed by the American Psychiatric Association. They contain listings and descriptions of psychiatric diagnoses, analogous to the International Classification of Diseases manuals. The DSMs have changed as the prevailing concepts of mental disorder have changed. DSM-I (1952) reflected Adolf Meyer's influence on American psychiatry, and classified mental disorders as various "reactions" to stressors. DSM-II (1968) dropped the reactions concept, but maintained a perspective strongly influenced by psychodynamic theory. DSM-III (1980) marked a watershed in the development of the classification system, in that it outlined a research-based, empirical, and phenomenologic approach to diagnosis, which attempted to be atheoretical with regard to etiology. DSM-IV continues this tradition, which may be characterized as the "biologic" or "syndromal" approach to diagnosis.

2. What is the purpose of the multiaxial system?

The five-axis classification system was developed to provide a systematic framework for the thorough, descriptive assessment of a patient's psychiatric condition and overall functioning. The axes are:

- Axis I: Clinical disorders
- Axis II: Personality disorders,
      mental retardation
- Axis III: General medical conditions
- Axis IV: Psychosocial and environmental problems
- Axis V: Global assessment of functioning

3. What are the characteristics of axis I disorders?

Axis I diagnoses comprise those clinical syndromes that generally develop in late adolescence or adulthood. Schizophrenia, bipolar disorder, panic disorder, posttraumatic stress disorder, and alcohol abuse are diagnoses coded on axis I. One can think of axis I diagnoses as illnesses, as opposed to the persistently maladaptive behavior patterns that characterize personality disorders.

4. How do axis I disorders differ from axis II disorders?

Axis II comprises personality disorders and mental retardation. Maladaptive personality traits and behavior problems also are noted on axis II (see Question 7 below).

5. Can one make multiple diagnoses on axes I and II?

Definitely. A patient with well-controlled schizophrenia may develop a problem with alcohol abuse, and would therefore warrant both diagnoses on axis I. A patient with mental retardation may also meet criteria for obsessive-compulsive personality disorder, and would therefore receive both diagnoses on axis II. Several diagnoses can be included on each axis.

6. What if a patient's signs and symptoms don't fit neatly into one or more categories?

Several ways exist to deal with this very common situation. On axis I, most clinical syndromes described have one variant called [syndrome name] *not otherwise specified* (NOS). Psychosis NOS, adjustment disorder NOS, and bipolar disorder NOS are diagnoses for when not all criteria characterizing a given syndrome are met, but that syndrome seems closest to describing the patient's difficulties.

If the clinical picture is even less clear, you can defer the diagnosis on either axis I or II until you are able to gather the information for a more definitive diagnosis. The code for a deferred diagnosis on either axis I or II is 799.90.

Finally, you can make a *provisional* diagnosis if enough information is available to make a reasonable formulation, but some doubt or uncertainty remains. Simply write "provisional" after the suspected diagnosis.

7. Do these issues apply to personality disorders as well?

Yes. If a patient seems to have several of the characteristics of, for example, antisocial personality disorder, but does not meet all criteria for that diagnosis, you can record that the patient has antisocial *traits*. Likewise, a patient may have traits of more than one personality disorder; in this situation, you would make a diagnosis of, for example, mixed personality disorder with borderline and histrionic traits.

8. How does axis III function?

Axis III primarily records medical problems *relevant to the ongoing treatment* of the patient. Examples are glaucoma in a patient requiring antidepressants, asthma in a patient with anxiety who is taking theophylline, AIDS in a patient with new-onset psychosis, and cirrhosis of the liver in a patient with alcohol dependence.

9. What about axes IV and V?

Axis IV records psychosocial stressors encountered by the patient within the previous 12 months that have contributed to (1) the development of a new mental disorder; (2) the recurrence of a previous mental disorder; or (3) the exacerbation of an ongoing mental disorder. The stressor should be described in as much detail as needed to indicate how it affects the patient's functioning. Even mild stressors should be noted if they figure into the clinical presentation.

Axis V records the patient's global level of functioning both at the time of evaluation and during the past year. The clinician consults the **Global Assessment of Functioning (GAF) scale** in the manual and determines the patient's current GAF score as well as the highest one obtained during a relatively prolonged period within the past year.

Global Assessment of Functioning Scale

Consider psychological, social, and occupational functioning on a hypothetical continuum of mental health–illness. Do not include impairment in functioning due to physical or environmental limitations.

Code (Note: Use intermediate codes when appropriate, e.g., 45, 68, 72.)

100	**Superior functioning in a wide range of activities, life's problems never seem to get out of hand, is sought out by others because of his or her many positive qualities.**
91	**No symptoms**
90	**Absent or minimal symptoms** (e.g., mild anxiety before an exam), **good functioning in all areas, interested and involved in a wide range of activities, socially effective, generally satisfied with life, no more than everyday problems or concerns** (e.g., an occasional argument with family
81	members.)
80	**If symptoms are present, they are transient and expectable reactions to psychosocial stressors** (e.g., difficulty concentrating after family argument); **no more than slight impairment in social,**
71	**occupational, or school functioning** (e.g., temporary falling behind in schoolwork).
70	**Some mild symptoms** (e.g., depressed mood and mild insomnia) **OR some difficulty in social, occupational, or school functioning** (e.g., occasional truancy, or theft within the household), **but**
61	**generally functioning pretty well, has some meaningful interpersonal relationships.**
60	**Moderate symptoms** (e.g., flat affect and circumstantial speech, occasional panic attacks) **OR moderate difficulty in social, occupational, or school functioning** (e.g., few friends, conflicts
51	with peers or co-workers).
50	**Serious symptoms** (e.g., suicidal ideation, severe obsessional rituals, frequent shoplifting) **OR any serious impairment in social, occupational, or school functioning** (e.g., no friends, unable
41	to keep a job).

Table continued on following page.

Global Assessment of Functioning Scale (Cont.)

40	**Some impairment in reality testing or communication** (e.g., speech is at times illogical, obscure, or irrelevant) **OR major impairment in several areas, such as work or school, family relations, judgment, thinking, or mood** (e.g,. depressed man avoids friends, neglects family, and is
31	unable to work; child frequently beats up younger children, is defiant at home, and is failing at school).
30	**Behavior is considerably influenced by delusions or hallucinations OR serious impairment in communication or judgment** (e.g., sometimes incoherent, acts grossly inappropriately, suicidal preoccupation) **OR inability to function in almost all areas** (e.g., stays in bed all day; no job,
21	home, or friends).
20	**Some danger of hurting self or others** (e.g., suicide attempts without clear expectation of death; frequently violent; manic excitement) **OR occasionally fails to maintain minimal personal hy-**
11	**giene** (e.g., smears feces) **OR gross impairment in communication** (e.g., largely incoherent or mute).
10	**Persistent danger of severely hurting self or others** (e.g., recurrent violence) **OR persistent inability to maintain minimal personal hygiene OR serious suicidal act with clear expectation**
1	**of death.**
0	Inadequate information.

The rating of overall psychological functioning on a scale of 0–100 was operationalized by Luborsky in the Health-Sickness Rating Scale (Luborsky L: Clinicians' judgments of mental health. Arch Gen Psychiatry 7: 407–417, 1962). Spitzer and colleagues developed a revision of the Health-Sickness Rating Scale called the Global Assessment Scale (GAS) (Endicott J, Spitzer RL, Fleiss JL, Cohen J: The global assessment scale: A procedure for measuring overall severity of psychiatric disturbance. Arch Gen Psychiatry 33:766–771, 1976). A modified version of the GAS was included in the DSM–III–R as the Global Assessment of Functioning (GAF) Scale.

10. Does the DSM system provide a good way to diagnose psychiatric disorders?

Compared to what? This is a thorny question. So long as psychiatry lacks definitive tests to diagnose illness, arguments about which criteria should form the basis of the diagnostic system will continue to flourish. The publication of DSM-III in 1980 was widely hailed both inside and outside the field for at last providing diagnoses that relied on what people *observed* rather than what they *believed* on the basis of theory. A wide variety of mental health (and general medical) practitioners found that DSM-III provided a straightforward, comprehensible, and user-friendly tool for making sense of (or at least classifying) psychopathology.

The DSM system has some clear shortcomings, however, and some well-regarded clinicians have called it parochial, reductionistic, adynamic (i.e., not sensitive to the dynamic hypothesis mentioned above), and clumsy in its difficulty distinguishing between "state" and "trait" behaviors. The DSM system was designed to have high reliability among different raters; that is, it was fashioned so that two different clinicians would likely arrive at the same diagnosis for a given patient. Yet it is clear that *reliability* and *validity* of diagnosis remain distinct. Some would say that the DSM system favors the former at the expense of the latter; others would reply that so long as validity remains elusive, we should do our best to at least improve reliability, which can be empirically tested in field trials. DSM-IV creates some problems and helps to solve others. A nondogmatic, open-minded, and pragmatic approach to this complicated issue probably serves *patients* best.

BIBLIOGRAPHY

1. American Psychiatric Association: Diagnostic and Statistical Manual–IV. Washington, D.C., American Psychiatric Association, 1994.
2. Klerman GL, Vaillant GE, Spitzer RL, Michels R: A debate on DSM-III. Am J Psychiatry 141:4, 1984.

II. Diagnostic Procedures

5. PROJECTIVE TESTING

Judith E. Fox, Ph.D.

1. What are projective tests?

Projective tests are individually administered tests generally used to obtain information about **emotional functioning**. Projective tests are founded on the idea that in ambiguous, unstructured, and open-ended situations aspects of the individual's internal, emotional world are projected onto the environment to influence his or her perception and experience of it. Test responses are understood as samples of the individual's emotional life.

Murray was one of the first psychologists to offer a description of how the process of projection works. Murray's ideas about projection were derived largely from Freud: To cope with what is felt to be personally threatening, individuals defensively turn what they experience internally to be dangerous into external dangers. Once the experienced dangers are perceived to be external, they are easier to cope with. Rather than viewing this process of projection necessarily as a defensive maneuver, Murray view it more as people's tendency to be influenced in the cognitive mediation of perceptual inputs by their needs, interests, and overall psychological organization.[4] The label *projective methods* is applied to various techniques that present the examinee with such psychological activity.

2. What are the most commonly used projective techniques?

Among the many projective tests, the Rorschach, Thematic Apperception Test (TAT), and Draw-A-Person Test are perhaps the most commonly used. Sentence completion tests, in which the patient is asked to complete sentences such as "my mother…" or "the best time I ever had was…" also are common. Although many tests have been developed to uncover inner thoughts and feelings, Lindzey[14] long ago suggested a way to classify projective tests on the nature of the projective activity:

• **Associations:** The patient is asked to verbalize a response to some stimuli. Examples include the Rorschach test, in which the subject views several ink blots and responds verbally to each, and the word association test, in which the patient is asked to indicate the word that comes to mind in response to another word.

• **Completions:** The patient completes an unfinished stimulus. Sentence completion tasks are an example.

• **Constructions:** The patient is required to form or develop a production out of a stimulus. The story-telling task of the TAT, for example, requires the patient to construct a story from a picture.

• **Choice or ordering:** Patients are asked to place objects in categories or rank order choices or preferences for items.

• **Self-expression:** The patient creates something without a stimulus to initiate the response. Drawing tasks or dramatic play are examples.

All of these projective methods are based on the assumption that the patient's responses and creations reflect some aspect of his or her inner world; thus they are viewed as vehicles that lend articulation to a person's inner experiences.

3. What are the differences between objective and projective personality tests?

"When the subject is asked to guess what the examiner is thinking, we call it an objective test; when the examiner tries to guess what the subject is thinking, we call it a projective device."[11]

The utility of dichotomizing "objective" and "projective" tests is controversial. This dichotomy sometimes refers to the way in which a test has been developed, the degree to which the results involve clinician subjectivity, and/or whether or not test questions are open-ended. If often is used to classify tests based on whether they were developed in accordance with fundamental principles of measurement. These principles increase the likelihood that a test is a reliable and valid indicator of the personality variables that it purports to measure.

Personality tests such as the Minnesota Multiphasic Personality Inventory (MMPI) may be termed objective when they do not require the clinician to exercise a great deal of individual judgment in ascertaining a subject's test score and personality profile. Even with objective tests, however, subjectivity of the examiner affects interpretation of the test profile. Exner, the developer of a major scoring and interpretation system for the Rorschach, notes that the objective-projective dichotomy is grossly over-simplified: "Any stimulus situation that evokes or facilitates the process of projection can be considered a projective method. This is quite independent of whether or not basic rules of measurement have been employed in developing or establishing the test."[4] Exner developed a comprehensive system of scoring and interpreting the Rorschach. This, then, is an example of a projective test that has been developed in a fashion similar to the objective test.

Regardless of the type of test, contemporary psychologists generally interpret the findings in the context of history, behavior, and interpersonal relationships.

Personality Tests

OBJECTIVE	PROJECTIVE
Structured to elicit a specific class of responses (e.g., true-false inventories)	Elicit open-ended responses
Questions direct; answers self-evident	Questions unstructured; answers obscure
Clinician individual judgement less exercised	Tend to require clinician subjectivity
Developed through lengthy empirical testing and group comparison	?
Individual scores can be graphed and compared with scores obtained from a normative sample	?

4. Describe the Rorschach test.

The Rorschach, one of the most widely used projective tests, was developed in 1921 by Hermann Rorschach. It consists of a set of ten ink blots. Each block is sequentially presented to the patient, who is asked to describe what the ink blot suggests. The examiner then asks about the various details of the perceptions to understand the key factors associated with their creation.

Of the numerous scoring systems developed for Rorschach data, many involve looking at least three general categories: (1) the location or area of the ink blot on which the response is based; (2) the specific aspects or determinants of the blot used to form the percept (e.g., shape, color, shading), and (3) the content of the percept (e.g., whether it is human or animal). Some systems also attempt to capture the fashion by which the individual organized the response. The degree to which a percept represents an integrated and/or well-formed response often is one indicator of the intactness of the person's thinking.

The major premise of the Rorschach is that a person organizes stimuli from the environment based on needs, motives, conflicts, and perceptual processes. Ambiguous stimuli, like ink blots, promote cognitive disorganization and represent the fashion and ease by which the individual draws from internal resources to organize and confront ambiguous situations.

5. What are the assets and limitations of the Rorschach?

Since its initial development, the Rorschach has been a controversial psychological testing instrument. Criticisms of the Rorschach, as is true of most projective tests, focus on the validity and reliability of the test instrument and the conclusions based on test results. Although both reliability and validity have reached acceptable levels on the Rorschach, more objective psychological tests reach superior levels of validity.

The most contemporary, data-based system of scoring and interpreting the Rorschach is the Exner Comprehensive System,[5] which provides many scores and formulas of varying reliability and validity. The examiner must be aware of the differences among scores in terms of psychometric properties to interpret test productions adequately.

The Rorschach is a complex test. Extensive training in required to evaluate its findings, and some graduate school programs lack such training. Furthermore, the Rorschach may have limited value as an assessment tool for children, in whom its reliability may be adequate for short-term evaluation but limited for longer-term predictions. Lastly, because its administration and interpretation are relatively complex compared with some other psychological tests, it allows an increased possibility for error.

On the positive side, highly trained Rorschach clinicians can describe a person's characteristics accurately based on responses to the test.[10] The Rorschach also is thought to assist in the evaluation of underlying personality structure because its ambiguity bypasses conscious awareness and defensiveness. It often is used to evaluate an individual who outwardly presents as well-adjusted but inwardly may experience psychopathology. Edell[3] has shown, for example, that individuals with borderline personality disorder may perform normally on structured tests, but demonstrate psychopathology on the less structured Rorschach. Lastly, the Rorschach is relatively easy to administer.

6. Describe the Thematic Apperception Test (TAT) and discuss its assets and limitations.

The TAT is a projective test developed by Henry Murray in the mid 1930s. It consists of 20 cards that depict a variety of ambiguous scenes. The subject is instructed to make up a story about each card and to include a beginning, middle, and end to the story as well as to describe the thoughts and feelings of the characters.

Unlike the Rorschach, the TAT presents more structured test stimuli. It requires a different kind of organization and verbal response. Its interpretation is largely based on Murray's theory of personality, which emphasizes both biologic and socioenvironmental determinants of behavior. Murray believed that the way in which individuals deal with their environment involves both how their environment affects them and how their unique set of needs, attitudes, and values affects their reaction to the environment. The TAT grew from Murray's motivation to assess individuals psychological needs.

Generally, the interpretation of TAT responses is based on content analysis of the story. Quantitative analysis of the TAT generally is not attempted, even though some scoring systems have been successfully applied.[15] Because scoring systems generally are not applied, the reliability and validity of the measure are difficult to ascertain. The effectiveness of the technique often depends more on the clinician's skill than on the quality of the test.

On the positive side, the TAT provides material related to various aspects of psychological functioning, including mood, interpersonal themes, problem-solving style, and motivational variables. Patients generally find the test interesting and nonthreatening, and it is easy to administer. Like all projective techniques, the TAT may bypass conscious defenses and facilitate self-revelation.

7. What are projective drawings? How are they used?

One common assumption of projective drawing tests of personality is that individuals symbolically create themes, dynamics, and attitudes that project images, feelings, and thoughts vital to understanding the individuals.

Projective drawings were most popular during the 1950s and 1960s when psychoanalytic theory was dominant. Goodenough's Draw-A-Man Test, developed in 1926,[7] was the first projective drawing test; it was used to estimate a child's level of intellectual maturity. Machover[16] extended projective drawings into the area of personality assessment. Such characteristics as size of drawing and placement on the page were interpreted as indicators of self-esteem and/or mood. Koppitz[12] expanded the developmental and personality aspects of human figure drawings by creating scoring systems reflecting various cognitive and emotional attributes. The House-Tree-Person Test was concurrently by Buck. In 1987 Burns developed the Kinetic House-Tree-Person Test, in which the patient is asked to make the person in the drawing "do something." This is probably the most popular form of projective drawings used today. Similarly, the Burn's Kinetic Family Drawing, in which the patient draws his family "doing something," has been used to assess interpersonal relationships and family dynamics.

In interpreting drawings, clinicians tend to depend on clinical intuition, judgment, and experience. In a review of projective drawings, Grath-Marnat[8] concludes that projective drawings have been used most successfully as a rough measure of intellectual maturation. They are moderately successful in measuring global estimates of adjustment, impulsivity, and anxiety. They are least successful in assessing specific aspects of personality or in making clear diagnoses.

8. How is the efficacy of results produced by projective testing evaluated?

• **Test reliability.** Many projective tests have been criticized for results that are not highly stable, consistent, and predictable. Reliability refers to the extent to which an individual will achieve the same score if the test is administered again. Although some variability between scores is expected, a test is thought to be most reliable when variability is at a minimum. In evaluating the reliability of a test, higher reliabilities are obtained when stable variables are measured (e.g., stable personality traits), and lower reliabilities when unstable aspects (e.g., current emotional states) are measured.

Some projective tests (e.g., the TAT) lack normative data; the clinician must rely on his or her own experience to interpret the responses. The effectiveness of the technique often depends more on the clinician's skills than on the quality of the test. Patient responses to projective tests also have been found to be affected by such variables as mood, stress, sleep deprivation, and differences in instruction. Such variables may limit a reliable measure of personality traits. Furthermore, when a personality test does not use standardized administration and scoring, its reliability is severely reduced.

• **Test validity.** Projective tests also have been criticized for the degree to which they actually measure what they intend to measure. Validity involves the relationship between the test and some external, independently observed event. Thus, a score on impulse control on a particular projective test should correlate highly with some observed criterion of impulse control, i.e., how the patient behaves when experiencing strong emotions. Validity data on projective tests are limited.

• **Test-taking factors.** Projective techniques generally are viewed as less susceptible to "faking," because they present the subject with an ambiguous situation in which the underlying concepts are covert or unknown. Individuals, therefore, are less able to manipulate their responses to be viewed in a particular light. Projective tests also are nonthreatening to most subjects because they are intrinsically interesting and have no "wrong" answers.

9. When should patients be referred for projective testing?

In general, projective testing is used to address questions about emotional functioning. Examples include the nature and level of depression, anxiety, and/or anger; level and style of impulse control; quality and clarity of thinking (e.g., does the patient experience disordered thinking and/or psychosis); coping styles and capacities; style and capacity for relatedness to others; experience of others; style of solving problems; originality and integrative capacities; emotional responses to stress; emotional reactivity; defensiveness and style of defense; level of personal adjustment or ego functioning; ability to tolerate stress; adequacy of daily functioning; reality testing; level of self-esteem; and experience of family dynamics.

Although some psychologists may use projective testing alone to answer some of the above questions, it is more often used as part of a battery of tests and interpreted in the context of responses to several tests, history, and present described functioning. Projective tests are viewed as often versatile and rich in their findings but not as self-sufficient. Several authors, such as Anastasi,[1] have emphasized that projective tests give optimal results when used in a battery of tests and/or as a type of structured clinical interview. Others have noted, however, that test results have not been shown to increase in validity with the addition of other tests.[6]

10. In what specific situations is projective testing especially valuable?

Personality tests often are used to identify the patient's verbal responses to structured vs. unstructured situations. Such information may be invaluable to understand how someone who generally appears to function well in a structured interview would handle an ambiguous situation that may be more stressful and disorganizing. Individuals with borderline personality disorder, for example, may perform well on structured tests but evidence disorganized thinking on ambiguous, projective tests. Projective tests may address certain diagnostic questions pertaining to the intactness of thinking and reality testing.

Projective testing also may be useful in gaining information about emotional functioning in situations in which the individual is highly defensive and/or motivated to appear in particular ways during interview or on more direct, objective tests. Such an approach to test-taking may be part of patients' overt personality style or related more to their situation, e.g., feeling a need to present well because of a pending legal situation. In such instances, the ambiguity of projective testing may bypass the patient's reluctance to provide personal material.

BIBLIOGRAPHY

1. Anastasi A: Psychological Testing, 6th ed. New York, Macmillan, 1988.
2. Bellak L: The TAT, CAT and SAT in Clinical Use, 4th ed. New York, Grune & Stratton, 1986.
3. Edell WS: Role of structure in disordered thinking in borderline and schizophrenic disorders. J Pers Assess 51:23–41, 1987.
4. Exner JE: Rorschach assessment. In Weiner LB (ed): Clinical Method in Psychology. New York, John Wiley & Sons, 1983.
5. Exner JE: The Rorschach: A Comprehensive System, vol 1, 2nd ed. New York, John Wiley & Sons, 1986.
6. Garb HN: The incremental validity of information used in personality assessment. Clin Psychol Rev 4:641–655, 1985.
7. Goodenough F: Measurement of Intelligence by Drawings. New York, World Book, 1926.
8. Grath-Marnat G: Handbook of Psychological Assessment, 2nd ed. New York, John Wiley & Sons, 1990.
9. Handler L: The clinical use of the Draw-A-Person Test (DAP). In Newmark CS (ed): Major Psychological Assessment Instruments. Newton, MA, Selyn & Bacon, 1985.
10. Karon BP: Projective tests are valid. Am Psychol 33:764–765, 1978.
11. Kelly GA: The theory and technique of assessment. Annu Rev Psychol 9:325–352, 1958.
12. Koppitz EM: Psychological Evaluation of Human Figure Drawings by Middle School Pupils. New York, Grune & Stratton, 1984.
13. Leiter E: The role of projective testing. In Wetzler S, Katz M (eds): Contemporary Approaches to Psychological Assessment. New York, Brunner/Mazel, 1989.
14. Lindzey G: Projective Techniques and Cross-Cultural Research. New York, Appleton-Century-Crofts, 1961.
15. McClelland DC: The Achieving Society. NJ, Van Norstrand, 1961.
16. Machover K: Personality Projection in the Drawings of the Human Figure. Springfield, IL, Charles C Thomas, 1949.
17. Oster GD, Gould P: Using Drawings in Assessment and Therapy. New York, Brunner/Mazel, 1987.
18. Rabin I (ed): Assessment with Projective Techniques. New York, Springer, 1981.
19. Weiner IB: Conceptual and empirical perspectives on the Rorschach assessment of psychopathology. J Pers Assess 50:472–479.

6. NEUROPSYCHOLOGICAL TESTING

Laetitia L. Thompson, Ph.D.

1. What is neuropsychological testing?

Neuropsychological testing uses **behavioral measures** to assess skills and abilities that relate to brain functioning. Most neuropsychological tests have been developed to measure "higher cerebral functioning," so they usually focus on **cognitive skills and abilities**. These tests have been developed to help diagnose brain damage or brain dysfunction in some patients and to help ascertain the behavioral effects of brain damage in others. Such evaluation can provide information about cognitive strengths and weaknesses within an individual and the areas in which an individual's functioning may differ from that of the normal population. This type of evaluation is most commonly conducted on patients with neurologic disorders.

2. How does it differ from clinical psychological evaluation?

Clinical psychological evaluation uses tests designed to provide information about the **personality** and **emotional functioning** of patients. Measures may include objective personality tests or so-called projective techniques such as the Rorschach or the Thematic Apperception Test. Procedures used in clinical psychological evaluations generally differ from those used in neuropsychological evaluations, although occasionally there may be some overlap. For example, clinical evaluations frequently include an intelligence test, which is essentially a measure of cognitive function, and many neuropsychological evaluations have a personality measure to screen for emotional difficulties. The focus of the two types of evaluations differs, however, so the referring person must think about the goal of the evaluation in deciding where to refer.

3. What is neuropsychological testing like for the patient? (or, How to prepare your patient for a neuropsychological evaluation.)

Neuropsychological tests are behavioral. They are not invasive and present no physical risk to the patient. Typically the patients works with one or two testing examiners (sometimes, all or part of the testing is done by the neuropsychologist).

The tests may require reading or listening to verbal information, viewing nonverbal visual information, or palpating stimuli. Some tasks require pencil and paper, whereas others need only verbal responses from the patient. Some tasks require manipulation of objects, puzzle assembly, drawing of objects, or writing. If a patient has impaired vision or hearing, testing usually can be modified; it is helpful to discuss this with the neuropsychologist at the time of the referral.

The testing *can* be fatiguing, and precautions should be taken to administer the tests in an order that: (1) intersperses easier and harder tests; (2) begins the testing with tasks that reduce rather than increase anxiety; and (3) places tests with demanding attentional/speed requirements when the patient is fresh and well rested, yet past the initial anxiety.

In referring a patient for neuropsychological evaluation, it can be reassuring to talk briefly with the patient about the type of situation to be encountered. Patients sometimes telephone or arrive for their appointments wondering if they are going to be "stuck with needles or probed with electrodes." After they realize the testing is behavioral, they frequently are quite relieved.

4. What issues are addressed by neuropsychological testing?

First, it can help with diagnostic issues in certain cases, as when there are considerations of depression or dementia. In addition to overall level of performance, the neuropsychologist can look at patterns of test performance. For example, some patterns are associated more frequently with depression, whereas others are more likely to be seen in dementia. Of course, in some individuals, elements of *both* depression and dementia may co-exist, and neuropsychological evaluation may confirm this. Another type of diagnostic situation might involve a psychiatric patient for whom there is also a suspicion of a neurologic problem, such as early dementia or traumatic brain injury.

Second, as views about psychopathology change and more psychiatric conditions are found to have biologic components, more interest exists in understanding the neuropsychological characteristics of psychiatric disorders. The psychiatric disorder that has received the most attention to date has been schizophrenia, but now there are also studies of neuropsychological functioning in patients with bipolar, obsessive-compulsive, panic, post-traumatic stress, attention-deficit-hyperactivity, and conduct disorders, among others. It may be helpful to obtain information about the neurocognitive strengths and weaknesses of individual patients with these disorders and to learn whether their pattern of performance is similar to those of other patients with the same disorder.

Third, a practical area of concern is the everyday implications of neurocognitive function (or dysfunction) for psychiatrically ill patients. Neuropsychological evaluation helps clarify these issues and provides important information about long-term planning.

5. What are appropriate questions to consider in referring a psychiatric patient for neuropsychological testing?

When referring a patient for evaluation, the referring person ought to communicate the major question(s) to the neuropsychologist rather than simply indicating "neuropsychological testing" on a referral form. This facilitates a more useful battery of tests, as well as a more focused report. Some specific referral questions are listed in the table.

Examples of Common Referral Questions

1. Is the patient depressed, demented, or both?
2. Does this patient with schizophrenia have cognitive impairment? Is the impairment typical of that seen in schizophrenia?
3. A 59-year-old patient has a history of schizophrenia. Is there also evidence for early dementia?
4. The patient complains of memory problems. Is there objective evidence of memory problems or other cognitive deficits?
5. Does the patient have the cognitive capabilities to: live independently? comply with a medication regimen? work in a competitive or sheltered capacity?
6. The patient does not follow through with treatment planning. Is this related to memory or other cognitive deficits?

6. What should a neuropsychological evaluation and report include?

The neuropsychologist can select from many tests. The numerous options may confuse the referring person, who sees little apparent rhyme or reason to the specific tests used. It may be helpful, in determining the comprehensiveness of a particular evaluation, to keep in mind areas of cognition that usually are covered.

Major Cognitive Areas Assessed in a Comprehensive Evaluation

General intelligence	Perceptual functioning
Attention and concentration	Spatial analysis
Learning and memory	Sensory motor functioning
Language	Psychological/emotional status
Executive function	

Psychological/emotional status may be assessed during an interview and/or through formal testing.

Most neuropsychologists stress the use of standardized measures with high reliability and validity as well as normative guidelines to assist interpretation. Most emphasize that level of performance is only part of the process of interpretation, and that the pattern of performance across several tests is important. Some psychologists emphasize the quality of the patient's performance or the types of errors made.

In addition to the formal testing, the evaluation ought to include history taking, either from the patient, family, physician, and/or records, paying particular attention to background information and any medical history relating to possible neuropsychological risk factors.

The report should include discussion of the history, a report and discussion of the patient's behavior during testing, and an assessment of whether the test results are considered valid measures of the patient's neurocognitive functioning. Most reports also include a test-by-test description of the results, followed by conclusion(s), recommendations, and/or discussion of the overall meaning and implications of the results for the patient.

7. When is it appropriate to refer a patient for a neuropsychological *screening* rather than a comprehensive evaluation?

Many times, psychiatrists and other referrers hope that a screening evaluation will suffice for their patients. In some cases, relatively brief screening (i.e., a 1- to 2-hour battery) can adequately answer the question and, in some cases, a brief evaluation will be all a patient can tolerate because of acute psychiatric symptoms.

When there are questions regarding an in-patient with acute psychiatric symptoms, limited testing may be the only feasible alternative. Such testing provides information about the general level of intellectual functioning or presence of clear dementia, but it is unlikely to answer more specific questions, especially in younger adults in whom relatively subtle neurocognitive deficits may exist. Complex questions indicate the need for more comprehensive testing, and it may be better to defer testing until the patient is as stable as possible in terms of medication and psychiatric symptoms.

Screening may be appropriate to answer questions about presence or absence of neurocognitive dysfunction. More intensive evaluation is necessary if there are specific questions about nature, localization, or the functional implications of deficits.

Describing the patient to the neuropsychologist and discussing the issues and questions often is the best way to determine the most appropriate battery of tests to be given.

8. What are the effects of depression on neuropsychological testing?

The former answer to this question was that patients presenting with depression but without any "organic" dysfunction would show few, if any, deficits on classic neuropsychological batteries of tests such as the Halstead-Reitan. More recent studies, however, using newly developed measures of attention, information processing speed, and learning have shown that depression can cause slowing of information processing, decreased attention and concentration abilities, and learning inefficiency. Research findings are inconsistent about the existence of a high correlation between severity of depression and test performance. Groups of severely depressed patients are likely to perform more poorly than mildly depressed patients, but these findings are not sufficiently consistent to enable the clinician to predict the degree of cognitive inefficiency by knowing severity of depression.

In many cases, deficits in depressed individuals are subtle, but they may still affect interpretation of results. For example, in a patient with a clinical depression who has had a mild traumatic brain injury (TBI), it can be very difficult to know whether mild deficits in areas of concentration and/or learning are caused by the TBI, the depression, or a combination. Frequently, the practical approach to such a case is to treat the depression and then reevaluate the patient for any residual neurocognitive deficits. Other areas of cognition generally are not impaired in depressed patients (language, problem solving, visual spatial analysis, executive functioning, visual or auditory perception, for example), but, of course, individual patients may present as exceptions to the rule.

In a few instances, severe depression may render the patient untestable. If the patient has severe agitation or psychomotor retardation, he or she may not be able to comply with test requirements and fail to put forth sufficient effort to yield valid results. In my experience, this is not a common occurrence, but it does happen. In such instances, neuropsychological evaluation must be postponed until the acute depression improves.

9. What are the effects of anxiety on neuropsychological testing?

Most people who undergo neuropsychological testing experience some anxiety about the process. Part of a good testing procedure involves establishing rapport with the patient and providing a reassuring atmosphere to minimize anxiety. In most situations, this will suffice to allow valid testing. Very little systematic investigation has been done, however, to explore the effects of especially high levels of anxiety on test performance. The few existing studies have found little in the way of specific effects. Clinically, neuropsychologists rely on behavioral observation of the patient to help determine whether unusual levels of anxiety interfere with the patient's effort on the testing. Occasionally, undue anxiety may produce an invalid result (which should, of course, be noted), but in my experience, most patients can control their anxiety sufficiently to produce valid results. Frequently, putting the tests in an order to minimize stress to the patient is enough to permit the patient to complete the evaluation. Whether or not a particular evaluation is valid must be determined by the neuropsychologist.

In some cases, patients with formal anxiety disorders may be referred for neuropsychological evaluation. Research into the effects of formal anxiety disorders is currently at an early stage, and few definite conclusions can be drawn, but the following provides a brief summary of select diagnoses.

10. How do specific anxiety disorders affect cognitive functioning?

Patients with **panic disorder** typically have been found to fall below normative guidelines for impairment on a few tests, but across studies, cognitive deficits have been inconsistent. Currently, more evidence exists for memory problems than for other cognitive deficits, suggesting possible involvement of the temporal regions of the brain in panic disorder, but additional research is needed to replicate previous findings.

A few studies have assessed neurocognitive functioning in patients with **obsessive-compulsive disorder** (OCD). Results showing impaired memory and executive functioning suggest possible bilateral frontal and temporal involvement, with considerable disagreement from study to study as to whether the left or right hemisphere is more implicated.

Post-traumatic stress disorder (PTSD) is another anxiety disorder that has received attention, mostly in individuals with combat-related PTSD. Most studies have not included well-matched control groups, but rather have compared patient performance to available normative guidelines. Such studies have not found large deficits in groups of patients, but have shown that individuals may perform in the below average to borderline range on some tests of memory and attentional function.

Good neuropsychological testing involves administration of the tests in a supportive way to minimize state anxiety and behavioral observation of the patient to determine whether efforts to minimize anxiety have been successful. In patients with panic disorder, OCD, or PTSD, careful analysis of the pattern of test results can help determine: (1) whether deficits appear related to the anxiety disorder alone; and (2) the extent to which any cognitive deficits will have an impact on the patient's everyday life.

11. Is neuropsychological testing indicated in schizophrenia? How do patients with schizophrenia perform?

Schizophrenia is now thought to be a brain disorder, and many, but not all, patients show neurocognitive impairment. Research on the neuropsychological profiles of patients with schizophrenia has revealed considerable heterogeneity. Some patients perform normally on testing, whereas others are quite diffusely impaired. Commonly, the individual earns mildly impaired scores on a number of measures, but looks somewhat more impaired on verbal learning measures. This more pronounced verbal learning deficit superimposed upon diffuse mild impairment has now been found in several studies evaluating groups of schizophrenic patients, but specific individuals do not always, or even routinely, produce this profile. Little evidence exists for a decline in general intellectual functioning following the onset of symptoms, and it is rare for schizophrenic patients to have severe impairment without the presence of some coexisting dementia.

Because of the lack of a unique neuropsychological profile in patients with schizophrenia, interest has evolved in understanding patterns of deficits in subgroups of schizophrenic patients. Groups of paranoid patients generally perform better on neuropsychological testing than groups of non-para-noid patients. Studies of groups of patients with either predominantly positive or negative symptoms have produced similar results, with those patients showing more negative symptoms having much more significant impairment. Finally, patients with early-onset schizophrenia show more deficits than patients whose symptoms develop after adolescence.

Neuropsychological test results may be useful in predicting functional outcome in patients with schizophrenia. Walker et al. looked at patients 1.5 years after assessment and found that cognitive test scores were more powerful predictors of outcome measures than were ratings of psychiatric symptoms.[11] Therefore, extent of cognitive impairment may be important in predicting everyday functioning parameters such as treatment compliance, independent living, and employability.

12. What effects do medications have on testing?

This is obviously a very complex question, the answer to which depends on what medication or medications at what dosages. Medications that have central nervous system effects may, in some cases, affect neuropsychological test results.

A few guidelines exist to help determine when testing is best done. If a patient has just started a new medication and is experiencing temporary side effects, it is not a good time to evaluate the patient. If a patient is toxic or is approaching a toxic level, performance may be significantly affected.

Examining specific medications is beyond the scope of this chapter. However, most studies have shown that the acute symptoms of the disease are more deleterious for cognitive performance than the medications, if the patient is taking an optimal dose. Antidepressants have not been found to cause significant adverse effects on test performance in individuals with good clinical response who are not experiencing acute side effects. Generally speaking, neuroleptics also have not been found to cause significant problems on tests of cognitive function; thus, stopping medication in an individual who is obtaining clinical benefit is not advantageous. Lithium may cause some modest decrements in upper extremity motor performance, but has not been found to produce changes in neuropsychological test scores that would result in diagnostic or interpretive error.

13. What does it mean when neuropsychological testing and the results of neuroimaging disagree?

Relationships between neurobehavioral measures and neuroimaging techniques have changed dramatically over the past 25 years and likely will continue to, primarily as a result of the evolution of neuroradiologic technology. Furthermore, as the development of functional imaging advances, more opportunities will become available for understanding brain-behavior relationships. For example, research studies using functional MRI and neuropsychological testing have increased knowledge about localization of higher cerebral functions in the brain, but such research also has shown how difficult it is to make broad generalizations about localization of function for individual patients.

Clinical evaluation still employs structural imaging in most cases, and in individual cases, apparent discrepancies or contradictions may exist between neurobehavioral measures and neuroimaging results. These differences may be in either direction (more abnormality on imaging than seen in behavior or vice versa). Reasons include:

1. There may be long-standing, probably congenital, abnormalities, but the patient has relatively normal neurocognitive functioning because the brain organized with the abnormality already in place.

2. The physiological changes associated with brain lesions identified by computed tomography or magnetic resonance imaging may exceed the boundaries of the structural abnormality.

3. Individual differences in functional brain organization are complex and not yet completely understood.

4. Neurobehavioral measures may be incorrectly interpreted, e.g., interpreting errors on sensory or motor tests resulting from peripheral nervous system injury as central nervous system impairment.

5. Changes at a microscopic level may cause behavioral change, but may not be visible with current imaging technology.

As functional imaging becomes more common in clinical practice, differences between neuropsychological performance and neuroimaging may diminish. The use of functional imaging already is advancing our knowledge of brain-behavior relationships.

BIBLIOGRAPHY

1. Bigler ED: Frontal lobe damage and neuropsychological assessment. Arch Clin Neuropsychol 3:279–297, 1988,
2. Bigler ED, Yeo RA, Turkheimer E (eds): Neuropsychological Function and Brain Imaging. New York, Plenum Press, 1989.
3. Grant I, Adams KM (eds): Neuropsychological Assessment of Neuropsychiatric Disorders. New York, Oxford Press, 1996.
4. Heinrichs RW, Zakzanis KK: Neurocognitive deficit in schizophrenia: A quantitative review of the evidence. Neuropsychology 12:426–445, 1998.
5. Hill CD, Stoudemire A, Morris R, Matino-Saltzman D, Markwalter HR: Similarities and differences in memory deficits in patients with primary dementia and depression-related cognitive dysfunction. J Neuropsychiatry Clin Neurosci 5:277–282, 1993.
6. Lezak MD: Neuropsychological Assessment, 3rd ed. New York, Oxford University Press, 1995.
7. Newman PJ, Sweet JJ: Depressive disorders. In Puente AE, McCaffrey RJ (eds): Handbook of Neuropsychological Assessment: A Biopsychosocial Perspective. New York, Plenum Press, 1992.
8. Orsillo SM, McCaffrey RJ: Anxiety disorders. In Puente AE, McCaffrey RJ (eds): Handbook of Neuropsychological Assessment: A Biopsychosocial Perspective. New York, Plenum Press, 1992.
9. Reitan RM, Wolfson D: The Halstead-Reitan Neuropsychological Battery: Theory and Interpretation, 2nd ed. Tucson, AZ, Neuropsychology Press, 1993.
10. Sweet JJ, Newman P, Bell B: Significance of depression in clinical neuropsychological assessment. Clin Psychol Rev 12:21–45, 1992.
11. Walker E, Lucas M, Lewine R: Schizophrenic disorders. In Puente AE, McCaffrey RJ (eds): Handbook of Neuropsychological Assessment: A Biopsychosocial Perspective. New York, Plenum Press, 1992.

7. SELF-REPORT QUESTIONNAIRES

Garry Welch, Ph.D.

1. What are the potential uses of self-reporting psychiatric and personality tests?

There are many potential clinical and research uses, although interpretation of scores and profiles often requires a high level of expertise. These tests are helpful in:

- History taking and formulating clinical hypotheses
- Screening and diagnosis of clinical problems and mental disorders
- Determining appropriate referral to specialty services
- Monitoring change and response to treatment interventions
- Conducting research into factors associated with the disorders
- Auditing and assessing clinical services

2. What is reliability?

Reliability is whether the measure provides repeatable or reproducible test scores that accurately reflect the patient's true status and contain little influence from unimportant extraneous factors. For example, if a test is supposed to detect current anxiety state, it is reliable if it mostly measures current anxiety and does not take into account other factors—such as the individual's recall of the answers given the last time the test was administered—and does not include unclear questions or poorly worded instructions.

3. What is the role of reliability in psychiatric and personality tests?

Reliability of measurement is important because it sets an upper limit on the validity, or clinical usefulness, that the measure will likely have when applied to various individuals and in various settings. Unreliable measures cannot be highly valid, and results obtained from them may cloud the true meaning of test scores, thereby undermining clinical decision-making.

4. How do I determine if a test is reliable?

Reliability indices used to describe psychiatric and personality questionnaires range in value from 0 (no reliability) to 1 (perfect reliability) and are of two types: (1) the test-retest index, which indicates how stable the test scores are over a short period, with individuals assumed not to have changed much on the topic of interest, and (2) the internal reliability index, which shows whether the questions are all highly intercorrelated and are therefore likely to be measuring the same thing.

Test-retest reliability typically is measured by the correlation coefficient or (preferably) the intraclass correlation coefficient. Test-retest reliability coefficients can be difficult to interpret if they are not high (i.e., around 0.8). Lower reliability values may indicate that the test is unreliable, or that the individuals tested have changed in status over the period of testing. Test-retest coefficients obtained for known fluctuating variables (e.g., depressed mood or anxious mood) are expected to be lower than those for a relatively stable personality trait, such as extroversion, which may demonstrate test-retest reliability of around 0.9.

Internal reliability indices are easier to interpret than test-retest and typically involve the use of Cronbach's alpha index. Results should range from 0.7 to 0.8 if the test is to be used to compare groups of people, but the upper range should be higher (preferably around 0.9) if the test is to be used to classify individuals.

Ideally, both test-retest and internal reliability information should be available for a test. Reliability information obtained from different settings may vary. For example, data gathered in a heterogeneous general population study may not directly apply to a highly selected hospital-based patient population. Typically, reliability coefficients will be somewhat lower in the latter case for technical reasons related to the narrower range of scores obtained.

5. What is validity?

Validity is whether a test adequately measures what it is supposed to measure, to allow specific conclusions to be drawn. There are several types of validity: *content, predictive, convergent,* and *discriminant.*

6. What is the role of validity in psychiatric and personality tests?

Although reliability analyses can establish that a test is measuring *something* in a reproducible fashion, validity analyses can help establish exactly *what* is being measured. Validity analyses can determine whether the test can satisfactorily perform an important clinical task, such as early screening for problems, making a diagnosis, monitoring response to treatment, and directing research into the causes of particular disorders.

Validity studies usually involve (1) calculating correlations between the test and other related measures or individual attributes, and (2) looking at the size of difference in mean scores for selected study groups.

7. How do I determine if a test is valid?

The fundamental question in considering the validity of a test is "Do the test scores have biologic or clinical meaning for the specific task I have in mind and for the particular individuals?" One of the difficulties in assessing validity in psychiatry and psychology is that there often is no absolute standard against which to judge the validity of a test. Although this creates headaches for clinicians and researchers in many branches of medicine, it is a particular problem in mental health, where psychosocial phenomena that can be neither readily observed nor easily described are of interest. Ideally, the validity of psychiatric and personality tests is determined by weighing the evidence from a variety of validity studies that show that the test measures what it was designed to measure.

Checklist for Reliability and Validity Issues Related to Questionnaires

---

Reliability

Test retest reliability—

    Are temporal reliability coefficients around 0.8 over 2-day to 2-week periods?

    Are values lower for fluctuating variables like mood and higher (approximately 0.9) for stable variables such as personality traits?

Internal reliability—

    Are Cronbach alpha values around 0.7–0.8 for group comparisons or about 0.9 for individual screening or classification uses?

Validity

Content

    Is the breadth of the conceptual domain adequately covered?

    Is critical content covered?

Predictive

    Does the test predict future behavior?

Convergent

    Does the test correlate well with existing similar measures?

    Are similar findings obtained from different sources, e.g., from subject, clinician, or spouse?

Discriminant

    Do the scores of selected groups differ in their mean as predicted?

    Are low correlations found with theoretically unrelated variables, or are negative correlations found where these are theoretically expected?

    For a screening test, does it have 100% sensitivity and high positive-predictive power?

    Does a measure of treatment response have good responsiveness (see Question 12)?

Construct

    This term represents a judgment, based on an accumulation of related validity studies performed over time, that the test measures its intended topic.

---

8. What is *content* validity?

It is essentially a subjective judgment, based usually on expert consensus and/or a review of the literature, that the breadth of the conceptual domain the test is aiming to measure is adequately covered or that the most clinically significant areas of the domain (i.e., critical content) are well covered. Generally, when a new psychiatric or personality test appears in the literature it has some practical or theoretical advantage over the older ones. For example, a new test may be briefer and quicker to administer, have better worded questions, or have new questions that reflect recent changes in theory or clinical practice. Or it may be a companion measure to be used as a screening device, replacing a longer questionnaire or clinical interview in special situations in which the use of the latter is impractical (e.g., community surveys).

9. What is *predictive* validity?

This term indicates interest in predicting some important behavior at a point in the future. For example, scores of a screening test of depressive symptoms might be expected to correlate highly with later suicidal behavior or later antidepressant drug use.

10. What does *convergent* validity show?

It verifies that the test correlates highly with measures to which it is thought to be theoretically related. For example, one measure of depression would be expected to have high correlations with other measures of depression. Another approach may be to establish that test scores obtained from different sources are at least moderately correlated, e.g., those from patient, therapist, and family members.

11. What does the term *discriminant* validity establish?

That the test is *not* correlated with measures to which it is theoretically *un*related, e.g., that depressed scores are not correlated with those measuring intelligence. Also, that test scores are significantly different for groups theoretically expected to differ, e.g., depressed patients should score higher than either normal controls or successfully treated patients on a measure of depression that is under scrutiny.

12. Define responsiveness.

The term describes the ability of a test to detect true change in patient clinical status over time (usually in the context of treatment). For example, scores for a depression test should be lower on retesting of a depressed patient group that has received a drug treatment or psychotherapy of known efficacy. Deyo et al. provide a good discussion of responsiveness and examples of suitable indices.

13. Which indices are most useful in diagnosis and screening?

Diagnostic and screening discriminant validity allows screening and classification of illness. The most useful validity indices for this purpose are **positive predictive power** (PPV), which indicates the proportion of high scorers (using a given cut-off score) on a test who were found to be clinically ill by clinical interview, and **sensitivity**, which indicates the proportion of truly ill individuals who scored high on the test. Typically they are expressed as percentages. For a good screening measure, ideally there should be 100% sensitivity at the recommended cut-off score, to ensure no potential true cases are missed, and as high a PPV as possible to minimize the number of false positives (high scorers who are in fact not ill) interviewed. Psychiatric and personality measures rarely are used alone to determine diagnosis, but are used commonly in screening and as an adjunct to the diagnostic interview.

14. Explain construct validity.

This umbrella or summary term involves judging how well a given test fulfills its aim in measuring an underlying concept. Construct validity is programmatic and requires the gradual accumulation of evidence through a wide range of appropriate validity studies that measure different aspects of the test's validity. It may include information from all of the types of validity plus data from **factor analytic studies**. These statistical studies examine the pattern of correlations among scores for individual questions in a test to determine whether groups of conceptually similar terms intercorrelate highly.

15. Will following the reliability and validity checklist (see Question 7) ensure that I use self-report questionnaires successfully?

Remember, *no measure is reliable and valid for all purposes*, and red flags should be raised if a test is uncritically described as "reliable and valid" in a clinical or research article you have read. Available information on the potential usefulness of a given test should be considered in light of your specific purpose, the characteristics of the patients or subjects to be tested, and the setting they are to be drawn from. Again, many psychiatric and personality tests require a high level of training and clinical expertise, and interpretation and appropriate professional help should be sought if necessary.

16. What is a valid questionnaire to measure depression?

The Beck Depression Inventory (BDI) is the most widely used and validated self-report questionnaire for measuring the symptoms of depression. It has 21 questions and is straightforward to administer and score. Information on its reliability and clinical usefulness (and normative data) is available for many different medical, psychiatric, and general population samples to aid the interpretation of an individual or group BDI score.

17. What are the potential clinical uses of the BDI?

The BDI is used mostly to monitor change in the severity of depressive symptoms over time in individuals receiving treatment for depression or taking part in research studies of depression. It is not recommended as a diagnostic tool, although cut-off scores for nondepressed (< 10), mildly depressed (10–14), moderately depressed (15–22), and severely depressed (23 +) categories have been recommended by the original authors based on validity studies. Among medically ill patient groups, physical symptoms common to depression become problematic when interpreting BDI scores. In patients with renal failure, for example, a cut-off of 15 best discriminates clinically depressed patients from the nondepressed, although only 40% of individuals scoring above 15 will, in fact, be clinically depressed on subsequent full psychiatric interview. Common confounding somatic symptoms in renal failure include fatigue, anorexia, and sleep and bowel dysfunction that result from problems such as elevated blood urea nitrogen levels, acidemia, electrolyte imbalances, and problems with calcium metabolism.

18. Is there a valid questionnaire to measure anxiety?
    The State Trait Anxiety Inventory is the most widely used and well validated self-report measure of the symptoms of anxiety. It has 20 questions that measure state (i.e., situation-specific) anxiety and 20 that measure trait (i.e, resulting from enduring personality style) anxiety. The test is simple to administer and score and takes only 10 minutes to complete. The state scale has been widely used in the assessment of current anxiety in general population, psychiatric, and medical settings. As expected, both scales have good internal reliability, and the state scale has lower reported test-retest reliability (0.16–0.62) than the trait scale (0.65–0.82). The state scale correlates well with other similar anxiety measures and is a responsive measure of treatment outcome in clinical trials involving psychotropic drugs, medical procedures, and psychotherapy. Evaluation of potentially confounding somatic State Trait Anxiety Inventory items has yet to be carried out in suitable medical settings.

19. What are the practical uses of the normative data provided for psychiatric and personality tests?
    Normative data can be very useful in interpreting individual or group scores because they provide yardsticks against which the clinical or other significance can be judged. They typically are presented as mean test scores plus standard deviations (SD; the variability of the scores) for selected groups and are to be found in test manuals and research papers. Norms may be available for a wide range of groups, and the test user must select the most appropriate. Medically or psychiatrically ill groups, general populations groups, or groups based on specific demographic factors (such as age or sex) typically are provided.
    To compare the score of an individual with others, it often is useful to transform individual scores to **standard or Z scores** recalculated in SD units. Individuals scoring at the group mean are then converted to a score of 0, and those scoring above or below one SD from the mean are converted to a score of 1 and –1, respectively. This is handy because 68% of people are expected to always fall within one SD of the mean. For example, if an individual scores 76 on a test and the comparison group has a mean score of 65 and an SD of 8, the individual's new Z score will be 1.4 (i.e., his or her score is 1.4 SDs above the group mean).
    Z scores often are converted to **T scores**, so that all values are positive, because some people prefer not to work with negative numbers. With T scores, the group mean and SD are reset to some other, more convenient value, although the relative value of any individual's score is unchanged. For example, in intelligence testing, T-score means and SDs commonly are reset from 0 and 1 to 100 and 15, respectively, and in personality testing they are reset to 50 and 10.

20. How is human personality broadly conceptualized and measured today?
    Although this is a complex area with a long history of debate among competing schools of thought, a broad general acceptance now exists that the **Five-Factor Model** of personality provides the most comprehensive description. The model suggests that personality can be best described in general terms by five concepts (with aspect of personality involved in parentheses):

- neuroticism (emotional)
- extroversion (interpersonal)
- openness to experience (experiential)
- agreeability (attitudinal)
- conscientiousness (motivational)

21. Elaborate on the Five-Factor Model.
    This model is a major advance in the field of personality assessment, helping to integrate widely varying and historically conflicting schools of thought (e.g., behaviorism, humanism, social

learning, cognitive-developmental, and psychoanalysis). It also provides a conceptual basis for organizing the wide array of currently available personality tests. The Five-Factor Model is important because it promises to provide a broad conceptual framework for the several hundred specific personality factors described to date, and empirical support exists for its cross-cultural generalizability.

Critics of the Five-Factor Model note that some important concepts (such as impulsivity) are not included and that it is essentially atheoretical and descriptive, rather than explanatory.

Typical usage has entailed close association with the revised NEO Personality Inventory in general population studies. However, wide application is occurring in psychiatry, to provide a broad dimensional assessment of a personality and to complement the familiar "case/non-case" categorical or diagnostic approach typically used for personality disorders. The Five-Factor Model also has application in behavioral medicine and industrial psychology.

22. What are some more specific measures of personality?

A wide range of specific personality measures are available to assess more finely grained concepts of personality than those measured in the Five-Factor Model. The more common of these include: the Eysenck Personality Questionnaire, the 16PF, the California Personality Inventory, and the Minnesota Multiphasic Personality Inventory. Such measures help generate useful clinical hypotheses, but generally are not good diagnostic tools for psychiatric problems. Commonly, patient profiles are generated from test scores and the overall profile pattern is interpreted, rather than individual subscale scores examined. For example, many clinically useful profiles have been suggested using the Minnesota Multiphasic Personality Inventory subscales, and literally thousands of studies have been carried out with this test and its applications.

Another measure, the Personality Research Form, is a valuable research tool, and its 22 dimensions fit the Five-Factor Model.

23. What are good questionnaires to use in evaluating eating disorders?

Two measures of the symptoms of anorexia nervosa and bulimia nervosa are available to screen for clinical and subclinical eating disorders, to describe fully if eating disorder symptoms are present, and to detect changes in symptom status over time. They also are widely used in research to improve understanding of the nature and treatment of eating disorders. The two recommended measures are the Eating Disorder Inventory-2 (EDI-2) and the Bulimia Test–Revised (BULIT–Revised). These are *not* diagnostic measures, but principally are useful adjuncts to clinical assessments and decision making.

24. Describe the EDI-2.

The EDI-2's 91 questions assess a wide range of behaviors, feelings, and symptoms found in eating disorders. It has three core clinical subscales related to eating and weight and shape concerns, and eight more that provide information on general problems often present with eating disorders. The Drive for Thinness, Bulimia, and Body Dissatisfaction subscales are the most important clinically. The Drive for Thinness subscale has been applied with a cut-off score of 14 to identify any potential eating disturbance. The scores for all 11 subscales are presented as individual patient profiles and the overall pattern compared with normative profiles provided in the EDI-2 manual. The EDI-2 subscales are:

Core clinical subscales
1. *Drive for thinness*—excessive fear of weight gain, preoccupation with weight and dieting
2. *Bulimia*—frequent bouts of uncontrollable eating binges and thoughts about binges
3. *Body dissatisfaction*—about body size and shape

General subscales
1. *Ineffectiveness*—feelings of insecurity, worthlessness, and inadequacy
2. *Perfectionism*—high expectations for personal performance and achievement
3. *Interpersonal distrust*—feelings of alienation, avoidance of close relationships
4. *Lack of interoceptive awareness*—inability to identify accurately one's own emotional states and bodily sensations related to eating and hunger

5. *Maturity fears*—desire to retreat or regress to the relative safety and security of childhood

6. *Asceticism*—belief in the virtue of self-discipline, control of bodily urges, and self-denial

7. *Lack of impulse regulation*—a tendency toward impulsivity, self-destructive behavior, and recklessness

8. *Social insecurity*—perceptions of self-doubts and insecurity in social relationships

25. How is the EDI-2 used?

Typically a patient profile is compared with those given for available norms to clarify the nature and severity of the problems. The EDI-2 can be most helpful in providing information to understand the patient, planning treatment, and assessing progress.

26. What is the function of the BULIT–Revised?

The BULIT–Revised was designed to screen for bulimia nervosa (BN) and to monitor changes in related bulimic symptom severity over time. It is composed of 28 core questions, plus 8 others used for descriptive purposes but not scored. The BULIT–Revised test includes questions on the nature and frequency of binge eating, loss of control during binges, use of purging behaviors, and dissatisfaction with bodily shape. The internal reliability of the BULIT–Revised is high and has been found to correlate well with related measures.

As a community screening measure, Welch and colleagues showed that a cut-off score of 98 is optimal among young women (i.e, clinically important cases will not be missed). However, many false-positive cases will be included (about 30%) because of technical problems related to the low base rate of BN among females in community samples (approximately 2–3% prevalence). This problem also occurs in screening for anorexia nervosa.

Nevertheless, both the EDI-2 and BULIT–Revised can reduce the subsequent interviewing workload in community studies. Also, in the clinical setting, individual BULIT–Revised questions and the total score can help in assessment and in monitoring response to treatment.

27. What tests are good options for measuring general psychiatric distress or probable psychiatric caseness by questionnaire?

Two useful tools are the General Health Questionnaire, which is designed for research use in community and nonpsychiatric settings, and the Symptom Check List–90, designed for use in psychiatric and medical populations.

28. Describe the General Health Questionnaire.

The General Health Questionnaire comes in short, intermediate, and long versions; the intermediate 30-question version is probably the most commonly employed. Its principal use is in identifying probable nonpsychotic psychiatric illness.The General Health Questionnaire is simple to administer and score, although long-standing patient problems may be missed, because the test asks how the patient feels relative to "usual." The test manual recommends two additional questions that can be added to adjust for this problem ("use of psychiatric drugs" and "history of nervous problems"). The General Health Questionnaire has been found to correlate highly with similar screening measures, and the 30-question version has an overall sensitivity of 74% and a specificity of 82%. Patients with physical health problems may score higher because of the presence of somatic anxiety symptoms.

29. Describe the Symptom Checklist–90 (SCL-90).

The SCL-90 assesses nonpsychotic psychiatric symptoms in nine different symptom areas: somatization, obsessive-compulsion, paranoid ideation, psychoticism, phobic anxiety, depression, anxiety, interpersonal sensitivity, and hostility. It offers a global score related to the intensity of perceived psychological distress and the number of psychological symptoms (Global Severity Index). The nine subscales generally have good internal and test-retest reliability, and the Global Severity Index has been found to correlate well with similar measures and have good responsiveness to detect changes in psychological distress. A standardized (T-score) cut-off score of 63 has been suggested for the Global Severity Index to detect probable psychiatric illness.

Note that norms for the General Health Questionnaire and the SCL-90 are available for a range of medical, psychiatric, and general population groups.

30. Are computer programs available to help score and interpret some of the psychological tests mentioned here?

Yes. This is a burgeoning field with many new programs coming onto the market each year. Stoloff and Couch provide a recent listing of useful, currently available computer programs to help score and interpret commonly used tests. The measures covered include the BDI, the Spielberger State-Trait Anxiety Inventory, the 16PF, the Minnesota Personality Inventory, the California Personality Inventory, and the Personality Research Form.

31. The phrase "quality of life" pops up everywhere. What is it?

Health-related quality of life is a complex, patient-centered, and dynamic description of the changes in patient functioning and well being over time that are related to the patient's illness, treatment, and complications. A general consensus now exists that, in its fullest sense, quality of life encompasses four distinct areas that cover the patient's total experience of illness: (1) physical health and symptoms, (2) functional status and activities of daily living, (3) mental well-being (including existential and spiritual aspects of living), and (4) social health, i.e., social role functioning and social support (including the patient's relationship to the medical team and hospital environment).

32. What measures can be used to assess health-related quality of life?

Quality-of-life measures can be used to compare individual patient profiles with those of a similar patient group or to compare quality of life across different patient groups. These measures commonly are termed "generic" and include the SF-36, the Sickness Impact Profile, and the Nottingham Health Profile. Another measure of quality of life is the disease-specific. This type is tailored to the specific issues of a given illness and provides greater sensitivity to detect subtle changes in quality of life than more generic measures. Selection of the appropriate generic or specific measure depends on the research goal or clinical issue. Note, however, that the SIP and NHP are better suited for severely ill patients.

Patient-focused self-reporting is the preferred mode of assessment of the subjective aspects of quality of life such as psychological and social functioning, not only because self-reporting measures are inexpensive and easy to administer, but also because they provide the most important information: the patient's perspective. Some potential applications of quality-of-life measurement include:
- Screening and monitoring for psychosocial problems in individual patient care
- Population surveys of perceived health problems for medical audit
- Outcome measures for use in health services or evaluation research
- Outcome measures in clinical trials
- Cost/utility analyses

BIBLIOGRAPHY

1. Bowling A: Measuring health: A Review of Quality of Life Measurement Scales. Philadelphia, Open University Press, 1991.
2. Costa PT, McCrae RR: Revised NEO Personality Inventory and the NEO Five-Factor Model. Odessa, FL, Psychological Assessment Resources, 1992.
3. Deyo R, Kiehr P, Patrick DL: Reproducibility and responsiveness of health status measures: Statistics and strategies for evaluation. Controlled Clinical Trials 12:142s–158s, 1991.
4. Garner DM: Eating Disorder Inventory-2 Professional Manual. Odessa, FL, Psychological Assessment Resources, 1991.
5. Patrick D, Deyo R: Generic and disease-specific measures in assessing health status and quality of life. Med Care 27:S217–S232, 1989.
6. Proceedings of the International Conference on the Measurement of Quality of Life as an Outcome in Clinical Trials. Controlled Clinical Trials 12:243s–256s, 1991.

7. Stoloff M, Couch J: Computer Use in Psychology: A Directory of Software, 3rd ed. Washington, DC, American Psychological Association, 1992.
8. Streiner D, Norman GR: Health Measurement Scales: A Practical Guide to Their Development and Use. Oxford, Oxford University Press, 1989.
9. Thelen M, Farmer J, Wonderlich S, Smith M: A revision of the bulimia test—the BULIT–R. Psychological Assessment 3:119–124, 1987.
10. Thompson C: The Instruments of Psychiatric Research. Chichester, 1989.
11. Welch GW, Thompson L, Hall A: The BULIT–R: Its reliability and clinical validity as a screening tool for DSM–III R bulimia nervosa in a female tertiary education population. Int J Eating Dis 14:95–105, 1993.
12. McCrae RR, Costa PT, Pedroso de Lima M: Age differences in personality across the adult life span: Parallels in five cultures. Develop Psychol 35(2):466–477, 1999.

8. STANDARDIZED PSYCHIATRIC INTERVIEWS

Jacqueline A. Samson, Ph.D.

1. When should I use a standardized interview?

Standardized interviews are necessary when collecting data for research and for comparing your own patients with those reported in the psychiatric literature. They also are valuable as a systematic means of evaluating patients that is less subject to bias or incomplete assessment.

In clinical practice, it's easy to spend a lot of time discussing the problems volunteered by the patient, but fail to ask about other problems that are less apparent but no less important. Patients are particularly reticent when they feel symptoms are embarrassing or socially unacceptable. Alcohol or drug abuse, sexual compulsions, or symptoms related to trauma often are missed because clinicians don't probe. Standardized interviews enhance understanding of specific syndromes and pinpoint the questions most useful in eliciting psychiatric information. In this way, they are valuable training devices.

2. How is a standardized interview different from a clinical interview?

In a standardized interview, there are **specific guidelines** that define the areas of questioning to be covered and the kind of information to be elicited from a patient. The interviewer is expected to cover all the areas included in the guidelines and to ask for a sufficient amount of detail to complete ratings in each area. The format of the interview is also specified to insure that the interview is conducted in a comparable fashion by all clinicians both within and across institutions.

3. What is the difference between a fully structured and a semi-structured interview format?

A fully structured interview specifies the wording of questions and the order in which questions are asked. The format is defined and must not be altered by the interviewer in any way. In a semi-structured interview, the wording of questions and ordering are specified but may be modified by the interviewer to suit the needs of a particular patient, as long as all areas are covered in the interview. Fully structured interviews provide a high degree of consistency from one interview to another, and have been used extensively in epidemiologic studies that involve many raters. Semi-structured interviews are less standardized but allow for clarifications and probes that can improve the validity of responses from atypical or severely impaired patients.

4. What kinds of standardized interviews are available?

The two most common types are interviews to assess the psychiatric diagnosis (**diagnostic interviews**) and interviews to assess the severity of certain types of symptoms at a specific point in time (**cross-sectional symptom severity rating scales**).

Summary of Diagnostic Interviews

INTERVIEW	DIAGNOSTIC SYSTEM	FORMAT	INTERVIEWER
Schedule of Affective Disorders and Schizophrenia (SADS)	Research Diagnostic Criteria (RDC)	Semi-structured	Clinician
Diagnostic Interview Schedule (DIS)	DSM-III	Fully structured	Lay person
Structured Clinical Interview for DSM Diagnosis (SCID)	DSM-III-R, DSM IV	Semi-structured	Clinician
Composite International Diagnostic Interview (CIDI)	DSM-III-R, ICD-10	Fully structured	Lay person

5. Which fully structured diagnostic interview is used most commonly?

The Diagnostic Interview Schedule (DIS). The DIS was developed for use in large-scale epidemiologic surveys and for administration by specially trained nonclinicians.[15] It is structured to obtain both lifetime and current diagnoses (within the last year). Questions are organized by symptoms, and patients are asked first whether the symptom has ever occurred in their lifetime, and second whether the symptoms occurred within the last 1-month, 6-month, or 12-month period. Probes are included for each symptom to determine whether alcohol or drugs were involved, the patient sought treatment, and occupational or social functioning was impaired. Symptoms are coded as present if they are independent of alcohol or drug use and resulted in either treatment or impairment of functioning. Diagnoses are assigned by computer on the basis of algorithms applied to coded interview data.

A modified version of the DIS called the Composite International Diagnostic Interview has been created to allow for assignment of diagnoses according to the International Classification of Diseases (ICD-10) system.[25]

6. Which semi-structured diagnostic interviews are used most commonly?

The **Schedule for Affective Disorders and Schizophrenia** (SADS) interview contains 82 scales to assess symptoms of depression, mania, psychosis, and anxiety.[7] Multiple questions are provided for each rating scale, and the interviewer may select those that work best with a particular patient. Supplementary information based on observation, clinical report, or chart review may be incorporated into interview ratings. At the completion of the interview, specific inclusion and exclusion criteria are applied to the symptom ratings, and diagnoses are assigned by the rater. The SADS comes in two parts: part I documents symptoms associated with the current episode; part II documents symptoms during previous episodes. A diagnostic system called Research Diagnostic Criteria (RDC) was developed for use with the SADS questions. The RDC system and SADS interview were created before the DSM-III systems (in fact, the DSM-III systems were modeled to a degree on the RDC), but are easily modified to obtain DSM-III or DSM-IV diagnoses.

The **Structured Clinical Interview for DSM-III-R Diagnosis** (SCID) obtains an accurate psychiatric diagnosis relatively quickly (unlike the SADS, which is for more comprehensive research use).[21] Thus, certain questions can be skipped as soon as it is apparent that the patient does not meet the necessary diagnostic criteria. Symptoms are scored as absent, present, or subthreshold. Unlike the SADS, current and past diagnoses are assessed in the same interview. This strategy may be modified for patients who have difficulty shifting mental set from present to past and back to present. The questions in each section follow the diagnostic criteria outlined in DSM-III-R, and the interviewer notes at the conclusion of each module whether or not the patient meets full diagnostic criteria.

Versions of the SCID are available with questions worded so as to assume that the patient is currently symptomatic (patient version) and also with questions worded with no assumption of present or past patient status (nonpatient version).

7. How do the various interviews accommodate the diagnoses found in the DSM-IV?

At this point in time, the SCID has been revised and field tested for DSM-IV.

While changes in the standard system of diagnoses allow updating of clinical methods to reflect state-of-the-art knowledge about psychopathology, they also create difficulties for researchers in long-term studies due to problems comparing results based on different diagnostic systems. Thus, many researchers continue to use the interviews in the original form to maintain consistency of data collection over time and across studies.

8. How much time is required to complete the diagnostic interview?
The duration of the interview depends on the amount of psychopathology presented by the patient and the ability of the patient to give a concise history. A completed interview with a good informant who shows a moderate amount of psychopathology (for example, a current episode of major depression, dysthymic disorder, and a past episode of panic disorder) requires about 1.5 hours.

9. When should I use a symptom severity rating scale instead of a diagnostic interview?
Symptom severity rating scales are designed to measure the severity of specific symptoms at a particular point in time. They are used to measure symptom severity once a diagnosis has already been made. Typically, symptom assessments are repeated to monitor response to treatment. For example, a psychiatrist might administer a Hamilton Depression Rating Scale, which measures the severity of depressive symptoms, before starting a drug, and then repeat the assessment each time the patient comes in. The initial score is compared with the followup scores to determine whether there is a significant improvement in symptoms over time.

Cross-Sectional Symptom Severity Rating Scales

RATING METHOD	SYMPTOMS			FUNCTIONING
	Depression	*Anxiety*	*General*	
Interview:	Hamilton Depression Rating Scale Inventory for Depressive-Symptomatology (IDS) Montgomery-Asberg Scale Raskin Scale	Hamilton Anxiety Rating Scale	Brief Psychiatric Rating Scale (BPRS)	Global Assessment of Functioning (GAF) Clinical Global Impression Scale (CGI)
Self Report:	Beck Depression Inventory Inventory for Depressive Symptomatology (IDS-SR) Zung Inventory	Beck Anxiety Inventory State-Trait Anxiety Inventory	Symptom Check-list-90 (SCL-90) Profile of Mood States (POMS)	Social Adjustment Scale (SAS)

10. What if I don't have time to administer the assessment? Are there any questionnaires that the patient can fill out that will provide the same information?
Presently, there are no widely used self-report questionnaires for assessing psychiatric diagnosis. Valid diagnostic assessment requires a clinician who can interpret signs and symptoms against a standard and consider them in assigning a differential diagnosis. Some success has been reported by researchers who created an interactive computer program to assign a diagnosis based on the fully structured method used in the DIS.

Many self-report questionnaires are available to assess symptom severity. Some of these questionnaires are general and cover a wide variety of symptoms, while others focus on one symptom dimension, such as depression (see table above).

11. Symptom assessment does not tell me whether or not a person is functioning in the community. Are there any measures that monitor improvement in actual functioning?
Yes. Several simple scoring systems are widely used by clinicians to document functioning. **The Global Assessment of Functioning Scale** (see Chapter 4) provides descriptions of possible levels of functioning along a continuum ranging from functioning in all areas to persistent inability to maintain personal hygiene. **The Clinical Global Impression Scale** (see chart on next page) asks the clinician to rate the overall severity of the illness compared with all other psychiatric patients. The

ratings range from "normal, not at all ill" (a score of 1) to "among the most extremely ill patients." In addition, there are self-reported questionnaires that ask patients to assess their own functioning across a number of social roles. **The Social Adjustment Scale**[22] has been widely used for this purpose, and published norms for scoring are available.

One drawback with self-reported instruments is that questions usually are based on the patients' experience of satisfaction with their role performance. Thus, ratings do not directly assess actual functioning against an external standard.

CLINICAL GLOBAL IMPRESSIONS

1. Severity of Illness

Considering your total clinical experience with this particular population, how mentally ill is the patient at this time?

```
0 = Not Assessed              4 = Moderately ill
1 = Normal, not at all ill    5 = Markedly ill
2 = Borderline mentally ill   6 = Severely ill
3 = Mildly ill                7 = Among the most extremely
                                  ill patients
```

2. Global Improvement – Rate total improvement whether or not, in your judgment, it is due entirely to drug treatment.

Compared to his condition at admission to the project, how much has he changed?

```
0 = Not Assessed              4 = No change
1 = Very much improved        5 = Minimally worse
2 = Much improved             6 = Much worse
3 = Minimally improved        7 = Very much worse
```

3. Efficacy Index – Rate this item on the basis of DRUG EFFECT ONLY. Select the terms which best describe the degrees of therapeutic effect and side effects and record the number in the box where the two items intersect.

THERAPEUTIC EFFECT		SIDE EFFECTS			
MARKED:	Vast improvement. Complete or nearly complete remission of all symptoms	01	02	03	04
MODERATE:	Decided improvement. Partial remission of symptoms.	05	06	07	08
MINIMAL:	Slight improvement which doesn't alter status of care of patient.	09	10	11	12
UNCHANGED OR WORSE		13	14	15	16
	Not Assessed = 00				

BIBLIOGRAPHY

1. American Psychiatric Association: Diagnostic and Statistical Manual of Mental Disorders–III. Washington, DC, American Psychiatric Association, 1980.
2. American Psychiatric Association: Diagnostic and Statistical Manual of Mental Disorders–III-R. Washington, DC, American Psychiatric Association, 1987.
3. American Psychiatric Association: Diagnostic and Statistical Manual of Mental Disorders–IV. Washington, DC, American Psychiatric Association, 1994.
4. Beck AT, Brown G, Epstein N, Steer RA: An inventory for measuring clinical anxiety: Psychometric properties. J Consult Clin Psychol 55:893–987, 1988.
5. Beck AT, Ward CH, Mendelson M, et al: An inventory for measuring depression. Arch Gen Psychiatry 4:561–571, 1961.
6. Derogatis LR: SCL-90-R Administration, Scoring and Procedures Manual—II. for the Revised Version. Towson, MD, Clinical Psychometric Research, 1983.
7. Endicott J, Spitzer RL: A diagnostic review. The Schedule for Affective Disorders and Schizophrenia. Arch Gen Psychiatry 35:837–844, 1978.
8. Guy W: ECDEU Assessment Manual for Psychopharmacology, Revised, 1976. Rockville, MD, DHEW Publication No. (ADM) 76-338, 1976, pp 217–222.
9. Hamilton M: The assessment of anxiety states by rating. Br J Med Psychol 32:50–55, 1959.
10. Hamilton M: The development of a rating scale for primary depressive illness. Br J Soc Clin Psychol 6:278–296, 1967.
11. Lipman RS: Differentiating anxiety and depression in anxiety disorders: use of rating scales. [description of Raskin and Covi scales]. Psychopharm Bull 18:69–105, 1982.
12. McNair DM, Lorr M, Droppleman LF: Manual for the Profile of Mood States. San Diego, Educational and Industrial Testing Service, 1971.
13. Montgomery SA, Asberg ML: A new depression scale designed to be sensitive to change. Br J Psychiatry 134:382–389, 1979.
14. Overall JE, Gorham DR: The Brief Psychiatric Rating Scale. Psychol Rep 10:799–812, 1962.
15. Robins LN, Helzer JE, Croughan JL, Ratcliff KS: National Institute of Mental Health Diagnostic Interview Schedule: Its history, characteristics and validity. Arch Gen Psychiatry 38:381–389, 1981.
16. Robins LN, Wing J, Wittchen H-U, Helzer JE: The Composite International Diagnostic Interview: An epidemiologic instrument suitable for use in conjunction with different diagnostic systems and in different cultures. Arch Gen Psychiatry 45:1069–1077, 1988.
17. Rush AJ, Giles DE, Schlesser MA, et al: The Inventory for Depressive Symptomatology (IDS): Preliminary findings. Psychiatry Res 18:65–87, 1986.
18. Skodol AE, Bender DS: Diagnostic interviews. In APA Taskforce for Handbook of Psychiatric Measures (eds): Handbook of Psychiatric Measures. Washington, DC, American Psychiatric Association, Inc., In Press.
19. Spielberger CD: Manual for the State-Trait Anxiety Inventory. Palo Alto, CA, Consulting Psychologists Press, 1983.
20. Spitzer RL, Endicott J, Robins E: Research diagnostic criteria. Rationale and reliability. Arch Gen Psychiatry 35:773–782, 1978.
21. Spitzer RL, Williams JBW, Gibbon M, First MB: The structured clinical interview for DSM-III-R (SCID). I: History, rationale and description. Arch Gen Psychiatry 49:624–629, 1992.
22. Weissman MM, Bothwell S: Assessment of social adjustment by patient self-report. Arch Gen Psychiatry 33:1111–1115, 1976,
23. Williams JBW, Gibbon M, First MB, et al: The structured clinical interview for DSM-II-R (SCID). II: Multisite test-retest reliability. Arch Gen Psychiatry 49:630–636, 1992.
24. Wittchen H-U, Robins LN, Cottler LB, et al, and Participants in the Multicentre WHO/ADAMHA Field Trials: Cross-cultural feasibility, reliability and sources of variance in the Composite International Diagnostic Interview (CIDI). Br J Psychiatry 159:645–653, 1991.
25. World Health Organization: Composite International Diagnostic Interview (CIDI), Version 1.0. Geneva, World Health Organization, 1990.
26. Yonkers KA, Samson JA: Mood disorders. In APA Taskforce for Handbook of Psychiatric Measures (eds): Handbook of Psychiatric Measures. Washington, DC, American Psychiatric Association, Inc., In Press.

9. BRAIN IMAGING IN PSYCHIATRY

Russell G. Vasile, M.D.

1. Which brain imaging techniques commonly are employed in the clinical practice of adult psychiatry?

Computed axial tomography (CT) and magnetic resonance imaging (MRI) are used to assess brain *structure*. Single photon emission computed tomography (SPECT) and positron emission tomography (PET) are used to assess brain *function*. SPECT scans provide a measure of regional cerebral blood *flow* in the brain, while PET scans indicate localized metabolic activity by measuring regional glucose utilization. Since metabolic rates and localized regional blood flow are closely linked in the brain in most circumstances, the results of SPECT and PET often are comparable.

Another technique to assess brain function is afforded by electroencephalography (EEG), which provides an instantaneous, localized measure of electrophysiologic activity of the brain. Recently, computer-assisted techniques have been developed to summarize and present EEG data in a topographic format; this technique is termed quantitative EEG, or brain electrical activity mapping (BEAM).

2. What is the clinical role for brain imaging in the assessment of psychiatric patients?

The primary purpose of brain imaging studies is to detect or exclude organic factors that could be contributing to psychiatric symptomatology. Symptoms such as cognitive dysfunction, mood disturbance, and psychotic manifestations may be caused by occult organic disorders influencing brain function. These studies play a complementary role in the overall clinical assessment of psychiatric patients.

Brain Disorders Presenting with Psychiatric Symptoms* and Imaging Techniques
That May Assist in Diagnosis

Dementia
- MRI (structural assessment of atrophy)
- SPECT (blood flow patterns may identify Alzheimer's disease)
- EEG (characteristic increase in slow wave activity in dementia)

Tumor
- MRI (anatomic assessment)
- SPECT (useful to assess tumor vascularization)
- EEG (may reveal focal slowing)

Stroke
- MRI and CT (useful after infarction)
- SPECT (may identify early ischemic changes before CT and MRI)
- EEG (identifies extent of functional disruption of electrophysiologic activity)

Parkinson's disease
- MRI (identifies characteristic defects in neuroanatomy)

Temporal lobe epilepsy
- EEG (characteristic abnormal spikes a key to diagnosis)
- SPECT (hyperperfusion of seizure focus during seizure, hypoperfusion interictally)

Multiple sclerosis
- MRI (can reveal subtle neuroanatomic defects)

Table continued on following page

Brain Disorders Presenting with Psychiatric Symptoms and Imaging Techniques
That May Assist in Diagnosis (Continued)*

Huntington's disease
- MRI (subtle neuroanatomic defects demonstrable)

AIDS
- SPECT (emerging reports suggest SPECT abnormalities characterized by diffuse focal hypoperfusion)

Toxic metabolic conditions and delirium
- EEG (disruption in usual EEG coherence, excessive for fast wave activity)

Head trauma
- CT (excellent to assess bone fracture, possible subarachnoid bleeds, other hemorrhagic events)
- MRI (superior resolution of subtle anatomic defects, but CT studies may be easier to obtain in urgent situations)

---

* Including depressive symptoms, cognitive dysfunction, and psychosis

3. Which disorders are detected by imaging?

The structural imaging techniques, CT and MRI, assess conditions that manifest tangible anatomic defects. They play an important role in the differential diagnosis of dementia and the detection of space-occupying lesions such as tumors, subdural hematomas, and brain tissue defects secondary to stroke. SPECT scanning identifies characteristic patterns of regional cerebral blood flow in multi-infarct and Alzheimer's dementia, and is contributory in the early assessment of strokes and cerebrovascular defects, providing evidence of defects in cerebrovascular perfusion before they are discernible by MRI or CT scanning. PET scans are far more expensive to obtain than SPECT studies, and are less readily available to clinicians. PET studies do not, as yet, have significant clinical applicability, but show great promise as a research tool.

EEG and quantitative EEG, which measure the amount and location of different brain wave forms, can detect seizure disorders and also can contribute to the assessment of dementia. Both of these conditions exhibit characteristic patterns on EEG. Toxic states including drug intoxication and metabolic encephalopathies also exhibit characteristic patterns on EEG.

4. What are the most important indications for CT and MRI scanning in psychiatry?

Consider the evaluation of brain structures in psychiatric practice:
- To confirm or rule out the presence of structural lesions that may be contributing to psychiatric symptoms. Such lesions require specific management and may be reversible. Examples include subdural hematoma, tumor, and multiple sclerosis.
- To assess psychiatric symptoms that could have, in part, a defined neuropathological basis. For example, confusion in an elderly depressed patient might be related to multi-infarct dementia that could be demonstrated by a brain imaging study.
- To rule out or confirm other diagnostic possibilities that could be contributing to a patient's psychiatric symptoms. For example, to exclude organic pathology in a patient suffering from a conversion disorder.

5. Compare MRI and CT.

MRI has largely supplanted CT scanning in the assessment of brain structures. MRI is a technique based on the phenomena of nuclear magnetic resonance and computer-based image reconstruction techniques. CT studies reflect the attenuation of x-rays through tissue, while MRI provides information about the interaction of protons with their environment (T1 images) and interaction with other protons (T2 images).

The superior spatial resolution of MRI allows detection of small obstructions in the aqueductal system, which could allow discrimination between communicating and noncommunicating hydrocephalus. MRI with gadolinium contrast affords detailed assessment of breakdown in the integrity of the blood brain barrier, which might result from stroke, inflammation, or tumor.

Comparison of CT and MRI

MRI	CT
Superior tissue resolution	Superior bone imaging
Visualization in coronal, sagittal, transverse planes	Transverse plane only
No radiation risk; multiple studies feasible	Radiation risk present
Superior spatial resolution	Differentiates acute parenchymal hemorrhage from edema
Discrimination between gray and white matter	
Reveals more anatomic detail	Reveals calcifications, meningeal abnormalities, and certain hemorrhagic events
Can detect small lesions (e.g., glioblastoma)	
Posterior fossa, temporal lobes, cerebellum, and brainstem accessible	Areas are inaccessible due to bony artifacts
	Superior detection of subarachnoid hemorrhage
Superior study of demyelinating diseases (e.g., multiple sclerosis, basal ganglia, and periventricular areas)	Evaluation relatively simple, quick
	Patients with mental implants can be scanned with CT
Superior assessment of brain injury 48–72 hours after trauma*	
Evaluation logistically complex and slow**	
Patients with metal implants cannot be subjected to MRI	

* Especially nonhemorrhagic intracranial injuries ** In addition to time expenditure, possible claustrophobic reaction by patient

6. What is functional MRI?

This technique uses MRI to evaluate measures such as changes in regional cerebral blood *volume* and can be used in experiments involving activation paradigms that measure changes in blood volume in resting and activated states. Functional MRI is the focus of increasing research interest and likely will play a role in clinical practice in the future.

7. Are there any MRI or CT findings that specifically characterize depression, mania, or schizophrenia?

CT and MRI investigations have been directed toward the assessment of patients with primary affective disorders. CT scanning has proven of limited value, due to low resolution in the brain and bony artifact obscuring potentially important structures. Some, but not all, studies found larger ventricles in patients with affective disorders compared to controls. Increased ventricular size was associated with psychotic symptoms, psychomotor retardation, and elevated urinary free-cortisol levels in the depressed patient populations studied.

MRI studies of patients with primary affective disorder, such as major depressive illness or mania, have not yielded consistent results. "Hyperintensities"—bright white areas on MRI images—have been described in the periventricular white matter of young bipolar and elderly depressed patients. Hyperintensities located deep in left frontal white matter and left putaminal regions have been correlated with geriatric depression. Subcortical hyperintensities also have been described in demented patients and have been associated with hypertension and vascular disease. Their pathophysiologic significance, if any, remains uncertain.

The MRI research on schizophrenic patients has generated much data on subtle neuroanatomic abnormalities, particularly in ventricular and temporolimbic structures, but no consistent pathognomonic neuroanatomic abnormality has been demonstrated. Structural changes in the brains of schizophrenics appear to be located primarily in frontal and temporal lobes more than posterior brain regions. Increased lateral ventricular and third ventricle size, and abnormalities involving alteration of the circuitry of the limbic system, have been described. Hypofrontality has been observed repeatedly in schizophrenia in response to various cognitive tasks.

In summary, neither MRI nor CT scanning demonstrates characteristic neuroanatomical abnormalities diagnostic of schizophrenia or affective illness, but accumulating evidence points to brain abnormalities in both conditions.

8. What are the most significant indications for SPECT scanning in psychiatry?
- Differential diagnosis of dementia: Alzheimer's disease versus multi-infarct dementia
- Cerebrovascular disease: assessment of infarction versus ischemia
- Focal epilepsy: identification of seizure focus
- Brain tumor: assessment of blood supply of tumor tissue; necrosis of tumor tissue versus recurrence

SPECT is particularly useful in the acute assessment of blood flow to the brain and is commonly used in neurologic settings to assess stroke patterns. Of note, acute changes in cerebral blood flow may not result in structural defects for several hours; hence, structural changes following stroke may be evident only over time.

Recent studies have suggested that Alzheimer's disease can be differentiated from multi-infarct dementia on the basis of the pattern of regional cerebral blood flow in these conditions. The perfusion defects in Alzheimer's disease are almost always bilateral, involve the association cortex, and are most severe in the posterior temporoparietal lobes. The hypoperfusion exhibited in these lobes often is present in the early phases of the disease, with frontal lobe hypoperfusion being a later manifestation. Multi-infarct dementia has a more patchy, diffuse pattern of hypoperfusion, with widely scattered, focal perfusion defects.

SPECT also may play a role in the localization and assessment of epileptic seizure foci in patients with focal epilepsy. Post-ictal SPECT has been used to identify unilateral temporal foci as regions of increased activity (e.g., increased regional cerebral blood flow) and can be used to confirm the presence of the epileptic focus in those patients who have reduced uptake in the same location on interictal SPECT.

In focal seizure disorders, SPECT images reveal a sharp increase in regional cerebral blood flow during the acute seizure; by contrast, interictally, the seizure focus is commonly hypoperfused relative to normal nonirritable tissue. This has been of value in assessing temporal lobe disorders and focal lesions giving rise to complex partial seizures. This use of SPECT provides an alternative to more invasive techniques, such as depth EEG.

9. Describe the mechanisms of PET and SPECT.
Both PET and SPECT scanning use computer-assisted techniques for the reconstruction of cross-sectional images of radiotracer distributions. A typical reconstruction resolution value for PET is 4–6 mm, and for SPECT 6–8 mm. The commonly used PET radionuclides are ^{15}O, ^{13}N, ^{11}C, ^{18}F, which have short half-lives, ranging from 2 minutes to 2 hours. The SPECT imaging radiotracers technetium 99m and ^{123}I have half-lives of 6 hours and 13 hours, respectively. SPECT studies can be performed several hours after injection of the radiotracer. The half-life of the particular radionuclide employed in a study is of importance in that it impacts flexibility in study design. A longer half-life radionuclide facilitates studies of longer duration, affording more time for data acquisition as, for example, when utilizing a cognitive activation paradigm such as the Wisconsin Card Sort.

10. Which is the more practical tool: SPECT or PET?
SPECT. The cost of a PET system, which requires a cyclotron for radioisotope production, is 1–3 million dollars, while that of a SPECT system is 0.3–0.6 million dollars. The cost per study for a SPECT ranges from $500–1000, while PET studies cost $1500–2000.

Due to the extraordinary expense associated with developing and maintaining a PET scanning facility, PET imaging has remained primarily a technique of major research interest, not widely employed in clinical practice. SPECT scans, by comparison far less expensive, are increasingly available to clinicians.

11. Are there any SPECT or PET findings that specifically characterize depression, mania, schizophrenia, or anxiety disorders?
SPECT scans cannot be considered diagnostic of depressive disorders or mania at this time. Several noteworthy SPECT studies demonstrate specific regions of hypoperfusion in depressed

patients that resolve upon successful treatment of depression. The frontal and temporal brain regions have been implicated, but other brain regions, such as the caudate nucleus, have been implicated as well; the literature does not reveal a consensus "gold standard" finding as yet.

Studies of schizophrenic patients have implicated the frontal lobes as regions of hypoperfusion, specifically in relation to activating tasks such as the Wisconsin Card Sort.

Increased frontal lobe blood flow has been shown in obsessive-compulsive disorder, and a few studies have demonstrated a return to normal levels following treatment with serotonergic antidepressant agents.

PET studies of schizophrenia generally have reported lower metabolic rates in the frontal regions, particularly in response to cognitive tasks designed for frontal lobe activation. Hypofrontality appears to be associated with the negative symptoms of schizophrenia. Temporal lobe abnormalities also have been reported. PET research on obsessive-compulsive disorder has indicated an increase in frontal lobe and basal ganglia metabolism. Several PET studies of major depressive disorder have observed reduction in metabolic rate, particularly in the frontal lobes; this hypofrontality appears to be more marked in bipolar as compared to unipolar patients, and in some studies appears to be most prominent in the left lateral frontal region.

Future Application of PET and SPECT Imaging

Neuroreceptor mapping
- Identify neuroreceptor patterns in primary psychiatric disorders such as depression and schizophrenia

Identification of pathways of normal cerebral function
- Assess pathways of sensory function, including visual and auditory
- Identify neuroanatomical sites of affective and cognitive function

Quantification of metabolism in specific brain regions in primary psychiatric disorders
- Analyze subtypes of affective illness, bipolar versus unipolar depression
- Obsessive compulsive disorder
- Panic disorder

Further understanding of medical disorders that contribute to psychiatric symptomatology
- AIDS dementia
- Chronic fatigue syndrome
- Substance abuse (cocaine)

12. Describe the mechanism of EEG.

EEG affords a continuous measure of brain electrical activity with a chronological resolution in milliseconds. Recent advances in computer software technology have given rise to *quantitative* EEG techniques that provide color-coded topographic displays of EEG data. Quantitative EEG employs conventional, standard EEG, but organizes and presents the data in a fashion that facilitates visuospatial interpretation.

EEG data provides information about the amount and spatial location of various EEG frequencies, ranging from fast activity (alpha) to slow wave activity (delta). Additionally, EEG assesses discontinuities in electrical activity, characterized by spike and wave formations consistent with seizures. Finally, evoked responses to auditory and visual stimulation can be assessed in relation to established norms.

Patterns of the amount and location of the various EEG frequencies can be of diagnostic value. For example, an increased amount of topographically diffuse delta activity is commonly encountered in dementia. Drug-induced toxic states are associated with increased alpha activity. The diagnosis of seizure disorder may be established by the characteristic spike and wave formation demonstrated on the EEG.

EEG provides instantaneous data, and 24-hour EEG studies now can be obtained on an ambulatory basis to facilitate the documentation of seizure activity and its correlation to behavioral phenomena.

13. What is the role of EEG and quantitative EEG in psychiatry?

EEG has been used to assess brain function in a range of settings, including dementia, in which slow wave activity is prominent; toxic states, typically characterized by fast activity; and seizure disorders, noteworthy for spike and wave patterns characteristic of seizure activity. EEG is consistently abnormal in patients with delirium and often is employed in monitoring the course of that condition.

EEG is particularly helpful in the assessment and differential diagnosis of **cognitive dysfunction.** Dementia often is characterized by increased slow wave activity. The evaluation of unusual behavioral presentations, which may reflect an occult underlying seizure disorder, is another potential role for EEG. For example, a patient with marked obsession and quasi-philosophical preoccupations may be exhibiting behaviors consistent with the interictal personality features of patients with temporal lobe dysfunction.

Currently, active research efforts are underway to describe patterns of EEG activity that might distinguish depression from the early stages of dementia. As yet, there are no definitive EEG characteristics that consistently discriminate these disorders.

14. How might brain imaging be useful in assessing the patient with cognitive dysfunction?

Brain imaging studies can identify reversible causes of cognitive dysfunction, such as subdural hematoma or meningioma. EEG could be helpful in discriminating between toxic-metabolic states, which could contribute to cognitive dysfunction, and incipient dementia. SPECT scanning reveals a typical pattern of blood flow in Alzheimer's dementia, and a different pattern in other dementias such as multi-infarct dementia. Transient ischemic disorders and cerebrovascular insufficiency also can be assessed by the SPECT modality.

15. How might brain imaging studies be useful in assessing a patient with depression?

A variety of conditions that cause apathy, lethargy, trouble concentrating, and sad mood can be confused with primary depression. Indeed, the concept of "secondary" depression, or depression secondary to a discrete medical cause, is well established. Examples include certain post-stroke depressions and depression secondary to Parkinson's disease, multiple sclerosis, or other neurologic conditions. Post-stroke depression is particularly common following left anterior frontal lobe infarctions, whether they are cortical or subcortical lesions. Additionally, differentiating dementia and depression may be difficult without the data available through brain imaging.

MRI and CT reveal structural defects in certain conditions such as stroke; EEG shows typical patterns in dementia and seizure activity, and also may show asymmetries following strokes. SPECT scans can confirm the diagnosis of stroke, dementia, or underlying seizure foci.

Imaging studies may be of particular value in the treatment of the refractory depressed patient or the depressed patient with atypical features. The possibility of an occult neuropathologic condition contributing to the depressive disorder should be seriously considered in these patients.

16. Are brain imaging studies indicated for assessing a patient with psychosis?

Yes. Several organic conditions, including subdural hematoma and stroke, may result in psychotic symptoms that could be confused with schizophrenia. Occult frontal or temporal lobe tumor, unusual seizure disorders, or drug-induced psychosis may need to be ruled out in the assessment of psychotic conditions. MRI or CT can assess organic states and determine the cause of unusual behavior. EEG can help exclude toxic-metabolic conditions that could be contributing to psychotic symptoms. SPECT scanning could assess the possibility of cerebrovascular insufficiency as a contributory factor in altered mental status.

17. What are the main currents in brain imaging research that could prove clinically relevant in the near future?

The major advances in brain imaging research involve the development of new ligands for specific receptor sites. These new ligands enable researchers to more precisely assess neuroreceptor function in specific psychiatric conditions, and to evaluate change in receptor function following psychotropic medication treatment. Ligands currently are available for use with PET and SPECT to assess cholinergic, benzodiazepine, and dopaminergic receptors. Mapping receptor distribution and assessing interaction with pharmacological probes are becoming increasingly feasible.

Ongoing developments in software technology will facilitate the integration of anatomic and physiologic techniques through the coregistration of MRI and SPECT images. The precise neuroanatomic superimposition of these different modalities will allow more exact localization of pathophysiologic dysfunction in brain disorders.

Physiologic functional MRI techniques are now contributing heavily to studies of brain activation in health and disease, and clinical application may be found for these tools in the near future.

BIBLIOGRAPHY

1. Ames D, Chiu E (eds): Neuroimaging and the Psychiatry of Late Life. Cambridge, United Kingdom, Cambridge University Press, 1997.
2. Krishnan KR, Doraiswamy PM (eds): Brain Imaging in Clinical Psychiatry. New York, M. Dekker, 1997.
3. Vasile RG: Single-photon emission computed tomography in psychiatry: Clinical perspectives. Harv Rev Psychiatry 4:27–38, 1996.
4. Lewis S: Structural brain imaging in biological psychiatry. Br Med Bull 52(3):465–473, 1996.
5. Wright DC, Bigler ED: Neuroimaging in psychiatry. Psychiatr Clin North Am 21(4):725–759, 1998.
6. Buckley PF: Structural brain imaging in schizophrenia. Psychiatr Clin North Am 21(1):77–92, 1998.
7. Krausz Y, Bonne O, Marciano R, et al: Brain SPECT imaging of neuropsychiatric disorders. Eur J Radiol 21(3):183–187, 1996.
8. Waldemar G, Hugh P, Paulson OB: Functional brain imaging with single-photon emission computed tomography in the diagnosis of Alzheimer's disease. Int Psycholgeriatr 9 Suppl 1:223–227, 1997.
9. Levin JM, Ross MH, Renshaw PF: Clinical applications of functional MRI in neuropsychiatry. J Neuropsych Clin Neurosci 7(4):511–522, 1995.
10. Dougherty D, Rauch SL: Neuroimaging and neurobiological models of depression. Harv Rev Psychiatry 5:138–159, 1997.
11. Saxema S, Brody AL, Schwartz JM, Baxter LR: Neuroimaging and frontal-subcortical circuitry in obsessive-compulsive disorder. Br J Psychiatry Suppl (35):26–37, 1998.
12. Keshaven MS, Krishana RR: New frontiers in psychiatric neuroimaging. Prog Neuropsychopharmacol Biol Psychiatry 21(8):1181–1183, 1997.
13. Gur RE, Chin S: Laterality in functional brain imaging studies of schizophrenia. Schizophr Bull 25(1): 141–156, 1999.
14. Kegeles LS, Mann JJ: In vivo imaging of neurotransmitter systems using radiolabeled receptor ligands. Neuropsychopharmacology 17(5);293–307, 1997.
15. Schmitz EB, Moriarty J, Costa DC, et al: Psychiatric profiles and patterns of cerebral blood flow in focal epilepsy: Interactions between depression, obsessionality, and perfusion related to the laterality of the epilepsy. J Neurol Neurosurg Psychiatry 62(5):458–463, 1997.

III. Principal Clinical Disorders and Problems

10. SCHIZOPHRENIA AND SCHIZOAFFECTIVE DISORDERS

Herbert T. Nagamoto, M.D.

1. Define schizophrenia.
Schizophrenia is a complex illness or group of disorders characterized by hallucinations, delusions, behavioral disturbances, disrupted social functioning, and associated symptoms in what is usually an otherwise clear sensorium.

2. What are the symptoms of schizophrenia?
Schizophrenia involves at least a 6-month period of continuous signs of the illness. Active symptoms may include:

• **Delusions**, which are false beliefs that (1) persist despite what most people would accept as evidence to the contrary and (2) are not shared by others in the same culture or subculture.

• **Hallucinations**, which are perceptions that appear to be real when no such stimulus is actually present. Hallucinations may involve any of the five normal senses, but in schizophrenia they are usually auditory.

• **Disorganized speech.**

• **Grossly disorganized or catatonic behavior**. Catatonia, a syndrome characterized by stupor with rigidity or flexibility of the musculature, may alternate with periods of overactivity.

• **Negative symptoms**, such as (1) affective flattening or decreased emotional reactivity; (2) alogia or poverty of speech; (3) avolition or lack of purposeful action. Usually work performance, social relations, and self-care decrease below the highest previous levels.

3. What are some additional clinical features?
Prodromal or residual phases may include social isolation or withdrawal, peculiar behavior, digressive overelaborate speech, odd beliefs such as ideas of reference (thinking that others' words, actions, or expressions are in reference to oneself when this is not the case) or magical thinking, unusual perceptual experiences, or marked lack of initiative, interests, or energy.

Age of onset is usually during adolescence or early adulthood. The course is highly variable, but generally involves significant functional impairment.

Violent acts sometimes receive significant attention. While it has been generally accepted that violent acts are no more frequent in schizophrenic patients than in the general population, recent epidemiologic data have shown a link between mental illness and violence. The percentage of violence in the U.S. attributed to schizophrenic patients, however, is minimal—and much less than that due to alcohol abuse.

Some schizophrenic patients have various **somatic complaints** as part of their illness, but they also may be medically ill and not complain or incorporate symptoms into their delusional system.

Life expectancy is reduced by death from suicide and other causes. Approximately 40% of schizophrenics attempt suicide at some point in their lifetime, and 10–20% succeed.

4. How common is schizophrenia?

The lifetime incidence of schizophrenia is approximately 1%. This figure is remarkably stable across racial, cultural, and national lines.

5. What medical conditions may induce psychosis and be mistaken for acute schizophrenia?

Psychosis, which is characterized by a disturbance in or loss of contact with reality, may include symptoms of schizophrenia, including delusions, hallucinations, bizarre behavior, ideas of reference, paranoia (irrational suspiciousness or false beliefs of persecution), disorganized speech, and illogical thinking. A number of medical conditions can induce psychosis:

- Substance abuse and drug toxicity (see Question 6)
- Space-occupying central nervous system lesions—tumor (especially limbic and pituitary), aneurysm, abscess
- Head trauma
- Infections—encephalitis, abscess, neurosyphilis
- Endocrine disease—thyroid, Cushing's, Addison's, pituitary, parathyroid
- Systemic lupus erythematosus and multiple sclerosis
- Cerebrovascular disease
- Huntington's disease
- Parkinson's disease
- Migraine headache and temporal arteritis
- Pellagra and pernicious anemia
- Porphyria
- Withdrawal states, including alcohol and benzodiazepines
- Delirium and dementia
- Sensory deprivation or overstimulation states can induce psychosis, such as psychosis induced in the intensive care unit

6. Which street drugs and prescription medications may induce psychosis?

Street drugs	Prescription drugs
Cocaine	Metronidazole and other antibiotics
Phencyclidine	Antidepressants
Lysergic acid diethyl- amide (LSD)	L-dopa
	Bromocriptine
Mescaline	Amantadine
Psilocybin	Ephedrine
Marijuana	Phenylpropanolamine
Morning glory seeds	Idomethacin and other nonsteroidal antiinflammatory agents
Alcohol	Cimetidine and other antihistamines
	Disulfiram
	Carbamazepine and other anticonvulsants
	Digoxin, propranolol, and other cardiac medications
	Thyroid hormones
	Various medications with strong anticholinergic effects

Note that routine urine toxicology screens usually monitor for only a limited number of substances.

7. Which tests should a screening medical work-up of psychosis include?

Complete blood count
Serum electrolytes, glucose, blood urea nitrogen, creatinine, calcium, and phosphate
Liver function tests
Thyroid function tests
VDRL or RPR, HIV antibody test in high-risk patients*
Electrocardiogram
Urinalysis and urine toxicology screen

Chest x-ray
Sleep-deprived EEG
Head CT or MRI scan
Blood levels of therapeutic medications, when appropriate
Lumbar puncture, when appropriate
* VDRL = Venereal Disease Research Laboratory test, RPR = rapid plasmin reagin test, HIV = human immunodeficiency virus.

8. How is schizophrenia differentiated from manic-depressive illness and other psychiatric conditions?

The differential diagnosis of schizophrenia and other psychiatric conditions that may manifest psychotic symptoms is difficult and best done from a longitudinal perspective on the course of the illness. Such a differential is crucial, because effective treatments vary depending on the conditions. In **affective disorders** (manic depressive illness and major depression), the duration of psychotic symptoms is relatively brief in relation to the affective symptoms. **Schizophreniform disorder**, by definition, involves the symptoms of schizophrenia with a duration of less than 6 months. Patients with **obsessive-compulsive disorder** may have beliefs that border on delusions but generally recognize that their symptoms are at least somewhat irrational. **Brief reactive psychoses** may be seen in patients with borderline or other personality disorders as well as dissociative disorders. **Post-traumatic stress disorder** may involve visual, auditory, tactile, and olfactory hallucinations during flashbacks. Beliefs or experiences should not be considered delusional or psychotic if they are in the context of a person's religion or culture.

9. What causes schizophrenia?

This question thus far has eluded an answer. A number of factors, however, have been implicated in the pathogenesis of schizophrenia, which often is conceptualized as a group of disorders with common symptoms.

Factors Implicated in the Etiology of Schizophrenia

Genetic factors (see Question 10)	Endocrine factors
Brain structural changes	Viral and immune factors
Neurochemical changes	
Neurophysiological changes	

Brain structural studies have failed to find a pathognomonic lesion in schizophrenia, but have consistently found a number of abnormalities. CT, MRI, and postmortem studies have found changes in frontal, temporal, limbic, and basal ganglia areas, as well as in brain symmetry, in schizophrenic patients. Some of these findings have been corroborated by changes in regional cerebral blood flow, functional MRI, and positron emission tomographic (PET) studies.

Multiple neurochemical changes also have been implicated in schizophrenia. It has been long noted that an excess in dopaminergic activity in the central nervous system is central to the development of schizophrenic symptoms. Compelling data also implicate norepinephrine, serotonin, and cholinergic (muscarinic and nicotinic), glutamatergic, GABAergic, and neuropeptide systems.

Neurophysiological changes have been shown through various neuropsychologic and physiologic measures.

Schizophrenic patients have shown abnormal informational processing on such measures as the Continuous Performance Test. They also have shown abnormal sensory processing on skin conductance habituation, backward masking, smooth pursuit eye movements, prepulse inhibition of acoustic startle, and evoked potentials, such as P300, P1, mismatched negativity, and failure to decrement the P50 auditory response in a conditioning-testing paradigm.

Endocrine factors have long been suspected. Females tend to develop schizophrenia later and often have less severe symptoms than males. In males, the onset of schizophrenia typically is during puberty. Changes in prolactin, melatonin, and thyroid function have been found in schizophrenia.

Viral and immune factors also have been implicated. Although the search for a causative virus in schizophrenia has thus far been unfruitful, various factors point to this possibility. For example, a number of immune changes have been found, including IgA, IgG, and IgM. Furthermore, a larger than expected number of schizophrenic patients are born in late winter and early spring, leading to the hypothesis that perinatal viral infections may be involved in causing schizophrenia.

Psychosocial factors are no longer felt to be causative in schizophrenia but clearly play a role in the course of the illness.

10. What is the role of genetics in schizophrenia?

Genetic factors play a significant role, but are not sufficient alone to account for the development of schizophrenia. Compelling data have come from family studies. In the general population, the lifetime risk of developing schizophrenia is approximately 1%. A child born with one schizophrenic parent has about a 14% chance of developing schizophrenia. The risk rises to approximately 25% if both parents are schizophrenic. Another approach has looked at siblings with varying degrees of genetic similarity. Nontwin siblings of a schizophrenic patient have about an 8% chance of developing schizophrenia. For nonidentical (dizygotic) twins, if one twin is schizophrenic, approximately 10% of the other twins develop schizophrenia. This risk, or concordance rate, rises to 40–50% in identical (monozygotic) twins.

Genetic linkage studies to date have implicated chromosomes 5, 6, 8, 10, 13, and 15 in schizophrenia. Although such data support a strong role for genetics in the etiology of schizophrenia, they also clearly show that other factors play a significant role in determining who does and does not develop schizophrenia.

11. What are the treatments for schizophrenia?

Antipsychotic medications are the cornerstone of the treatment of schizophrenia (see Chapter 48). Inpatient treatment in a therapeutic milieu may be crucial in the early and acute phases. Residential treatment settings, group homes, and day hospital programs may help patients to remain outside the hospital. Supportive **individual and group psychotherapy** can help patients to understand and come to terms with their illness and need for treatment, to identify factors that influence symptoms, and to develop strategies to deal more effectively with the illness. **Family therapy sessions** also may help families of schizophrenic patients to understand the illness and to help the patient. Families may have a negative impact if they are high in expressed emotion, hypercritical, or overtly hostile toward the patient. Schizophrenic patients often have extremely poor social skills. **Social skills training** has been shown to be highly effective in helping to improve quality of life. **Vocational rehabilitation** helps some stabilized patients to return to more productive roles in society.

12. List the positive prognostic signs in schizophrenia.

Improved prognosis in schizophrenia is associated with:
• Good premorbid functioning, late onset, female gender, clear precipitating events, acute onset.
• Mood disturbances, brief active phase, good interepisode functioning, marriage, decreased residual symptoms, fewer chronic negative symptoms.
• Decreased structural brain abnormalities, normal neurologic functioning.
• Family history positive for mood disorder, negative for schizophrenia.

13. What is schizoaffective disorder?

Schizoaffective disorder has been defined in numerous ways, but essentially it is an illness that combines symptoms of schizophrenia with a major affective disorder, i.e., major depression or manic-depressive illness.

14. How is schizoaffective disorder different from schizophrenia or manic-depressive illness?

Mood disturbance is common in all phases of schizophrenia, and psychotic symptoms are common during acute phases of manic-depressive illness (bipolar affective disorder). Accurate diagnosis often requires a clear longitudinal history of symptoms. In schizophrenia, the total duration of affective symptoms is brief relative to the total duration of the illness. In manic-depressive illness, delusions and hallucinations primarily occur during periods of mood instability.

A DSM-IV diagnosis of schizoaffective disorder requires an uninterrupted period of illness during which there is either a major depressive, manic, or mixed (manic and depressive) episode that is concurrent with active symptoms of schizophrenia. In addition, during the same period of illness, there are delusions or hallucinations for at least 2 weeks in the absence of prominent mood symptoms, and mood episode symptoms are present for a substantial portion of the active and residual phases of the illness.

It is important to make as clear a diagnosis as possible, as the cornerstone of treatment for schizophrenia is antipsychotic medications, whereas mood stabilizers and antidepressants are crucial in treating affective disorders.

15. Does significant depression rule out schizophrenia?

Although the diagnosis of schizophrenia emphasizes that psychotic symptoms predominate over mood symptoms, schizophrenic patients may suffer significant depression, which strongly contributes to their increased suicide risk. Increased suicide risk may extend even after an episode of depression resolves, and may result from the patient's inability to come to terms with the debilitating effects of schizophrenia.

Pharmacologic treatment of depression in schizophrenia is somewhat controversial, because antidepressants apparently reduce the efficacy of antipsychotic medications in acutely ill schizophrenic patients. On the other hand, adjunctive antidepressant medications have been shown to be effective in the acute maintenance treatment of depression in schizophrenic and schizoaffective patients.

BIBLIOGRAPHY

1. Adler LE, et al: Schizophrenia, sensory gating, and nicotinic receptors. Schizophr Bull 24:189–202, 1998.
2. American Psychiatric Association: Diagnostic and Statistical Manual of Mental Disorders, 4th ed. Washington, DC, American Psychiatric Association, 1994.
3. Buckley PF (ed): Schizophrenia. Psychiatr Clin North Am 21(1), 1998.
4. DeLisi LE (ed): Depression in Schizophrenia. Washington, DC, American Psychiatric Press, 1990.
5. Hales RE, Yudofksy SC, Talbott JA (eds): The American Psychiatric Press Textbook of Psychiatry, 3rd ed. Washington DC, American Psychiatric Press, 1999.
6. Kaplan HI, Sadock BJ (eds): Comprehensive Textbook of Psychiatry, 6th ed. Baltimore, Williams & Wilkins, 1995.
7. Tamminga CA (ed): Schizophrenia in a Molecular Age. Ann Rev Psychiatry 18(4), 1999.
8. Yudofsky SC, Hales RE (eds): The American Psychiatric Press Textbook of Neuropsychiatry, 3rd ed. Washington DC, American Psychiatric Press, 1997.

11. PARANOID DISORDERS

Theo C. Manschreck, M.D.

1. What are paranoid disorders?

The term paranoid disorders refers to a variety of conditions characterized by **delusions** and related behavior. One of the earliest described of these disorders was paranoia, now called delusional disorder, which is of unknown cause. The cardinal psychopathologic feature is the delusion. Paranoia actually is uncommon; other forms are seen frequently.

There are two broad categories of paranoid disorders: **disorders with known causes** (medical and substance disorders) and **idiopathic disorders**, which include delusional disorder, paranoid personality disorder, shared psychotic disorder, atypical psychosis (psychotic disorders not otherwise specified), schizophrenia and schizophreniform disorder, mood (psychotic forms of mania and depression) disorder, and schizoaffective disorder.

2. How did the term paranoia originate?

The Greeks used the term *paranoia* (meaning beside one's self) to designate a symptom that we regard now as a nonspecific and general feature of many mental disorders. The term was not used for almost 2000 years until it was revived by Karl Kahlbaum, who in 1863 identified a disorder he called paranoia. He described this condition as "a form of partial insanity, which, throughout the course of the disease, principally affected the sphere of the intellect." Emil Kraepelin, a contemporary of Kahlbaum, was influenced by these observations. He retained the concept of paranoia as a separate disorder in his groundbreaking classification of mental illnesses.

3. What is the current meaning of "paranoid"?

In recent years *paranoid* has referred to a multitude of behaviors, from ordinary suspiciousness to persecutory delusions. It also has been used to characterize grandiose, litigious, hostile, jealous, and even angry behavior, regardless of the fact that these behaviors may be within the normal spectrum. The key principles for understanding the current meaning of paranoid are:

1. *It is a clinical construct* used to describe various subjective and objective behavioral features which are deemed to be psychopathologic. These features are interpreted to be abnormal based on evidence accumulated from patients and other informants. This judgment requires some humility and care. It is supported by the occurrence of specific features (see table) as part of a behavior pattern which is extreme, intense, based on false assertions, inappropriate, disturbing to others, and possibly bizarre or dangerous. Often the patient is convinced and resolute in his or her belief; counter evidence and argument fail to persuade.

2. *It refers to no specific condition.* For example, the presence of paranoid features does not mean that a schizophrenic condition is present.

Features of Paranoid Disorders

Objective Features		
Anger	Hate	Obstinacy
Critical, accusatory behavior	Hostility	Resentment
Defensiveness	Humorlessness	Seclusiveness
Fragile self-esteem	Hypersensitivity	Secretiveness
Grandiosity or excessive self-importance	Inordinate attention to small details	Self-righteousness
	Irritability, quick annoyance	Sullenness
Grievance collection	Litigiousness (letter writing,	Suspiciousness
Guardedness, evasiveness	complaints, legal action)	Violence, aggressiveness

Subjective Features*
Delusions of self-reference, persecution, grandeur, infidelity, love, jealousy, imposture, infestation, disfigurement, and disease

* Part of private mental experience. The patient often discloses these features during the clinical interview, but may not do so, even with specific questioning.

4. How common are paranoid conditions?

Paranoid *features* are among the most common and serious manifestations of psychopathology. They occur in a variety of psychiatric and medical illnesses and are, perhaps, the most frequently encountered symptoms of severe psychopathology. However, the frequency of some of the idiopathic *conditions* is less clear. Delusional disorder may be uncommon; shared psychotic disorder is considered rare. Atypical psychosis, because of its lack of specificity, is difficult to estimate. The incidence of organic delusional syndrome (medical and substance disorders) is presumed to be common.

The essential strategy in evaluating conditions in which paranoid features are present is a competent and thorough differential diagnosis.

5. What is the etiology of paranoid disorders?

The etiology of paranoid disorders is largely unknown except, of course, in those cases for which an organic factor can be isolated. Paranoid features, including the types of delusions that are encountered in delusional disorder, occur in a large number of medical and psychiatric conditions. Many theories exist about the origin of delusions, but evidence to support them is limited.

6. Is there a neuropathology for the paranoid disorders?

Except for those conditions in which a specific organic factor can be identified, determining a specific neuropathology or brain pathology to correlate with the psychopathology of the delusional experience is more hope than reality. Nevertheless, clues based on neuropsychiatric studies suggest where we might find some neuropathologic evidence. For example, patients who have severe cortical disorders, such as Alzheimer's disease, tend to experience simple and transient persecutory delusions. Delusions of a more systematized, elaborate, and complex character tend to be more chronic and resistant to treatment and have been associated with subcortical neurologic conditions that generally produce greater cognitive impairment than the typical idiopathic disorders.

7. Define delusional disorder.

In recent years delusional disorder has become a better-recognized form of paranoid presentation. The term *delusional disorder* refers to a condition of unknown cause whose chief feature is a nonbizarre delusion present for at least 1 month. The diagnosis of delusional disorder corresponds closely to an older concept, paranoia, as formulated by Kraepelin and others over a century ago. There are several types of such delusions, and the predominant type is identified to make the diagnosis. Minimal deterioration in personality or function and the relative absence of other psychopathologic symptoms have been considered important evidence for distinguishing this disorder from schizophrenia and other psychotic conditions.

8. What are the clinical features of delusional disorders?

The core feature is persistent, nonbizarre delusions not explained by other psychotic disorders. The delusion may emerge gradually and become chronic, and sometimes is associated with a precipitating event. Behavioral, emotional, and cognitive responses generally are appropriate, and neither mood disorders nor schizophrenic illness is present.

Delusional Disorder (DSM-IV)

• Nonbizarre delusion(s) (i.e., involving situations that occur in real life, such as being followed, poisoned, infected, loved at a distance, being deceived by spouse or lover, or having a disease) of at least 1-month duration.

• The symptom criteria for schizophrenia have never been met. Note: Tactile and olfactory hallucinations may be present in delusional disorder if they are related to the delusional theme.

• Apart from the impact of the delusion(s) or its ramifications, functioning is not markedly impaired and behavior is not obviously odd or bizarre.

• If mood episodes have occurred concurrently with delusions, their total duration has been brief relative to the duration of the delusional periods.

• The disturbance is not caused by the direct physiologic effects of a substance (e.g., a drug of abuse or a medication) or a general medical condition.

From the Diagnostic and Statistical Manual of Mental Disorders, 4th ed. American Psychiatric Association, 1994; with permission.

9. What is a nonbizarre delusion?

Nonbizarre means that the delusion concerns situations that can occur and are possible in real life, such as being followed, having a disease, being secretly in love, and the like.

10. List the types of delusional disorder.

There are five main types and two residual ones.
  • **Erotomanic:** the predominant theme of the delusion is that a person, usually of higher status, is in love with the subject.

- **Grandiose:** the theme is one of inflated worth, power, knowledge, identity, or special relationship to a deity or important famous person.
- **Jealous:** one's sexual partner is unfaithful.
- **Persecutory:** the person is being malevolently treated or conspired against in some way.
- **Somatic:** the person has some physical defect, disorder, or disease.
- **Mixed:** more than one of the above types are present but no one theme is predominant.
- **Unspecified:** the delusions do not fit into any of the categories.

11. Why is it difficult to recognize delusional disorder?

Delusional disorder is at best uncommon; many clinicians probably have encountered one or two cases, but many have not. It is difficult to recognize because one of its hallmarks is an absence, or modest occurrence, of psychopathology other than delusions. Such patients, if they are patients at all, are in all likelihood misdiagnosed, perhaps as having mild cases of schizophrenia. Because they may seek out internists, dermatologists, lawyers, or the police, they may never be diagnosed at all.

12. Which is the most common type of delusional disorder?

Persecutory, which is also the classic form of the condition. Such individuals frequently are highly litigious and their delusions often are highly systematized (elaborate and detailed).

13. What features are characteristic of the jealous type?

This type, sometimes referred to as the Othello syndrome or conjugal paranoia, is common and associated with dangerousness. Jealousy is a powerful emotion. Individuals with this delusion may resort to assault, homicide, even suicide in response to their delusional concerns about a lover's unfaithfulness. It generally affects males, often with no history of psychiatric difficulty. The delusions may appear suddenly and serve to "explain" a host of remote and recent events involving the spouse's fidelity. This type is particularly difficult to treat, often diminishing only upon separation, divorce, or death of the spouse.

14. What is morbid jealousy or pathologic jealousy?

These terms are used in relation to other disorders. Jealousy is a common symptom and may derive from several conditions, such as epilepsy, mood disorder, schizophrenia, or substance abuse.

15. What is another name for the erotomanic type?

The erotomanic type is called De Clerambault's syndrome when the symptom occurs in other disorders, such as schizophrenia.

16. Describe the characteristic features of erotomania.

It is the delusion of secret love, usually from an individual of higher social standing. Although erotomania may occur in both sexes, it is more common in females. Such patients usually pester, and possibly harass, the object of their love with letters, phone calls, or unexpected visits. The delusion typically concerns a more "spiritual union" or romantic love, rather than sexual attraction.

17. What behavior might a patient with the grandiose type of delusional disorder exhibit?

These patients suffer from megalomania. They are inclined to join cults, preach on the street corner, proselytize their beliefs, or attempt to associate with popular or eminent individuals.

18. List other names for the somatic type of delusional disorder.

Monosymptomatic hypochondriac psychosis, monodelusional psychosis, delusional parasitosis, delusion of infestation, and epidermozoophobia.

19. What are the characteristics of the somatic type?

Somatic patients seek out professional attention for diseases they believe they have. When individual tests fail to detect their "diseases," they often move on to other physicians, unable to respond to reassurance and the evidence collected in their evaluations. There are several patterns: (1) patients concerned about parasites or insect infestation; (2) patients convinced that their body, nose, face, or hair has been altered; and (3) patients concerned that they emit foul bodily odors. Patients with such disturbances are more likely to seek help from dermatologists, exterminators, plastic surgeons, and dentists than psychiatrists. Somatic conditions differ from simple hypochondriasis because of the degree of reality impairment associated with them.

20. Define organic delusional syndrome.

Organic delusional syndrome or disorder refers to delusional illness for which a specific etiology can be determined. It is a DSM-III term that has been replaced in DSM-IV by "psychotic disorders due to a general medical condition" or "substance-induced psychotic disorder." In general, many conditions arising from infectious, neurologic, toxicologic, metabolic, or even genetic or chromosomal sources can be causative. They have been described in both case reports and other observations for many years. For the clinician, of course, it is important to be aware of the most common causes, so that these can be identified and diagnosed rapidly.

21. What are the most common sources of organic delusional disorder?

The most common forms of organic delusional disorder result from substance intoxication and withdrawal. Usual substances are alcohol, stimulants (e.g, cocaine, amphetamine), sympathomimetic agents, antihistamines, steroids, marijuana, and phencyclidine.

Common Causes of Organic Delusions

Alcohol abuse
Drug abuse (especially CNS stimulants)
Iatrogenic: anticholinergic poisoning, steroid poisoning, diet pills, sedative-hypnotic withdrawal
Delirium
Dementia
Other neurologic sources: human immunodeficiency virus (HIV) syndromes, brain tumors, epileptic disorder, especially complex partial seizure disorder

22. What are the features of organic delusional syndrome?

The essential feature is prominent delusions resulting from a specific organic factor. The diagnosis is not made if the delusions occur in the context of difficulties in the maintenance of attention or orientation, as in confusion (a syndrome referred to as *delirium*). The nature of the delusions is variable and, to some extent, depends on the etiology of the disorder. Persecutory delusions are probably the most common type.

Amphetamine use, as well as that of cocaine and other stimulants, has been associated with the development of organic delusional syndrome, but other sources are unrelated to substance abuse. It has been found in temporal lobe epilepsy (complex partial seizure disorder), as an interictal syndrome often indistinguishable from schizophrenia, and in cases of Huntington's disease. Additionally, cerebral lesions of the right hemisphere have resulted in this disorder.

Hallucinations may be present, but they are usually not the prominent characteristic. Associated features include mild cognitive impairment and the presence of various symptoms, many of them found in schizophrenia, such as perplexity, unusual dress and behavior, abnormalities of psychomotor activity, unusual speech, and dysphoric mood. In contrast to delusional disorder in which impairment is uncommon or modest, these conditions are associated with impairments in social, cognitive, and occupational functioning.

23. What is shared psychotic disorder?

Also called induced paranoid disorder, double insanity (*folie a deux*), and other terms, it was first described by Lasegue and Falret in 1877. It is believed to be rare, but accurate incidence and prevalence figures are not available. The literature consists almost entirely of single case reports.

The delusion is characterized by its transfer from one individual to another. Involved persons may have been intimately associated for a long time and typically live in relative social isolation from other people. In its most common form, the individual who first has the delusion is chronically ill and is the influential member of a close relationship with a more suggestible person; the weaker partner becomes the induced psychotic disorder patient. Typically the latter is less clever, more gullible, submissive, and passive, and lower in self-esteem.

Old age, low intelligence, impairment of sensory function, alcohol abuse, and cerebrovascular disease have been among the factors that have been associated with this peculiar disorder. A genetic predisposition to idiopathic psychosis has been suggested as a possible risk factor.

There is some question as to whether such people are truly delusional or merely highly impressionable. Frequently, there is passive acceptance of the delusional beliefs of the dominant person, until they are separated, at which point the unusual belief may remit spontaneously. The criteria for the diagnosis require an absence of psychotic disorder before onset of the induced delusion.

24. What is paranoid personality disorder?

Paranoid personality disorder is a nonpsychotic condition involving a marked change in personality traits as the individual becomes a young adult. These traits include a pervasive and unwanted tendency to interpret the actions of other people as demeaning or threatening. Behaviors include expecting to be exploited, questioning the loyalty or trust of friends or associates, reading hidden meanings into benign remarks or events, bearing grudges, not confiding in others because of fear that the information will be used against the person, tending to be easily slighted and quick to react with anger, questioning the fidelity of spouses or sexual partners, and intense changes in mood. Little is known about this disorder's prevalence, association with familial transmission patterns, and predispositions. Its relationship to schizophrenia and even to other paranoid disorders is also unclear. It is an interesting clinical phenomenon about which we need considerably more information.

25. What is Capgras syndrome?

In 1923, Capgras and Reboul-Lachaux described a syndrome consisting of the delusion that doubles of important or significant others and of oneself exist. For example, the patient may claim that his or her spouse has been replaced by an impostor. The syndrome is not related to hallucinations, simple misrecognition, or illusions. It is a delusion. In 1983, Berson summarized 133 cases of this syndrome reported in the literature. His conclusions were that the disorder appears in both men and women, over a wide range of ages, and with a wide range of other mental disorders. The most common diagnosis in such cases has generally been schizophrenia (about 60%); 23% of patients identified with this disorder suffered from diagnosable brain disorder.

26. How important is the differential diagnosis?

It is the most important process in the evaluation of patients with paranoid disorders. Most of these disorders are, at the very least, uncommon, and they are idiopathic. In addition, they have features characteristic of many medical and psychiatric conditions. Diagnosis of paranoid disorders requires the exclusion of other conditions and the matching of the features of a particular case to the appropriate criteria.

27. What are the steps in forming a differential diagnosis for paranoid disorders?

First, recognize, characterize, and judge as pathologic those features that are identified as possibly paranoid. Be sensitive to the range of subjective and objective characteristics frequently found in paranoid conditions. This step is critical as well as difficult because of the patient's unwillingness to reveal him- or herself in the process of the interview or to cooperate with clinical investigation. Careful interviewing of the patient and other informants is usually the basis for determining that the behavior is psychopathologic.

Second, having determined that a paranoid condition is present, evaluate premorbid characteristics, the course of the disease, associated symptoms, and so on. Important in this process is the discovery of confusion, perceptual disturbances, mood and motor disturbances, signs of physical illness, or confusing symptoms that may suggest different causes for paranoid features. Isolated acute symptoms of paranoid behavior often are present in early stages of medical conditions.

Third, conduct a compete medical and psychiatric history, with special attention to alcohol and drug use. A thorough physical examination includes neurologic and mental status exams and appropriate laboratory studies—particularly serologic, toxic, endocrinologic, and microbiologic features—as well as radiographic and electroencephalographic investigations. Where possible, CT and possibly MRI studies should be performed to identify structural brain disease (e.g, a tumor, or multi-infarct dementia) associated with psychopathologic changes.

28. What are the most important conditions to consider in the differential diagnosis?

Certain conditions with delusional features should be routinely considered in a differential diagnosis because of their seriousness or frequency and because they are the most likely sources of delusional presentations.

• **Medical diseases and syndromes:** typically feature a disturbance of perception, especially of visual or auditory functioning. **Drug intoxications** are particularly relevant; abused drugs and even prescribed drugs, such as steroids and L-dopa, have been known to cause delusional syndromes, often without cognitive impairment. Among elderly people, **dementia** should be considered. Mental status exam should uncover the characteristic cognitive changes that generally do not occur in delusional disorder. **Delirium**, for example, has a fluctuating course, with confusion, memory impairment, and *transient* delusions that contrast with the *persistent* delusions in most idiopathic paranoid disorders.

• **Schizophrenia:** should be considered when the delusions are bizarre; affect is blunted or incongruent with thinking; thought disorder, if present, is pervasive; and role functioning is impaired. Paranoid schizophrenic patients may have somewhat less bizarre delusions than patients with other types of delusions; however, their role functioning is impaired, and auditory hallucinations are prominent.

• **Mood disorders:** in particular, depression and mania. Profound changes in mood suggest depression. In paranoid disorders, mood may be depressed, but the change usually is not as overwhelming and pervasive as in depression. Delusions in depression frequently are related to the mood of depression, the so-called mood congruent delusions. The key is to consider the associated psychopathologic features. Depression refers to a group of signs and symptoms, such as changes in appetite, sleep, libido, concentration, decisiveness, interest, and energy. Depression often is cyclical, and may follow a fluctuating course. It also may be associated with a positive family history.

Manic delusions often are grandiose and, therefore, to some extent mood-congruent. They usually occur during severe stages of mania and are relatively easy to recognize as part of the manic syndrome. Marked instability of mood, intense euphoria or irritability, reduced need for sleep, increased energy, lack of inhibition, and increased activity levels distinguish mania from paranoid disorder.

29. Name other conditions that should be considered in the differential.

• **Other personality disorder:** paranoid features can occur in schizoid and schizotypal personality disorders as well as in paranoid personality disorders. The decisive distinction with most of the other paranoid disorders is the presence of clear-cut delusions, hallucinations, and other psychotic features.

• **Obsessive-compulsive disorder:** delusions and hallucinations typically are absent in these disorders. Fears, rituals, rumination, and preoccupation are generally more pervasive and more likely to influence functioning than in delusional or paranoid disorders.

• **Somatoform disorder:** Body dysmorphic disorder may be difficult to distinguish. The degree of conviction about imagined disfigurement may be helpful in making this distinction. Other psychopathologic features are more likely to be present in somatoform disorders as well. Hypochondriasis may present some difficulty in differential diagnosis. Patients almost always retain, however, some degree of uncertainty about their health concerns.

30. What principles apply to the differential diagnosis of elderly paranoid patients?

In the elderly, the differential diagnosis is, if anything, even broader due to **disorders associated with aging**. Although it is possible for idiopathic paranoid disorders *to begin* late in life, the likelihood is low. There is, however, a high risk for paranoid features *to recur* in depression, schizophrenia, and as a result of organic factors. The sudden onset of paranoid features should be considered a sign of medical illness, possibly cerebrovascular disease, and an acute onset may be a harbinger of acute organic delusional syndrome. The incidence of many medical diseases associated with paranoid features increases with age. Other sources of increased risk for paranoid disturbance among older individuals include a lack of stimulating company, physical illness, aging itself, and reductions in sensory functioning, such as visual acuity and hearing.

31. Are laboratory tests of value in the assessment of paranoid disorders?

Yes, they often are critical to reaching a proper diagnosis. A range of assessments usually is necessary, but some are more likely to detect key factors in particular cases. **Drug screening** measures (urine toxicology) are essential. Check for commonly abused substances such as alcohol, marijuana, stimulants such as cocaine and amphetamine compunds, and hallucinogens sush as phencyclidine; substance-induced delusional responses are frequent. Prescribed substances such as sedatives and hypnotics also can be detected. Other **routine laboratory tests** (e.g., blood counts, HIV assays, thyroid, liver functions, electrolytes, blood sugar) as well as EEG and brain radiography (CT scan) often help to disclose the presence of pathology (e.g., temporal lobe seizure disorders, mass lesions) that can be related to paranoid presentations. **Neuropsychological assessment** may help disclose evidence of impaired intellectual functioning and suggest brain abnormalities. Assessment of intelligence through I.Q. testing may show discrepancies between verbal and performance scores as well as scatter in overall performance, suggesting the need for further assessment of medical disorders.

32. What is the treatment for paranoid disorders?

No set treatment guidelines apply to all cases of paranoid disorders. Each of the conditions is sufficiently different to require a separate approach. Consider paranoid personality, which, in addition to being uncommon, is unlikely to come to the attention of clinicians. Such patients may, because of depressive symptomatology or anxiety, eventually fall into the care of psychiatric professionals. But generally speaking, these patients maintain an arm's-length distance from any health care, and specifically psychiatric, facility. Symptomatic therapies and supportive counseling frequently are attempted in such cases. Success is, at best, modest.

Organic delusional syndrome, on the other hand, may be treatable so long as the treatment focuses on the underlying organic factor that initiated and perpetuated the delusional presentation. For example, in substance abuse, removal of the initiating factor may result in a rapid improvement in the patient's mental state. Often such patients also require treatment with antipsychotic medication (e.g., risperidone, haloperidol), which may have the added effect of reducing the agitation, suspiciousness, and even the delusional thinking associated with these conditions. However, if the original initiating factor remains, the prognosis is likely to be poor unless symptomatic treatment is continued. With progressive disorders, such treatment may only serve to delay severe deterioration.

33. Is delusional disorder treatable?

Delusional disorder *may* be treatable. Due to the condition's very nature, the patient may have difficulty admitting a psychiatric illness exists and is not likely to seek care. Psychotherapy, medication, and even hospitalization can be important components of care, but in refractory conditions the delusion will not remit with these interventions.

34. Is psychotherapy helpful?

Psychotherapy creates a therapeutic alliance that can allow patients with delusional disorder to deal with whatever stressors and concerns contribute to the overall impairment associated with the delusional experience. For example, if the patient is dysphoric and finds it difficult to work, a chance to share some of these concerns with a sympathetic clinician may provide considerable relief.

35. What role does pharmacology play in the treatment of delusional disorder?

Medications have been promoted recently, but the data concerning their use is limited. Certainly there is value in considering an antipsychotic: delusion is, after all, a major symptom of psychosis, and it stands to reason that an antipsychotic agent might have some role in treatment. In practice, however, the success of such interventions as well as other somatic treatment is meager. Hypochondriacal delusions of the somatic type have been reported to respond to pimozide, a potent dopamine blocking agent and antipsychotic medication. These observations have been based on a small series of cases and are uncontrolled. Antidepressants have been promoted by some individuals who have treated patients with delusional disorder. Again, the observation is that patients who have dysphoric mood in association with presence of the delusions respond nicely.

36. When is hospitalization advisable?

Hospitalization is recommended in circumstances in which the patient's behavior has become dangerous or self-destructive. Hospitalization may be a satisfactory temporary solution, allowing the patient to be confronted with the impact of the behavior and the need for greater restraint.

37. Have there been any advances in the somatic treatment of delusional disorder?

For years psychiatrists have reported limited success and often negative results from somatic treatment of delusional disorder. A recent examination of some 200 cases reported in the literature since 1961, consistent with DSM-IV criteria and with sufficient detail to make comparisons, showed that approximately 80% of patients either recovered fully or partially with the treatment. The most frequently reported treatment was **pimozide**, which produced full recovery in 69% and partial recovery in 22%; typical neuroleptics produced full recovery in 23% and partial recovery in 45%.

No specific conclusions were drawn regarding treatment with antidepressants, although a number of reports were favorable. The most commonly treated subtype was somatic, but meta-analysis suggested that patterns of response were similar across subtypes of delusional disorder. Reports that included followup indicated that persistent use of medication is necessary to maintain remission.

Results of treatment with newer atypical antipsychotic medicines, i.e., clozapine, risperidone, olanzapine, and quetiapine, are preliminary but promising. Several case reports indicate risperidone and clozapine effectiveness.

The review concluded that antipsychotic drugs may be effective, and a trial, possibly of pimozide or an atypical agent, is warranted. Certainly trials make sense when the agitation, apprehension, and anxiety that accompany delusions are prominent.

Treatment with antipsychotic medication is, of course, not a substitute for treatment of the underlying factor in an organic delusional syndrome. Antipsychotic medication usually is for temporary symptomatic relief.

38. Is there treatment for shared psychotic disorder?

Little is known about treatment for this condition. Observations have had a tantalizing quality in suggesting that separation (e.g., divorce, death) of the two parties may lead to dimunition of the delusion in the induced psychotic partner, even to the point that the patient can no longer be considered delusional. Apart from this, there are no systematic controlled observations about intervention in the literature.

39. What is the therapy for atypical psychosis?

Patients who have these conditions must be dealt with individually, identifying the symptoms that constitute the basis of their complaint. If a specific, or particularly prominent, delusional form of thinking is present, antipsychotic medications may be helpful. Again, very little systematic literature is available for this condition, and general guidelines are not possible.

40. Has there been any progress in identifying the cause(s) of delusional disorder?

The cause of delusional disorder is unknown. However, factors such as advanced age, sensory impairment, family history of delusional psychopathology, and recent immigration are associated with increased risk. Of these, perhaps the best supported is the **familial psychopathology**. If delusional disorder is merely a form of schizophrenia or mood disorder, then the incidence of these conditions in family studies of delusional disorder patients should be higher than that of the general population. However, this is not the consistent finding. In addition, a recent study concluded that patients with delusional disorder are more likely to have family members who exhibit paranoid symptoms (e.g., suspiciousness, jealousy, secretiveness) or have paranoid illness themselves than families of controls. Other studies show that paranoid personality disorder and avoidant personality disorders are more common among relatives of delusional disorder patients than among relatives of normal controls or schizophrenic patients. There is recent evidence for increased risk of alcoholism among relatives of delusional disorder patients compared to those of patients with schizophrenia, other psychotic disorders, and schizophreniform disorder.

41. How dangerous are paranoid conditions?

It depends. Factors associated with the presentation of paranoid symptoms often are decisive in permitting inference of risk. For example, the intensity of the delusional thinking and its associated mood qualities (such as increased expression of anger and hostility in association with the delusion) are particularly relevant. Other important factors are the presence or likelihood of substance abuse and organized thinking and behavior. Greater personality intactness can increase the risk of dangerousness in individuals afflicted by delusional features. Erotomania and jealousy create powerful emotional energy and have been associated with violent behavior frequently enough to warrant heightened awareness when these symptoms are prominent.

Delusional disorder subtypes associated with these delusions occasionally present problems of dangerousness. Notably, of the delusional disorder subtypes, the somatic subtype is low-risk. These patients generally do not show intense anger, hostility, or enraged responses associated with their delusional thinking.

42. What is stalking?

Stalking is uninvited and unwelcome pursuit or following, often with harassment and pestering of the victim, who feels threatened and often fearful. It is a behavior in which the stalker directs intense emotions toward the victim. Stalkers may have a variety of psychiatric difficulties, but may be free of psychiatric illness. Of the paranoid conditions, the erotomanic subtype of delusional disorder and other disorders with erotomanic symptomatology are the most likely to be associated with stalking behaviors. These behaviors are known to be particularly onerous to deal with because of their pronounced refractoriness. However, if the delusion can be adequately treated, it is unlikely that these behaviors will persist.

BIBLIOGRAPHY

1. American Psychiatric Association: Diagnostic and Statistical Manual of Mental Disorders, 4th ed (DSM-IV). Washington DC, American Psychiatric Association, 1994.
2. Berson RJ: Capgras syndrome. Am J Psychiatry 140:969–978, 1983.
3. Cummings JL: Psychosis in neurologic disease: Neurobiology and pathogenesis. Neuropsychiatry Neuropsychol Behav Neurol 5:144–150, 1992.
4. Gawin FH, Ellinwood E: Cocaine and other stimulants. N Engl J Med 318:1173–1182, 1988.
5. Howard RJ, Almeida O, Levy R, et al: Quantitative magnetic resonance imaging volumetry distinguishes delusional disorder from late-onset schizophrenia. Br J Psychiatry 165:474–470, 1995.
6. Kraepelin E: Manic Depressive Insanity and Paranoia. Edinburgh, Livingstone Press, 1921.
7. Krakowski M, Volavka J, Brizer D: Psychopathology and violence: A review of literature. Compr Psychiatry 27:131–148, 1986.
8. Manschreck TC, Petri M: The paranoid syndrome. Lancet 2:251–253, 1978.
9. Manschreck TC: Delusional disorder and shared psychotic disorder. In Kaplan H, Sadock B (eds): Comprehensive Textbook of Psychiatry, 7th ed. Baltimore, Lippincott, Williams & Wilkins, 2000.
10. Manschreck TC: Pathogenesis of delusions. Psychiatr Clin North Am 18:213–230, 1995.
11. Manschreck TC: The assessment of paranoid features. Compr Psychiatry 20(4):370–377, 1979.
12. McAllister T: Neuropsychiatric aspects of delusions. Psychiatr Ann 22:269–277, 1992.
13. Meloy JR (ed): The Psychology of Stalking. San Diego, Academic Press, 1998.
14. Munro A: Delusional Disorder. New York, Cambridge University Press, 1999.
15. Munro A, Mok H: An overview of treatment in paranoia/delusional disorder. Can J Psychiatry 40:616–622, 1995.

16. Opler LA, Klahr DM, Ramirez PM: Pharmacologic treatment of delusions. Psychiatr Clin North Am
    18:379–391, 1995.
17. Serreti A, Lattuada E, Cusin C, Smeraldi E: Factor analysis of delusional disorder symptomatology. Compr
    Psychiatry 40(2):143–147, 1999.
18. Stoudemire A, Riether A: Evaluation and treatment of paranoid syndromes in the elderly. Gen Hosp
    Psychiatry 9:267–274, 1987.
19. Webb W: Paranoid conditions seen in psychiatric medicine. Psychiatr Med 8:37–48, 1990.

12. BIPOLAR DISORDERS

Marshall R. Thomas, M.D.

1. What is bipolar disorder? How is it different from manic-depressive illness?

Bipolar disorder encompasses a heterogeneous group of disorders characterized by cyclical disturbances in mood, cognition, and behavior. The diagnosis requires a history of mania for at least 1 week or hypomania for at least 4 days. **Bipolar I disorder** refers to patients who have had at least one episode of mania. **Bipolar II disorder** refers to patients with a history of hypomania and major depressive episodes. **Cyclothymia** refers to patients with chronic (at least 2-year duration) mood swings that fluctuate between hypomania and minor but not major depression.

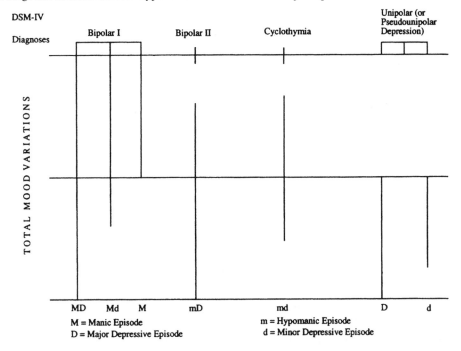

Modified from Goodwin F, Jamison K: Manic-Depressive Illness. New York, Oxford University Press, 1990.

In 1921, the German psychiatrist Emil Kraepelin introduced the term manic-depressive insanity, which included patients with recurrent unipolar depression as well as bipolar disorder and distinguished both groups from schizophrenia, which he termed dementia praecox. Kraepelin emphasized the similarities in course and outcome between patients with highly recurrent mood disorders, regardless of polarity. In 1962, Leonard introduced the term bipolar and emphasized differences between unipolar and bipolar patients.

Many researchers argue that modern adherence to Leonard's bipolar/unipolar dichotomy, although clarifying certain issues, has caused clinicians to overlook the similarities between bipolar and many unipolar patients, who share a common pattern of recurrence, remission, and exacerbation. The modern concept of bipolar spectrum disorder encompasses patients with bipolar I and II disorders, cyclothymia, hyperthymia (chronic hypomania), and **pseudounipolar depression**. Pseudounipolar depressives are patients with a highly recurrent unipolar illness, a positive family history for bipolar disorder, and a positive therapeutic response to antibipolar treatments.

2. Describe the epidemiology of bipolar disorder.

The lifetime risk for bipolar I disorder is 0.6–0.9% in industrialized nations, with no apparent gender differences; unipolar depression, however, is twice as common in women as it is in men. Differing criteria for what constitutes hypomania have made it difficult to determine the prevalence of bipolar II and cyclothymic disorders. Bipolar II disorder is probably at least as common as bipolar I, and the lifetime prevalence of cyclothymia is estimated at 0.4–1.0%. Over the last 50 years, all mood disorders have increased in prevalence, with an earlier age of onset in each successive generation—a phenomenon referred to as the **cohort effect**.

Family studies find that if one parent has a major affective disorder the risk to the offspring is 25–30%, whereas if both parents have an affective disorder the risk to the offspring may be as high as 50–75%. Suicide is common in untreated bipolar disorder; 25–50% of patients attempt suicide at least once. Seasonal variations exist; depression is more common in the spring (March through May) and autumn (September through November), whereas mania is more common in the summer. The peak incidence of suicide occurs in May, with a second peak in October.

3. How is mania recognized?

Manic states range in severity from milder hypomania to psychotic or delirious manic states. The symptomatology evolves as the episode becomes more severe. The mood in mania may be elated or euphoric, but as severity increases the mood is more likely to become irritable, labile, and dysphoric. Thoughts may race; as mania progresses, thinking becomes disorganized, expansive, and grandiose. Behavior increases from early physical hyperactivity, pressured speech, and decreased need for sleep to later manifestations of hypersexuality, increased impulsivity, and risk taking.

Manic Episode: Diagnostic Criteria

• Distinct period of elevated, expansive, or irritable mood:
At least 1 week
Or hospitalized
• Three of the following: four if mood only irritable:

Inflated self esteem or grandiosity	Distractibility
Decreased need for sleep	Increased activity
Pressured speech	Excessive involvement in pleasurable activities
Flight of ideas or thoughts racing	with high risk of painful consequences

• Marked impairment, psychosis, or hospitalization
• Not due to direct effect of substance or medical condition

From American Psychiatric Association: Diagnostic and Statistical Manual of Mental Disorders, 4th ed. Washington, DC, American Psychiatric Association, 1994, with permission.

Hypomanic Episode: Diagnostic Criteria

• Distinct period of elevated, expansive, or irritable mood (at least 4 days)
• Three additional symptoms: four if mood only irritable
• Unequivocal change in functioning
• Change observable by others

Table continued on following page

Hypomanic Episode: Diagnostic Criteria (Continued)

• Episode not severe enough to cause:
  Marked impairment
  Hospitalization
  Psychosis
• Not due to direct effects of a substance or general medical condition

From American Psychiatric Association: Diagnostic and Statistical Manual of Mental Disorders, 4th ed. Washington, DC, American Psychiatric Association, 1994, with permission.

4. What is a "mixed state"?

A mixed state is diagnosed when the patient simultaneously meets criteria for mania and major depression. Mixed states are common, occurring in approximately 40% of manic patients. Mixed states are sometimes difficult to distinguish from or are misdiagnosed as agitated depressions and borderline conditions. Mixed states are more common in patients with substance abuse and neurologic disorders (e.g., head injury) and are associated with increased suicidality, chronicity, and poorer response to lithium.

5. What is the clinical significance of bipolar II disorder?

Bipolar II (BP II) disorder is diagnosed in patients with episodes of hypomania interspersed with episodes of major depression. Clinically, patients usually present during periods of depression. Often the diagnosis is not clear, because both hypomania and depression may be associated with irritability, and the psychomotor symptoms of hypomania may be subtle. BP II disorder is more common in women. BP II tends to run in families (breeds true), and patients who present as BP II tend to stay in the same category; they have subsequent episodes of hypomania but not mania.

Bipolar II disorder should not be viewed as a minor form of BP I, because psychosocial morbidity, substance abuse, and suicide attempts are at least as common in BP II. What constitutes the best treatment course for patients with BP needs further study. Patients with BP II show a predominance of depression, but antidepressant treatments may induce rapid cycling and mixed states, as they do in BP I disorder. Patients with BP II also may be biologically heterogeneous. For example, severe environmental stressors such as prolonged abuse or neglect may cause forms of mood disregulation that phenotypically resemble BP II (referred to as *bipolar II phenocopy*) in patients without family histories of affective disorders.

6. How are bipolar and unipolar depression differentiated?

About 10–20% of hospital first admissions for depression later develop a bipolar disorder. Careful scrutiny of the patient's history for episodes of mania or hypomania may help to make the diagnosis in some cases. The clinical course of **bipolar depression** is characterized by premorbid cyclothymic temperament; recurrences; and early-age, rapid, and postpartum onsets. Symptomatically bipolar depressives are more likely to demonstrate psychosis, hypersomnia, anergia (low energy), and severe shut-down depressions that are immobilizing. Bipolar depressives also are more likely to have family histories of bipolar disorder and familial loading for affective disorders in general. In the absence of a premorbid history of **mania**, **hypomania**, or **cyclothymia**, no single associated finding is pathognomonic for bipolar disorder, but clusters of such factors make the diagnosis more likely.

7. Describe the course of illness issues in bipolar disorder.

In the past there has been a tendency to underestimate the rate of recurrence and to overestimate the age of onset of bipolar disorder. **Many bipolar adolescents are misdiagnosed** as conduct-disordered or schizophrenic, because they may demonstrate labile mood, abnormal thinking, and disturbed behavior several years before their first recognizable major affective episode. For bipolar patients, the mean age of first impairment due to psychiatric symptoms is 18.7 years; the mean age of first treatment is 22 years; and the mean age of first hospitalization is 25.8 years. *The lag between age of first impairment and age of first treatment is cause for concern* in light of data suggesting that early intervention and treatment may prevent the development of a more malignant course of illness.

The rate of cycling increases with each successive episode. The average free interval between the first and second episode is 5 years, but by the fourth episode cycles are occurring at least yearly. Although duration of episodes demonstrates interindividual variability, the average untreated manic episode lasts 4 months and the average depressive episode 6–9 months. Manic episodes often begin abruptly over hours to days. Bipolar depressions usually take weeks to develop, but they still have a more rapid onset than unipolar depression.

Approximately 20% of bipolar patients demonstrate rapid cycling. Rapid cycling is more common in women, patients with BP II, and patients who have received antidepressant treatments. Rapid cyclers may have a poorer response to lithium and a higher rate of hypothyroidism.

In clinical cohorts, another 20% of bipolar patients have a chronic course with no free interval between episodes. A history of chronicity, substance abuse, and mixed states is associated with poorer outcome.

8. Describe the relationship between stress and onset of affective episodes in bipolar disorder.

At times it is difficult to sort out whether stress has led to an episode, or the prodromal symptoms of an episode have led to the stress. Investigations suggest that stressors are statistically more likely to be associated with the onset of episodes early in the course of illness. This finding, along with the finding of increasing cycling, have suggested that **the illness may kindle itself** and become increasingly endogenous over time. In kindling, a model borrowed from neurology, a subthreshold stimulus applied at a regular interval over time becomes capable of inducing seizure activity.

Interpersonal and work difficulties are common precipitants associated with mood destabilization. Sleep reduction may be a final common pathway that leads to mania in a variety of situations, including stress-induced sleep disruption, parturition, and travel. There also is a high rate of bipolarity in patients whose moods demonstrate seasonal variation.

9. List medical conditions that may cause, mimic, or exacerbate bipolar disorder.

Organic factors can cause or exacerbate both mania and depression. The DSM-IV provides a separate diagnostic category for organically derived mood disorders: mood disorder due to . . . [indicate the general medical condition]. Historically, the term "secondary mania" has been used to designate manic states that arise from neurologic, endocrinologic, metabolic, infectious, or other medical conditions. Many organic factors may contribute to depression or mania individually, but few can engender a true bipolar syndrome with cycling between two states.

Organic Causes of Bipolar Mood Syndromes

Drugs	Isoniazid, steroids, disulfram
Neurologic factors	Multiple sclerosis, closed head injury, CNS tumors, epilepsy, Huntington's disease, cerebrovascular accident
Metabolic factors	Thyroid disorders, postoperative states, adrenal disorders, vitamin B12 deficiency, electrolyte abnormalities
Infection	AIDS dementia, neurosyphilis, influenza

Modified from Goodwin F, Jamison K: Manic-Depressive Illness. New York, Oxford University Press, 1990.

Patients with an **organic affective disorder** are less likely to have a positive family history and may respond to treatment of the underlying condition. Other organic affective syndromes, such as those associated with brain trauma and multiple sclerosis, are not reversible but benefit from antibipolar treatments. Patients with a genetic predisposition to bipolarity may have a lower threshold for developing organic affective syndrome secondary to organic stressors.

10. What psychiatric conditions are commonly comorbid with bipolar disorder?

Bipolar disorder is the axis I disorder most likely to be associated with comorbid **substance abuse** or dependence; 60% of bipolar patients demonstrate abuse or dependence in one form or another. A study by the National Institutes of Mental Health (NIMH) found that 46% of bipolar patients abused or were dependent on alcohol, and 41% abused or were dependent on marijuana, cocaine, opiates, barbiturates, or hallucinogens. All forms of substance abuse are more common in manic or mixed phases of the illness. Comorbid substance abuse is associated with significantly poorer outcomes and increased rates of suicide.

Anxiety symptoms, **axis II disorders**, and **certain psychotic conditions** are found more commonly in patients with bipolar disorder. During mixed manic states and depressive episodes, bipolar patients may experience extreme anxiety that may remit with control of the affective disorder. Some bipolar patients may appear character-disordered (borderline or narcissistic), because their mood disorder is inadequately treated, whereas others demonstrate a comorbid axis II diagnosis in the absence of mood disregulation. Up to 50% of bipolar patients have psychotic symptoms such as delusions or hallucinations at some point in the course of their illness.

The presence of psychotic symptoms only during periods of prominent mood disturbance distinguishes psychotic affective disorders from schizophrenia and schizoaffective disorder, in which psychotic symptoms exist outside of periods of mood disturbance.

11. What are the advantages and disadvantages of using lithium in the treatment of bipolar disorder?

Advantages: Lithium has been in clinical use for over 40 years. It appears to be highly effective for mild manic symptoms and classic euphoric mania. Although lithium is less effective in treating bipolar depression, approximately 50% of bipolar patients with mild-to-moderate depression respond to treatment if given enough time. Lithium appears more effective in treating with mania-depression-interval (MDI) as opposed to depression-mania-interval (DMI) sequences. One distinct advantage of lithium for some patients is the fact that its standard preparations are significantly less expensive than other antimanic drugs.

Disadvantages: Despite lithium's remarkable efficacy in euphoric mania, 30–50% of bipolar patients either are unable to tolerate or fail to respond to lithium. Even for patients who benefit the rate of response is slow: 10–14 days for mania and 4–8 weeks for depression. Gastrointestinal distress, cognitive dullness, polyuria, and tremor represent common acute effects. Weight gain is a common cause of discontinuation over the long term; 25% of patients gain 10 pounds or more. Approximately 10% of patients develop hypothyroidism. Elderly patients with compromised renal function require careful dosage adjustment. Patients with mixed states, severe mania, psychosis, substance abuse, and a history of neurologic insults are less likely to respond to lithium monotherapy.

12. What are the advantages and disadvantages of using anticonvulsants in the treatment of bipolar disorder?

Although lithium is considered by many clinicians to be the first-line drug in the treatment of mania and bipolar mood cycling, many patients either are unable to tolerate or fail to respond to lithium. As a result, in the last 15–20 years, there has been increasing interest in the use of anticonvulsants, particularly valproic acid and carbamazepine, to treat bipolar mood disorders. Controlled trials have demonstrated the efficacy of both drugs in acute mania, and studies of valproic acid have suggested a more rapid onset of antimanic action compared with lithium. Valproic acid, like lithium, is FDA-approved for the treatment of acute mania. More recently, investigators and clinicians have looked at the use of lamotrigine, gabapentin, and topiramate for patients with bipolar disorder.

The disadvantages of these agents are mainly related to side effects. Valproic acid usually is well tolerated, although weight gain is an issue of concern for some patients. Rapid loading at 500 mg 3 times/day can be accomplished in hospital settings for many acutely agitated patients. Carbamazepine is more difficult to dose and requires a more gradual upward titration. Carbamazepine also autoinduces its own metabolism and heteroinduces the metabolism of other drugs. As a result, careful drug level monitoring is required, and other drugs, such as antipsychotics and birth control pills, may be rendered less effective unless dosage adjustments are made. Lamotrigine is associated with a potentially life threatening rash, especially in pediatric patients. Gabapentin is relatively well tolerated, but is of questionable efficacy. A common side effect of topiramate is weight loss, which is an advantage for some patients.

13. **How does stage of illness affect treatment strategy in bipolar disorder?**

The treatment strategy in bipolar disorder depends on the current stage of the illness, dimensional assessment of the illness, and knowledge of past treatment. The treatment of *acute mania* (described in Chapter 49) includes the use of antimanic drugs and, depending on the severity of illness, adjunctive agents such as sedative-hypnotics, benzodiazepines, and antipsychotic agents. The treatment for *acute depression* (discussed in more detail in the controversies section below) is complicated in bipolar patients by the need to minimize the use of antidepressant agents.

Preventive treatment with antibipolar agents usually is indicated, because bipolar disorder almost always is recurrent. The high rate of suicide attempts in all phases of illness dictates an ongoing assessment of safety issues throughout the course of treatment. Recent studies suggest that many patients may do better long-term with antibipolar combination treatments (e.g., lithium plus valproic acid) instead of more traditional antimanic monotherapy strategies (e.g., lithium or valproic acid used alone).

CONTROVERSIES

14. **What is the treatment for bipolar depression?**

Issue. All antidepressants appear capable of inducing mania, mixed states, and mood cycling, thus worsening the long-term course of the illness.

Discussion. Patients with mild-to-moderate bipolar depression may respond to antimanic agents such as lithium alone, although there is often a significant lag time of up to 8 weeks before a full antidepressant response. Tricyclic antidepressants (TCAs) should be avoided, because they may be more likely than other antidepressants to induce cycling and also appear to be marginally effective in the treatment of bipolar depression. Bupropion also can induce mania, at least in some patients. Recent data suggest that selective serotonin reuptake inhibitors (SSRIs), such as fluoxetine, sertraline, and paroxetine, may be less likely to induce mania and hypomania than TCAs and monoamine oxidase inhibitors (MAOIs). MAOIs appear to be particularly effective in patients with anergic depressions or atypical symptoms (mood reactivity, hypersomnia, hyperphagia, leaden fatigue, and rejection sensitivity), many of whom may be bipolar.

Currently, most clinicians attempt to treat mild-to-moderate bipolar depression without an antidepressant. Some clinicians prefer augmentation with a second antimanic agent before adding an antidepressant. If an antidepressant is required, a short-acting SSRI (sertraline or paroxetine) or bupropion is the first choice. If these are ineffective, an MAOI or electroconvulsive therapy may be used. Patients with rapid cycling depressions or mixed states of mania and concurrent depression require cessation of antidepressant agents and treatment with anticonvulsant combination strategies.

15. **What is the role of antipsychotic agents in the treatment of bipolar disorder?**

Issue. Traditional antipsychotic agents (neuroleptics) frequently have been prescribed to patients with bipolar disorder. Many patients begin these agents when hospitalized for acute mania, but then continue on antipsychotics post hospital discharge after the acute symptoms have resolved. Clinicians should avoid unnecessarily exposing patients to these agents since the older class of antipsychotics is associated with risks of drug-induced extra pyramidal symptoms, neuroleptic-induced dysphoria, and potentially irreversible tardive dyskinesia.

Discussion. 60% of patients with bipolar disorder experience psychotic symptoms at some time during the course of their illness. The high historical use of antipsychotic agents in bipolar patients may relate to the fact that clinicians and patients have found that antipsychotic agents are helpful in obtaining and maintaining a clinical response. The side effects of the older antipsychotic agents, however, meant that this therapeutic advantage was purchased at a potentially high cost to the patients.

In recent years, a new generation of antipsychotics has been developed that is much less likely to cause drug-induced parkinsonism and tardive dyskinesia. The newer atypical antipsychotic agents, which include clozapine, risperidone, olanzapine, and quetiapine (with additional agents in the pipeline) combine 5 HT_2 post synaptic antagonism with D_2 receptor blockade. In addition to fewer neurologic side effects, these newer agents have positive effects on mood, anxiety, impulsivity, and aggression.

Clozapine, olanzapine, and, to a lesser extent, risperidone have all been studied in patients with bipolar mood disorders. Clozapine appears to have a powerful anti-manic and mood stabilizing effect and is useful in treatment resistant bipolar disorder. Olanzapine and risperidone may have stronger anti-depressant effects, but appear to induce mania in some patients. Nevertheless, controlled trials of olanzapine have shown its efficacy in treatment of acute mania and have resulted in FDA approval for use in acute mania.

BIBLIOGRAPHY

1. American Psychiatric Association: Diagnostic and Statistical Manual of Mental Disorders, 4th ed. Washington, DC, American Psychiatric Association, 1994.
2. Baldessarini RJ, et al: Pharmacological treatment of bipolar disorder throughout the life cycle. In Shulman KI, Tohen M (eds): Mood Disorders Across the Life Span. New York, Wiley-Liss, 1996, pp 299–338.
3. Calabrese JR, et al: Spectrum of activity of lamotrigine in treatment-refractory bipolar disorder. Am J Psychiatry 156(7):1019–1023, 1999.
4. Freeman MP, Stoll AL: Mood stabilizer combinations: A review of safety and efficacy. Am J Psychiatry 155(1):12–21, 1998.
5. Ghaemi S, et al: Use of atypical antipsychotic agents in bipolar and schizoaffective disorders: Review of the empirical literature. J Clin Psychopharmacol 19(4):354–361, 1999.
6. Goodwin F, Jamison K: Manic-Depressive Illness. New York, Oxford University Press, 1990.
7. McElroy S, et al: Clinical and research implications for the diagnosis of dysphoric and mixed mania or hypomania. Am J Psychiatry 149:1633, 1992.
8. Nathan PE, Gorman JM (eds): A Guide to Treatments that Work. New York, Oxford University Press, 1998.
9. Post RM, et al: A history of the use of anticonvulsants as mood stabilizers in the last two decades of the 20th century. Neuropsychobiology 38(3):152–166, 1998.
10. Schou M: The effect of prophylactic lithium treatment on mortality and suicidal behavior: A review for clinicians. J Affective Disorders 50(2–3):253–259, 1998.
11. Tohen M, et al: Olanzapine versus placebo in the treatment of acute mania. Am J Psychiatry 156(5):702–709, 1999.

13. DEPRESSIVE DISORDERS

Lawson R. Wulsin, M.D.

1. What are the seven secrets of depression?

Depression is (1) common, (2) often missed, (3) not hard to diagnose if you look for it, (4) often severe, (5) often recurrent, (6) costly, and (7) highly treatable. These facts are "secrets" in the sense that they are not well understood by the American public or by many physicians.

Depression is among the five most common disorders seen in a primary care physician's office. Unrecognized and untreated depression has been acknowledged as a major public health problem in the United States for the past 20 years. As many as half of the cases of depressive disorders go unrecognized by the patient or the doctor, and among those recognized most will remain untreated. The reasons for such neglect include stigma, misunderstandings about the seriousness and treatability of depression, and preferential attention by patient and doctor to somatic complaints.

The disability caused by depressive disorders rivals that of coronary artery disease and is greater than the disability resulting from chronic lung disease or arthritis, according to the Medical Outcomes Study.[15] The cost of depressive disorders in terms of treatment, work missed, and loss of function approximates $43 billion annually in the U.S. Depression is associated with 80% of suicides. Yet it is highly treatable, with 80% of patients responding to antidepressant therapy, psychotherapy, or both, when treated by qualified professionals. The cost of diagnosis and treatment is small, relative to other common severe medical disorders, whereas the cost of *not* treating a depressive disorder is great.

2. What does the term "depressive disorders" include?
The following DSM-IV diagnoses:
  • Major depressive disorder, single episode
  • Major depressive disorder, recurrent
  • Dysthymic disorder
  • Depressive disorder not otherwise specified
  • Adjustment disorder with depressed mood
  • Mood disorder due to general medical condition
  • Substance-induced mood disorder
Major depressive disorder, particularly when recurrent, is the most severe of these subtypes.

3. List the criteria for diagnosing a major depressive episode.
  • At least five of the following symptoms present in a 2-week period (including either depressed mood or anhedonia):

Depressed mood	Fatigue, loss of energy
Loss of pleasure or interest (anhedonia)	Increased sense of worthlessness or guilt
Significant weight (appetite) loss or gain	Decreased concentration
Insomnia or hypersomnia	Recurrent morbid thoughts or suicidal
Agitation or retardation	ideation

  • Not due to substance abuse, medical illness, or bereavement
  • Significant distress or impairment of functioning
  • Not due to medication or general medical condition
  • Not better accounted for by bereavement

Guidelines for application of these criteria are useful and easily available in the mood disorders module of *Prime MD*,[13] the *Structured Clinical Interview for DSM-IV*,[14] and in the pocket-sized *Diagnosing DSM-IV Psychiatric Disorders in the Primary Care Setting*.[17] They provide questions that best assess whether the patient meets a given criterion, and provide directions on how to score the patient's responses when information is ambiguous or insufficient.

Specifiers describe the severity, the current phase of the disease (remission, recurrence), and some salient features such as seasonal pattern or rapid cycling.

4. What is the difference between major depression and dysthymia?
A diagnosis of dysthymia requires only three of the nine symptoms listed in Question 3, and they must be present for 2 years. Dysthymia can be a primary disorder, but it often is secondary to chronic medical problems (e.g., chronic pain, cancer) or psychiatric illness (recurrent major depression, schizophrenia). Depressive disorder not otherwise specified (NOS) includes minor depression (a few symptoms for less than 2 years) and recurrent brief depression (severe episodes which last less than 2 weeks).

5. True or false: Dysthymia is a mild, rare disorder, and treatment is unnecessary.
False. Dysthymia, because of its co-occurrence with medical conditions, is common in patients followed regularly in primary care settings. It is a more frequent finding than major depressive disorder. While seemingly less severe than other some other subtypes, chronicity can decrease quality of life and impair work and social functioning. Dysthymia is easily overlooked and attributed to the "normal" effects of illness. Treatment with psychotherapy and/or medications may be warranted.

6. How common is major depression?
The point prevalence in Western industrialized nations is 2.3–3.2% for men, and 4.5–9.3% for women. The lifetime risk is 7–12% for men, 20–25% for women. In primary care settings 6–10% of patients have current major depression. These figures make major depression as common in primary care practices as upper respiratory tract infections and hypertension.

7. How serious an illness is major depression?

Major depression is as serious as diabetes or heart disease. In a 1989 study of 11,242 primary care outpatients, the "poor functioning uniquely associated with depressive symptoms, with or without depressive disorder, was comparable with or worse than that uniquely associated with eight major chronic medical conditions (such as advanced heart disease, diabetes, gastrointestinal disorders, back problems, arthritis)."[15] In 1990, the Global Burden of Disease study found that the leading cause of disability worldwide was unipolar major depression, more than twice as disabling as the second most disabling disorder (iron deficiency anemia.).[9] These data suggest that the depressive disorders (not only major depression, but dysthymia and depressive symptoms) are associated with poor physical and social functioning. Depression increases mortality significantly through suicide, accidents, and exacerbation of medical illness.

8. What percentage of the medically ill have a depressive disorder?

Rates vary depending on the measures used to assess depression and the population studied. Rates rise with severity of medical illness, so that hospitalized patients have higher rates (20–33%) of depression than primary care clinic patients (5–20%). The depressed person often initially presents a somatic complaint (pain, insomnia, or fatigue), and the diagnosis of depression often is missed by either patient or clinician. Recent studies estimate that only half of the people with recognized major depression get any treatment.

Although no single intervention has improved recognition and treatment of depression, a combination of efforts results in good treatment outcomes: physician training, patient education, convenient mechanisms for screening at-risk patients, convenient methods for establishing a diagnosis of depression, well-tolerated and effective antidepressants, short-term psychotherapy focused on depression recovery and prevention, convenient methods for monitoring response to treatment, and access to consultation for complicated cases. Until 15 years ago, these resources were not available to most physicians, but today most primary care physicians can obtain access at minimal cost.

9. What are some easy bedside measures for evaluating depression?

The Beck Depression Inventory is a 21-item self-report questionnaire that patients usually find easy to understand and complete in 5 minutes. Scoring and interpretations are simple, providing a tool for screening and monitoring progress. Another self-report questionnaire commonly used in primary care settings is the General Health Questionnaire. Clinician rating scales, such as the Hamilton Depression Rating Scale, require specific training for administration and scoring but can be learned easily with a structured interview guide. The best translation of the DSM-IV criteria into conversational English that is precise and clear can be found in the modules for major depression and dysthymia of the *Prime MD*,[13] *Structured Clinical Interview for DSM-IV*[14] or in *Diagnosing DSM-IV Psychiatric Disorders in the Primary Care Setting*.[17]

10. How do you diagnose depression?

After the index of suspicion for depressive disorders is raised by the history, physical examination, mental status exam, or response to a screening measure, the clinician should then proceed to interview the patient carefully to establish which criteria the patient meets for any of the depressive disorders. Ask about duration, persistence, and severity of each symptom. Collaborative sources, such as relatives and past records, will help when the patient's responses are ambiguous, insufficient, or distorted by depression. Include your own observations when assessing the patient's agitation, energy level, concentration, and hopelessness.

Because the vegetative signs of depression may be caused by medical illnesses and medications, the diagnosis of depression in the medically ill should not rest solely on the presence of such factors as fatigue, insomnia, and anorexia. Look also for the cognitive and affective criteria such as poor concentration, a sense of hopelessness or worthlessness, depressed mood, and anhedonia. When in doubt about the overlap between medical illness and depression (Is the anergia and retardation caused by cancer and pain medications or depression?), it usually is preferable to treat a suspected depression in a medically ill person to relieve the suffering from depression and to reduce the exacerbations of the medical illness caused by the depression.

11. What is the effect of depression on medical illness?

Depressive disorders complicate the course of medical illness through a variety of possible mechanisms: magnifying pain, impairing adherence to regimens, decreasing social supports, and dysregulating humoral and immunologic systems. Untreated depression has been shown to increase rates of death dramatically in nursing home patients and in patients with myocardial infarctions. Depressed patients with chronic medical conditions show significantly more disability than nondepressed patients. Note that the former are bearing the burden of two independent diseases.

12. What percentage of depressed patients commit suicide? What percentage try?

About 15% of hospitalized depressed patients eventually commit suicide. About 10 times as many make suicidal acts. Depressive disorders are associated with about 80% of suicidal events. Other factors that increase the risk of suicide for the depressed person include alcohol and drug abuse, panic disorder and other states of intense anxiety, family history of suicide, medical illness, hopelessness, few social supports, recent personal loss, and unemployment. Treatment of the factors which contribute to suicide risk dramatically reduces both the immediate and chronic risks.

13. After the first episode, how likely is a patient to have a second major depressive episode?

More than 50% of those who have a first major depressive episode will have a recurrence. Untreated episodes generally last 6–24 months, with two thirds achieving a spontaneous full recovery. Risk factors for recurrences include incomplete recovery, previous recurrences, a strong family history of recurrent affective disorders, and a history of "double depression," i.e., a major depression superimposed on dysthymia.

14. What are the important subtypes of major depression?

• **Psychotic features.** Requires treatment with an antipsychotic medication as well as an antidepressant. Generally represents a more severe form of major depression warranting aggressive treatment and prevention.

• **Seasonal pattern.** Requires at least two episodes of major depression at the same season in successive years. Clear seasonal patterns allow some predictability and preventive treatment with phototherapy, or antidepressants in combination with psychotherapy.

• **Melancholia.** Severe vegetative signs of anergia, insomnia, and anorexia with diurnal worsening in the morning. These signs of melancholia often are the first to respond to antidepressant trials, with cognitive and affective signs following.

• **Atypical features.** In contrast to melancholia, this subtype features overeating, oversleeping, weight gain, and overreactive moods. It often responds better to monoamine oxidase inhibitors than to tricyclics.

• **Postpartum onset.** Has a 10–15% prevalence within 6 months after delivery of the child. A previous episode of depression or bipolar disorder may justify preventive treatment at the time of the next delivery.

These subtypes often are described as specifiers in listing the formal diagnosis of major depression.[2] They are important in some cases for their implications for treatment (e.g., psychotic features), in others simply for research purposes, and in some cases for prevention (e.g., seasonal pattern, postpartum onset).

15. What is the best biologic marker of major depression?

There are no "good" (cheap, easy, accurate) biologic markers for any of the depressive disorders. The most accurate diagnostic marker of major depression is the following profile on sleep electroencephalography (EEG): decreased total sleep, increased sleep latency, decreased rapid eye movement (REM) latency, increased REM density, and decreased stage 4 sleep. However, the sleep EEG is not yet a practical tool for the diagnosis of depression in primary care settings. The key to diagnosis is a **careful depression history** and the **mental status exam**.

16. What is the differential diagnosis of a major depressive episode?
- Mood disorder resulting from a medical condition
- Substance-induced mood disorder
- Dementia
- Bipolar disorder
- Attention deficit/hyperactivity disorder
- Adjustment disorder with depressed mood
- Bereavement
- Sad mood

Attribution of depression to a **medical disorder** depends on the timing of the two disorders, the severity of the medical problem, and, sometimes, the patient's eventual response to treatment of the underlying medical disorder. The same applies to **substance-induced** mood disorders.

Dementia's extensive overlap of symptoms with depression has led to the term *pseudo-dementia* for depression in elderly people who appear demented but respond to antidepressants. The onset of depression generally is faster than dementia and accompanied by more cognitive and affective distress (guilt, hopelessness, and poor concentration that improves transiently with extreme effort).

Diagnosis of the depressive phase of **bipolar disorder** rests on a previous history of mania or hypomania, or sometimes on identifying a mixed state of simultaneous depressed and manic symptoms.

Attention deficit/hyperactivity disorder can be complicated by a secondary depression or present some symptoms of depression (poor concentration, restlessness, insomnia, or sense of worthlessness). School history, course of illness, and response to treatment clarify this differential diagnosis. **Adjustment disorder** and **bereavement** are temporally linked to identifiable events with specific durations, beyond which these diagnoses may evolve into major depression.

The common experience of **sad mood** is not by itself sufficient for any diagnosis, even when the sad mood lasts for a few days. However, clusters of depressive symptoms that last 10–13 days and are sometimes severe, though not qualifying for major depressive disorder, should be diagnosed depressive disorder NOS and should, in most cases, be treated as a major depressive disorder.

17. What are the options for treating a major depressive episode?
Every patient who receives the diagnosis of major depression should learn the options for treatment. They consist of antidepressant medications, psychotherapy, electroconvulsive therapy, or some combination of these. A substantial body of research has established the efficacy of each of these methods of treatment. Furthermore, with systematic trials of treatment by qualified clinicians, 80–90% of people with major depression recover.

No set guidelines exist for an adequate trial of **psychotherapy**, but 1 hour a week for 20 weeks is a substantial trial if the therapy is focused on managing the depression (e.g., cognitive therapy for depression, or interpersonal therapy for depression). Significant symptom relief often occurs within 4–6 weeks.

An adequate trial of an **antidepressant** is 4–6 weeks on a therapeutic level. The antidepressants for which the level/response relationship has been well studied include impiramine, desipramine, amitriptyline, and nortriptyline. For selective serotonin reuptake inhibitors (fluoxetine, citalopram, paroxetine), an adequate trial is 4–6 weeks on 20 mg/day; for sertraline, 50 mg/day.

18. When is a person considered "refractory" to antidepressants?
Failure of two or more *full* trials (maximum tolerable dose for 6 weeks) may suggest refractoriness to those medications. However, close scrutiny of most drug failures often reveals inadequate trials, intolerance of side effects, or complicating medical or psychosocial factors. Additional carefully selected therapy trials usually result in recovery (see Chapters 47 and 54).

19. When should a depressed person be referred to a psychiatrist?
Refer in the following situations:
- Suicidal risk
- Psychosis

• Need for hospitalization
• Failure of an adequate antidepressant trial
• Complicated medical or psychiatric comorbidity
• Suspected need for combined medication and psychotherapy
• Evaluation for pharmacotherapy

The psychiatrist may manage the acute episode and refer the patient back to the primary care physician for maintenance treatment. Alternatively, the two clinicians may choose to work collaboratively with patients who have complicated medical and psychiatric comorbidity.

BIBLIOGRAPHY

1. Agency for Health Care Policy and Research: Depression in Primary Care. Rockville, Maryland, U.S. Department of Health and Human Services, 1993.
2. American Psychiatric Association: Diagnostic and Statistical Manual IV. Washington, DC, American Psychiatric Association, 1994.
3. Beck AT: Depression Inventory. Philadelphia, Center for Cognitive Therapy. 1978.
4. Eisenberg L: Treating depression and anxiety in primary care. N Engl J Med 326:1080–1084, 1992.
5. Frasure-Smith N, Lesperance F, Talajic M: Depression following myocardial infarction: Impact on 6-month survival. JAMA 270:1819–1825, 1993.
6. Goldberg DP, Hillier VF: A scaled version of the General Health Questionnaire. Psychol Med 9:139–145, 1979.
7. Kaplan HI, Sadock BS (eds): Comprehensive Textbook of Psychiatry, 6th ed. Baltimore, Williams & Wilkins, 1995.
8. Katon W: Depression: Relationship to somatization and chronic medical illness. J Clin Psychiatry 45:4–11, 1984.
9. Murray CJL, Lopez AO: The Global Burden of Disease, Summary. Geneva, World Health Organization, 1996.
10. Regier DA, Hirschfield RMA, Goodwin FK, et al: The NIMH depression awareness, recognition, and treatment program: Structure, aims, and scientific basis. Am J Psychiatry 145:1351–1357, 1988.
11. Rovner BW, German PS, Clark R, et al: Depression and mortality in nursing homes. JAMA 265:993–996, 1991.
12. Schulberg HC, Burns BJ: Mental disorders in primary care: Epidemiologic, diagnostic, and treatment research directions. Gen Hosp Psychiatry 10:79–87, 1988.
13. Spitzer RL, Williams JBW, Kroenke K, et al: Utility of a new procedure for diagnosing mental disorders in primary care. The PRIME-MD 1000 Study. JAMA 272:1749–1756, 1994.
14. Spitzer RL, Williams JBW, Gibbon M, First M: Structured Clinical Interview for DSM-IIIR–Nonpatient version (SCID-NP, version 1.0). Washington, DC, American Psychiatric Press, 1990.
15. Wells KB, Stewart A, Hays RD, et al: The functioning and well-being of depressed patients: Results from the Medical Outcomes Study. JAMA 262:914–919, 1989.
16. Williams J: A structured interview guide for the Hamilton Depression Rating Scale. Arch Gen Psychiatry 45:742–747, 1988.
17. Zimmerman M: Diagnosing DSM-IV Psychiatric Disorders in the Primary Care Setting. Philadelphia, Psychiatric Press Products, 1994.

14. PANIC ATTACKS AND PANIC DISORDER

Robert D. Davies, M.D.

1. List the common symptoms that constitute a panic attack.

A panic attack is defined as a discrete episode of intense discomfort or fear during which there is a sudden onset of at least four of the following symptoms:

- palpitations
- sweating
- tremulousness
- a sense of smothering or shortness of breath
- a sensation of choking
- chest pain
- nausea or abdominal distress
- dizziness or lightheadedness
- paresthesias
- chills or flushing
- feelings of unreality (derealization) or being detached from oneself (depersonalization)
- a fear of losing control or of going crazy
- a fear of dying

The development of these symptoms must reach a peak within 10 minutes.

2. What differentiates a panic attack from panic disorder?

A panic attack is not considered to be a psychiatric disorder in and of itself. Panic attacks may occur infrequently in some people without being part of any clinical syndrome—as much as 15% of the population report having had at least one panic attack in their lifetime. Panic attacks also occur in many psychiatric disorders other than panic disorder.

Panic disorder is a distinct clinical disorder consisting of recurrent, unexpected panic attacks. People with panic disorder experience at least a month of worrying about having another panic attack or about the possible implications of such an attack (such as dying, crashing their car, being unable to function). Often it is the anxiety and worry between panic attacks (called *anticipatory anxiety*) that becomes the most disabling feature of the disorder. People with panic disorder often begin associating their attacks with certain situations (such as being a traffic or being in crowds) and may fuel future panic attacks by anticipating exposure to those situations. They may begin avoiding those situations that they believe are eliciting their attacks. In many cases of panic disorder, the attacks occur randomly, without any precipitant; in some, attacks occur during sleep ("nocturnal" panic attacks).

3. List other psychiatric disorders in which panic attacks might occur.

- Specific phobias
- Social phobia
- Major depression
- Post-traumatic stress disorder
- Obsessive-compulsive disorder
- Stimulant intoxication
- Substance withdrawal syndromes

4. Are there any medical conditions that might cause panic-like symptoms?

Absolutely. Take that cup of coffee in your hand, for instance. Caffeine use, as well as the use of other psychostimulants (e.g., amphetamines, cocaine) can cause panic symptoms. Asthma (and other pulmonary diseases), angina, cardiac arrhythmias, hyperthyroidism, hyperparathyroidism, vestibular dysfunction, transient ischemic attacks, and seizure disorders all can cause panic-like symptoms. This may explain why only about 35% of patients seeking treatment for panic initially go to a mental health setting. In fact, many people with panic disorder seek out numerous medical evaluations (including repeated trips to the emergency department) before seeking psychiatric care. For this reason it is clear that a detailed medical history and focused medical work-up are important when evaluating panic attacks.

5. How common is panic disorder?

Estimates from epidemiologic surveys show a 3.5% prevalence in the general population, with women being twice as likely as men to experience panic disorder (5% and 2%, respectively). Onset is typically before the age of 30 (often starting in adolescence), although the disorder may develop in some people later in life. In these late-onset cases, it is particularly important to look for medical causes. The course of panic disorder varies: approximately one-third of patients go into a stable remission; 45% have a more unremitting, chronic course of their symptoms; and the remaining 24% have an intermittent course, with remissions and relapses throughout their lifetime.

6. Do people with panic disorder ever have other psychiatric disorders as well?

Comorbidity in psychiatric illness is exceedingly common—it is estimated that 48% of people with a psychiatric disorder actually have more than one. Panic disorder is certainly no exception. Estimates of comorbidity in panic disorder range from 24% to as high as 91%. Clearly the most common comorbid diagnosis is **depression**, with as many as 50% of people with panic disorder experiencing depression at some point. The longer the history of panic disorder in an individual, the more likely depression is to develop.

Proper diagnosis and treatment of panic disorder often are delayed, as people tend to seek out medical explanations of their symptoms. By the time they are appropriately diagnosed and treated, depression may already be present. The presence of anxiety or panic in depressed individuals increases the risk of suicide. For this reason, among others, *early recognition and treatment of panic disorder is imperative.*

Substance abuse also is common, as people with panic attacks (as well as other anxiety disorders) try to self-medicate. Tolerance to the brief anxiolytic effect of alcohol leads them to gradually increase the amount of alcohol they consume as they attempt to regain the initial effect. As many as 15% of people who seek treatment for alcoholism also have an anxiety disorder.

Other anxiety disorders, such as simple phobias, social phobia, or generalized anxiety disorder, can co-occur with panic disorder as well.

7. What is agoraphobia?

Agoraphobia is the fear of being in a place or situation from which escape would be difficult or embarrassing, or where it might be difficult to get help should panic symptoms arise. The anxiety caused by this fear is so great that such situations are avoided or tolerated only with extreme distress.

Agoraphobia may occur in panic disorder or it may occur in the absence of panic. People with agoraphobia tend to limit their activities (e.g., not go to stores or, in extreme cases, not leave their homes) or they may pursue such activities only when accompanied by someone with whom they feel safe (such as a spouse).

8. What causes panic disorder?

Panic disorder rates are 3 to 6 times higher in the families of people with panic disorder than in the general population. Studies have shown that children raised by mothers with panic disorder end up having higher rates of anxiety disorders than do children whose mothers do not have panic disorder. It is not clear whether this represents a genetic factor at play, a learned anxiety response, or a combination of the two.

The biological basis of panic disorder is not fully understood. **Serotonin** is widely considered to be involved in the pathogenesis of panic. However, theories suggesting both serotonin excess as well as serotonin deficits have been proposed. It is known that several brain regions are involved in the production of panic symptoms. The serotonergic inputs to the periaqueductal gray matter may be involved in the mediation of an unconditioned fear response. It is hypothesized that a deficit of serotonin blunts this mediation, resulting in panic symptoms. The amygdala is believed to be involved in the development of a conditioned fear response that could equate to anticipatory anxiety and phobic avoidance. Increased levels of serotonin in this area may actually induce anxiety. The effectiveness of selective serotonin reuptake inhibitors (SSRIs) does not help clarify the precise role of serotonin in panic, as they may increase serotonin levels initially, through reuptake inhibition, as well as decrease serotonin later on, through down-regulation of postsynaptic receptors.

9. What medications are beneficial in the treatment of panic disorder?

Several classes of medications have been shown to be beneficial in the treatment of panic disorder. **Benzodiazepines** have long been a mainstay of treatment, although worries about tolerance and abuse have made some clinicians leery about using them. Benzodiazepines with short onsets of action (such as alprazolam) are useful in quickly reducing the intensity of panic symptoms. Those with longer onsets of action and longer half-lives (such as clonazepam) may be beneficial in preventing future attacks—particularly when taken on a regular, scheduled dose. **Monoamine oxidase inhibitors** (MAOIs) (particularly phenelzine) and **tricyclic antidepressants** (TCAs; imipramine, clomipramine) decrease the frequency and the intensity of panic attacks. SSRIs (fluoxetine, sertraline, paroxetine) are efficacious as well.

SSRIs have become the first-line treatment option for many clinicians because of the preferential side-effect profile when compared to either MAOIs or TCAs. Care must be taken, however, to start at very low doses to aid patients in tolerating these medications, as they may experience some initial agitation or anxiety which may trigger panic symptoms. This initial agitation and the delayed onset of the beneficial effect from the antidepressants point to short-term use of a benzodiazepine to offer some immediate relief of symptoms. Rapid symptoms relief can help decrease the formation of avoidance patterns.

10. Are there other treatments available for panic disorder?

Medications alone are sometimes used to treat panic disorder. Relapse rates following discontinuation of medications may exceed 50%. Although medications are clearly beneficial in decreasing the frequency of attacks and the severity of symptoms, they are not particularly beneficial in decreasing anticipatory anxiety or the phobic avoidance that often develops. **Cognitive behavioral therapy** (CBT), used alone or in combination with medications, is particularly useful in treating these aspects of panic disorder—which often are the most disabling symptoms.

CBT is usually a short-term (12–20 sessions) therapy that incorporates relaxation skills, such as diaphragmatic breathing and progressive muscle relaxation, with the examination of catastrophic and distorted thought processes. Patients are taught to challenge these thought processes, which helps to decrease their anticipatory anxiety. Then they gradually are exposed to the anxiety-producing situations that are linked to their panic attacks in an effort to extinguish their anxious response and decrease their phobic avoidance. CBT helps people successfully taper off medications like benzodiazepines without an immediate re-emergence of symptoms, thereby improving the overall outcome of treatment. When patients do have an eventual recurrence of symptoms, a brief refresher of the techniques of CBT often is useful in limiting the severity and length of the recurrence.

BIBLIOGRAPHY

1. American Psychiatric Association: Diagnostic and Statistical Manual of Mental Disorders, 4th ed. Washington, DC, American Psychiatric Association, 1994.
2. Ballenger JC: Panic disorder in the medical setting. J Clin Psychiatry 58 (Suppl 2):13–17, 1997.
3. Davidson JR: The long-term treatment of panic disorder. J Clin Psychiatry 59(Suppl 8):17–21, 1998.
4. den Boer JA, Slaap BR: Review of current treatment in panic disorder. Int Clin Psychopharmacol 13(Suppl 4):S25–S30, 1998.
5. Eaton WW, Kessler RC, Wittchen HU, Magee WJ: Panic and panic disorder in the United States. Am J Psychiatry 151(3):413–420, MARCH 1994.
6. Gelder MG: Combined pharmacotherapy and cognitive behavior therapy in the treatment of panic disorder. J Clin Psychopharm 18(6 Suppl 2):2S–5S, 1998.
7. Goddard AW, Charney DS: SSRIs in the treatment of panic disorder. Depress Anxiety 8(Suppl 1):114–120, 1998.
8. Katshnig H, Amering M: The long-term course of panic disorder and its predictors. J Clin Psychopharm 18(6 Suppl 2):6S–11S, 1998.
9. Otto MW, Whittal ML: Cognitive-behavior therapy and the longitudinal course of panic disorder. Psychiatr Clin North Am 18(4):785–801, 1995.
10. Nutt DJ: Antidepressants in panic disorder: Clinical and preclinical mechanisms. J Clin Psychiatry 59(Suppl 8):24–28, 1998.
11. Spiegel DA, Bruce TJ: Benzodiazepines and exposure-based cognitive behavior therapies for panic disorder: Conclusions from combined treatment trials. Am J Psychiatry 154(6):773–781, 1997.

15. SOCIAL PHOBIA AND SPECIFIC PHOBIAS

Robert D. Davies, M.D.

1. What is the difference between fear and a phobia?

Fear is a normal psychological and physiological reaction to an actual threat or danger, or to the anticipation of an actual threat or danger. A phobia is an excessive and *unreasonable* degree of fear triggered either by exposure to or anticipation of a specific object or circumstance. People with specific phobias realize that their level of fear is excessive, but they still try to avoid any exposure to the feared object or circumstance. These avoidance attempts and the anxiety that results when avoidance is unsuccessful cause a significant disruption in normal functioning.

Common Phobias

Animal type	Insects	Blood/injury type	Injections/blood draws
	Snakes		Seeing blood
	Dogs		Seeing an injured person
Nature type	Storms	Situational type	Driving
	Heights		Tunnels
	Water		Bridges
			Flying
			Elevators

2. How do people develop phobias?

Good question. It is not clear why some people develop specific phobias. Many phobias begin in childhood—particularly those of the animal and nature type. Very often there has never been an exposure to the feared object or situation. In fact, if there has been a traumatic exposure (for instance, an attack by a dog), then future avoidance more accurately reflects the type of avoidance seen in post-traumatic syndromes. People with phobias tend to overestimate the degree of danger that a given situation or object represents. Again, if the level of fear is reasonable and appropriate, then the individual is not considered to have a phobia.

3. How do you treat a specific phobia?

Cognitive behavioral therapy is probably the most effective treatment for a specific phobia. Through a process of graded exposure called **systematic desensitization**, individuals with a phobia are able to extinguish or control their response. They are first instructed in techniques to decrease anxiety, such as diaphragmatic breathing and progressive muscle relaxation. They then develop a hierarchy of exposure to the feared situation or object, based on the amount of anxiety they estimate each degree of exposure would elicit. For example, someone with a phobia of venipuncture might place "talking about having blood drawn" at the low end of their hierarchy, eliciting an anxiety response rated at "1." Seeing a blood drawing kit might elicit an anxiety response of "5," while actually having his or her blood drawn would be a "10." The therapist exposes the patient to these situations, starting at the least anxiety provoking and working up to the actual fear situation. At each stage the patient practices calming down and tolerating the exposure, until the phobic situation or object can be experienced without an excess of anxiety.

When the phobia is of a specific situation that can be anticipated, such as a fear of flying, the use of low-dose benzodiazepines prior to the experience also can be effective. The medication allows them to tolerate the exposure, but generally does not affect future exposures to the feared situation.

4. What is social phobia?

Social phobia is a form of phobia—distinct from specific phobias—in which an individual has an excessive and persistent fear of a given social situation where they might be exposed to the scrutiny of others. The exposure to, or anticipation of, the feared situation causes a marked anxiety response, and the individual either avoids those situations or endures them with significant discomfort. The person usually recognizes that the fear is excessive. Avoidance attempts and/or the anxiety disrupts social or occupational functioning.

When there is only one situation that is feared, the person is considered to have a **specific social phobia**. The most well-known specific social phobia is "performance anxiety"—the fear of public speaking. When more than one situation is feared, it is called **generalized social phobia**. People with generalized social phobia tend to be more disabled, as almost all social settings and interpersonal contacts elicit anxiety and avoidance. Someone with a specific social phobia may be able to structure his or her life in such a way as to avoid or limit exposure to the particular situation that causes anxiety.

The most common fears seen in social phobia include speaking before a group or being the center of attention, eating in public, writing in public, and using public lavatories. For many people, the fear of scrutiny and anxiety is the result of a physical condition such as a tremor, Tourette's syndrome, scarring, obesity, or physical deformity. In these situations, however, the individual is not considered to have social phobia (as his or her assessment of being negatively scrutinized by others may well be accurate).

5. How common a problem is social phobia?

Social phobia is now known to be one of the most common psychiatric disorders in the general population. Epidemiologic researchers have found that there is a 13.3% lifetime prevalence of social phobia, with a higher prevalence existing in women (15.5%) than in men (11.1%). Unfortunately, it is estimated that only 2% of the people with social phobia actually seek treatment for it. Many people end up structuring their lives to avoid whatever situation triggers their anxiety. This may work for some people with specific social phobias, but for those individuals with generalized social phobia, their ability to lead a full life often is significantly impaired.

Alcohol commonly is utilized in an attempt to decrease the anxiety and allow the individual to tolerate the feared social situation. In approximately 85% of the people with both social phobia and alcohol abuse, the social phobia precedes the alcohol problem.

6. What are the cognitive processes involved in social phobia?

People with social phobia tend to *overestimate* their own symptoms of anxiety—for instance, if they are feeling anxious and flushed, they may assume that they are beet red. They also *misinterpret* the responses of others in negative ways. They overestimate the degree to which other people are paying attention to them, and the likelihood that they will be embarrassed or rejected. Finally, they tend to *overemphasize* any perceived or actual failures, while discounting their achievements and positive feedback.

7. What other conditions might be confused with social phobia?

The differential diagnosis for social phobia includes agoraphobia, panic disorder, generalized anxiety disorder, depression, body dysmorphic disorder, avoidant or schizoid personality disorders, and nonpathological shyness.

8. Can medications help in social phobia?

Absolutely. For individuals with specific social phobia, such as performance anxiety, **β-blockers** (e.g., propranolol) can be beneficial. These drugs target the physiologic symptoms of anxiety (such as increased heart rate) rather than the emotional experience. This ends up having an indirect effect on the cognitive component of the anxiety—as the physiologic "feedback" to the cognitive aspect of the anxiety is blocked. **Benzodiazepines** (e.g., alprazolam, lorazepam, clonazepam) also are effective in these individuals and can be used on an as-needed basis. For those people with generalized social phobia, both **monoamine oxidase inhibitors** (e.g., phenelzine, tranylcypramine) and **serotonin specific reuptake inhibitors** (e.g., paroxetine, sertraline, fluoxetine) can be effective treatments. The use of these antidepressants also has the benefit of treating comorbid depression when it occurs.

Other medications that are showing some promise in treating social phobia include venlafaxine (which inhibits the reuptake of both serotonin and norepinephrine) and gabapentin (which works at the GABA receptor complex). Tricyclic antidepressants, however, have not been shown to be efficacious.

9. Are there other types of treatment for social phobia?

An important form of treatment for social phobia is **cognitive behavioral therapy** (CBT). This type of therapy involves cognitive restructuring by helping the individual with social phobia identify his or her cognitive distortions and challenge the accuracy of their perceptions. They also learn how to decrease their physiologic response of anxiety with various techniques including deep-breathing and progressive muscle relaxation. Graded exposure to the feared situation also is employed as they learn to tolerate increasingly greater exposure to the feared situation. Eventually, the anxious response is extinguished.

Group CBT also is helpful in the treatment of social phobia. This form of treatment includes social skills training and role-playing, and allows individuals to get direct, immediate feedback on their perceptions of how others view them.

BIBLIOGRAPHY

1. American Psychiatric Association: Diagnostic and Statistical Manual of Mental Disorders, 4th ed. Washington, DC, American Psychiatric Association, 1994.
2. Goisman RM, Allsworth J, Rogers MP, et al: Simple phobia as a comorbid anxiety disorder. Depress Anxiety 7(3):105–112, 1998.
3. Heimberg RG, Juster HR: Treatment of social phobia in cognitive-behavioral groups. J Clin Psychiatry 55(Suppl):38–46, 1994.
4. Jefferson JW: Social phobia: A pharmacologic treatment overview. J Clin Psychiatry 56(Suppl 5):18–24, 1995.
5. Keck PE, McElroy SL: New uses for antidepressants: Social phobia. J Clin Psychiatry 58(Suppl 14):32–38, 1997.
6. Kessler RC, McGonagle KA, Zhoa S, et al: Lifetime and 12-month prevalence of DSM-III-R psychiatric disorders in the United States: Results from the National Comorbidity Survey. Arch Gen Psychiatry 51:8–19, 1994.
7. Schneier FR, Johnson J, Hornig CD, et al: Social phobia: Comorbidity and morbidity in an epidemiologic sample. Arch Gen Psychiatry 49:282–288, 1992.

16. GENERALIZED ANXIETY DISORDER

Robert D. Davies, M.D., and Leslie Winter, M.D.

1. What is generalized anxiety disorder?

Anxiety and worry are commonly experienced responses to the stress of day-to-day life. We all worry at times about various aspects of our lives—particularly the unknown or novel. This is absolutely normal. However, when worry and anxiety are the predominate approach to life, it is not normal. People with generalized anxiety disorder (GAD) experience excessive levels of anxiety and worry most of the time and have great difficulty controlling their worry. The excessive level of anxiety they experience causes significant distress and often impairs their ability to function in various areas of their life (such as socially or occupationally). Many people with GAD become preoccupied with the physical symptoms associated with anxiety (such as gastrointestinal distress and fatigue) and worry about their health. This worry may lead them to repeatedly seek out medical evaluations and reassurance. Thus, GAD typically is seen in primary care settings rather than in mental health settings.

2. List the physical symptoms of generalized anxiety disorder.
- Physical restlessness (feeling "on edge")   • Irritability
- Fatigue   • Muscle tension
- Difficulty concentrating or mind going blank   • Sleep disruption

The diagnosis of GAD is made only when at least three of these symptoms are present.

3. What is the prevalence of GAD?

Estimates from epidemiologic surveys estimate that the lifetime prevalence of GAD in the general population is 5.1%, with a higher prevalence in women (6.6%, versus 3.6% in men). It is a chronic condition that may demonstrate periodic episodes of acute worsening throughout its course. GAD often begins in childhood and persists throughout life. For some individuals it may consist of chronic, yet mild symptoms; for others it may cause significant levels of impairment in social settings, interpersonal relationships, and occupational functioning.

GAD is seen most often in primary care rather than in psychiatric settings. This may be related, in part, to the myriad physical symptoms that are typically present in people with GAD. Chronic medical conditions such as irritable bowel syndrome and headaches often occur along with GAD.

4. What other psychiatric illnesses are likely to occur with GAD?

It has been estimated that 50–90% of people with GAD also have at least one other psychiatric condition. This high degree of comorbidity has caused some researchers to call into question the validity of the diagnosis of GAD as a distinct clinical entity. It is possible that what we call GAD may be a predisposing condition that leads to other anxiety and mood disorders. Major depression and dysthymia frequently are seen in individuals with GAD. Some believe that this cluster of symptoms reflects a mixed anxiety–depressive state. Other anxiety disorders such as panic disorder, simple phobias, social phobia, and obsessive-compulsive disorder also can occur in an individual with GAD. Substance abuse is likely—just as it is with all other anxiety disorders. Personality disorders also may be seen in these individuals, and it can be difficult to sort out the effects of chronic anxiety from those of maladaptive personality traits.

5. Which psychiatric conditions might be confused with GAD?

The differential diagnosis of GAD is extensive because worry and anxiety are seen in so many conditions. Depression, particularly when there is a prominent degree of guilty rumination, may look like GAD. Conditions involving anxiety triggered by specific situations (such as specific phobias, social situations in social phobia, or exposure to trauma-related situations in post-traumatic stress disorder) may be confused with GAD. Panic disorder, particularly when there is a great deal of anticipatory anxiety, may be confused with GAD—as can the excessive worry about weight or body image seen in anorexia nervosa and bulimia. People with GAD may be mistakenly diagnosed as having somatization disorder due to their tendency to become focused on physical symptoms and preoccupied with their health. Personality disorders (particularly avoidant personality disorder) may look like GAD. Finally, substance use disorders (including nicotine and caffeine) and substance withdrawal also can elicit symptoms of excessive anxiety.

6. List the medical conditions that can cause anxiety.
- Hyperthyroidism or hypothyroidism   • Seizure disorders
- Hypoglycemia   • CNS tumors
- Diabetes mellitus   • Strokes
- Pheochromocytoma   • Traumatic brain injuries
- Chronic obstructive pulmonary disease   • Cardiac arrhythmias
- Asthma   • Mitral valve prolapse
- Pulmonary emboli   • Substance intoxication and/or withdrawal

7. Can certain types of medications cause anxiety symptoms?

Yes. Many classes of drugs used for medical as well as psychiatric conditions can cause symptoms of anxiety. Anxiety is a common side effect of some drugs (such as bronchodilators, psychostimulants, and corticosteroids); with other drugs (e.g., meperidine, antihistamines, and benzodiazepines), anxiety may represent an idiosyncratic response to the medication. Rapid discontinuation may precipitate anxiety in a patient as well (reported with corticosteroids, benzodiazepines, some SSRIs, and venlafaxine). Toxicity may result in symptoms of anxiety (seen with theophylline). Almost all classes of antidepressants cause anxiety in some patients, particularly during the initiation of treatment. Antipsychotics commonly cause akathisia—a markedly distressing level of internal agitation. When evaluating a patient with anxiety, care must be taken to review the types and dosages of all current or recently discontinued medications.

8. What are the pharmacologic treatments used in GAD?

Benzodiazepines, which decrease the severity of anxiety symptoms, have long been the mainstay of treatment for GAD. However, when a chronic condition is treated with a medication that only suppresses symptoms, the medication itself becomes chronic. Although benzodiazepines offer the benefit of rapid symptom relief, their chronic use can lead to tolerance (the need for escalating dosages to maintain efficacy) and dependence.

Buspirone, the $5HT_{1A}$ agonist, is effective in treating GAD. Its biggest benefit over benzodiazepines is that no dependence develops with chronic administration. Likewise there is no risk of abuse, which makes it a good consideration for individuals with comorbid GAD and substance use disorders. A major drawback, however, is that the onset of symptom relief may be delayed for several weeks after initiating treatment. This delay can have an adverse effect on medication compliance in the anxious patient, who may quickly decide that the medication is not working.

Tricyclic antidepressants (TCAs) are beneficial in some cases of GAD. Their side-effect profile and lethality in overdose, however, tend to limit their use. The use of selective serotonin reuptake inhibitors (SSRIs) in treating GAD is increasingly widespread. SSRIs offer a more agreeable side-effect profile for most patients. Both SSRIs and TCAs have the added benefit of treating comorbid depression when it occurs.

9. What other treatments are used to treat GAD?

Management of anxiety symptoms through relaxation training, exercise programs, and stress reduction are all important aspects of treatment. These interventions help people to feel more in control of the degree of their anxiety and worry. Cognitive behavioral therapy has been shown to decrease the physiologic aspects of GAD and alter the cognitive distortions that fuel the anxiety. As GAD tends to be a chronic condition, therapies that aid the patient in understanding the precipitants to their anxiety, the connection between physical symptoms and psychological "worry," and the cognitive processes that keep them focused on worrying, as well as help affect lifestyle changes tend to have the most long-lasting benefit.

BIBLIOGRAPHY

1. American Psychiatric Association: Diagnostic and Statistical Manual of Mental Disorder, 4th ed. Washington, DC, American Psychiatric Association, 1994.
2. Beck AT, Emery G, Greenberg RL: Anxiety Disorders and Phobias: A Cognitive Perspective. New York, Basic Books, Inc., 1985.
3. Brauman-Mintzer O, et al: Psychiatric comorbidity in patients with generalized anxiety disorder. Am J Psychiatry 150:1216–1218, 1993.
4. Elliston JM: Integrative Treatment of Anxiety Disorders. Washington, DC, American Psychiatric Press, Inc., 1996.
5. Lader MH: The nature and duration of treatment for GAD. Acta Psychiatr Scand 98(Suppl 393):109–117, 1998.
6. Harvey AG, Rapee RM: Cognitive-behavior therapy for generalized anxiety disorder. Psychiatr Clin North Am 18(4):859–870, 1995.
7. Kendler KS: Major depression and generalised anxiety disorder: Same genes, (partly) different environments—revisited. Brit J Psychiatry 168(Suppl 30):68-75, 1996.
8. Kessler RC, McGonagle KA, Zhao S, et al: Lifetime and 12-month prevalence of DSM-III-R psychiatric disorders in the United States: Results from the national comorbidity study. Arch Gen Psychiatry 58:8–19, 1994.
9. Maser JD: Generalized anxiety disorder and its comorbidities: Disputes at the boundaries. Acta Psychiatr Scand 98(Suppl 393):12–22, 1998.
10. Rickels K, Schweizer E: The treatment of generalized anxiety disorder in patients with depressive symptomatology. J Clin Psychiatry 54(Suppl):20–23, 1993.

17. OBSESSIVE-COMPULSIVE DISORDERS

Richard L. O'Sullivan, M.D., and Michael A. Jenike, M.D.

1. Define obsessive-compulsive disorder.

Obsessive-compulsive disorder (OCD) is classified in DSM-IV as an anxiety disorder manifested by either obsessions and/or compulsions that cause significant distress or dysfunction in social or personal areas. Obsessions are **thoughts** and are defined as "recurrent, persistent ideas, images, or impulses that are a significant source of distress or interfere with social or role functioning." Compulsions are **behaviors** or **mental acts** that are "repetitive, purposeful, and intentional and performed in response to an obsession or according to certain rules or in a stereotypical fashion." The thoughts or behaviors cause distress, are resisted at least initially, do not form part of a psychosis, and are recognized as senseless. **Anxiety** is a central feature of OCD, and the repetitive behaviors or mental acts are often a means to neutralize the distress associated with obsessions.

2. Define obsessive-compulsive personality disorder.

Obsessive-compulsive personality disorder (OCPD) may be misdiagnosed as OCD or comorbid with OCD. OCPD tends to be a chronic, pervasive condition embodying several traits, such as obsessive attention to detail, inflexibility, and perfectionism. Such characteristics differ from but may be confused with the compulsive rituals found in OCD. Obsessive-compulsive personality disorder can be distinguished from OCD by the lack of obsessions, compulsions, rituals, and severe anxiety that are common to OCD. The cognitions and behaviors typical of OCD usually are very disturbing, or dystonic, to the patient, whereas the personality traits of OCPD generally are not dystonic. The symptoms of OCD frequently wax and wane in intensity; OCPD traits are relatively enduring.

FEATURES OF OBSESSIVE-COMPULSIVE DISORDER*

Either obsessions or compulsions

Obsessions
Recurrent and persistent ideas, thoughts, impulses, or images that are experienced as intrusive and senseless and cause marked anxiety or distress.
Thoughts, impulses are not simply excessive worries about problems.
Person attempts to ignore or suppress such thoughts or to neutralize them.
Person recognizes that the obsessions are the product of his or her own mind.

Compulsions
Repetitive behaviors or mental acts performed in response to an obsession or rigidly applied rules.
Behaviors are designed to neutralize or prevent distress or some dreaded event or situation, but are excessive or not realistically connected with what they are meant to neutralize.
Persons recognizes his or her behavior is excessive or unreasonable (except children).
Obsessions/compulsions cause marked distress, are time-consuming (more than 1 hr/day), or significantly interfere with the person's normal routine.
If another axis I disorder is present, the content of the obsessions or compulsions is not restricted to it.
Disturbance is not due to the direct physiologic effects of a substance or general medical condition.

FEATURES OF OBSESSIVE-COMPULSIVE PERSONALITY DISORDER•

A pervasive pattern of perfectionism and inflexibility, beginning by early adulthood, present in various contexts

plus

At least 4 of the following:
Preoccupations with details, rules, lists, order, organization, and schedules.
Perfectionism that interferes with task completion.
Excessive devotion to work and productivity to the exclusion of leisure activities and friendships.
Overconscientious, scrupulous, and inflexible about matters of morality, ethics, or values.
Unable to discard worn-out or worthless objects even when they have no sentimental value.
Unreasonable insistence that others submit to his or her way of doing things.
Miserly spending style toward self and others; money is viewed as something to be hoarded.
Rigidity and stubbornness.

---

* DSM-IV criteria.
Reprinted with permission from the Diagnostic and Statistical Manual of Mental Disorders, 4th ed. Copyright 1994 American Psychiatric Association.

3. How is obsessive-compulsive personality disorder treated?

Care should be taken to distinguish OCD from OCPD because treatments differ. Little evidence suggests that behavioral or pharmacologic treatments, which are effective for OCD, are useful in treating OCPD. Traditional psychodynamic psychotherapy is often the treatment of choice for OCPD and may be helpful over the long term, but controlled data about effective treatments for OCPD are lacking.

4. When do everyday habits or idiosyncrasies cross the line to become OCD or require treatment?

Habits, idiosyncrasies, and compulsiveness are common human behaviors. Thoughts or behaviors become maladaptive or may require treatment when they are sufficiently distressing or so time-consuming that they interfere with functioning.

5. Is OCD a common problem?

Yes. It affects 1–3% of populations in cross-cultural studies. It may begin at any age but most commonly becomes evident in early adulthood. Childhood cases are more common in boys than girls, but overall in adults the disorder is more common in women.

The clinical presentation in children and the elderly generally is similar to that in adults but may require more diagnostic acumen for practitioners not familiar with OCD. For example, a child who is a slow learner because he or she has to keep rereading a sentence (a form of checking) may be misdiagnosed as having a primary learning problem instead of OCD. Another example is a child who appears to have a bladder problem because of frequent trips to the bathroom, when in fact contamination obsessions drive the child to wash his hands compulsively. In older patients, anxious preoccupations with physical symptoms, sometimes misinterpreted as "ruminations," may actually be obsessions.

6. When and how does OCD start?

Obsessive-compulsive behaviors usually have existed for many years before they come to professional attention. Onset of symptoms generally is gradual but occasionally is abrupt. The mean age of onset is approximately 22 years.

OCD may start as intrusive thoughts that seem odd and frightening, such as violent images that enter the mind. Such images are distressing and are resisted, at least initially. In addition, the thoughts do not feel as though they are voluntarily created, but are intruding into consciousness. OCD also may begin as repetitive, ritualized behaviors that need to be done in the same way over and over. Frequently patients show more than one obsession or compulsion, and these may change over time.

7. Describe some common OCD preoccupations and behaviors.

Common obsessions include contamination, aggression, bodily fears, concerns about safety or harm, and need for exactness, completeness or symmetry. Compulsions frequently include checking, washing, repeating, counting, collecting, and hoarding. Compulsions usually are paired with obsessions. Performance of a compulsion may temporarily relieve some of the anxiety generated by an obsession. For example, after shaking hands or touching doorknobs, a person with contamination obsessions may need to wash the hands repeatedly until he or she feels clean and the anxiety associated with the obsession lessens, at least temporarily. If a person has concerns about safety or harm to others, he or she may need to recheck that nothing terrible has happened; for example, by repeatedly calling people or checking behind the car to see that no one has been run over. Such behaviors can be extremely time-consuming, sometimes taking up much of a person's day, and may have a severe, deleterious impact on functioning of the individual and family.

8. When is misdiagnosis likely to occur in patients with OCD?

A particularly important clinical problem is the development of postpartum OCD, which may be acute and severe in onset. It is easily confused with or dismissed as normal anxieties of motherhood. In addition, severe or bizarre obsessions may be misdiagnosed as psychotic symptoms, particularly in people with a psychotic disorder. Attention should be paid to the potential for misdiagnosis in this population as well. (See Question 14.)

9. What are current theories about the pathophysiology of OCD?

Whereas early literature referred first to demons, then to psychodynamic influences as the genesis of OCD, growing evidence suggests a **neurobiologic basis**. Family studies suggest that at least some forms of OCD have a familial predisposition. Neuropsychological assessments of groups of patients with OCD demonstrate abnormalities. Structural and functional neuroimaging studies implicate basal ganglia structures, especially the striatum, as well as orbitofrontal hyperactivity in the pathophysiology of OCD. A failure of brain development has been suggested by the findings of increased gray matter and decreased white matter in OCD patients compared with normal controls. The role of environmental influences in the development and expression of OCD is not clear.

10. What disorders possibly are related to OCD?

Several disorders bear some similarities to OCD and are commonly considered within a spectrum of OCD disorders:

- Trichotillomania (compulsive or repetitive hair pulling)
- Body dysmorphic disorder (obsession with an imagined or exaggerated defect in appearance)
- Tourette's syndrome (motor and vocal tics)
- Globus hystericus (episodic fear of choking and inability to breathe, often with sensation of a lump in the throat)
- Compulsive skin picking or nail biting
- Bowel and bladder obsessions
- Olfactory reference syndrome (belief that one is emitting an offensive odor)

11. How do I screen for OCD and related disorders?

Patients frequently are secretive about symptoms because of shame about their obsessions and compulsions. They consider their thoughts and behaviors to be disturbed and embarrassing, and therefore are reluctant to disclose them. The degree of shame, coupled with a reluctance to discuss symptoms, often results in misdiagnosis or undertreatment of the full range of suffering. Thus the first step is to ask screening questions in *every* initial evaluation. Patients may have symptoms of more than one disorder, such as both OCD and trichotillomania, or body dysmorphic disorder and skin picking. They may not realize that the conditions are treatable.

Screening Questions for Obsessive-Compulsive and Related Disorders

---

Do you have thoughts, ideas, or mental images that come into your mind that you cannot seem to get rid of?
Are these thoughts troubling to you in some way—do they make you anxious or upset?
Are there any behaviors or habits that you do over and over that seem excessive or unusual?
Is your life negatively affected by an inflexible need to do things "just right" or in a ritualized, repetitive way?
Do you find that you tend to collect things excessively or have trouble throwing things out so that your home becomes cluttered?
Do you find yourself touching, rubbing, or picking at parts of your body repeatedly?
Do you ever pull out your hair?
Are there any aspects of your appearance that you find yourself troubled by or preoccupied with?
Have others commented on behaviors or actions you perform that seem unusual or excessive to them or to yourself?

---

12. How often is psychosis associated with OCD?

Although patients frequently report that they feel "crazy" as a result of symptoms, frank psychosis, delusions, and hallucinations are relatively uncommon in patients with OCD. If psychosis is present, it generally should not be considered as part of OCD, and other diagnoses or comorbid conditions should be considered. However, some people with body dysmorphic disorder are preoccupied with the perception of a defect to delusional proportions, and most patients with olfactory reference syndrome have delusional perceptions of odor.

13. Do patients with OCD act on their obsessions?

Although patients often are fearful that they may act on their obsessions, it is important to reassure them that this is extremely rare.

14. How is OCD misdiagnosed?

OCD may be misdiagnosed as a psychotic disorder, depression, or other anxiety disorder (see Question 8). OCD also may be *under*diagnosed when it occurs in people with developmental disorders, mental retardation, or Tourette's syndrome. The differential diagnosis should include such disorders.

Neuroleptic medications have been used incorrectly to treat OCD when obsessions are misdiagnosed as psychotic symptoms or schizophrenia. Misdiagnosis generally occurs because the clinician has not inquired about the full range of symptoms, has considered "spectrum" disorders to be typical OCD, or has mistaken OCD symptoms as indicative of another disorder. Diagnosis may be complicated by the reluctance of some patients to disclose fully their range of symptoms, particularly with obsessions that are sexual or violent in nature, related to bodily function, or blasphemous.

15. Does routine brain imaging have a role in OCD?

Although research applications of neuroimaging have shown structural and functional brain abnormalities in people with OCD, clinical brain imaging generally is not indicated, with a few exceptions. Because obsessive-compulsive symptoms may occur as a result of various illnesses, new onset of OCD symptoms in patients over age 55 may be an indication for a magnetic resonance imaging or computed tomography scan of the brain to assist in the differential diagnosis and to rule out other pathology. In atypical patients; patients with systemic autoimmune, inflammatory, vascular, or neoplastic diseases in which brain lesions also may arise; and patients with cognitive difficulties or focal neurologic abnormalities, neurologic consultation and brain imaging may be indicated.

16. How does one begin treatment for OCD?

After the diagnosis is made, the patient should be educated about the disorder. Options for behavioral and medication treatment should be reviewed. Social supports, such as self-help groups for patients and families, should be considered. Education may include several excellent patient-oriented books. Decisions about pharmacologic and behavioral interventions typically are made on a case-by-case basis. The severity and types of symptoms as well as the resources and motivation of the patient are important factors in treatment planning.

17. What are effective treatments for OCD?

Clinical experience and research support two primary modes of treatment for OCD: behavioral and pharmacologic. The majority of patients report a significant improvement in symptoms with these treatment modalities. Inadequate empirical support justifies the use of psychodynamic psychotherapy as treatment for OCD. However, patients with OCD may have other problems that respond to psychotherapy. In addition, patients with early-onset OCD may benefit from psychotherapy, because they are likely to have missed a number of developmental milestones. Psychoeducational support groups may be helpful for patients with OCD and also for their families. Excellent sources of information about local resources include the following:

Obsessive Compulsive Foundation, 9 Depot Rd., Milford, CT 06460 (203-878-5669).

Trichotillomania Learning Center (TLC), 1215 Mission St., Suite 2, Santa Cruz, CA (831-457-1004).

Tourette Syndrome Association, Inc., 42-40 Bell Blvd., Bayside, NY 11361-2874 (718-224-2999).

Anxiety Disorders Association of America, 6000 Executive Blvd., Suite 513, Rockville, MD 20852 (301-231-8368).

18. What are the components of behavioral treatment for OCD?

Behavioral therapy generally is effective for checking and washing rituals. It is symptom-focused and goal-directed and may be accomplished in as few as a dozen sessions, depending on symptom severity. Motivation and compliance are important factors in success. Results vary, but many patients maintain their response over extended periods. Virtually all patients with OCD should be offered a course of behavior therapy.

Treatment typically begins with a behavioral analysis, identifying the various target behaviors and associated cognitions that are problematic. The environmental context for the behaviors is identified, with recognition of internal and external cues and reinforcers important in symptoms maintenance. Primary treatment for compulsive rituals consists of exposure and response prevention. Such techniques involve a graded progressive exposure to the anxiety-inducing stimulus, with prevention of the associated ritualistic response.

Behavioral therapy is less effective for patients with obsessions and no rituals. Thought-stopping has been used with limited success.

19. What are the first-line medications for OCD treatment?

A number of medications have demonstrated efficacy in treating OCDs. All are potent serotonin reuptake inhibitors (SRIs) and effective antidepressants: clomipramine (Anafranil), fluoxetine (Prozac), sertraline (Zoloft), paroxetine (Paxil), and fluvoxamine (Luvox). Although chemically distinct, they have similar efficacy in treating patients with OCD. Tolerance and response to each agent may vary with individuals. The medications also differ in pharmacokinetics, side effects, and interactions. It is believed that their antiobsessional effects result in part from blocking serotonin reuptake. It is still unclear, however, exactly how serotonin fits into the pathophysiology of OCD.

Initial drug choice should be an SRI, and if the first choice is not successful or if side effects limit use, the other agents, including clomipramine, should be tried. Patients who do not respond to one medication may benefit from another in the same class. Dosage may be increased as tolerated to the upper end of recommended doses, and a trial usually should last for 10 days before medication is changed or augmentation strategies are begun. Response times vary. Rare patients report a quick reduction in symptoms, but maximal response may take several months.

Note that tolerance and side effects are important factors in choice of agent, because pharmacotherapy for OCD may be long-term for some patients.

20. Should behavioral therapy or medications be started first? Should they be started together?

Absolute guidelines for when to begin which type of treatment are lacking, but some general principles may help to guide clinical decision making. In general, medications should be avoided as a first-line treatment in children or pregnant women, until the patient has not responded to behavioral therapy and the severity of the illness dictates pharmacotherapy. Medications have been successfully used in the elderly as well as in patients with other serious medical problems, but care should be exercised about side effects and interactions. Many patients receive combined medication and behavioral therapy. The two treatments complement each other. Some patients have great success with medications or behavioral therapy alone. Patients with significant comorbid DSM-IV axis I or II illnesses, poor motivation or compliance, chaotic social situations, or only obsessions tend to do poorly in behavioral therapy alone. Behavioral therapy for compulsive rituals yields improvement in about two-thirds of patients, with lasting gains over several years of follow-up. Treatment with SRIs alone generally results in moderate improvement.

21. How does one gauge response to OCD treatment?

The Yale-Brown Obsessive Compulsive Scale (YBOCS) is a quick and simple clinician-administered scale that gives reliable ratings of symptom severity for obsessions and compulsions. In addition, assessment of anxiety and depressive symptoms with self-report instruments is useful. Clinical global assessments of severity and improvement also are frequently used. Treatment refractoriness may be defined as less than 25% decrease in OCD symptoms on the YBOCS or persistent significant symptoms despite adequate trials of first-line behavioral therapy or medications. Complete resolution of symptoms is rare, but the great majority of patients get considerable relief. Strategies for pharmacologic approaches to the approximately 20% of patients who are refractory to standard treatments are shown below.

Pharmacologic Strategies for Refractory Obsessive-Compulsive Disorder

AGENT	DOSE	DURATION
First-line: SRIs		
Clomipramine	Up to 250 mg/d	> 10 wk
Fluoxetine	Up to 80 mg/d	> 10 wk
Fluvoxamine	Up to 300 mg/d	> 10 wk
Sertraline	Up to 200 mg/d	> 10 wk
Paroxetine	40 to 60 mg/d	> 10 wk
Augmentation		
Clonazepam	Up to 5 mg/d	> 4 wk
Neuroleptics		
Pimozide	Up to 3 mg/d	> 4 wk
Buspirone	Up to 60 mg/d	> 8 wk
Alternative Monotherapy		
Clonazepam	Up to 5 mg/d	> 4 wk
Phenelzine	Up to 90 mg/d	> 10 wk
Tranylcypromine	Up to 60 mg/d	> 10 wk
Buspirone	Up to 60 mg/d	> 6 wk

Adapted from Jenike MA, Rauch SL: Managing the patient with treatment-resistant obsessive compulsive disorder: Current strategies. J Clin Psychiatry 55(Suppl):11–17, 1994.

22. What conditions frequently coexist with OCD? How does this affect treatment planning and response?

Common comorbid conditions include major depression, simple and social phobia, eating disorders, substance abuse, panic disorder, and Tourette's syndrome. Comorbid axis I conditions may need to be treated first, concomitantly, or after treatment of OCD, depending on the relative clinical severity of the comorbid condition. Avoidant and dependent personality disorders are among the most common in OCD probands. Schizotypal, borderline, and avoidant personality disorders may negatively affect response to pharmacotherapy. Conversely, patients who appear to have a personality disorder while they have significant OCD symptoms may no longer meet criteria for a personality disorder once their OCD is effectively treated.

23. What is the relationship between OCD and Tourette's syndrome?

Symptoms in OCD and Tourette's syndrome may overlap: Tourette's patients frequently have OCD symptoms, and tics are common in OCD patients. Family and genetic studies and other current evidence suggest a common pathophysiology with a different phenotypic expression in some forms of Tourette's syndrome and OCD. Treatment of OCD comorbid with Tourette's syndrome generally requires neuroleptics (or clonidine) and an SRI. Behavioral therapy for tics is not highly successful overall, but may be useful for compulsive rituals. The clinical and phenomenologic overlap between OCD and spectrum disorders is an exciting area of current research.

24. What is the role of neurosurgery in treatment of OCD?

Severe, disabling, treatment-refractory OCD symptoms have been successfully treated with various neurosurgical procedures, including frontal leucotomy, limbic leucotomy, anterior capsulotomy, and cingulotomy. Such procedures are reserved for patients who have failed extensive trials of behavioral and pharmacologic interventions and are literally disabled and dysfunctional as a result of OCD. Risks are those associated with any neurosurgical procedure, including infection, seizure, and potential loss of normal functioning. Neurosurgery should be considered only after everything else has failed.

25. How long does OCD last? Is treatment lifelong?

OCD tends to be a chronic disorder. There may be episodic or continuous forms, and in occasional patients acute episodes do not recur. Duration of active treatment varies. Some patients have chronic low levels of symptoms by which they are not severely affected, except at times of increased stress or when a concomitant axis I disorder, such as depression, occurs. Such patients may benefit from periodic use of medication or booster sessions of behavioral therapy.

Development of behavioral skills is important in all patients with OCD, to help minimize symptoms and interference. Some patients require only relatively short-term use of mediations (6–12 months), whereas others need medication for an extended period. Current research is attempting to determine which patients need long-term treatment.

BIBLIOGRAPHY

1. American Psychiatric Association: Diagnostic and Statistical Manual of Mental Disorders, 4th ed. Washington, DC, American Psychiatric Association, 1994.
2. Baer L: Getting Control: Overcoming Your Obsessions and Compulsions. Boston, Little Brown, 1991.
3. Baer L, Rauch SL, Ballantine T, et al: Cingulotomy for intractable obsessive-compulsive disorder. Arch Gen Psychiatry 52:384–392, 1995.
4. Black DW, Noyes R, Goldstein RB, Blum N: A family study of obsessive compulsive disorder. Arch Gen Psychiatry 49:362–368, 1992.
5. Goodman WK, Price LH, Rasmussen SA, et al: The Yale-Brown Obsessive Compulsive Scale. II: Validity. Arch Gen Psychiatry 46:1012–1016, 1989.
6. Grados MA, Labuda MC, Riddle MA, Walkup JT: Obsessive compulsive disorder in children and adolescents. Int Rev Psychiatry 9(1):83–97, 1997.
7. Greist JH, Jefferson JW, Kobak KA, et al: Efficacy and intolerability of serotonin transport inhibitors in obsessive-compulsive disorder: Meta-analysis. Arch Gen Psychiatry 52:53–60, 1995.
8. Insel TR, Winslow JT: Neurobiology of obsessive compulsive disorder. Psychiatr Clin North Am 15:813–824, 1992.
9. Jenike MA, Baer L, Minichiello WE (eds): Obsessive-Compulsive Disorders: Practical Management, 3rd ed. Chicago, Mosby-Year Book, 1998.
10. Jenike MA, Baer L, Ballantine T, et al: Cingulotomy for refractory obsessive-compulsive disorder. Arch Gen Psychiatry 48:548–555, 1991.
11. Jenike MA, Rauch SL: Managing the patient with treatment-resistant obsessive compulsive disorder: Current strategies. J Clin Psychiatry 55(Suppl):11–17, 1994.
12. King RA, Leonard H, March J, et al: Practice parameters for the assessment and treatment of children and adolescents with obsessive-compulsive disorder. J Am Acad Child Adolesc Psychiatry 37(Suppl 10): 27–45, 1998.
13. Orloff LM, Battle MA, Baer L, et al: Long-term follow-up of 85 patients with obsessive-compulsive disorder. Am J Psychiatry 151:441–442, 1994.
14. O'Sullivan RL, Keuthen WJ, Christenson GA, et al: Trichotillomania: Clinical symptom or behavioral syndrome. Am J Psychiatry 154:1442–1449, 1997.
15. Pauls DL, Towbin KE, Leckman JF, et al: Gilles de la Tourette's syndrome and obsessive compulsive disorder: Evidence supporting a genetic relationship. Arch Gen Psychiatry 43:1180–1182, 1986.
16. Phillips KA: The Broken Mirror: Understanding and Treating Body Dysmorphic Disorder. New York, Oxford, 1996.
17. Pitman RK, Green RC, Jenike MA, Mesulam MM: Clinical comparison of Tourette's disorder and obsessive-compulsive disorder. Am J Psychiatry 144:1166–1171, 1987.
18. Potenza MW, McDougle CJ: Potential of atypical antipsychotics in the treatment of nonpsychotic disorders. CNS Drugs 9(3):213–232, 1998.
19. Ricciardi JN, Baer L, Jenike MA, et al: Changes in DSM-III-R axis II diagnoses following treatment of obsessive-compulsive disorder. Am J Psychiatry 149:829–831, 1992.
20. Stein DJ, Christenson GA, Hollander E (eds): Trichotillomania. Washington, DC, American Psychiatric Press, 1999.
21. Swerdlow WR, Zinner S, Farber RH, et al: Symptoms in obsessive-compulsive disorder and Tourette syndrome: A spectrum? CNS Spectrums 4(3):21–26, 29–33, 1999.
22. Wilhelm S, Keuthen WJ, Dekkersbach T, et al: Self-injurious skin-picking: Clinical characteristics and comorbidity. J Clin Psychiatry 60(7):454–459, 1999.

18. POSTTRAUMATIC STRESS DISORDER

John J. Kluck, M.D.

1. What is posttraumatic stress disorder (PTSD)?

PTSD is caused by experiencing severe psychic trauma. Psychic trauma is defined as an inescapable event that overwhelms an individual's existing coping mechanisms. The seven cardinal features of PTSD are:

- The trauma must be of life-threatening magnitude, and the person must respond with intense fear, helplessness, or horror. The person may either personally experience or witness the trauma.
- The trauma is reexperienced in the following ways:
    Frequent intrusive memories of the event (the patient complains that he or she cannot stop thinking about the trauma)
    Frequent nightmares concerning the event
- The person acts or feels that the event is recurring; for example,
    "Reliving" the event
    Flashbacks
- Any reminders of the event are persistently avoided, and general responsiveness is numbed by:
    Avoidance of all conversations, places, people, or events that might remind the person of the event
    Feeling detached from others, being emotionally restricted, or having a sense of a foreshortened future
- The person experiences persistent and intense autonomic arousal, including hypervigilance and an exaggerated startle response.
- Symptoms must last more than 1 month.
- Symptoms must cause significant distress and impairment in major areas of human functioning.

2. What are the subtypes of PTSD?

There are three subtypes:
    Acute PTSD has been present 1–3 months.
    Chronic PTSD symptoms have been present > 3 months.
    With delayed onset, the symptoms appear > 6 months after the trauma.

3. List associated features of PTSD.

- Survivor's guilt
- Disturbed interpersonal relationships
- Impaired ability to modulate feelings
- Self-destructive behavior
- Impulsive behavior
- Dissociative symptoms
- Somatic complaints
- Shame
- Social withdrawal
- Changes in personality characteristics

4. List disorders often associated with PTSD.

There may be an increased risk of the following disorders:
- Panic disorder
- Agoraphobia
- Obsessive-compulsive disorder
- Social phobia
- Major depression or bipolar disorder
- Somatization disorder

- Substance-related disorders
- Dissociative identity disorder and other dissociative disorders
- Borderline personality disorder

5. Do young children present differently from adults?
The symptoms of PTSD for young children differ from adults in the following ways:

Adults	Young Children
• Respond to trauma with intense fear, helplessness, or horror	• Respond to trauma with disorganized or agitated behavior
• Reexperience the trauma with intrusive images, thoughts, and perceptions	• Engage in repetitive play in which themes or aspects of trauma are expressed
• Have recurrent distressing dreams of the trauma	• Have nonspecific nightmares; e.g., monsters
• Act or feel as if trauma were recurring	• Reenact the trauma

6. What are some associated features in children?
- The younger the child, the more vulnerable they are, and the fewer psychic resources they have.
- Children develop pessimistic expectations for the future, including a foreshortened life span.
- A child's developmental phase contributes to their specific presentation.
- Younger children tend to withdraw and may even become mute.
- Latency-age children may use obsessive defenses to repetitively discuss the trauma, but with isolation of affect.
- Latency-age children can use fantasy; i.e., to fantasize what they might have done.
- Adolescents develop a syndrome more like adults.
- Adolescents are more prone to act out, through truancy, sexual behavior, substance abuse, or delinquency.

7. What is the differential diagnosis of PTSD?
In **adjustment disorder**, the stressor can be of any severity. Diagnose adjustment disorder when there is insufficient criteria to diagnose PTSD and the stress is not extreme, but the patient's symptoms meet the criteria for PTSD.

Acute stress disorder is distinguished from PTSD because it must resolve in a 4-week period.

In **obsessive-compulsive disorder**, recurrent, intrusive thoughts are experienced as inappropriate and are not related to a specific trauma.

Flashbacks in PTSD must be distinguished from illusions and hallucinations found in psychotic disorders, such as **schizophrenia, mood disorders with psychotic features, other psychotic disorders, delirium, substance use disorders, and psychotic disorders due to a general medical condition**.

Consider malingering whenever there is a significant secondary gain, such as avoiding prosecution, avoiding work, and getting financial remuneration.

8. Is PTSD a normal response to a horrible event?
PTSD has long been thought of as a normal response to a severe stressor that continues long after the stressor has resolved. There are two major problems with this hypothesis. Most survivors of even horrific trauma, such as combat, the Holocaust, or torture, do not develop long-lasting PTSD. Further, several recent studies have shown that PTSD can result from mild stressors that commonly occur, such as motor vehicle accidents, medical procedures, and myocardial infarcts.

9. Discuss the psychophysiology of PTSD.
First and foremost, PTSD is a *physical* experience. Extremely intense, simultaneous stimuli of auditory, visual, olfactory, gustatory, and kinesthetic origin can overwhelm the brain's ability to integrate them into a meaningful experience; i.e., the construction of a story of the trauma that integrates the trauma with the self, and integrates the trauma with pre-existing schema. All layers of the brain, brainstem/hypothalamus, limbic system, and neocortex usually are affected. There is considerable evidence that neurons can be physically and permanently changed.

There are at least four lasting psychobiological abnormalities in PTSD:

Psychophysiological effects
- Extreme autonomic responses to stimuli reminiscent of the trauma
- Hyperarousal to intense but neutral stimuli (loss of stimulus discrimination)

Neurohormonal effects
- Elevated catecholamines (NE)
- Decreased glucocorticoid levels
- Decreased serotonin activity
- Increased opioid response to stimuli reminiscent of trauma

Neuroanatomical effects
- Decreased hippocampal volume
- Activation of the amygdala (implicated in evaluating the emotional meaning of incoming stimuli) and right visual cortex during flashbacks
- Decreased activation of Broca's area during flashbacks (possibly explaining why the PTSD patient has difficulty putting the experience into words)
- Marked right-hemispheric lateralization

Decreased immunological response

10. What are the risk factors for developing PTSD?

Pretrauma vulnerability: Genetic biological, and environmental factors can influence vulnerability to PTSD. Examples include family history of mental disorders, especially alcoholism; history of child abuse; early separation from parents; parental poverty; lower education; and previous traumatization by a similar event.

Age: Children are much more susceptible to the effects of trauma than adults.

Magnitude of the stressor: In general, the more intense and threatening the trauma is (serious injury or death), and the longer the duration or the more repetitive the trauma is, the greater the risk of developing PTSD. Green has proposed seven categories of generic traumas that "cut across different types of traumatic events":

1. Threat to one's life and body integrity
2. Severe physical harm or injury
3. Receipt of intentional injury/harm
4. Exposure to the grotesque
5. Witnessing or learning of violence to loved ones
6. Learning of exposure to a noxious agent
7. Causing death or severe harm to another

Preparation for the event: The less the preparation, the higher the risk of developing PTSD.

Immediate and short-term responses: The likelihood of developing PTSD can be correlated to the individual's response to a trauma, or peritraumatic response. Predictive of the development of PTSD are dissociation, freezing/surrender, disorganization, agitation, and severe anxiety and panic. *Coping styles* also have been found to be predictive of PTSD in one study, but not another. Intuitively, one would expect that the more successful a person is in coping, such as taking some action to lessen the effects of the stressor, the less likely he or she would be to develop PTSD.

Posttrauma responses: Nearly all victims of severe trauma demonstrate distress immediately following the trauma. PTSD-like symptoms are so frequent that their presence alone is not a good predictor of developing PTSD. While the literature is mixed concerning what factors are good predictors, in general, the more a victim's behavior and cognition are *adaptive* following a trauma, and the more they are able to assimilate and or accommodate the trauma into their experience, the less likely they are to develop PTSD.

11. Discuss the role of memory in PTSD.

The person with PTSD usually cannot construct a full, coherent story of the trauma because:
- Too much happened too fast to record memories
- Dissociative phenomena

• The brain has a fundamental difficulty integrating the trauma with other past life events. Ordinary declarative memories (the conscious awareness of past events) fade in intensity with time. Traumatic memories retain their intensity, even after many years, as if the event always just happened yesterday. Thus, the trauma seems to be a recent experience, rather than an event from the past.

Reminders or "triggers" of the trauma can precipitate the spectrum of intrusive symptoms, flashbacks, intrusive thoughts, and nightmares. Sometimes, the trigger is only remotely related to or symbolic of the trauma. With the passage of time, the person with PTSD can activate intrusive phenomena with a neutral stimulus.

When there has been more than one unresolved trauma, the activation of PTSD memories of one may activate memories of the other. This is especially true for people with histories of child abuse. For instance, the helplessness felt in an automobile accident may activate memories of helplessness during childhood sexual or physical abuse.

12. How are compulsivity and avoidance factors in PTSD?

Victims with PTSD frequently demonstrate **compulsive reexposure** to the trauma through hurting others, hurting themselves, or placing themselves in a position to become revictimized. Violent criminals have a high incidence of childhood abuse. Self-destructive behaviors include cutting, burning, suicide attempts and completions, and starvation (anorexia). Rape victims are more likely to be raped again; victims of childhood physical abuse are more likely to be abused by a spouse; and victims of childhood sexual abuse are much more at risk to become prostitutes.

Avoidance of triggers becomes the principal activity of the person, who would do anything to not remember the trauma and not have the associated feelings. But since, with time, the person becomes more and more sensitized to cues in the environment, they necessarily must avoid more and more events. The side effect of this process is that more time is spent thinking about the trauma and less time is spent thinking about present-day life.

The more intense the emotions experienced during the trauma, the more **emotional numbing** takes place. All emotions shut down, positive and negative alike. This leads to social isolation and detachment from loved ones, with resultant conflict and eventual disruption or ending of relationships. Alcohol and drugs may be used to assist in the numbing process, and they may become problems in their own right.

13. How are perceptions skewed by PTSD?

The body of a person with PTSD is in a state of chronic hyperarousal of the autonomic nervous system. As in panic disorder, the brain and body are sending the message that there is a **constant state of danger**. Thus, the individual reacts with hypervigilance, an exaggerated startle response, and agitation. The most insignificant of stimuli can rapidly elicit intense negative emotions. The victim's prior belief that the world is basically a safe place is shattered. Victims of PTSD are always on emotional overload; thus, they do not have the benefit of using emotions as signals and guides in relationships or to determine when and what action to take.

Studies in adults and children reveal that fantasy tends to break down the barriers against remembering the trauma. Thus, **elimination of fantasy** is systematic. Since fantasy is necessary for planning and considering options, the PTSD victim has great difficulty with these functions in everyday life. This, in turn, leads to impulsivity and inflexibility.

One common defense mechanism, especially in children, is to **blame themselves** for the trauma. Women frequently blame themselves for being raped. Feelings of helplessness are overridden with feelings of guilt. It is better to feel responsible and in control (even falsely) than to feel helpless. Vulnerability and humiliation usually are present in severe traumas. The victim's self-confidence goes down, and he or she begins to feel defective and/or inadequate in all aspects of life. This produces profound shame and, if severe enough, may be dissociated away from consciousness.

14. What is the core psychological effect of trauma?

Like everyone, trauma victims have developed their own theory about themselves, the world, and the relationship between themselves and the world. Within their reality are strongly held assumptions. These commonly include:

- Belief in their own personal invulnerability
- Perception of the world as meaningful and comprehensible
- View of themselves in a positive light.

Whenever a person experiences a severe trauma, these unconscious assumptions are challenged. If the trauma cannot be assimilated into preexisting experience, then the person experiences severe anxiety. The stress response syndrome may be largely attributable to the **shattering of basic assumptions** about the self and the world.

15. Describe the general principles of treatment.

The principle treatment modality for PTSD is some type of psychotherapy, such as supportive, psychodynamic, cognitive behavioral, and others, with medication used to augment the psychotherapy and help reduce symptoms.

The goals of treatment are:

- To help patients regain a sense of being worthwhile
- To again feel in control of themselves and their lives (the opposite of the feelings of helplessness experienced in the trauma)
- To re-work their shattered assumptions.

16. How is treatment conducted?

Many authors, such as Herman, Chu, Van Der Kolk, and others, use a phase-oriented model to conceptualize treatment. While there are differences, most have three phases:

Phase I   Establishing safety, stabilization, symptom reduction and the therapeutic alliance

Phase II   Dealing with the traumatic event; e.g., through remembering and abreaction, desensitization, deconditioning, mourning, etc.

Phase III Restructuring personal schema and integrating the trauma into a meaningful life narrative; i.e., putting the trauma into perspective and moving forward in developing a positive life.

The first phase is devoted to **establishing safety**—in the actual environment as well as in memories. For instance, if the patient with PTSD is living with the perpetrator of violence, plans should be made to ensure safety; i.e., developing a safety plan, arranging alternate housing, or learning how to avoid provoking the abuser. Encourage the patient to improve self care and to reduce self-destructive behaviors, e.g., by abstaining from alcohol and drugs of abuse. Educate early about the signs and symptoms of PTSD, and teach various coping mechanisms for mastering intrusive memories and flashbacks. Address social supports, and inform patients that important people in their lives also should learn about the symptoms of PTSD. Finally, encourage patients not to let their symptoms stop them from functioning in everyday life.

In the second phase, the main task is **"story" construction**. Frequently, information is needed from collateral sources, such as other victims' accounts, eye-witnesses, police records, hospital records, etc. Affects should be identified as they are attached to elements of the story. Many people have great difficulty talking about a trauma because the feelings are so intense, and Broca's area "turns off" during the trauma. Other approaches include desensitization to the trauma memories, controlled exposure and memory reactivation, and restructuring of trauma-related cognitive schemes. Patients must restructure their personal schema and integrate the trauma into a meaningful narrative within the continuum of their life, while putting the trauma into perspective.

In the third phase of treatment, patients must **assimilate the trauma(s)** into their belief system, or accommodate their beliefs to better fit reality. Their basic assumptions about themselves and the world need to be re-thought. This will necessitate adjusting their sense of self and identity. They are forever changed, and as such need to re-negotiate relationships and make new ones. Patients need to become involved in activities that provide them with feelings of mastery and pleasure.

17. How are medications used to treat PTSD?

The principal reasons for using medications are to:

- Reduce PTSD specific symptoms

Frequency and/or severity of intrusive symptoms
Interpreting incoming stimuli as recurrences of the trauma
Developing hyperarousal to stimuli reminiscent of the trauma, as well as in generalized hyperarousal
Becoming avoidant
Developing numbing
- Treat depression and/or mood swings
- Treat anxiety
- Reduce psychotic or dissociative symptoms
- Reduce impulsivity and aggression against self and others.

Although almost every class of psychiatric medication has been used to treat PTSD, very few medications have been systematically studied. Additionally, the findings of most studies may not be applicable, because they have been done with male combat victims with chronic PTSD.

Antidepressants such as fluoxetine, amitriptyline, desipramine, and phenelzine may decrease symptoms of PTSD in addition to their benefits for depressive disorder. Anticonvulsants such as carbamazepine and valproic acid also could be beneficial in treating chronic PTSD. Propanolol and benzodiazepines such as alprazelam and clonazepam appear to decrease the autonomical arousal associated with PTSD. Finally, clonidine, an Alpha$_2$-adrenergic agonist, may be useful in treating PTSD symptoms. Lithium, neuroleptics, and cyproheptadine have been studied only sparsely.

Perhaps the best approach is to choose a medication based on the more problematic target symptoms. This may require a combination of medications, e.g., an SSRI to decrease numbing and depression, and a benzodiazepine and a beta blocker to decrease autonomic hyperarousal.

BIBLIOGRAPHY

1. American Psychiatric Association: Diagnostic and Statistical Manual of Mental Disorders, 4th ed. Washington, DC, American Psychiatric Association, 1994.
2. Chu JA: Rebuilding Shattered Lives: The Responsible Treatment of Complex Posttraumatic and Dissociative Disorders. New York, John Wiley & Sons, Inc., 1998.
3. Eth S, Pynoos RS: Developmental perspective on psychic trauma in childhood. In Figley CR (ed): Trauma and Its Wake, Volume I. New York, Brunner/Mazel, 1985.
4. Herman JL: Trauma and Recovery. New York, Harper-Collins, 1992.
5. Janoff-Bulman R: The aftermath of victimization: Rebuilding shattered assumptions. In Figley CR (ed): Trauma and Its Wake, Volume I. New York, Brunner/Mazel, 1985.
6. Pynoos RS, Steinberg AM, Goenjian A: Traumatic stress in childhood and adolescence: Recent developments and current controversies. In van der Kolk BA, McFarlane AC, Weisaeth L (eds): Traumatic Stress: The Effects of Overwhelming Experience on Mind, Body, and Society. New York, The Guilford Press, 1996.
7. Shalev AY: Stress versus traumatic stress: From acute homeostatic reactions to chronic psychopathology. In van der Kolk BA, McFarlane AC, Weisaeth L (eds): Traumatic Stress: The Effects of Overwhelming Experience on Mind, Body, and Society. New York, The Guilford Press, 1996.
8. van der Kolk BA: The body keeps score: Approaches to the psychobiology of posttraumatic stress disorder. In van der Kolk BA, McFarlane AC, Weisaeth L (eds): Traumatic Stress: The Effects of Overwhelming Experience on Mind, Body, and Society. New York, The Guilford Press, 1996.
9. van der Kolk BA, McFarlane AC, van der Hart O: A general approach to treatment of posttraumatic stress disorder. In van der Kolk BA, McFarlane AC, Weisaeth L (eds): Traumatic Stress: The Effects of Overwhelming Experience on Mind, Body, and Society, New York, The Guilford Press, 1996.
10. van der Kolk BA, McFarlane AC: The black hole of trauma. In van der Kolk BA, McFarlane AC, Weisaeth L (eds): Traumatic Stress: The Effects of Overwhelming Experience on Mind, Body, and Society, New York, The Guilford Press, 1996.
11. van der Kolk BA, van der Hart O, Marmar CR: Dissociation and information processing in posttraumatic stress disorder. In van der Kolk BA, McFarlane AC, Weisaeth L (eds): Traumatic Stress: The Effects of Overwhelming Experience on Mind, Body, and Society, New York, The Guilford Press, 1996.

19. PSYCHOACTIVE SUBSTANCE USE DISORDERS

Jane A. Kennedy, D.O.

1. Define psychoactive substance abuse disorder, addiction, and dependence.

Terms used to define substance use disorders are varied and confusing. For the most part, loss of control, compulsion to use, and continued use despite adverse consequences are indicative of *psychoactive substance use disorder*. To many, the term *addiction* implies the psychological compulsion to use a substance, whereas the term *dependence* implies the physiologic components of withdrawal or tolerance.

However, the Diagnostic and Statistical Manual, 4th edition (DSM–IV), of the American Psychiatric Association expands the definition of dependence. For a diagnosis of **psychoactive substance dependence**, three or more criteria, which may or may not include physiologic tolerance or withdrawal, must be met. Other criteria include persistent efforts to cut down or stop use; using more or for a longer time than intended; filling one's time with drug or alcohol activities, such as intoxication or drug procurement; giving up important life activities, such as work or family; and continued use despite knowledge that it will cause or worsen physical or psychological problems.

For a diagnosis of **psychoactive substance abuse disorder**, only one criterion is needed: repeated failure to fulfill significant role obligations; recurrent use in physically hazardous situations, such as driving when intoxicated; repeated substance-related legal problems; or continued substance use despite related social or interpersonal problems. For both abuse and dependence, such maladaptive behaviors must have a duration of at least 1 month.

2. Does addiction run in families?

Yes. The risk of addiction is 3–4 times higher for children of substance abusers than for children of non-substance abusers. The cause may be genetic, environmental, or a combination of factors. Familial patterns have been studied primarily in alcoholic families. Twin studies reveal a higher concordance of alcoholism in monozygotic than dizygotic twins, and adoption studies show that twins raised apart have a similar increase in prevalence of alcoholism, whether raised in non-alcoholic or alcoholic families. However, because the concordance in monozygotic twins is not 100%, environmental factors may play an equally important part in the development of alcoholism.

3. How should a physician ask about drug and alcohol problems?

Most patients with alcohol or drug problems are fearful of negative reactions from their physician if they tell the truth. Start by asking questions about tobacco, alcohol, and marijuana in a matter-of-fact, nonjudgmental manner. Questions should address how much (not whether) the patient drinks, blackouts, drunk driving, and whether *the patient* thinks that he or she ever drinks more than appropriate. Similar questions should be asked about each category of drugs, including routes of administration.

Several screening questionnaires have been found to be useful in primary care. The Michigan Alcohol Screening Test (MAST) has 25 questions to be answered by the patient, but may be too lengthy in the primary care setting. The CAGE questionnaire, which has 4 questions, is easier to use for taking a history:

1. Have you tried to **C**ut down on alcohol?
2. Have you been **A**nnoyed when someone criticized your drinking?
3. Have you felt **G**uilty about your drinking?
4. Have you used alcohol as an **E**ye-opener by having a drink in the morning?

Two or more positive answers suggest alcohol problems with high sensitivity and specificity. The physician may substitute or add the word drug to get a similar screen of drug problems.

4. What is the relationship between substance use disorders and psychiatric illnesses?

Dual diagnosis of substance use disorder and psychiatric illness is a complex issue. In primary substance use disorders, **chronic use may induce psychiatric symptoms**; for example, psychosis from stimulants or hallucinogens or depression from alcohol dependence. In substance use disorders secondary to psychiatric illnesses, **patients may self-treat their symptoms**; for example, alcohol may be used to relieve anxiety or to decrease manic symptoms. In addition, patients may have independent syndromes of substance abuse and major mental illness.

The diagnosis of comorbid psychiatric and substance use disorders is significant, and the reported prevalences may depend on the populations surveyed. In the general population, 27% have a diagnosis of substance abuse or dependence at some time during their lifetime. On the other hand, nearly half of patients with schizophrenia have a substance use disorder, and substance abuse or dependence is found in 84% of patients with antisocial personality disorder. Substance abuse or dependence is seen in 24% of patients with anxiety disorders and 32% of patients with affective disorders; in patients with bipolar illness, the prevalence of substance use disorder is 56%. In addition, comorbid substance use disorders are seen in approximately 90% of prisoners who have schizophrenia, bipolar disorder, or antisocial personality disorder. About 50% of patients admitted to public psychiatric hospitals and 40–50% of hospitalized medical patients have comorbid substance abuse or dependence.

It is best to wait 2–3 weeks after a patient becomes abstinent before diagnosing a psychiatric disorder; often the symptoms of depression, anxiety, or psychosis disappear as the patient clears. However, in patients with a definite history of psychiatric disorder before onset of substance abuse or during periods of abstinence, treatment should be initiated immediately.

5. Does treatment work?

Yes, but no one treatment works for all patients. Some people stop alcohol use without formal treatment or with brief interventions, such as advice from their physician. Many types of formal treatment modalities are discussed in the following chapters about specific substances. In general, substance use disorders are chronic and relapsing; the treatment goal is to decrease the frequency and duration of relapses as well as morbidity and mortality. Like other chronic diseases such as hypertension or diabetes, the aim is **management** rather than cure.

Stopping the substance use must be the primary goal. In the early phases of treatment, patients need external controls, such as urine or breath monitoring, behavioral contracting, and involvement of family or employer to help them stop. Once the patient is abstinent, the focus is prevention of relapse, which includes reducing accessibility of the substance, identifying stimuli that may trigger cravings, understanding feelings, and developing coping responses and improved social skills. Relapse is high during the first year of treatment, but as periods of abstinence lengthen, the likelihood of relapse decreases. Ongoing treatment should involve a biopsychosocial model, attending to health and psychiatric problems as well as marital, occupational, legal, financial, and social functioning. For any substance use disorder, a worse prognosis is associated with unemployment, lack of social support system, and presence of psychopathology, especially antisocial personality disorder.

6. Is inpatient treatment better than outpatient treatment?

The long-term benefit of inpatient hospitalization vs. outpatient treatment has not been documented. Patients with complicated medical or psychiatric problems, severe withdrawal, suicidality, or risk of seizure require inpatient treatment, but extended hospital stays have not been associated with increased long-term abstinence.

7. Should patients be completely abstinent? Or can they learn to control their use?

At this time little evidence suggests that controlled use can be achieved; abstinence should be the goal for most patients. Some patients want to abstain from their drug of abuse but use other substances in moderation; this practice is a potential trigger for relapse. Not infrequently, patients switch substances (quit heroin and become dependent on alcohol) or develop a second dependence (continue alcohol and add benzodiazepines).

8. Should all patients attend a self-help group?

Self-help groups can be extremely beneficial. Alcoholics Anonymous (AA), Narcotics Anonymous (NA), Cocaine Anonymous (CA), Rational Recovery (RR), and other such groups provide structure and support, decrease stigma, and offer hope as patients see others recover. However, outcome research shows that the drop-out rate in the first year of AA attendance is high (50–75%) and that although AA is helpful to those who stay, others may need to seek professional treatment. Self-help programs can be used in combination with professional treatment.

9. What is a therapeutic community?

Therapeutic community refers to residential, long-term (6–12 months) treatment, usually with gradual re-entry into society. In general, the approach is based on milieu therapy and is highly confrontive, with strict limits and structure. Graduates of the program often become staff members, having increased their level of responsibility as they progressed through the program. The drop-out rate in the first few months of treatment is high (75–80%), but graduates have improved outcome in terms of drug use, crime, and employment.

10. Should family members be included in alcohol or drug treatment?

Yes. Behavior associated with substance use disorders significantly affects family members, who may participate indirectly or directly in maladaptive patterns. They should be included in the patient's treatment, both for themselves and to help monitor and provide external control for the patient. Part of relapse prevention should be an agreement that the spouse will contact the treatment provider if concern develops about relapse.

Note that family members can find personal support as well as education through groups such as Al-Anon.

BIBLIOGRAPHY

1. American Psychiatric Association: Diagnostic and Statistical Manual of Mental Disorders, 4th ed. Washington, DC, American Psychiatric Association, 1994.
2. Arif A, Westemeyer J: Manual of Drug and Alcohol Abuse. New York, Plenum, 1988.
3. Ciraulo DA, Shader RI: Clinical Manual of Chemical Dependence. Washington, DC, American Psychiatric Press, 1991.
3a. Frances RS, Miller ST: Clinical Textbook of Addictive Disorders. New York, Guilford Press, 1998.
4. Friedman LS, Fleming NF, Roberts DH, Hymen SE: Source Book of Substance Abuse and Addiction. Baltimore, Williams & Wilkins, 1996.
5. Galanter M, Kleber HD: Textbook of Substance Abuse Treatment., 2nd ed. Washington, DC, American Psychiatric Press, 1999.
6. Institute of Medicine: Broadening the Base of Treatment for Alcohol Problems. Washington, DC, National Academy Press, 1990.
7. Kessler RC, McGonagle KA, Zhao S, et al: Lifetime and 12-month prevalence of DSM-III-R psychiatric disorders in the United States. Arch Gen Psychiatry 51:8–19, 1994.
8. Lowinson JH, Ruiz P, Millman RB, Langrod JG: Substance Abuse: A Comprehensive Textbook. Baltimore, Williams & Wilkins, 1997.
9. Milhorn HT Jr: Chemical Dependence: Diagnosis, Treatment, and Prevention. New York, Springer-Verlag, 1990.
10. Miller NS: Comprehensive Handbook of Drug and Alcohol Addiction. New York, Marcel Dekker, 1991.
11. Regier DA, Farmer ME, Rae DS, et al: Comorbidity of mental disorders with alcohol and other drugs. JAMA 264:2511–2518, 1990.

20. ALCOHOL USE DISORDERS

Jane A. Kennedy, D.O.

1. Who drinks alcohol?

About 75% of the population in the United States drinks, and about 23% reported alcohol abuse or dependence in the National Comorbidity Survey reported in 1994. Men are 2–3 times more likely than women to be problem drinkers, although women may hide their drinking more frequently.

2. Does alcoholism run in families?

Good evidence suggests a genetic link, and the strongest vulnerability appears to be for sons of alcoholic fathers. Several studies, including twin and adoption studies, show that children of alcoholics are about 4 times more likely to develop alcohol problems. Specific biologic abnormalities have been noted, such as decreased brain-wave reactivity (P300, a measure of visual evoked response) in children of alcoholics and decreased intensity of reaction to alcohol in sons of alcoholics.

3. What are the signs and symptoms of alcohol intoxication?

A person intoxicated by alcohol may have ataxia, slurred speech, mood lability, decreased concentration and memory, poor judgment, facial flushing, enlarged pupils, and nystagmus. Although alcohol initially has a stimulant effect, increasing levels result in depression of respiration, reflexes, blood pressure, and body temperature, potentially followed by stupor, coma, and death.

Blood alcohol levels are measured in grams percent (g%) or milligrams per 100 milliliters (mg/dl); in most states drivers are said to be "impaired" at levels of 0.05 g% (50 mg/dl) and "under the influence" at levels of 0.1 g% (100 mg/dl). Lack of intoxication at a level of 100 mg/dl is evidence of tolerance, and alcohol dependence disorder should be suspected.

4. What are the usual symptoms and time course of alcohol withdrawal?

In someone dependent on alcohol, stopping or suddenly decreasing the amount of alcohol intake may result in withdrawal symptoms, which reflect central nervous system and autonomic hyperactivity. Symptoms begin to appear in 4–24 hours, usually peak at 36–48 hours, and subside in about 5 days. Symptoms typically are in proportion to duration of drinking, but the presence of medical illness may increase the severity.

Mild withdrawal may manifest as insomnia, irritability, anxiety, and mild gastrointestinal problems that start a few hours after stopping alcohol and last up to 48 hours. Symptoms may progress first to tremor, sweating, tachycardia, elevated blood pressure, nausea, vomiting, and diarrhea and then to fever, hallucinations, delusions, confusion, agitation, and grand mal seizures. Hallucinations may appear within 24–96 hours and may be auditory, tactile, or visual (most common). Delirium tremens usually appears between 24 and 72 hours and may have a mortality rate of 5–15%; this syndrome, which is characterized by extreme agitation, delirium, psychosis (delusions and hallucinations), and fever, may last up to 5 days.

5. What about alcohol withdrawal seizures?

Alcohol withdrawal seizures ("rum fits") most often occur 6–48 hours after stopping or reducing alcohol and may occur in 5–10% of patients in alcohol withdrawal. The seizures generally stop within 6–12 hours; they may be multiple and are usually grand mal. If a patient has a past history of alcohol withdrawal seizures, the risk of recurrence is increased 10-fold.

Because < 5% of alcohol withdrawal seizures are focal, other causes, such as subdural hematoma, should be evaluated. Seizures that occur beyond 48 hours may be due to causes such as withdrawal from sedatives. Many alcoholics have chronic obstructive pulmonary disease, and seizures may be related to theophylline toxicity. Seizures also may be caused by metabolic disorders such as hypoglycemia or hypomagnesemia, which are not uncommon in alcoholics.

6. What is the treatment of alcohol withdrawal?

Removal of alcohol leads to a state of hyperexcitability. Most patients are able to withdraw without medication, but patients with moderate-to-severe symptoms are best treated with a sedative. Overall, the **benzodiazepines** have been found to be the most useful and the most practical. The long-acting benzodiazepines, such as chlordiazepoxide, diazepam, and chlorazepate, are used in decreasing doses to prevent seizure and to decrease the other symptoms of hyperexcitability. For patients with severe liver disease, who may encounter problems with accumulation of long-acting benzodiazepines and their metabolites, oxazepam is recommended because of its lack of active metabolites and its independence of liver metabolism. Oxazepam and lorazepam may be given intramuscularly, whereas other benzodiazepines are poorly absorbed with intramuscular administration.

Other agents have been examined for treatment of alcohol withdrawal, with various success:

- Alpha$_2$ adrenergic agonists: clonidine and lofexidine reduce noradrenergic symptoms, but have no anticonvulsant effects and may cause hypotension.
- Antipsychotics: haloperidol in low doses may be useful in patients with hallucinations and agitation that do not respond to benzodiazepines, but they should not be used alone. Antipsychotics do not prevent seizures and may lower seizure threshold. Thorazine, which may cause severe hypotension and lower seizure threshold, should not be used.
- Barbiturates: effective anticonvulsants but narrow therapeutic index and greater tendency to induce respiratory depression.
- Anticonvulsants: both carbamazepine and divalproex have been used effectively in small studies. In particular, divalproex seems to have considerably less effect on cognition and psychomotor performance.
- Ethanol: contraindicated because of toxicity and potential to cause high fluid load.
- Propranolol: contraindicated because it does not prevent seizures, may obscure withdrawal signs, and is contraindicated in various conditions seen in chronic alcoholics, such as lung diseases with bronchospasm, congestive heart failure, hypotension, and insulin-dependent diabetes.

7. What is the treatment of alcohol withdrawal seizures?

Benzodiazepines should be used for the treatment of withdrawal seizures—most commonly, the long-acting drugs such as chlordiazepoxide, diazepam, or chlorazepate. Some clinicians avoid the use of diazepam, because it may cause euphoria. For elderly patients or patients with compromised liver function, short-acting benzodiazepines, such as oxazepam or lorazepam, avoid accumulation of metabolites and may be administered parenterally.

8. Do patients need phenytoin for prophylaxis of alcohol withdrawal seizures?

Little evidence supports the use of phenytoin for the treatment or prophylaxis of alcohol withdrawal seizures unless the patient has a preexisting seizure disorder.

9. What is Wernicke-Korsakoff syndrome?

Wernicke's disease, or Wernicke's encephalopathy, is characterized by confusion and drowsiness, ataxia, and ocular disturbances (usually due to weakness or paralysis of the sixth cranial nerve), including nystagmus. Wernicke's syndrome may have acute onset or develop slowly over 1 week or so.

Korsakoff's psychosis is a state of amnesia that usually follows Wernicke's syndrome; patients have anterograde amnesia (inability to retain new memories, even their physician's name) and possibly retrograde amnesia (inability to recall the past). Otherwise they appear alert, responsive, and normal and may try to cover their memory problem by fabricating answers or "confabulating." In the string test, which has been used in diagnosis of Korsakoff's psychosis, the physician asks the patient to take an imaginary string in his or her hands, and the patient complies, as though the string were real.

Treatment with **thiamine** may reverse the ocular abnormalities and ataxia almost completely, but the confusion and amnestic problems may not respond as well. Rapid treatment of Wernicke's syndrome may prevent the onset of Korsakoff's psychosis; if treatment is delayed, the patient may become demented and unable to care for him- or herself. Thus, *Wernicke's encephalopathy is a medical emergency*.

10. When is thiamine needed?

Chronic alcoholics often are malnourished. Thiamine deficiency is common and may cause Wernicke-Korsakoff syndrome. The treatment is immediate administration of thiamine, 100 mg intramuscularly, followed by 100 mg intramuscularly or orally for the next 2 days. Because administration of glucose may deplete already deficient B-vitamins, thiamine should be given before glucose is administered.

11. What are the medical complications of chronic alcohol use?

Gastrointestinal complications. Gastrointestinal problems include gastritis, peptic and gastric ulcer, esophagitis, esophageal varices, alcoholic hepatitis, cirrhosis, and pancreatitis. Except for cirrhosis, these conditions are often reversible with abstinence from alcohol. Although a minority of alcoholics (15–20%) develop cirrhosis, the majority of patients with cirrhosis are alcoholics (50–80%). Therapeutic doses of acetaminophen are associated with hepatoxicity in alcoholics.

Neurologic complications. Wernicke-Korsakoff syndrome is a medical emergency (see Question 9). Hepatic encephalopathy may occur because the liver is no longer able to metabolize and detoxify substances. Asterixis, or "liver flap," appears late; early symptoms include confusion, agitation, and personality changes. Peripheral neuropathy is usually symmetrical and in the lower extremities. With prolonged drinking, alcohol dementia may occur with memory defects and difficulty with abstract thinking and new learning. Cerebellar degeneration, which causes a wide-spread gait, may be associated with Wernicke-Korsakoff syndrome. Stopping alcohol intake and vitamin treatment can improve these conditions.

Cardiovascular complications. Hypertension is associated with excessive alcohol intake, and patients who continue to drink heavily may not respond as well to antihypertensive medication. With abstinence, many patients become normotensive. Alcoholic cardiomyopathy has a fairly nonspecific presentation, and the diagnosis is usually based on the alcohol history; it should be suspected in patients under age 50 who present with heart failure. Alcohol ingestion and alcohol withdrawal cause sinus tachycardia.

Pulmonary complications. Alcoholics show increased incidence of tuberculosis and bacterial pneumonias; in addition, aspiration pneumonia may occur with vomiting and altered levels of consciousness. Because at least 80% of alcoholics are smokers, the incidence of bronchitis, emphysema, and chronic obstructive pulmonary disease is increased.

Hematologic complications. Macrocytosis (enlarged red blood cells) is an early laboratory manifestation of chronic alcoholism. It may be caused by folate deficiency or the direct toxicity of alcohol (unrelated to vitamin depletion). Iron deficiency anemia may occur in alcoholics because of chronic gastrointestinal bleeding, but the associated low mean corpuscular volume may be hidden by concurrent macrocytosis. Alcohol impairs the production and function of white blood cells, both neutrophils and lymphocytes, and increases the risk of infection. Blood platelet production also may be suppressed, and platelet function may be impaired. In addition, splenic enlargement secondary to liver disease may cause thrombocytopenia through increased sequestration of platelets.

Endocrine complications. Alcohol suppresses testosterone levels in men by effects on the pituitary gland and the testicle, and impaired metabolism of estrogen by the liver increases estrogen levels. Both events may result in signs of feminization, such as gynecomastia and feminine fat distribution; decreased libido; testicular atrophy; and impotence. Women experience menstrual irregularities, ranging from cessation of menses to excessive bleeding.

12. Is smoking associated with drinking?

At the minimum, 80–90% of alcoholics are regular and often heavy smokers. Some of the medical complications of alcoholism may be caused by cigarette smoking, and increased mortality also may be due to complications from smoking. A higher rate of alcoholism should be expected in smoking populations, such as patients with chronic obstructive pulmonary disease.

13. How can the physician detect alcohol problems in patients?

The history and physical exam of a patient reveal a great deal. Certainly the diagnosis of alcohol abuse or dependence must be pursued in a patient who shows withdrawal symptoms such as tremors and diaphoresis or who is intoxicated and smells of alcohol. Symptoms of medical conditions associated with excessive alcohol use, such as diarrhea, anemia, or impotence, also should suggest the diagnosis. Patients have been known to receive an extensive work-up for diarrhea caused by alcohol withdrawal, because the physician did not ask about drinking. The physician should ask about alcohol intake without being accusatory; problem drinkers may be honest if they do not feel threatened.

14. What physical findings are common in chronic heavy drinkers?

Flushed facies	Dilated superficial veins on the abdomen
Parotid gland enlargement	Right upper quadrant tenderness
Gynecomastia in men	Hepatomegaly
Spider angiomata	Muscle wasting or tenderness
Abdominal distension from ascites	Paresthesias in feet and calves
Abnormal gait due to cerebellar degeneration	

15. Can laboratory tests diagnose alcohol abuse and dependence?

Verbal questioning is more sensitive than laboratory tests for detecting alcohol problems; no one test can prove their presence. Several tests evaluated together, however, are sometimes useful, although often in the later stages of disease. The gamma-glutamyltransferase (GGT) test has been used most commonly; although not specific (many other factors may cause increased GGT), abnormally high values are seen in most chronic alcoholics. An elevated mean corpuscular volume (MCV) may be a sign of chronic heavy alcohol consumption and is thought to be a direct effect of alcohol on bone marrow or folate metabolism; again, an elevated MCV may have many other causes. Aspartate aminotransferase (AST) and alanine aminotransferase (ALT) are nonspecific indicators of hepatic damage but are frequently elevated in alcoholic liver disease; an ALT/AST ratio of > 2 is especially suspicious. Other blood tests found to be elevated with chronic alcohol intake are alkaline phosphatase, high-density lipoprotein cholesterol, and uric acid. It is best to look at laboratory markers in combination; the more tests that are elevated, the more likely the patient will be a heavy drinker. The carbohydrate-deficient transferrin test, which is being evaluated as a state marker for alcoholism, appears promising.

16. What is fetal alcohol syndrome?

The fetus is affected by maternal alcohol intake, probably in a dose-dependent manner. *The minimal safe amount of alcohol that will not cause fetal problems is unknown*, but certainly the likelihood of fetal alcohol syndrome (FAS) increases with increasing amounts of alcohol intake. The early weeks of the first trimester are thought to be the time of greatest vulnerability. Infants with FAS are smaller, may have mental retardation, and have characteristic facial features, such as no philtrum (ridge between nose and upper lip), thin upper lip, low-set ears, and short palpebral fissures. Cigarette smoking, malnutrition, and drug use may be complicating factors in the spectrum of clinical problems seen in these infants.

17. Are there any useful pharmacologic approaches in the treatment of alcohol abuse and dependence *after* withdrawal?

Disulfiram (Antabuse) has been used as a deterrent to drinking; it inhibits aldehyde dehydrogenase, which breaks down acetaldehyde, a metabolite of alcohol. If a patient drinks while taking disulfiram, the increased level of acetaldehyde causes flushing, throbbing headache, nausea, vomiting, tachycardia, hypotension, and hyperventilation; rarely, cardiovascular collapse and death may occur. A large study showed marginal efficacy of disulfiram, but patients were not monitored. Results are improved if the patient is required to take the disulfiram under observation.

Naltrexone, an opioid blocker, has been approved for use in the treatment of alcohol problems; it decreases craving, and reduces likelihood of continued drinking if the patient relapses. Because the reinforcing property of alcohol seems to be attenuated for some drinkers, naltrexone is helpful as an adjunct to treatment of alcohol dependence. No studies have reported the use of naltrexone beyond 12 weeks. **Nalmefene**, an experimental oral opioid antagonist, appears as effective as naltrexone and possibly has less risk of liver toxicity.

Acamprosate, an analog of homocysteic acid, has produced higher continuous abstinence rates and fewer drinking days. It seems to affect excitatory amino acid neurotransmitters and possibly the GABA system. It is not yet available in the U.S.

Gamma hydroxybutyrate has been used to treat alcohol and opiate withdrawal outside the U.S., but it is an abusable drug.

BIBLIOGRAPHY

1. Brewer C: Combining pharmacological antagonists and behavioral psychotherapy in treating addictions. Br J Psychiatry 157:34–40, 1990.
2. Fuller RF, Branchey L, Brightwell DR, et al: Disulfiram treatment of alcoholism: A Veterans Administration cooperative study. JAMA 256:1449–1455, 1986.
3. Garbutt JC, West SL, Carey TS, et al: Pharmacological treatment of alcohol dependence: A review of the evidence. JAMA 281:1318–1325, 1999.
4. Johnston SC, Pelletier LL Jr: Enhanced hepatoxicity of acetaminophen in the alcoholic patient. Medicine (Baltimore) 76:185–191, 1997.
5. O'Connor PG, Schottenfeld R: Patients with alcohol problems. New Engl J Med 338:592–600, 1998.
6. O'Malley SS: Opioid antagonists in the treatment of alcohol dependence: Clinical efficacy and prevention of relapse. Alcohol Alcohol 31(Suppl 1):77–81, 1996.
7. Sass H, Soyka M, Mann K, Zieglgansberger W: Relapse prevention by acamprosate. Arch Gen Psychiat 53:673–680, 1996.
8. Stibler H: Carbohydrate-deficient transferrin in serum: A new marker of potentially harmful alcohol consumption reviewed. Clin Chem 37:2029–2037, 1991.

21. OPIOID USE DISORDERS

Jane A. Kennedy, D.O.

1. What are opioids?

Opioids include naturally occurring substances such as opium and morphine, semisynthetic drugs such as heroin and hydromorphone, and totally synthetic drugs such as methodone or meperidine. These substances act at specific opioid receptors in the brain and the body, as do the endogenous opioids (endorphins, enkephalins, and dynorphins).

2. Who abuses opioids?

Opioid abusers sometimes are divided into heroin addicts and prescription opioid abusers ("medical addicts"). In the United States, approximately one-half million people are dependent on heroin, but only about 140,000 are in methadone maintenance treatment. In 1995, there were 141,000 new users, and most were under age 26; in 1997, 2.1% of high school seniors reported using heroin at least once. Although most users are still injecting heroin, there is an increase in intranasal use and smoking, due to increased purity and fear of HIV transmission with needles. Prescription drug abusers frequently are patients with real or fabricated pain, or health professionals with access to medications by prescription or diversion.

3. Describe the signs and symptoms of opioid intoxication.

Soon after injecting heroin, the person may vomit because of activation of the chemoreceptor trigger zone in the medulla; for the heroin user, this reaction often indicates "good" heroin. Feeling sedation, warmth, and euphoria ("flush and rush"), the user "nods," with the head dropping toward the chest. Speech may be slurred, and attention and memory are impaired. The pupils are pinpoint, and the users may scratch as they nod because of histamine release. The feeling of warmth is probably due to peripheral vasodilation, and hypotension may occur; respiratory depression and suppression of the cough reflex are centrally mediated.

4. What other effects are seen with use of opioids?

Analgesia due to reduced perception of and reaction to pain is common; tolerance to analgesic doses of opioid has been shown experimentally to develop within 48–72 hours. Constipation, sweating, and decreased libido may be chronic side effects of opioid use, but no evidence suggests organ damage from long-term use of opioids. Derangement of the neuroendocrine system can result from chronic opioid administration, but it has been shown that neuroendocrine and immune functions improve in patients on methadone maintenance. Smooth muscle constriction may cause urinary retention and biliary colic.

High doses of meperidine and of propoxyphene are associated with a stimulant-like effect that may include seizures and pupillary dilation; such effects seem to be caused by nor-metabolites. Use of meperidine in the presence of monoamine oxidase (MAO) inhibitors may cause hypertensive crisis.

5. What about tolerance with opioids?

Tolerance to euphoria, sedation, respiratory depression, vomiting, and analgesia occurs with regular use, and increased amounts of the drug are needed to create the same effect; however, there is little or no tolerance to constipation or miosis. Exceptions include patients on methadone maintenance, who do not become tolerant to long-term doses once they have been stabilized, and many patients with chronic malignant and nonmalignant pain, who maintain analgesia at a constant dose without development of tolerance. It is possible for patients to build tolerance over time to extremely high doses of opioids that would cause death in nontolerant people.

As with alcohol, tolerance dissipates quickly with abstinence but increases rapidly with reintroduction of the drug, obtaining levels of past tolerance within days rather than years (which were required for its development).

6. What happens with overdose of opioids?

The main effect of overdose is respiratory depression, which is the most common cause of death. Patients usually are comatose, cyanotic, and hypotensive with pinpoint pupils, although pupils may dilate as hypoxia occurs. Pulmonary edema frequently is associated with overdose of heroin and seizures with overdose of meperidine.

7. How is overdose treated?

Opioid overdose in treated with injection of naloxone (Narcan), an opioid antagonist. In the presence of long-acting opioids such as methadone, repeated doses of naloxone are needed, and a long-acting ($T\frac{1}{2}$ = 11 hours) opioid antagonist, nalmefene, is now available parenterally.

8. What are the complications of opioid use?

Infections such as HIV, hepatitis, endocarditis, osteomyelitis, meningitis, septicemia, and abscesses may result from unsterile conditions and needle sharing during injection of opioids. Patients using acetaminophen or aspirin in high quantity over time are at risk of hepatic and renal toxicity; gastric irritation also may result from use of aspirin compounds. Two-thirds of heroin addicts have abnormal liver enzymes (which often normalize in methadone treatment); one-third to one-half are positive for hepatitis B, and nearly 80% of injection drug users are positive for hepatitis C. Tuberculosis is more common in heroin addicts than in the general population.

9. What are symptoms of withdrawal from opioids?

Early symptoms	Intermediate symptoms
Myalgia	Sweats
Nausea	Fever
Rhinorrhea	Chills

Lacrimation	Piloerection ("cold turkey")
Increased production of phlegm	Insomnia or restless sleep
	Muscle spasms, often in lower limbs ("kicking")
Yawning	Bone pain (often in thighs)
Late symptoms	**At any stage**
Vomiting	Dilated pupils
Diarrhea	Anxiety
Hypertension	Irritability
Tachycardia	
Hyperventilation	

Opioid withdrawal has been described as a severe flulike syndrome, and addicts use the term "sick" to mean withdrawal. With short-acting opioids, withdrawal starts 6–24 hours after the last dose, peaks in 1–3 days, and subsides in about 5–7 days. With longer-acting drugs such as methadone or 1-alpha acetyl methadol (LAAM), withdrawal starts after 1–3 days, peaks at 3–6 days, and may take 2 weeks to subside completely. Although withdrawal from the long-acting drugs may be less severe, the longer duration makes it seem worse to many addicts.

A syndrome of prolonged low-grade withdrawal (**protracted abstinence syndrome**) is described by many addicts, especially if they have stopped the drug abruptly; it may last weeks to months and is characterized by dysphoria, low energy, chronic sleep disturbance, and chronic gastrointestinal disturbance.

10. Describe the treatment for opioid withdrawal.

Opioid withdrawal does not cause seizures and is not life-threatening, although addicts may feel that it is. Addicts usually treat withdrawal with more opioid drugs; if they are not available, alcohol, barbiturates, or benzodiazepines may be used for sedation. Because cross-tolerance with such drugs is incomplete, the most effective way to alleviate opioid withdrawal is with an opioid drug; methadone is most commonly used, but there are several alternatives. Relapse rates after detoxification are high. Below are suggestions for short-term detoxification, but note that patients need long-term treatment to maintain abstinence.

Methadone. Treatment of opioid withdrawal with opioids requires a special license. Methadone may be used for short-term (days) detoxification in hospitalized patients as well as long-term detoxification (up to 6 months) in licensed treatment programs. It is hard to know the extent of a patient's addiction by self-report during withdrawal; the patient may exaggerate because of fear that the physician will not help at all. Generally the first dose should not exceed 20–30 mg, and the total dose on the first day should not exceed 40 mg. Because methadone has an average half-life of 24 hours, doses accumulate during the first 5 days; overdose is a risk without careful titration. For short-term withdrawal in the hospital, patients usually can be stabilized on 40 mg and tapered by 10–20% per day.

Clonidine. Withdrawal causes increased beta-adrenergic activity because opioids suppress the adrenergic neurons in the locus ceruleus. Clonidine, an alpha$_2$-adrenergic agonist used as an antihypertensive agent, suppresses some symptoms of withdrawal and provides some sedation. Usually the need for clonidine follows the same curve as the withdrawal symptoms; maximal doses for outpatients should not exceed 1.2 mg/day, usually prescribed as 0.1–0.2 mg every 3–4 hours. Hypotension may occur, and patients should be monitored after the first dose and daily. The hypotensive effect makes clonidine less useful for women, who generally have a lower baseline blood pressure than men.

Buprenorphine. Buprenorphine is not yet available in the U.S. except as a parenteral analgesic, but ongoing studies suggest its usefulness for opioid withdrawal as well as for maintenance treatment. It is a partial mu agonist, with a long-acting (24 hours) effect similar to that of methadone. It has several advantages over methadone: withdrawal from buprenorphine is mild and short-lived, risk of overdose is low, and induction on naltrexone is more rapid.

11. What is opioid maintenance/replacement treatment?

Although the most researched approach in the field, opioid maintenance treatment remains controversial. It has been shown repeatedly to decrease morbidity and mortality, reduce crime, and improve health and social functioning for opioid addicts. When opioid maintenance therapy is combined with adjuvant psychosocial services, outcomes are improved even further. In addition, nonopioid alternatives have not shown equal success. However, because it does not fit the "abstinence" philosophy in the treatment field, opioid maintenance treatment remains stigmatized and underused.

Opioid maintenance can be used only in specially licensed treatment programs. Federal regulations require that physiologic evidence of opioid dependence must be demonstrated before starting a patient on methadone; if a patient in seen in the emergency department or hospital, withdrawal symptoms must be carefully documented. Research has clearly shown that retention in treatment is improved and illicit opioid use is decreased if patient doses are stabilized at > 60 mg/day with an optimal range of 60–100 mg.

LAAM, a long-acting synthetic opioid, also is used in licensed treatment programs. It is taken every other day, thus reducing the need for "take-home" doses of medication. Also, buprenorphine will soon be released for use in opioid replacement treatment.

12. What complications or problems are associated with opioid maintenance treatment?

The most common side effects are constipation and sweating, but patients also may have problems with decreased libido, weight gain, fluid retention, and sexual dysfunction. Medications that induce liver enzymes may interfere with methadone metabolism; the most common examples are rifampin, carbamazepine, and dilantin. Valproic acid does not seem to interfere. Agonist-antagonist drugs such as Stadol, Talwin, or Nubain should not be prescribed for patients on methadone or LAAM, as the antagonists cause an abstinence syndrome. There is no known organ toxicity with long-term opioid administration.

13. How long should a patient stay on opioid maintenance?

Research has demonstrated that the longer a patient stays in methadone treatment, the better the prognosis and the less the risk of HIV infection. For some patients treatment may last 1 year; for others it may be life-long. Recent research showed that 80% of patients relapsed in the first year off methadone: because of the risk of HIV infection now associated with relapse, most patients are not encouraged to withdraw from methadone. "Medical maintenance" clinics have been developed to manage stable, long-term patients who receive monthly supplies of methadone at a doctor's office, similar to treatment of hypertension or other medical problems. These patients are monitored for drug use and diversion by random urine tests and random calls to bring in remaining medication for counting.

14. Should methadone maintenance be used to treat pregnant opioid addicts?

The fetus is highly affected by going in and out of withdrawal as the mother uses short-acting opioids, and the mother is less likely to obtain prenatal care. Both factors result in more complications of pregnancy and lower birth weights. Methadone maintenance is strongly indicated for the pregnant opioid addict; healthier infants are born.

Methadone doses should be high enough to keep the mother from using opioid drugs (to avoid both drug effect and risk of HIV for the fetus) but as low as possible to decrease withdrawal for the infant. Mothers already on methadone may want to decrease their dose, with slow tapering at 1–2 mg/week. Tapering is done most safely during the second trimester. Although there is no risk of seizure in adults who withdraw from opioids, it is a risk in infants, who should be closely monitored for withdrawal symptoms and treated with phenobarbital or paregoric if they occur. Note that LAAM has not been approved for use in pregnancy.

15. Describe the treatment of pain in opioid maintenance patients.

Most methadone-maintained patients develop tolerance to its analgesic effects. For injuries and surgical procedures, patients need their regular methadone dose for opioid dependence treatment as well as whatever short-acting analgesics are usually prescribed for other patients undergoing the same procedure.

Patients with chronic pain sometimes get long-term analgesia from methadone, as may patients with chronic pain and addiction problems. Few controlled studies have examined this issue in a systematic manner. Pain medications should not be withheld from any substance abuser due to fears of addiction, but relapse risk should be discussed with the patient, and a collaborative approach should be used whenever possible.

16. What is the role of naltrexone?

Naltrexone is an oral, long-acting opioid receptor antagonist that has been shown to be a successful, nonopioid treatment in certain populations. It works by blocking the opioid receptors; thus if a person tries to get high, the effect is blocked. Naltrexone has been quite successful in treating health professionals who may have easy access to opioids on the job, and it is often recommended for opioid addicts who have been incarcerated and are returning to areas where opioids are again accessible.

Patients cannot have any opioids in their system when starting naltrexone; otherwise, the drug precipitates an abstinence syndrome that may last over 24 hours. For many opioid addicts, this is the biggest difficulty with starting naltrexone: they must abstain from short-acting opioids for 5–7 days and from long-acting opioids for 10–14 days. Many patients withdraw from opioids using clonidine during this period. They then are given an injection of naloxone before starting the oral, long-acting antagonist to be sure that opioids are no longer present.

BIBLIOGRAPHY

1. Ball JC, Lange WR, Myers CP, Friedman SR: Reducing the risk of AIDS through methadone maintenance treatment. J Health Soc Behav 29:214–226, 1988.
2. Gerstein DR: The effectiveness of drug treatment. Res Publ Assoc Res Nerv Ment Dis 70:253–273, 1988.
3. McLellan AT, Arndt IO, Metger DS, et al: The effects of psychosocial services in substance abuse treatment. JAMA 269:1953–1959, 1993.
4. Novick DM, Pascarelli EF, Joseph H: Methadone maintenance patients in general medical practice. JAMA 259:3299–3302, 1988.
5. Romac DR: Safety of prolonged, high-dose infusion of naloxone hydrochloride for severe methadone overdose. Clin Pharmacol 5:251–254, 1986.
6. Wang DS, Sternbach G, Varon J: Nalmefene: A long-acting opioid antagonist. Clinical applications in emergency medicine. J Emer Med 16:471–475, 1998.

22. SEDATIVE-HYPNOTIC USE DISORDERS

Jane A. Kennedy, D.O.

1. What drugs are considered sedative-hypnotics?

Sedative-hypnotic drugs include the barbiturates, barbiturate-like drugs, and benzodiazepines. They are a diverse group of synthetic drugs with clear medical uses and may be prescribed as anxiolytics (tranquilizers), hypnotics (to induce sleep), anticonvulsant medications, and muscle relaxants. Short-acting and long-acting forms are available; all have the potential for abuse. Most are taken orally, but some may also be injected intramuscularly or intravenously. Sedative-hypnotics are extensively prescribed in the United States. Barbiturates were introduced in 1903 but for the most part have been replaced by the benzodiazepines, which were introduced in 1960.

2. Who abuses sedative-hypnotics?

Sedative-hypnotics are abused by both street addicts and patients who are receiving them by prescription. Street addicts may use them as adjuvants to boost the effect of drugs such as opioids, to take the edge off stimulants, or to help manage drug or alcohol withdrawal. Prescription addicts may use the drugs alone, seeking sedation or euphoria, but usually combine them with other substances. Community surveys estimate that about 5% of the general population have used sedative-hypnotics for nonmedical purposes; prevalence is markedly greater in certain populations, such as patients on methadone maintenance.

3. How may the physician recognize sedative-hypnotic intoxication?

Barbiturate and benzodiazepine intoxication appears similar to alcohol intoxication without the odor of alcohol on the breath. Signs and symptoms are sedation, impaired psychomotor performance, slurred speech, ataxia, nystagmus, poor memory and concentration, and labile emotions.

4. Are sedative-hypnotics lethal in overdose?

Benzodiazepines, when used alone, are remarkably safe in overdose, whereas barbiturates are quite dangerous. Barbiturates or benzodiazepines in combination with other central nervous system depressants such as alcohol may cause death via respiratory depression or hypotensive shock. Profound and protracted coma may be seen with glutethimide (Doriden), a sedative sometimes abused in combination with Tylenol #4 ("Dors and Fours").

5. Does use of sedative-hypnotics result in physiologic dependence, tolerance, and/or withdrawal?

With regular use of high doses of sedatives, **dependence** occurs after about 1 month. However, development of dependence on benzodiazepines in lower, therapeutic doses is controversial. It is now thought that dependence may occur with daily use of therapeutic doses, usually after 2–4 months, but only in a subset of patients. Low-dose dependence is primarily a withdrawal syndrome; most patients taking a therapeutic regimen do not require increasing doses for continued efficacy.

Tolerance to the sedation and the mood effects of sedative-hypnotics may lead to ingestion of larger and more frequent doses to achieve the desired psychoactive effects. However, overdoses of barbiturates can be lethal, because tolerance of respiratory depression does not occur. When benzodiazepines are taken alone, remarkably high doses are tolerated, but toxicity is significantly enhanced when other depressants are added. Most addicts are aware of the relative safety of benzodiazepines compared with barbiturates; thus, barbiturate dependence is infrequent.

Withdrawal syndromes may be severe and life-threatening. The onset varies from hours to days, according to the half-life of the drug. Signs and symptoms include tachycardia, tremor, restlessness and insomnia, diaphoresis, nausea, vomiting, anxiety and agitation, transient hallucinations, and grand mal seizure. The clinical symptoms of withdrawal from either high-dose barbiturates or benzodiazepines are similar. Less severe withdrawal may be seen with discontinuation of lower (therapeutic) doses of benzodiazepines, but the severity may be increased with the shorter-acting, more potent benzodiazepines.

6. Does regular use of sedative-hypnotics cause medical problems?

Unlike alcohol, sedative-hypnotics rarely cause direct organ toxicity. Paraldehyde and chloral hydrate, rapid-acting hypnotics, may be irritating to the throat and gastric mucosa, when taken orally, or cause necrosis if injected intramuscularly.

7. Are Quaaludes still abused?

Methaqualone was removed from the market in the U.S. around 1980, but it is still available on the street in certain regions. Marketed originally as a "nonaddictive" sedative, it was widely abused, produced dependence, and was associated with lethal overdose as well as serious withdrawal syndromes. Unusual overdose symptoms include muscular hypertonicity, shivering, myoclonus, seizures, and excessive salivation and bronchial secretions, which may compromise the airway. Methaqualone was falsely rumored to be an aphrodisiac; abusers felt a pleasant high along with contentment.

8. Are muscle relaxants addictive?

Muscle relaxants may be abused, usually for their sedative properties. Grand mal seizures have been seen in patients who abruptly discontinue carisoprodol (Soma), because a metabolite of Soma is meprobamate, a barbiturate-like drug.

9. What is the treatment for sedative-hypnotic withdrawal?

Some patients who take prescribed lower doses become physiologically dependent even without abusing the drug for psychoactive effects. This problem is *not* considered an addiction, and the drug can be tapered over several weeks on an outpatient basis, with careful monitoring and patient-physician communication.

Patients who abuse a sedative-hypnotic should be stabilized on an oral, long-acting barbiturate, such as phenobarbital, or benzodiazepine, such as chlorazepate (Tranxene). After stabilization, the dose is tapered. Optimally, the initial period of withdrawal should occur in the hospital. This approach allows supervision of the patient in case of intoxication or severe withdrawal symptoms, such as seizure, and prevents the patient from using other drugs or alcohol during withdrawal. Use of valproic acid or carbamazepine may allow a more rapid taper without fear of withdrawal seizures, and open trials appear promising.

Hospitalization is not always possible, and sometimes benzodiazepine detoxification is accomplished on an outpatient basis with strict monitoring. Patients must be well-motivated or have strong contingent consequences; they should be seen on a daily basis and receive medication daily. Whenever possible, avoid using the abused substance for the taper, because craving and other conditioned behaviors may create difficulties.

BIBLIOGRAPHY

1. Pages KP, Ries RK: Use of anticonvulsants in benzodiazepine withdrawal. Am J Addict 7(3):198–204, 1998.
2. Perry PJ, Alexander B: Sedative/hypnotic dependence: Patient stabilization, tolerance testing, and withdrawal. Drug Intell Clin Pharm 20:532–537, 1986.
3. Seivewright N, Dougal W: Withdrawal symptoms from high dose benzodiazepines in poly drug abusers. Drug Alcohol Depend 32:15–23, 1993.

23. COCAINE AND AMPHETAMINE USE DISORDERS

Jane A. Kennedy, D.O.

1. Who uses cocaine and amphetamine?

Cocaine use in the United States has escalated dramatically since the early 1970s, when about 5 million had tried the drug at least once—in the late 1980s, about 40 million had tried it. Cocaine typically is used by persons aged 18–30. In the 1990s, indicators suggested a drop in cocaine use among casual, recreational users, but sustained or increased prevalence among hard-core users.

Amphetamine use is highest among 18–25 year olds; in some parts of the country it is strongly associated with motorcycle gang members. Since tightened regulation of prescription amphetamine in the late 1970s, only about 25% of abused amphetamine is prescription drug; the other 75% is illicitly manufactured.

2. Do cocaine and amphetamine have the same effect?

In recent years attention has focused on cocaine dependence, because its use is more widespread than use of amphetamines. Both drugs, however, increase the central action of dopamine and both the central and peripheral action of norepinephrine. In theory, they should be quite similar in effect, but most users have a distinct preference for either cocaine or amphetamine. Both drugs are quite reinforcing. Animals will self-administer stimulants continuously until they die, forsaking food and water and suffering repeated seizures and exhaustion; for many humans, similar effects have been seen.

3. What forms are available? What are the routes of administration?

Amphetamine is available in oral prescription medication as dextroamphetamine and methamphetamine; it also is manufactured illicitly as powder or crystallized ("ice") methamphetamine. Cocaine hydrochloride is obtainable pharmaceutically for use as a local anesthetic; it is available illicitly in either powder or crystallized ("rock" or "crack") forms.

Cocaine and amphetamine are snorted, injected, and smoked; amphetamines also may be taken orally. "Crack" is the smokable form of cocaine, and "ice" is the smokable form of amphetamine. Smoking is the most rapid route of delivery to the brain and thus the most reinforcing; however, dependence can occur with all routes of administration. A stimulant and a depressant injected together, most frequently cocaine and heroin, is called a "speedball."

4. Do stimulants have approved medical uses?

Cocaine hydrochloride is used as a local anesthetic; use of amphetamines such as dexedrine or methylphenidate has been limited to treatment of attention deficit hyperactivity disorder, narcolepsy, and resistant depression.

5. What are the signs and symptoms of stimulant intoxication?

The most common signs and symptoms are enlarged pupils, tachycardia, hypertension, and hyperreflexia. The user feels euphoric, energetic, talkative, alert, and grandiose, with decreased appetite and need for sleep. Some people, however, feel anxious, agitated, tense, and dysphoric. Still others feel calmed, slowed down, and focused. Stomach cramps, nausea, vomiting, and diarrhea may occur. Many users clench and grind their teeth.

Higher doses and more chronic use frequently lead to psychosis, usually with a paranoid quality. Reactions may range from "tweaking," a sense of hypervigilance and fearfulness (small noises may be interpreted as police outside the door), to overt psychosis with auditory and visual hallucinations, ideas of reference, and full-blown delusions.

Stimulants often induce stereotypic behaviors such as repetitive counting or cleaning, prolonged sexual activity, or picking at the skin ("cocaine bugs") due to formication (a sensation of insects crawling on the skin).

6. What is the duration of effect from cocaine and amphetamine?

Cocaine's rapid, short-lived "rush" of 15–20 minutes contrasts with the sustained effect of amphetamine, which may last for hours. The high associated with "ice" (smokable amphetamine) may last up to 48 hours and can be associated with prolonged psychosis and aggression.

7. Does tolerance occur?

Tolerance occurs to euphoria, wakefulness, anorexia, and possibly to convulsant and cardiovascular effects. Users may increase frequency of dosing intervals and quantities as they try to reproduce the euphoria.

8. Discuss the complications of stimulant use.

Sympathomimetic responses include decreased gastrointestinal motility, bladder stimulation resulting in painful urination, tachycardia with tachyarrhythmias, hypertension (hypotension also has been reported), and fever. Increased stimulation of the central nervous system may cause seizure. Other complications include cardiac ischemia, coronary artery constriction with angina or myocardial infarction, stroke, and cardiac or respiratory arrest. Cerebral and renal vasculitis are more common with amphetamines.

Although psychosis usually clears within days of stopping stimulant use, in some instances the psychosis persists, or the user develops a sustained sensitivity to its recurrence, even with small doses of amphetamine or cocaine. Panic disorder also may be precipitated by cocaine and persist even after use is discontinued. Bipolar patients may become manic with use of stimulants.

Other complications depend on route of administration. Intravenous use is associated with transmission of the human immunodeficiency virus (HIV), hepatitis, and endocarditis. Nosebleeds, nasal septum irritation or perforation, and sinusitis may result from nasal insufflation, and pulmonary complications such as cough, bronchitis, and pneumothorax may result from smoking. In addition, marked weight loss and malnutrition may occur during a "run," when many users go for days without eating. Use of sedatives to help with insomnia and "crashing" may create a secondary drug dependence.

Sexual promiscuity, due either to increased sexual interest or to exchanging sex for money or drugs, may put the user at high risk for sexually transmitted diseases, especially HIV infection.

9. What happens with overdose?

Death may occur from seizures, severe fever, cerebrovascular hemorrhage, or cardiovascular arrest. Treatment of overdose is supportive; seizures respond to diazepam, and psychosis may require antipsychotic medication.

10. Is there a stimulant withdrawal syndrome?

Many users experience only fatigue and exhaustion, and sleep for 12–24 hours. For others, dysphoria may be severe and associated with suicidal ideation. Increased appetite, insomnia, vivid dreams, and psychomotor retardation or agitation also may be seen. Some users experience protracted depression, which may respond to antidepressants.

Treatment of withdrawal, especially the re-emergence of craving for the drug, has been attempted with the use of dopamine agonists such as bromocriptine or amantadine. Open studies looked promising, but controlled trials have reported marginal results or have not supported their efficacy. Similarly, amino acid precursors of catecholamines have not proved to be useful.

11. What are the effects of stimulant use in pregnancy?

Vasoconstrictive properties of stimulants lead to decreased blood flow to the placenta and thus decreased oxygen delivery to the fetus. At the very least, infants have low birth weights; children also have been reported to have central nervous system hyperactivity in the first year of life, with irritability, jumpiness, hyperreflexia, and decreased attention spans. The incidence of abruptio placentae, premature delivery, sudden infant death syndrome, and cerebral hemorrhage is increased. Lower IQ levels were found in 4-year-old children exposed to amphetamines in utero.

12. What are the pharmacologic treatments of cocaine dependence?

Multiple medications have been tried without success; open trials frequently appear promising, but controlled studies show no efficacy. Desipramine, which appeared to increase abstinence from cocaine in controlled trials, has not shown the same effectiveness in repeat studies. Carbamazepine also appeared promising in open trials but did not hold up under randomized, controlled conditions. Buproprion, fluoxetine, flupenthixol, imipramine, levodopa/carbidopa, maprotiline, and trazodone also have been tried without effect. Buprenorphine, an opiate agonist-antagonist, was found to decrease cocaine use in methadone maintenance patients, but a controlled study did not replicate this finding. A cocaine vaccine, administration of an enzyme that metabolizes cocaine, and catalytic antibodies are currently being investigated.

13. What other treatments are useful for cocaine addiction?

The most successful approach has been **behavioral contracting** with positive reinforcement for negative urine screens. Compared with patients randomized to 12-step group treatment, retention was significantly better (58% vs. 11%), as was abstinence (42% vs. 5%).[2] More frequent contact (at least twice weekly) has been associated with improved outcome, and Kang et al. showed that once weekly therapy was ineffective, whether it was group, family, or individual psychotherapy.

BIBLIOGRAPHY

1. Delaney-Black V, Roumell N, Shankaran S, Bedard M: Maternal cocaine use and infant outcomes [abstract]. Pediatr Res 25:242A, 1990.
2. Higgins ST, Budney AJ, Bickel WK, Foerg FE, Donham R, Badger MS: Incentives improve outcome in outpatient behavioral treatment of cocaine dependence. Arch Gen Psychiatry 51:568–576, 1994.
3. Higgins ST, Katz JL: Cocaine Abuse: Behavior, Pharmacology, and Clinical Applications. San Diego, Academic Press, 1998.
4. Kang S-Y, Kleinman PH, Woody GE, et al: Outcomes for cocaine abusers after once-a-week psychosocial therapy. Am J Psychiatry 148:630–635, 1991.
5. Weddington WW, Brown BS, Haertzen CA, et al: Comparison of amantadine and desipramine combined with psychotherapy for treatment of cocaine dependence. Am J Drug Alcohol Abuse 17:137–152, 1991.

24. MARIJUANA, HALLUCINOGENS, PHENCYCLIDINE, AND INHALANTS

Jane A. Kennedy, D.O.

1. What is marijuana?

Marijuana is obtained from the cut and dried upper leaves, flowers, and stems of the cannabis plant. Its main psychoactive ingredient is delta-9-tetrahydrocannabinol (THC). The potency of THC in marijuana cigarettes varies greatly (1–15%), but has increased 15- to 30-fold since the 1970s. Hashish is obtained from dried resin secreted on the flowering tops (10–20% THC), and hashish oil is extracted with the use of organic solvents (15–30% THC).

2. Who uses marijuana?

Marijuana, the most widely used illicit drug in the U.S., is often said to be a gateway drug for teens, but it also has been used socially for many years by adults. About one-third of the U.S. population has used marijuana, and in the age range of 18–25 years, about 60% have used it at least once.

3. How is marijuana taken?

Marijuana usually is prepared from dried leaves and flowers and smoked as a cigarette or in a pipe, although in some parts of the world it is taken in tea. It also may be eaten orally, commonly in brownies; the euphoria is less intense but longer lasting. Because extracts are not water-soluble, marijuana is not used intravenously.

4. What are the psychological and physical effects of marijuana?

A person may feel euphoric, giddy with uncontrollable laughter, talkative, or sedated, and sensory perceptions may be enhanced. Short-term memory, attention span, and judgment are impaired; difficulty with abstract thinking and time distortion also occur. Anxiety, panic, paranoia, and dysphoria can result, and daily users may have chronic depression, irritability, and lethargy. Cannabis-induced psychosis has been reported but may be secondary to underlying psychotic disorder. "Red eyes" or conjunctival injection are a good clue of recent marijuana use. Common physical symptoms are increased heart rate, increased appetite, and dry mouth. Motor performance may be impaired for up to 10 hours after use. The effect of smoking marijuana peaks within 10–30 minutes, and intoxication may last several hours, depending on the dose. The effect of oral ingestion peaks within 45–60 minutes.

5. What are the medical consequences of marijuana use?

Decreases in sperm count, testosterone levels, and luteinizing hormone have been reported. Pulmonary complications, such as chronic cough, bronchitis, and chronic obstructive pulmonary disease, are seen; however, because most marijuana smokers also are cigarette smokers, it is difficult to lay blame on marijuana. The carcinogens in cigarettes also are present in marijuana, but in *increased* amounts; thus the risk for malignancy may be increased.

6. What are the medical uses for THC?

THC has been used to treat glaucoma (by lowering intraocular pressure), nausea and vomiting caused by chemotherapy, weight loss problems in patients with acquired immunodeficiency syndrome, and muscle spasm in multiple sclerosis. In general, THC has not been shown to be more efficacious than available prescription medications, and many patients do not like the psychoactive effect. Medical use of cannabinoids is an active focus of research, including a delivery system other than smoking, which has known harmful effects.

7. Is tolerance or withdrawal associated with marijuana?

Most chronic users report tolerance to the euphoric effects and a need for increased frequency or increased amount of marijuana to get the same effect. A withdrawal reaction has been reported with chronic use of very high doses, but it is rare and is not listed as a diagnosis in DSM-IV.

8. How long does THC stay in the urine?

THC is fat-soluble and is excreted slowly. Casual users may have a positive urine screen for 5–10 days and chronic users for up to 30 days.

9. What is the amotivational syndrome?

The amotivational syndrome has been described in several countries and several age groups of marijuana users, but in the U.S. it has been applied mainly to adolescents. Symptoms are apathy, disinterest, fatigue, and decrease in goal-directed activities. The syndrome has not been well researched and may not exist.

10. Is marijuana a gateway drug that leads to other drug use?

Possibly. A study of young men in Manhattan noted that of those who had not smoked marijuana, < 1% progressed to cocaine or heroin, whereas of those who were heavy marijuana users (> 1000 times), 82% used cocaine and 33% used heroin. It is unlikely that marijuana *causes* further drug use, but it may expose the young users to drug experience, risk-taking behavior, and people who use other drugs.

11. What are hallucinogens?

Hallucinogens are said to produce sensory hallucinations without causing delirium or cognitive impairment; the hallucinations may be auditory, visual, olfactory, tactile, or gustatory. Often what is actually experienced is an illusion (distortion of an actual sensory perception) rather than a hallucination.

12. What is LSD?

Lysergic acid diethylamide (LSD) or "acid" is a synthetic hallucinogen.

13. Who uses LSD?

Data from the 1998 household survey revealed that about 10% of the population had used LSD at least once in their lifetime—1.6% in the last year, and 0.7% in the past month. Recent use was most common in 18–25 year olds. In 1997, 14% of high school seniors reported using at least once. Whites were twice as likely to use either drug as African-Americans, and 1992 data from emergency departments revealed that over half of the LSD-related emergency visits were adolescents age 10–19 years.

14. How is LSD taken?

LSD is usually taken orally, although it may be absorbed through the skin, dropped in the eyes, or injected intravenously.

15. What are the intoxication effects of LSD?

Onset of effects begins in about 30 minutes, peaks at 2–3 hours and lasts about 8–12 hours. Effects are dose related. Perceptual and psychic changes occur, although the person usually recognizes that such changes are drug-induced. Effects may include depersonalization and derealization, a dreamlike state, illusions (melting face), synesthesias ("hearing" a color), intensification of sound and color, and prolonged afterimages ("trails"). A person feels excitation, distorted sense of time, peacefulness, or delusions, such as being able to fly. Hallucinations often are visual geometric figures; auditory hallucinations are rare. "Bad trips," which include anxiety, fear of insanity, suicidal depression, and panic attacks, may occur in anyone (even people who have "good trips"). Injuries can occur from delusional behavior, such as trying to fly.

Physical symptoms such as dizziness, weakness, motor restlessness, or nausea may occur initially, along with stimulant-like signs such as increased blood pressure and heart rate, fever, and dilated pupils. Sweating, tremors, incoordination, hyperreflexia, and blurred vision also may be present.

16. Is tolerance or withdrawal associated with LSD?
Tolerance to euphoria and perceptual experiences occurs rapidly (within a few days) with daily use, and most users report that they must wait several days between "trips" because of tolerance. Cross-tolerance exists with mescaline and psilocybin, but not with PCP. A withdrawal syndrome has not been identified, and animal studies show that LSD is not a highly reinforcing drug. Users rarely report compulsion or loss of control with LSD.

17. What are "flashbacks"?
Called **hallucinogen persisting perception disorder** in DSM-IV, flashbacks are transient, distressful reexperiencing of hallucinogenic effects during abstinence. Usually the flashback is a visual distortion (illusion) or actual hallucination, such as shadows, colored or geometric objects, macropsia or micropsia, intensified color, halos, or afterimages. It generally is unpleasant and frightening. Flashbacks usually stop after several months of abstinence, but can last for years in some patients.

18. What are the adverse effects of LSD?
Overdose has not been a problem, but patients may present to the emergency department with a "bad trip" (agitation and fear) or with injuries secondary to impaired judgment or delusions, such as trying to fly out of a second-story window. Bad trips usually are treated with a quiet room, low sensory stimulation, and "talking down" with support and reassurance. A benzodiazepine may be useful, especially with extreme anxiety and panic.

A prolonged psychotic state may be associated with hallucinogens such as LSD and PCP, as well as with stimulants and even cannabis. Whether this state is drug-induced or an unmasking of preexisting psychotic illness remains controversial; sometimes it responds to antipsychotic medication. Persistent auditory or visual hallucinations also may respond to carbamazepine.

19. What other hallucinogens are abused?
Similar symptoms and problems are seen with other hallucinogens; many have both amphetamine and hallucinogenic actions. Morning glory seeds and Hawaiian baby woodrose contain LSD derivatives, and the spices nutmeg and mace contain a substance related to methylene dioxyamphetamine (MDA). Mescaline from the peyote cactus, psilocybin from Mexican mushrooms ("magic mushrooms"), and bufotenin from toad skin are other natural hallucinogens.

20. What is "ecstasy"?
3,4-Methylene dimethylamphetamine (MDMA) is a synthetic substance called ecstasy, E, XTC, X, or Adam. Along with other "designer drugs," ecstasy has been popular at "raves," which are all-night dances in large warehouses with high-tech music and videos. MDMA may be taken as a pill or suppository, snorted as powder, or injected intravenously. Physically it has amphetamine-like effects; psychoactive effects include feelings of euphoria, spirituality, personal insight, and desire for intimacy. Fatal overdose has occurred as well as severe psychotic reactions, and animal studies suggest direct toxicity to serotonergic neurons.

21. What is phencyclidine?
Phencyclidine (PCP), also called angel dust, sherm, or embalming fluid, was synthesized for use as a general anesthetic in the 1950s but was discontinued because of side effects such as delirium, agitation, hallucinations, and psychotic reactions. It also was used as an anesthetic for animals (thus the street names animal or horse tranquilizer), but this use also has been discontinued.

22. Who uses PCP?
PCP is most commonly used in large cities such as Los Angeles, St. Louis, New York, and Washington, DC. It is most popular with black or Hispanic men in their 20s.

23. How is PCP used? What are its effects?
Most frequently cigarettes (tobacco, marijuana, mint, oregano) are dropped in PCP and smoked, but PCP also may be taken orally, intravenously, or by nasal insufflation. Physical symptoms include

elevation in blood pressure and body temperature, muscle rigidity, decreased pain sensation, and dilated pupils with both horizontal and vertical nystagmus. The psychoactive effect is euphoria and sometimes aggressive behavior. "Bad trips" are best treated with diazepam or neuroleptics with low anticholinergic profiles; restraints should be avoided because rhabdomyolysis has been reported.

24. What is ketamine?

Ketamine is a dissociative anesthetic that is used medically; it is a derivative of PCP with similar chemical structure and activity. Ketamine is occasionally abused, usually by health professionals with easy access.

25. What are inhalants?

Volatile substances such as gasoline, glue, spray paint, solvents, and lighter fluids are inhaled ("sniffed, huffed"). They are inexpensive, easily accessible, and legal.

26. Who uses inhalants?

About 20% of high school seniors in the U.S. have tried inhalants, and increasing numbers of children age 9–12 have been reported to experiment with their use. Although inhalant abusers are usually under 20 years old, emergency department visits among people 26 years and older have increased to 38% of total visits for inhalants. Whites, Native Americans, and Hispanics tend to use inhalants more than African Americans, and users are predominantly male. Although many inhalant users are experimenters or polysubstance abusers, a recent study showed that inhalant abusers were more than 5 times more likely to become intravenous drug users than non-inhalant users.

27. What are the effects of inhalants?

A rapid-onset (seconds to minutes) and short-lived euphoria occurs with inhalation of volatile substances. The user feels excitement, disinhibition, light-headedness, and confusion. Hallucinations may occur as well as nausea, vomiting, headache, and blurred vision. There may be a rash around the nose and mouth, and the person's clothes, skin, or breath may smell of solvents.

28. What are the complications of inhalants?

- Risk of sudden death due to cardiac arrhythmia, laryngospasm or asphyxiation
- Neurologic damage (in chronic users), with abnormal electroencephalogram, cerebellar degeneration, intellectual impairment, and dementia
- Impaired motor responses
- Memory loss
- Renal and hepatic toxicity
- Bone marrow suppression
- Pulmonary complications (chemical pneumonitis and emphysema in chronic users)

29. What is GHB?

Gamma hydroxybutyrate is a neurotransmitter that affects a variety of systems, including sleep cycles, temperature regulation, and memory. Outside of the U.S., it has been used therapeutically in anesthesia, for narcolepsy, and to treat alcohol and opioid dependence. It also is a drug of abuse, as in low doses it gives mild euphoria, disinhibition, and increased libido, and in high doses, feelings of sedation. Aggression, judgment impairment, and violent combativeness have been seen, as well as ataxia, dizziness, nystagmus, respiratory depression, apnea, coma, and death.

30. Describe the treatment for abuse of marijuana, hallucinogens, PCP, inhalants, ecstasy, or GHB.

Treatments have not been well studied. Users rarely seek treatment on their own and are usually under court order. Currently, little knowledge is available to guide treatment of these drug disorders. Most patients are young, and family participation is strongly encouraged. Most treatment approaches have aimed at achieving abstinence through support, limit-setting, and reinforcement techniques. Relapse prevention includes decreasing availability and acceptability of drug use.

BIBLIOGRAPHY

1. Crowley TJ: Learning and unlearning abuse in the real world: Clinical treatment and public policy. NIDA Research Monograph No. 84. Washington, DC, U.S. Government Printing Office, 1988, pp 100–121.
2. Clayton RR, Voss HL: Young men and drugs in Manhattan: A causal analysis. NIDA Research Monograph No. 39. Washington, DC, U.S. Government Printing Office, 1981.
3. Dinwiddie SH: Abuse of inhalants: A review. Addiction 89:925–939, 1994.
4. Li J, Stokes SA, Woeckener A: A tale of novel intoxication: A review of the effects of γ-hydroxybutyric acid with recommendations for management. Ann Emerg Med 31:729–736, 1998.
5. Millman RB, Sbriglio R: Patterns of use and psychopathology in chronic marijuana users. Psychiatr Clin North Am 9:533–545, 1986.
6. Schutz CG, Chilcoat HD, Anthony JC: The association between sniffing inhalants and injecting drugs. Compr Psychiatry 35:99–105, 1994.
7. Solowij N: Ecstasy (3,4-methylenedioxymethamphetamine). Curr Opin Psychiatry 6:411–415, 1993.
8. Steele TD, McCann UD, Ricaurte GA: 3,4-Methylenedioxymethamphetamine (MDMA, "Ecstasy"): Pharmacology and toxicology in animals and humans. Addiction 89:539–551, 1994.

25. DUAL DIAGNOSIS: SUBSTANCE ABUSE AND PSYCHIATRIC ILLNESS

S. Tziporah Cohen, M.D., and Alan M. Jacobson, M.D.

1. What is meant by the term dual diagnosis?

It describes patients who have both a substance use disorder and another major psychiatric disorder. Examples include a cocaine-dependent patient with panic disorder and an alcoholic patient with major depression. The term is used to highlight the difference between such patients and patients with a single diagnosis; patients with a dual diagnosis have special diagnosis and treatment needs. Although dual diagnosis refers to all patients with concomitant diagnoses of substance abuse and other psychiatric illness, the population is highly heterogeneous. Both of the patients mentioned above, for example, have dual diagnoses, but their disorders may require very different treatments.

2. Is dual diagnosis common?

Yes. Dual diagnosis is extremely common and often unrecognized. Of patients with a substance use disorder, approximately 50% have at least one other psychiatric disorder, most commonly a mood or anxiety disorder. Conversely, almost 30% of patients with other psychiatric disorders also have a history of substance abuse.

3. Why is it important to determine whether a patient has both a substance use and another psychiatric disorder?

The importance of identifying substance abuse in a patient with a psychiatric disorder cannot be overstated. In general, patients with a dual diagnosis have higher morbidity, lower likelihood for initial treatment success, higher relapse rates, increased rates of hospitalization, and decreased adherence to treatment. They also are at increased risk for suicide. The presence of substance abuse makes diagnosis of both disorders more complicated. For treatment of either disorder to be successful, both must be identified and treated individually.

4. Do certain psychiatric conditions tend to be seen with substance abuse?

Yes. Antisocial personality disorder is highly correlated with substance abuse. In one extensive study, 84% of individuals with antisocial personality disorder also had a history of substance abuse. Mood disorders also are commonly associated with substance abuse; in the same study, 32% of individuals with a diagnosis of mood disorder were substance abusers. In addition, specific psychiatric disorders are associated with *specific* drugs of abuse, such as bipolar disorder with alcohol and panic disorder with sedatives and hypnotics.

5. What is the cause of dual diagnosis?

Many mechanisms have been proposed to explain the co-occurrence of a substance use disorder and another psychiatric illness, but no evidence suggests that any one mechanism is the only possible explanation.

• **Psychopathology may serve as a risk factor for addictive disorders or may affect the course of an addictive disorder.** For example, a 32-year-old woman with a severe social phobia found that alcohol relieved her anxiety enough to allow her to function at her job. With repeated use, however, she became dependent on alcohol. Withdrawal symptoms led to more anxiety, which led to more drinking, and eventually she developed full-blown alcohol addiction. A second example is a 26-year-old male alcoholic with bipolar disorder who had periods of abstinence for as long as 6 months. However, each time he entered a manic episode, he stopped going to Alcoholics Anonymous meetings and began drinking again.

• **There may be familial (genetic) links between certain psychiatric disorders and substance use disorders.** For example, a 40-year-old man with a history of alcoholism was diagnosed with major depression. Family history showed that his mother had been dependent on alcohol in her early thirties and had recently had a depressive episode. His maternal grandmother also had a history of depression. His maternal uncle had been an alcoholic and committed suicide at age 38. The patient's sister had been diagnosed with major depression in college.

• **Psychiatric symptoms may develop in the course of chronic intoxication with an abused substance.** For example, a 55-year-old man who had been smoking marijuana almost daily for several years developed depressive symptoms as well as paranoid ideation. The symptoms disappeared when he stopped using marijuana.

• **Psychiatric disorders may emerge as a consequence of substance use and persist after remission.** For example, a 30-year-old woman with no history of psychiatric illness began using cocaine. After almost a year of use, she began having occasional panic attacks when high. After several more months, the attacks occurred in between cocaine highs. Years later, despite having been drug-free for 6 months, the panic attacks continued. They were successfully treated with paroxetine.

• **The occurrence of both disorders in the same individual is pure coincidence.** Because both mental illness and substance abuse are highly prevalent in the general population, an individual may have both a substance use disorder and a psychiatric disorder by chance, just as one individual may have both asthma and migraine headaches.

6. What is the self-medication hypothesis?

The self-medication hypothesis holds that substance abuse occurs when an individual attempts to self-medicate his or her psychiatric symptoms. This hypothesis is based on a small group of drug abusers and has not been validated experimentally. The theory holds that patients do not abuse drugs randomly; rather, they discover a drug that relieves painful feelings and thereby serves as a coping mechanism. Repetitive use of the drug as self-medication eventually may lead to dependence. Even after treatment of the psychiatric disorder, the addiction may persist and require independent treatment. For example, a 24-year-old man, who describes himself as having been depressed all of his life, tried heroin at a party and said that for the first time he felt relief from emotional distress. Soon he was using heroin daily and needed increasing amounts to get the same relief.

7. Can certain psychiatric symptoms be confused with intoxication or withdrawal symptoms?

Absolutely. Many psychiatric symptoms can be caused by substance use or withdrawal. For example, depressive symptoms such as insomnia, decreased libido, anhedonia, and suicidality often are seen with chronic alcoholism and marijuana use and may be indistinguishable from a major depressive episode. Manic symptoms, such as euphoria, inflated self-esteem, and decreased need for sleep, may occur during cocaine intoxication.

Psychiatric Symptoms Associated with Substance Abuse

SUBSTANCE	PSYCHIATRIC SYMPTOMS DURING INTOXICATION	PSYCHIATRIC SYMPTOMS DURING WITHDRAWAL
Alcohol	Anxiety, depression, sudden mood changes, paranoia, suicidality, memory loss	Hallucinations (delirium tremens, alcohol hallucinosis) anxiety, insomnia, psychomotor agitation
Cocaine	Mania, acute paranoid ideation, panic attacks	Depression, anhedonia, anxiety
Stimulants	Mania, paranoia, nightmares	Dysphoria, psychomotor retardation, irritability, guilt, suicidality
Inhalants	Anxiety, personality changes	Anxiety, depression
Cannabis	Anxiety, paranoid ideation, suicidality	
Opioids	Panic reactions, lethargy	Depression
Depressants	Depression, anxiety, paranoia, psychosis	Insomnia, irritability, psychomotor agitation
Hallucinogens	Hallucinations, paranoia, depersonalization, confusion	Flashbacks (may occur years after last use)

8. Can substance abuse cause mental illness?

Yes. Substance abuse may induce psychiatric disorders that persist even after drug use is discontinued. For example, some cocaine abusers develop panic attacks. Initially the attacks occur solely during cocaine intoxication, but with time they may occur between cocaine highs and even persist after complete cessation of drug use. These attacks often can be treated successfully with SSRIs or other treatments for panic disorder. Certain hallucinogens, such as lysergic acid diethylamide (LSD), may cause perceptual disturbances or visual hallucinations that continue for years after last use. The term **posthallucinogen perceptual disorder** has been coined to describe the occurrence of such disturbances, traditionally called flashbacks. Substance abuse also may exacerbate another already present but unrecognized psychiatric disorder. In this case the substance abuse does not cause the disorder, but rather makes it clinically apparent.

9. How can I tell whether a patient's psychiatric symptoms are caused by substance abuse?

Timing, timing, timing! It is crucial to assess mental illness only after a period of abstinence, so that diagnosis is not confounded by drug intoxication mimicking psychiatric symptoms. How long the drug-free period must last before an accurate psychiatric diagnosis can be made depends on both the drug and the suspected disorder. Generally it is recommended that the patient be drug-free for 2–4 weeks. A good history, from both the patient and family members, is crucial to understanding the clinical picture. A good history or prior familiarity with the patient also can help sort out confusing symptoms and make quicker diagnoses.

10. Do patients with a dual diagnosis need special treatment?

Yes and no. The most important issue is the need to treat *both* disorders. Treatment that minimizes the importance of either diagnosis results in unnecessarily high rates of relapse. Patients should be educated about both diagnoses and how they interact.

Several treatment settings and methods are available to treat the substance-abusing psychiatric patient. **Inpatient hospitalization** may take place in a dual-diagnosis treatment unit, a substance abuse treatment unit, or a psychiatric treatment unit. **Dual-diagnosis units** are the ideal setting, but they are not always available. Patients can be adequately treated in other settings, provided that the clinicians involved in their care are knowledgeable about their special needs. **Outpatient programs** are becoming more common and may involve intensive treatment that includes medication management, support groups, psychotherapy, self-help groups, and social services.

Generally, patients leaving inpatient treatment should continue treatment as outpatients, as abstinence requires long-term monitoring and support. Patients referred to outpatient programs from inpatient treatment are likely to stay in treatment longer than those patients who are referred as outpatients.

11. What is the role of psychotropic medications?

Pharmacotherapy is not only appropriate in certain patients with dual diagnoses; it often is necessary (as in some patients with psychiatric illness alone). While most medications are directed at the coexisting psychiatric disorder, a few are directed at substance use disorder. Naltrexone hydrochloride, an opioid antagonist, has been shown to decrease relapse rates in alcohol-dependent patients by half as compared to placebo. Desipramine, a tricyclic antidepressant (TCA), has been used to decrease cocaine cravings in some patients.

12. What should be considered when prescribing medication for substance abusers?

Several issues require special attention. Many drugs of abuse interact with psychotropic medications. Abused substances may increase or decrease the metabolism of certain medications via the induction of hepatic enzymes or a change in plasma protein binding. They can lower or raise plasma levels, resulting in decreased efficacy or dangerous side effects. Such interactions must be considered when prescribing medications for a substance-abusing patient or a patient with substance-abusing potential.

Certain medications, such as benzodiazepines, are addictive in and of themselves, and their potential for abuse in patients with substance abuse histories is increased. Although such medications are often necessary, clinicians should prescribe the least habit-forming option that is efficacious. For example, a patient with panic disorder may be treated with a TCA rather than an anxiolytic, which has a higher addictive potential.

Interactions Between Drugs of Abuse and Psychotropic Medications

DRUG OF ABUSE	THERAPEUTIC AGENT	POSSIBLE INTERACTIONS
Alcohol	Disulfiram (Antabuse)	Flushing, hypotension, nausea, tachycardia; fatal reactions
	MAO inhibitors	Dangerous, possibly fatal hypertension due to impaired hepatic metabolism of tyramine
	TCAs	Additive CNS impairment
	Antipsychotics	Increased CNS impairment on psychomotor skills, judgment, and behavior; increased risk of akathisia and dystonia
	Anticonvulsants	Induction of hepatic microsomal enzymes, reducing phenytoin levels; seizure risk
Barbiturates	TCAs	Reduced efficacy of tricyclics; may potentiate respiratory depression
	MAO inhibitors	Inhibited barbiturate metabolism, prolonging intoxication
	Antipsychotics	Induced hepatic microsomal enzymes may reduce chlorpromazine levels
	Anticonvulsants	Valproic acid increases phenobarbital levels and toxicity; induced hepatic microsomal enzymes may reduce carbamazepine levels and result in unpredictable phenytoin levels
Benzodiazepines	Disulfiram	Enhanced benzodiazepine effects (oxazepam and lorazepam not affected)
	MAO inhibitors	Rare reports of edema with chlordiazepoxide
Opiates	MAO inhibitors	Meperidine—severe excitation, diaphoresis, rigidity, hyper/hypotension, coma; death
	Antipsychotics	Meperidine and chlorpromazine—hypotension and excessive CNS depression
	Anticonvulsants	Propoxyphene increases carbamazepine levels with risk of toxicity; methadone metabolism may be increased by carbamazepine or phenytoin, causing withdrawal

Table continued on following page

Interactions Between Drugs of Abuse and Psychotropic Medications (Continued)

DRUG OF ABUSE	THERAPEUTIC AGENT	POSSIBLE INTERACTIONS
Stimulants	MAO inhibitors	Hyperpyrexia, severe hypertension, death when used with cocaine or amphetamines
	Antipsychotics	Cocaine and amphetamines may cause delusions and hallucinations of chronic psychoses to break through antipsychotics

MAO = monoamine oxidase, TCAs = tricyclic antidepressants, CNS = central nervous system.
Adapted from Gastfriend DR: Pharmacotherapy of psychiatric syndromes with comorbid chemical dependence. J Addict Dis 12(3):155–170, 1993; with permission.

13. Is psychotherapy helpful in treating patients with a dual diagnosis?

Psychotherapy, particularly supportive-expressive or cognitive-behavioral models, has been shown to be useful in treating patients with substance use disorders and psychiatric illness, although its efficacy depends on the specific psychiatric disorder and the drug of abuse. Patients with comorbid mood and anxiety disorders tend to benefit from psychotherapy more than patients with personality disorders. In general, psychotherapy provides support for continued abstinence as well as adherence to medication regimens. It also addresses underlying emotional states, such as depression or anxiety, that may contribute to the maintenance of substance abuse.

14. What is the role of self-help groups, such as Alcoholics Anonymous or Narcotics Anonymous?

Twelve-step groups such as Alcoholics Anonymous, Cocaine Anonymous, and Narcotics Anonymous are known to contribute successfully to the maintenance of abstinence in substance-abusing patients. Although they may be helpful for patients with dual diagnoses, they do not address issues specific to this population, such as use of psychotropic medications or difficulties in living with mental illness. Self-help groups especially for patients with a dual diagnosis may better address such concerns, but because of the heterogeneity of the population, patients may not feel that they have much in common with other participants. For some patients, however, such groups are invaluable tools, and participation should be encouraged on an individual basis.

BIBLIOGRAPHY

1. Abraham HD, Aldridge AM: Adverse consequences of lysergic acid diethylamide. Addiction 83:1327–1334, 1993.
2. Bell CM, Khantzian EJ: Drug use and addiction as self medication: A psychodynamic perspective. In Gold MS, Slaby AE: Dual Diagnosis and Substance Abuse. New York, Marcel Dekker, 1991, pp 185–203.
3. Bogenschutz MP, Siegfried SL: Factors affecting engagement of dual diagnosis patients in outpatient treatment. Psychiatric Services 49:1350–1352, 1998.
4. Cohen ST: Substance abuse and mental illness. In Friedman L, et al: Sourcebook of Substance Abuse and Addiction. Baltimore, Williams & Wilkins, 1996.
5. Dackis CA, Gold MS:Psychopathology resulting from substance abuse. In Gold MS, Slaby AE: Dual Diagnosis and Substance Abuse. New York, Marcel Dekker, 1991, pp 205–220.
6. Giannini AJ, Collins GB: Substance abuse and thought disorders. In Gold MS, Slaby AE: Dual Diagnosis and Substance Abuse. New York, Marcel Dekker, 1991, pp 57–93.
7. Khantzian EJ: The self-medication hypothesis of addictive disorders: Focus on heroin and cocaine dependence. American Journal of Psychiatry 142:1259, 1985.
8. Meyer RE: How to understand the relationship between psychopathology and addictive disorders: Another example of the chicken and the egg. In Meyer RE: Psychopathology and Addictive Disorders, New York, Guilford Press, 1986, pp 3–15.
9. Mirin SM, Weiss RD, Griffin ML, Michael JL: Psychopathology in drug abusers and their families. Compr Psychiatry 32:36, 1991.
10. Norris CR, Extein IL: Diagnosing dual diagnosis patients. In Gold MS, Slaby AE: Dual Diagnosis and Substance Abuse. New York, Marcel Dekker, 1991, pp 159–184.
11. O'Connell DF: Dual Disorders—Essentials for Assessment and Treatment. New York, Haworth Press, 1998.
12. Reiger DA, Farmer ME, Rae DS, et al: Comorbidity of mental disorders with alcohol and other drug abuse: Results from the epidemiologic catchment area study. JAMA 264:2511, 1990.
13. Slaby AE: Dual diagnosis: Fact or fiction? In Gold MS, Slaby AE: Dual Diagnosis and Substance Abuse. New York, Marcel Dekker, 1991, pp 3–27.

14. Weiss RD, Mirin SM: The dual diagnosis alcoholic: Evaluation and treatment. Psychiatr Ann 19:261–265, 1989.
15. Weiss RD, Collins DA: Substance abuse and psychiatric illness. Am J Addict 1:93, 1992.
16. Weiss RD, Mirin SM, Frances RJ: The myth of the typical dual-diagnosis patient. Hosp Community Psychiatry 43:107, 1992.

26. DISSOCIATIVE DISORDERS INCLUDING DISSOCIATIVE IDENTITY DISORDER (FORMERLY MULTIPLE PERSONALITY DISORDER)

John J. Kluck, M.D.

1. What is dissociation?

Dissociation is a defense mechanism whereby some elements of the conscious experience are disconnected from other elements of the conscious experience. For instance, during a severe trauma, a person may dissociate the "observing self" from the "experiencing self," as if they were watching another person experience the trauma. As such, the "observing self" may not experience fear, horror, or pain.

2. What are the dissociative disorders?

Dissociative disorders are a spectrum of disorders that rely heavily on dissociation as a means of self-protection from extreme emotions. This coping mechanism leads to significant distress or impairment in social, occupational, or other important areas of functioning.

3. What are the specific dissociative disorders, and how are they characterized?

Dissociative amnesia (formerly psychogenic amnesia) is characterized by an inability to recall important personal information (usually of a traumatic or stressful nature), and the lack of memory is too extensive to be explained by ordinary forgetfulness.

Dissociative fugue (formerly psychogenic fugue) is characterized by sudden and unexpected travel away from home or one's customary place of work, accompanied by an inability to recall one's past and confusion about personal identity, or the assumption of a new identity.

Dissociative identity disorder (formerly multiple personality disorder) is characterized by the presence of two or more distinct identities or personality states that recurrently take control of the individual's behavior and are accompanied by an inability to recall important personal information. Individuals with this disorder experience frequent gaps in memory—"losing time" for personal history, both recent and remote.

Depersonalization disorder is characterized by a persistent or recurrent feeling of being detached from one's mental processes or body. It is accompanied by intact reality testing.

Dissociative disorder not otherwise specified is characterized by predominant dissociative symptoms, but does not meet the criteria for one of the other dissociative disorders.

4. What are the associated features and disorders of each dissociative disorder?

Dissociative Disorder	Associated Features	Associated Disorders
Dissociative amnesia	Depressive symptoms, depersonalization, trance states, analgesia, and spontaneous age regression	Conversion disorders, mood disorders, and/or personality disorders
Dissociative fugue	Depression, dysphoria, grief, shame, guilt, psychological stress, conflict, and suicidal and aggressive impulses	Mood disorders, posttraumatic stress disorder (PTSD), substance-related disorder

Table continued on following page

Dissociative Disorder	Associated Features	Associated Disorders
Dissociative identity disorder (DID)	History of severe physical and sexual abuse during childhood; PTSD symptoms of nightmares, flashbacks, and increased startle responses; self-mutilation; suicidal and aggressive behavior. May be a repetitive pattern of physical and sexual abuse by significant others and/or strangers.	Mood, substance-related, sexual, eating, sleep, personality disorders

5. What is the differential diagnosis of dissociative disorders?

Dissociative Disorder	Possible Similar Diagnosis	Distinguishing Features
Dissociative amnesia*	Amnestic disorder due to a general medical condition	Presence of a medical condition that could explain the condition
	Amnestic disorder due to a brain injury	Usually retrograde memory loss associated with a head trauma, as compared with anterograde memory with dissociative amnesia
	Seizure disorders	Motor abnormalities and EEG abnormalities
	Delirium and dementia	A broad spectrum of brain dysfunction
	Substance-induced, persistent amnesic disorder	A significant history of ongoing substance use associated with persistent memory loss
	Substance intoxication	A recent history of heavy substance use associated with memory loss
	Malingering	Dissociative amnesia disorder patients usually score high on hypnotizability and dissociative capacity
Dissociative fugue**	Direct physiological consequence of a specific general medical condition (e.g., head injury)	Objective evidence of such a medical condition
	Complex partial seizures (CPS)	Aura, motor abnormalities, stereotyped behavior, perceptual alterations, a postictal state, and abnormal findings on serial EEGs
	Direct physiological effects of a substance	A significant history of ongoing substance use
	Travel during a manic episode	Grandiose ideas and other manic symptoms
	Wandering episode in a schizophrenic person	Signs and symptoms of schizophrenia
	Malingering	Conduct is bizarre *without* secondary gain
Dissociative identity disorder (DID)†	Direct physiological consequence of a specific general medical condition (e.g., seizure disorder)	Objective evidence of such a medical condition
	Complex partial seizures	Aura, motor abnormalities, stereotyped behavior, perceptual alterations, a postictal state, and abnormal findings on serial EEGs
	Malingering	Obvious secondary gain
	Factitious disorder	A pattern of help-seeking or dependent behavior
	Direct physiological effects of a substance	A significant history of ongoing substance use

See notes next page.

Table notes:
* Dissociative amnesia is not diagnosed if it occurs exclusively during any of the following: dissociative fugue, dissociative identity disorder, depersonalization disorder, posttraumatic stress disorder, acute stress disorder, or somatization disorder.
** Dissociative fugue is not diagnosed if it occurs exclusively during the course of dissociative identity disorder, depersonalization disorder, posttraumatic stress disorder, acute stress disorder, or somatization disorder.
† Controversy exists concerning the differential diagnosis of DID as compared to a variety of other mental disorders, such as schizophrenia and other psychotic disorders, bipolar disorder, anxiety disorders, somatization disorders, and personality disorders.

6. Why has the prevalence of DID increased dramatically in recent years?

This issue is the source of great controversy. Some believe that mental health professionals are now aware of the diagnosis; therefore, previously undiagnosed cases are now being recognized. Others believe that some mental health professionals are overinvested in finding this disorder; thus, it is over-diagnosed in a population of people that are naturally suggestible.

7. Why is it difficult to diagnose DID?

- Many practitioners do not actively search for symptoms of DID in their patients.
- Many DID patients do not present with florid symptoms.
- Most DID patients present with moderate to severe depressive symptoms.
- Most DID patients usually do not present with complaints of amnesia ("lost time") unless asked directly. Even when asked, they may deny amnesia because of embarrassment.
- Alternate personalities (referred to as "alters") may not present themselves in the initial stages of treatment.

8. What is the etiology of DID?

The etiology of DID is complex and controversial, and not supported with strong empirical evidence. Currently, there are two main proposed pathways to the formation of DID. The traditional theory is that DID arises because of **severe, chronic inescapable childhood trauma** (physical and/or sexual). The child dissociates or "splits off" the experience from consciousness to protect the self from awareness of the event and the very intense feelings associated with it.

More recently, several authors have suggested that, in the face of severe trauma, the child must maintain an attachment or **bond with the perpetrator**. The child cannot predict, control, or escape the situation, leading to feelings and thoughts of helplessness and powerlessness. The biological imperative states that the child must be and stay attached to the perpetrator to stay alive. While the abuse dictates that the child break away, it would be impossible to do so. The child's solution is to dissociate into two parts: an unaware attachment part, and an unattached experiencing part.

Theoretically, with repeated trauma over many years, more splits in the self occur to maintain order, continuity, and organization. Some of these split-off additional selves, which may or may not become named, are experienced as separate individuals with separate consciousnesses.

9. What is the nature of traumatic memories of childhood abuse?

This is an area of major controversy. Since the early 1900s, psychological theorists (e.g., Janet and Freud) suggested that people developed "psychogenic amnesia for severe childhood abuse." However, in recent years, many scholars have questioned if it is possible to "forget" or "repress" memories of overwhelming trauma, and then later recall them. Part of the conflict is related to the fact that, until recently, the concepts of memory have been largely theoretical, with little real supportive data. Despite the fact that mental health professionals have depended on these concepts, the issues of whether there is an unconscious mind and if repression is possible have never been conclusively resolved.

Patients who have a history of severe childhood abuse commonly are very hypnotizable and suggestible, and often have an inordinate desire to please their therapists. Such patients can be quite sensitive to the reactions of the therapist, and may be easily influenced by the therapist's interests and belief systems. Thus, if a therapist is overzealous in finding and treating victims of severe childhood abuse, this urge can be transmitted to the patient, who may attempt to "accommodate" the therapist by "developing memories" of events that did not happen; i.e., the so-called pseudomemories.

In working with someone who might have DID, avoid leading questions and responses that could even subtly reveal an investment in finding histories of severe childhood abuse.

10. Summarize recent ideas concerning normal memory.

Normal memory is mediated by the hippocampus and the frontal lobe.

Explicit (declarative) versus implicit (non-declarative) memory

• Explicit memory is the recollection of past events with conscious or intentional effort, and has both visual and verbal components.

• Implicit memory is the development of various behaviors based on past experience of which one has no recall. This includes conditioned responses.

Sensory versus short-term versus long-term memory

• Sensory memory systems record and store stimuli of the five sensory systems.

• Short-term memories are the *active contents* of the mind. They are the result of a person's analysis of an experienced event, which is different from a recording of the actual event. What goes into short-term memory is largely voluntary, but unwanted associated events also can be stored with the voluntary memories. Short-term memory, also called *working memory*, is what one uses to process the immediate present.

• Long-term memory storage is vast and mostly voluntary. Like short-term memory, unwanted associated memories can accompany voluntary memories. Long-term memories may be transferred from short-term memory, but passing through short-term memory is probably not necessary. Rehearsing a memory in short-term memory does help, up to a point, to transfer a memory into long-term memory. Forgetting may be influenced by decay, the loss of intensity of a memory over time, and by associative interference (the storage of a similar memory to the event forgotten).

Normal memory is malleable.

• Memories are reliably *inaccurate*.

• Memory is not like a video camera, recording events or scenes and then storing them in a vast video library.

• Memory is a *dynamic process*. Each time one recalls an event, the memory changes. Current events influence and change memories. Bias and belief systems can also color memories.

• Memories are greatly influenced by the intensity of affect experienced at the time of the event.

• Memories are influenced by the context of the retrieval; i.e., suggestion and giving approval for a response can influence the response.

• Memory for ordinary events may be a combination of the actual event, similar events, and the individual's own enrichment (fantasy).

• Memories can be recovered for events that never happened; i.e., pseudomemories or false memories. This can include iatrogenic memories, created with the help of a therapist asking leading questions or making unwarranted suggestions to the patient. Other important figures also can induce false memories through similar processes.

11. Summarize recent ideas concerning traumatic memory.

Traumatic memory is largely mediated by the amygdala.

• Individual responses to trauma are dependent on several factors: premorbid temperament, interpersonal resiliency factors, and the presence or absence of preexisting or concurrent psychopathology.

• Traumatic memories generally are not influenced by the storage of other similar, associated events; i.e., interference.

• Traumatic memories *do not wane in intensity* over the passage of time; i.e., decay. "The memory (of a trauma) is just as vivid today as it was 20 years ago when it happened.")

• A traumatic memory may be recalled at any time if triggered by a reminder.

• The memories are mostly *sensory* and *emotional* and the subject may not be able to put words to them. This is very different from explicit memory. Trauma victims often cannot make up a story of what happened to them.

- Individuals may be amnesic for parts of a traumatic event, and memories of other aspects may become intensely fixed in the mind.
- Dissociation is believed to play a role in amnesia for a traumatic event.
- J. Freyd has theorized that the victim of ongoing childhood abuse by a caregiver *must* become amnesic regarding the abuse, because the child is so dependent on the caregiver for life-sustaining functions. Freyd has coined the term "betrayal trauma," and posits that these victims cannot allow themselves to remember the traumas until later in life when they are better able to take care of themselves. She calls this an evolutionary adaptive function.
- Delayed recall of very severe traumas has been and remains highly controversial between academic memory researchers and clinicians.

12. List factors associated with traumatic amnesia.

Age: the younger one is at the time of the trauma, then the greater the vulnerability.
Dose: the more severe and the longer the duration of the trauma, the greater the vulnerability.
Preexisting vulnerability
Head injury
According to several studies of childhood sexual abuse, women report the following:
- About 25–30% have total amnesia for the event(s)
- About 35–40% remember some of the event(s).
- About 30–40% say they always remembered the abuse.

13. How can these new understandings concerning memory apply clinically to a person with a dissociative disorder?

Normal memories are quite corruptible and must be understood in the context of the patient's life.

Traumatic memories, which are largely sensual and emotional, can be very accurate and intense, but the patient may not be able to put them into words. Thus, traditional talk therapies may not be effective.

False memories can be induced. Thus, the therapist must remain neutral and avoid asking leading questions or making unwarranted suggestions. For example, "Do you think you could have been satanically ritually abused?" "I have seen similar cases like yours. Your father may have sexually assaulted you."

14. What are the goals of treatment of a DID patient?

The treatment can be thought of as being divided into three phases: early, middle, and late-stage treatment. **The goals of early-stage treatment include:**
- Helping patients improve **self-care**. As children they were forced into the position of taking care of an adult's needs, and did not receive appropriate care themselves. Thus, they did not learn to take care of themselves.
- Establishing a better **sense of safety** by helping them to reduce their suicidal ideation and behaviors, as well as other self-destructive and self-defeating coping strategies.
- **Reducing symptoms** of PTSD, dissociation, anxiety, and depression. Medications may be very helpful.
- Acknowledging that trauma played a central role in the development of their current symptomatology and dysfunction. **Education** about their disorder and its treatment is essential.
- Helping patients to realize that they are *one person* with different parts and aspects to themselves, and not different people or personalities.
- **Improving functioning** in their everyday life, such as at work, in school, and in relationships.
- Teaching, training, and helping to practice better **coping mechanisms** to assist them in managing their PTSD and dissociative symptoms.
- Helping them to improve their relationships and shore up their **support systems**.
- Identifying the key alters: their roles, strengths and weaknesses, and needs. Helping the patient to develop as much "co-consciousness" as possible (i.e., each identity has an awareness of the other identities).

- Insisting that patient (host or executor) must be responsible for all of the alters' behaviors all of the time. Until this is achieved, this task must remain a top priority.
- Helping the patient understand that all of the alters are important parts of the self, and attempts should be made to meet the needs of each one, even the "bad" ones.
- Helping the patient and the alters learn to work cooperatively for the best interest of "them" all.

15. How are the goals of early-stage DID treatment achieved?

The approach to achieving these goals is largely directive in nature, using cognitive and behavioral techniques. Uncovering repressed traumatic memories, processing traumatic memories and nightmares, and experiencing abreactions of traumatic memories is counter-productive in this stage, and usually leads to profound regression and dysfunction. Depending on the ego strength of the individual, the first phase of treatment may require months to years. Many patients will either be satisfied with this level of improvement or incapable of going much farther.

16. What are the goals of mid-stage treatment for a DID patient?

The goals of mid-stage treatment include:

- **Talking about the traumas,** if the patient is able to put words to the traumatic experiences. Understanding the meaning of what happened, and correcting cognitive distortions are more important than the veracity of the memories per se. For instance, being beaten by a parent may mean to the patient, "I was to blame for the beating," "I am bad," "I am worthless," "I am not loveable," etc. The patient needs to construct as integrated a memory as possible of what happened to them and what it meant in reality, while experiencing the associated feelings. He or she needs to realize that the traumas happened a long time ago, were survived, and are not happening now. Patients need to realize that their mistreatment by their caretakers was *not* their (the patient's) fault. Then they need to put into perspective that *the traumas did not destroy their self-worth.*
- **Using nonverbal techniques,** if the patient cannot put words to their traumatic experiences. These techniques include eye movement, desensitization and restructuring (EMDR) techniques, deconditioning to the feelings associated with the traumas, and somatic therapies. Through the relationship with the therapist, patients need to learn that they must and can bear the associated pain. It is only through the controlled and coordinated experiencing of these intense trauma-related affects that the patient can decrease the intensity of their fear and pain. The therapist may then help the patient to find words to describe these experiences and to make meaning out of them. Nonverbal techniques also can be very helpful to patients who can describe their traumas in words.
- Having a secure, trusting, safe **relationship with a therapist**. It is only through the relationship with the therapist that the patient can face memories in a controlled and coordinated manner.
- **Reassessing former understanding** of how the real world operates. Before therapy, the patient's perceptions were fraught with misconceptions and distortions about themselves and the world. This can include issues regarding identity, competence, trust, power and control, autonomy, and value systems.
- **Fusing (disappearance) of alternate personalities.** Some patients fully integrate until there is only one personality. Others are pleased to reduce the number of alters, who have learned to function "together" cooperatively.

17. How are the goals of mid-stage treatment achieved?

The treatment during the mid-phase is extremely complex, and should not be attempted by neophyte therapists, or even experienced therapists, if they have not had specific training and supervision of several DID patients. This phase of treatment can take 1–3 years.

18. What are the goals of late-stage treatment for a DID patient?

The goals of late-stage treatment include:

- Coalesce a new sense of self, based on the patient's real strengths and weaknesses.
- Forgive, let go of, and grieve the past. The patient will never have the parents or the childhood that was wanted, and for this they must grieve.

• Make and maintain healthier relationships.
• Terminate therapy and grieve the loss of the therapist.
At the end of therapy, the patient should not be encumbered with memories and feelings from past traumas, allowing them to live in the here and now. They should be able to give up their preoccupation with their symptoms, and focus on the challenges of the outside world.

BIBLIOGRAPHY

1. Appelbaum PS, Uyehara LA, Elin MR: Trauma and Memory: Clinical and Legal Controversies. New York, Oxford University Press, 1997.
2. Bjork EL, Bjork RA: Memory Handbook of Perception and Cognition, 2nd ed. San Diego, Academic Press, 1996.
3. Chu JA: Rebuilding Shattered Lives: The Responsible Treatment of Complex Posttraumatic and Dissociative Disorders. New York, John Wiley & Sons, Inc., 1998.
4. Diagnostic and Statistical Manual of Mental Disorders (DSM–IV), 4th ed. Washington, DC, American Psychiatric Association, 1994.
5. Kluft RP, Fine CG: Clinical Perspectives on Multiple Personality Disorder. Washington, DC, 1993.
6. Pope KS, Brown LS: Recovered Memories of Abuse: Assessment, Therapy, Forensics. Washington, DC, American Psychological Association, 1996.
7. Putnam FW: Diagnosis and Treatment of Multiple Personality Disorders. New York, Guilford Press, 1989.
8. Ross CA: Dissociative Identity Disorder: Diagnosis, Clinical Features, and Treatment of Multiple Personality. 2nd ed. New York, John Wiley & Sons, Inc., 1997.

27. SEXUAL DISORDERS AND SEXUALITY

Harold P. Martin, M.D.

1. Name the three categories of sexual disorders.
Paraphilias
Gender identity disorders
Sexual dysfunction

2. What are paraphilias?
Paraphilia is defined by DSM-IV as a disorder in which a person experiences "recurrent, intense sexually arousing fantasies, urges, or behavior involving (1) nonhuman objects, (2) the suffering or humiliation of oneself or one's partner, or (3) children or non-consenting adults."

Patients may not be able to become sexually aroused unless involved with a paraphilia or may have an obsessive need to engage in the paraphiliac fantasy or behavior. According to DSM-IV, impairment in social or occupational functioning or significant emotional distress is necessary for a diagnosis. However, even if patients are comfortable with their paraphilia and have no apparent impairment of job or social life, the diagnosis can be made if the paraphiliacal behavior is obligatory for sexual arousal or recurrent, persistent, and obsessive. Behaviors may result in social or legal ramifications (e.g., pedophilia, exhibitionism). Indeed, for many paraphiliacs, the only emotional distress is the fear of discovery, legal punishment, or disapproval by persons they care about. Types of paraphilias include:

Exhibitionism: sexual arousal from exposing one's genitals to strangers.

Fetishism: use of nonliving objects—usually clothes—that the patient may hold, rub, smell, for sexual arousal.

Transvestic fetishism: cross-dressing, which usually is seen in heterosexual men, who find cross-dressing sexually arousing.

Pedophilia: fantasies, urges, or behaviors involving sexual activity with children.

Voyeurism: observing unsuspecting persons unclothed or involved in sex.

Sexual sadism: sexual arousal from inflicting suffering (physical or psychological on others).

Sexual masochism: sexual arousal from being hurt, humiliated, threatened, or made to suffer in some other way.

Frotteurism: touching or rubbing against a nonconsenting person.

The paraphilias are found almost exclusively in men. The difference between these and normal variations in sexual practices lies in the obligatory nature of the acts or thoughts or the recurring, unrelenting need for such behaviors with less and less interest in usual sexual behaviors.

3. Define gender identity disorder.

Gender identity disorder is a condition wherein a person experiences a strong, persistent desire to be of the opposite sex or insists that he or she is in actuality of the opposite sex. Patients experience persistent, strong discomfort in their assigned sex. Physical examination is essential to rule out the rare instances of intersex conditions (e.g., congenital ambiguous genitalia, hypogonadism, androgen insensitivity syndrome) and may require lab studies such as testosterone/estrogen blood levels or karyotyping for sex chromosomes.

This disorder is difficult to diagnose or understand in children. It is not a situation wherein girls act like tomboys or boys seem sissylike. It is a situation wherein a child wants to be of the opposite sex. Even then, ambivalence about sexual identity in childhood usually disappears in adulthood. Many homosexual men report feeling different from other boys when they were young but never wanted to be girls; rather, they found no interest in the stereotypical sexual roles of boys.

Depression, anxiety, substance abuse, and personality disorder are common comorbid conditions. Suicide attempts are not uncommon. Psychotherapy may be especially helpful when difficulties in interpersonal relationships, social isolation, or impaired self-esteem are paramount. A small percentage of patients seek sex-change surgery.

It is essential to differentiate this disorder from homosexuality. Homosexuality involves a sexual orientation to people of the same sex, not a wish for a man to become a woman or a woman to become a man. Sexuality includes sexual **identity**, sexual **roles**, and sexual **orientation** or choice. When individuals have different views on sexual roles or different sexual orientation, they are not considered pathologic or disordered. Only gender identity problems are considered a psychiatric disorder.

4. What are the sexual dysfunctions?

Sexual dysfunction refers to problems in sexual desire, sexual arousal, sexual orgasm, or pain with sexual activity.

Sexual desire disorders include hypoactive sexual desire and sexual aversion disorder.

Sexual arousal disorders include both female arousal disorder and male erectile disorders, both of which involve difficulties in becoming sexually aroused even if sexual desire is present and normal.

Orgasmic disorders include female and male orgasmic disorders, e.g., difficulties in having orgasms or premature ejaculation in men.

Dyspareunia or **vaginismus** are disorders involving pain with sexual intercourse and may plague female patients.

The final categories are **substance-induced sexual dysfunctions**, and **sexual dysfunction due to a medical condition**, which underline the fact that sexual dysfunction may be caused by either biologic or psychologic causes.

5. What types of questions about sexual functioning should be asked of all adult patients during a review of systems?

More important than specific questions is inclusion of questions about sexual functioning in a review of systems. Examples of questions include the following:

1. Are you currently sexually active? If so, with males, females, or both? With just one person or more than one person?
2. Do you have questions or concerns about your sexual life?
3. Do you use birth control? What and how do you use it?
4. Have you ever had a sexually transmitted disease?

   5. Has your medical problem affected your sexual functioning?

   6. For male patients the clinician may add:

      Do you have problems getting or keeping an erection?

      Do you have any problem with having an orgasm?

   7. For female patients the clinician may add:

      Do you have any problems having orgasms?

      Do you have any problem becoming physically aroused?

      Do you have any problem with pain or discomfort during intercourse?

Such questions need to be asked because sexual dysfunction is a common side effect of many medications and a not uncommon symptom of many medical conditions (e.g., diabetes, hypothyroidism, hypertension). If clinicians ask about sexual functioning, the chance of diagnosing a sexual problem increases by at least 10-fold.

Many physicians fail to ask screening questions about sexual function because they are uncomfortable. Yet they ask personal questions about other organ systems, such as bowel movements, menstrual periods, and alcohol intake. In addition, physicians may be afraid that they may find a sexual problem and not know what to do.

6. How common are sexual disorders or concerns?

In a recent data analysis of more than 3000 subjects ages 18 to 59 from the National Health & Social Life Survey, 43% of women and 31% of men described sexual dysfunction. In a survey of over 1200 men in Massachusetts ages 40–70, 48% had moderate or complete impotence. Even more common than sexual disorders or dysfunction are concerns and questions that our patients have about their sexual lives and practices. While the etiology of sexual dysfunction may be primarily biologic or primarily psychological, in most instances both factors are playing a significant role.

7. What are common sexual concerns of men?

Most common is concern over the size of the penis, followed by worry about whether they are adequate lovers. Rarely do such concerns reflect a true disorder. Men also commonly voice dissatisfaction with the frequency or types of sexual contact with their spouse. The common sexual dysfunctions include inability to get an erection when one wants it, inability to maintain an erection long enough for intercourse, and reaching orgasm too quickly or conversely taking too long to ejaculate.

8. What are women's concerns?

The most common concern of women revolves around orgasms, e.g., inability to achieve orgasms or not having orgasms with intercourse. The second most common area of concern is related to normalcy of sexual activities. Examples include whether it is permissible to have sex during menstruation; whether married people masturbate; or whether it is sick to have fantasies about someone other than one's partner during intercourse. Finally, as with men, women voice concerns about tension between themselves and their spouse or mate, such as differences in how frequently they have sex and what kind of sexual behavior each wants or does not want.

9. Why may a woman not have orgasms with sexual intercourse?

Twenty to thirty percent of normal women do not have orgasms with intercourse. This is not a disorder or dysfunction but reflects inadequate clitoral stimulation during intercourse. Direct stimulation of the clitoral area—before, during, or after intercourse—may be required for such women to have orgasms. Manual or oral stimulation before vaginal containment or manual stimulation of the clitoris during intercourse may solve the problem. The woman may need more genital stimulation before intercourse than she has received. It is important for the woman to know that this variant of sexual response is normal and that many women require more than just intercourse for orgasm.

10. What is the difference between global and situational sexual disorders?

A global problem occurs in any setting, with any partner, and during masturbation. It is not related to time of day, type of sexual activity, or other variables. A situational problem, in contrast, occurs only with a certain person, situation, place, or time.

Situational sexual dysfunctions are almost always psychological in etiology and are often relatively easy to treat. Global sexual dysfunctions may be either biologic or psychological in origin but are much more likely to be biologic and are often more difficult to treat.

11. What types of medications commonly cause sexual dysfunction?

The most common group are the psychotropic drugs. Antidepressants may interfere with desire, arousal, or orgasm. Selective serotonin reuptake inhibitors (SSRIs) have about a 30% incidence of sexual side effects. Antipsychotic drugs and lithium commonly cause sexual problems, although not as frequently as the SSRIs. Much less often sexual side effects occur with benzodiazepines, valproate, or carbamazepine. Indeed, sexual side effects are one of the most common reasons that patients stop taking psychotropic drugs.

Other medications frequently implicated for causing sexual side effects include antihistamines, alpha- or beta-adrenergic blockers, cimetidine, HIV drugs, chemotherapy, tamoxifen, digitalis, and steroids. When sexual problems are present, it is wise to check the side effects of all medications that the patient is taking.

12. What drug causes the most sexual dysfunction?

Alcohol. Although alcohol loosens sexual inhibitions in a few people, much more often the opposite effect occurs and sexual function deteriorates. Even 1 or 2 drinks or beers may interfere with sexual desire or arousal. Illicit street drugs also may interfere with sexual function, including cocaine, amphetamines, hallucinogens, narcotics, and marijuana.

13. What medical disorders commonly affect sexual functioning?

Any disease that affects the **circulation** may interfere with sexual arousal, including diabetes, hypertension, and atherosclerosis. Any disease that results in **neuropathy**, such as alcoholism, multiple sclerosis, or diabetes, may affect arousal and/or orgasm. **Injury, irradiation**, and **retroperitoneal surgery** may interfere with neuronal and vascular supply to the genitals and diminish or destroy arousal capability. Serious diseases that tax **energy**, such as congestive heart failure, chronic obstructive pulmonary disease, cancer, HIV with wasting, or chronic infections, diminish desire and arousal. **Depression** typically interferes with sexual desire; **mania** classically increases desire or interest; and **anxiety** may interfere with performance, primarily arousal. **Endocrinopathy** also may be a problem (e.g., thyroid disease, low testosterone or estrogen levels, prolactinemia, adrenal insufficiency).

14. When the patient complains of sexual dysfunction, what should the clinician do next?

A complete history and physical exam are essential, keeping in mind the medications and medical problems noted above.

A detailed sexual history needs to be obtained, noting when the problem started, whether it is global or situational, what the patient thinks is the cause, and what the patient has tried to remedy the problem.

Ideally the doctor should talk to the patient's partner. The partner usually views the sexual problem quite differently, giving quite discordant data. This interview also may clarify whether the partner is supportive or whether the problem is primarily an interpersonal conflict playing out as a sexual symptom.

When a biologic basis seems likely or possible, screening laboratory tests should include the following:

Complete blood count	Urinalysis
Liver function tests	Creatinine or blood urea nitrogen
Thyroid screen	Testosterone level in males
Prolactin level	Estrogen level in females

15. After a history, physical exam, and normal screening tests, what next?

Men should be referred to a urologist interested in sexual dysfunction. More sophisticated workup of endocrine function, genital circulation, and a nocturnal tumescence test may be indicated.

Women should be referred to an endocrinologist or gynecologist with a particular interest in sexual dysfunction. This is not always easy to find. Endocrine integrity needs to be evaluated in greater detail.

Both **men and women** benefit from psychiatric evaluation. Patients with a biologic cause of sexual dysfunction often have a secondary psychological reaction to sexual inadequacy that needs treatment and support.

16. What psychiatric disorders commonly interfere with sexual function?

Depression has as one of its hallmarks a lack of interest in activities that one used to enjoy. Sex is one of the most common activities in which the depressed patient has lost interest. Furthermore, anhedonia, or lack of pleasure in all activities, is a second common symptom of depression.

Anxiety disorders probably interfere with sexual function as commonly as depression. Increased anxiety interferes with normal function of the parasympathetic nervous system, which is required for sexual arousal.

Posttraumatic stress disorder can be accompanied by sexual dysfunction—decreased desire, decreased arousal, or aversion to sexuality, especially when the trauma was sexual in nature (such as rape or sexual abuse).

Many psychological bases for sexual dysfunction are not technically disorders or psychiatric diseases. Learned inhibition regarding sexuality and one's body is common. Sometimes decreased interest in sex or difficulties with arousal are the ways of expressing anger at one's mate. People who are ashamed of their body or feel unattractive may avoid sexuality. Patients may be afraid to have sex after myocardial infarction or stroke. Sexual disinterest not uncommonly starts during pregnancy or shortly after a child is born—for either the mother or father—and usually requires psychiatric treatment.

17. What is performance anxiety?

The classic patient with performance anxiety is the man whose anxiety about getting or maintaining an erection or having an orgasm causes the very problem about which he is so anxious. His sympathetic nervous system is so revved up from thinking and worrying that it prevents adequate sexual performance. The key to treatment is to get the patient to stop worrying, thinking, and becoming anxious about his anticipated sexual prowess or inadequacy and just to let it happen.

Women also may have performance anxiety. They may be anxious about whether they will become aroused, have an orgasm, or please their partner or whether the sexual experience will be unpleasant. The same principles apply in treatment.

18. What is the role of the primary care physician (PCP) in treating sexual problems?

The answer varies with the interest and comfort of the physician. The first principle of treatment is education of the patient, an important function for primary care physicians. Over 50% of the questions, concerns, or dysfunctions that patients have about their sex lives can be adequately answered or helped by the PCP. The PCP can answer questions about sex, prescribe bibliotherapy, and allay anxieties of most patients.

When the problem is due to medications, the PCP may change dosages or medications, advise the patient about side effects, and possibly suggest means of physical intimacy other than intercourse when the offending medication cannot be safely stopped. The PCP is in an ideal position to recommend changes in alcohol intake. Some patients find that if they refrain from alcoholic drinks until after sex, their desire, arousal, and general performance are greatly improved.

When the basis for the sexual problem seems to be marital or relationship discord, referral to a mental health professional is in order. Both depression and anxiety are frequently treated by primary care physicians. However, medication may not be enough, especially in anxiety disorders. The PCP also may need to talk to the couple about their concerns, give them reading materials about sex, and provide basic education and support. Referral to a psychiatrist may be required if this approach is not enough. In summary, the PCP can treat many if not most sexual problems that their patients present to them. At any time, however, it is perfectly appropriate to refer the patient or couple to a psychotherapist who has experience and interest in treating sexual problems.

19. Do any medications improve sexual function?

When there is a medical condition causing sexual dysfunction, the obvious path is to treat the etiological condition. Up until 1997, a host of medications including yohimbine, cyproheptadine, ritalin, and amantaine were tried, with very low success rates. In 1997, a large multicenter study reported a 40–45% success rate with transurethral Alprostadil in men with impotence. The following year, sildenafil (Viagra) became available. With the availability of these new therapies, a large percentage of men now are able to have erections suitable for intercourse—whether the cause of the impotence is organic or psychological.

Estrogen and testosterone replacement in post-menopausal women improves libido and arousal. Studies are currently in progress to study the effects of Viagra on women of all ages.

It is likely that other medications to improve sexual interest and performance will be released in the next few years.

20. If a medical disorder prevents sexual arousal, what can be done to help?

Try Viagra, transurethral Alprostadil, or the vacuum pump; injections such as papaverine; and penile implants in patients whose medical disorder precludes sexual arousal, such as post radical prostatectomy. When none of the above are successful, a therapist can help the couple find means of sexual pleasure and fulfillment without intercourse (e.g., cuddling, manual or oral stimulation of genitals, sensate focus). The therapist will need to help the patient and partner deal with the loss of usual sexual gratification.

21. How is Viagra used, and what are common side effects?

Debate will continue over whether most patients with sexual dysfunction should be medically evaluated before trying a drug such as Viagra, or whether it is safe and ethical to prescribe without a *complete* medical evaluation. Clearly, any condition that could be cured or helped by alternative treatment—e.g., endocrinopathy, vascular insufficiency, depression, marital discord—should not be overlooked. Moreover, Viagra can cause serious, even fatal, side effects in patients with cardiac disease. Thus, some medical assessment is required to rule out common, treatable causes of impotence, the presence of comorbid conditions, and cross-reactive medications. Common side effects include flushing of the face, headache, dyspepsia, and color vision changes. The primary critical cross-reaction is with any nitrates such as nitroglycerine (fatalities have been reported).

Viagra can be prescribed as 25, 50, or 100 mg; initial doses of 25 or 50 mg are typical. It should be taken about 1 hour before anticipated sexual intercourse. Effects usually last for about 4 hours.

Note that Viagra does *not* cause an erection. It may allow an erection to occur if there are physical or psychological stimuli that usually result in an erection. When a couple has adjusted and accommodated to not having intercourse, a sudden ability of the male partner to become aroused may provoke great tension in the relationship. Remind patients of the potential for pregnancy and about sexually transmitted disease prophylaxis.

22. Briefly discuss sexual development from birth to school age.

Infants are very much into exploring their bodies. They discover and explore feet, hands, ears, and genitals. They find that touching their genitals is a pleasant experience. This discovery may upset parents who may label such behavior as masturbation rather than exploration.

From 2–5 years of age children are interested in their genital anatomy and how it differs from people of the opposite gender. They are also quite interested in sexual roles, e.g., how males and females are similar and different in terms of games they play, what they enjoy, ways they talk. It is important to answer children's questions with accurate and simple explanations. Although it may be embarrassing at times, it is quite important to handle children's curiosity about sexuality in a matter-of-fact way, without heightening the feeling that the whole subject of sexuality is taboo.

23. What are children's concerns about puberty?

Children are concerned whether they experience the physical changes of puberty later or earlier than their peers. Girls are especially self-conscious about breast development, because it seems so obvious to others. Being like other children is the key: not to be too tall or too short, not to develop too soon or too late. Girls may be terrorized by their first menstrual period (especially if it occurs without prior discussion and appropriate information), worrying that they are bleeding to death or sick or that other people can smell or sense that they are having the "curse." A boy's first nocturnal emission may be frightening, because the boy may think that he has wet the bed or that something is terribly wrong. Anticipatory education from parents or physician helps to reduce such anxieties.

Children engage in sexual intercourse at increasingly younger ages. At a minimum the PCP has a role in discussing birth control, sexually transmitted diseases, and safe sex. PCPs should ask about sexual behavior in children from 10–12 years of age.

Adolescence is a time when defining one's identity is a key task. Adolescents typically try out different roles and identities and often provoke their parents. The PCP needs to be sensitive to adolescents (and their parents) who are unsure about sexual orientation, sexual attractiveness, and how to negotiate the whole world of sex and relationships. Counseling adolescents often involves listening with respect to their concerns and reassuring them.

24. Where do children get information about sex?

Most sexual information comes from friends and peers, not from parents, school, or books. Hence, their early sexual education is unreliable and often includes misinformation. PCPs provide a tremendous service by encouraging parents to give information about sex to their children. They also may be an important source of information about sex, sexual behavior, and sexual concerns.

25. Is it true that most people over 70 years old do not have sex?

No. Frequency of sexual intercourse decreases, but most couples, if unfettered by medical disease, continue to have intercourse 2–4 times a month. Self-stimulation also continues in senior citizens.

26. What changes in sexual functioning occur with aging?

There is no abrupt change in sexual functioning. Changes in sexual ability start when people are in their 40s. In men the changes include:
- A need for more physical stimulation of the penis to induce erection
- Slower, less firm erection
- Longer time to reach orgasm
- Decreased force of ejaculation
- Longer time to get an erection after orgasm
- Fewer spontaneous erections
- Erections that come and go even during intercourse

27. Why do such changes occur?

Such changes typically are due to less efficient blood supply to the genitals, wearing out of venous valves, pain from the vicissitudes of age, slower neuronal reflexes, and perhaps decreased testosterone. In addition, for psychological reasons a man may feel that he can or should no longer be as sexually active as in his youth.

28. How may sex improve with increasing age?

There are obvious advantages in taking longer to reach orgasm, taking more time for mutual caressing, and not feeling the need to have an orgasm. Sometimes inhibitions lessen with age, and less fear of pregnancy is a plus for men and women.

29. What common changes in women's sexuality occur with increasing age?

- Decreased vaginal lubrication and thinning of vaginal mucosa occur after menopause; for this reason, estrogen replacement should be considered. Local vaginal lubricants, including estrogen, may be helpful.
  - Sexual arousal occurs more slowly.
  - Irritation of the urethra is more common.

• Sex may be more pleasurable without concern for pregnancy or the need to use birth control; orgasm may be easier to achieve.

30. What may help with changes associated with aging?

The most essential aid is information and education. It is quite helpful for people to know what is happening to their bodies and why. Older patients should be reassured that sex does not have to disappear from their life.

Lubricants, estrogen replacement, and Kegel exercises should be discussed if not recommended for women after 50 years of age.

Older couples benefit from practical suggestions and advice to prevent changes in sexual function from discouraging an active sex life. The importance of spending more time in caressing, including genital stimulation needs to be stressed. Men need to know that even with a 50–75% erection vaginal containment is possible. Intercourse can be quite enjoyable even if the man does not have an orgasm. Men may view the ability to go longer before ejaculation as an asset rather than a liability.

31. Is the "use it or lose it" concept valid?

Despite the lack of good scientific data, most sex therapists are convinced that the longer a person goes without sex, the more difficult it is to resume sexual behavior. When one's partner is unable to engage in intercourse or if one's partner leaves or dies, sexual self-stimulation with some regularity is of value to keep the apparatus in good working order.

32. What are Kegel exercises?

The person volitionally and repeatedly tightens the muscles of the perineum for 3–4 minutes. The clinician may describe the exercise as the muscle tightening that holds in urine, bowel movements, or flatulence. Doing these exercises a few times a day helps to keep the muscle tone of the perineum taut and more satisfactory for both partners during sex. This exercise is valuable for both men and women.

33. What is safe sex?

Safe sex is the concept of having sex without fear of contracting a sexual disease from one's partner. In fact, there is only one method of truly safe sex—complete abstinence from sexual contact with another person. Other safe-sex practices are ways to decrease the risk of contracting a disease, but it is important to note that none is 100% safe. Nonetheless, decreasing the odds of disease transmission is especially important for people having sex with strangers or multiple partners, people at high risk of carrying sexually transmitted disease, or people with new partners whose past or current sexual history is unknown.

The underlying concept is to avoid contact with bodily fluids of the other person—especially genital fluids or blood. The use of a condom is essential, whether vaginal, anal, or oral sex is practiced. Condoms should be lubricated with a water-soluble lubricant; oil-based lubricants increase the risk of breakage. Using nonoxynol-9 or other spermicides with the condom may provide additional safety. Because heat or rough treatment may ruin condoms, patients should be advised not to carry them in a wallet or the glove box of a car.

Low-risk behaviors for transmission of sexually transmitted diseases include mutual masturbation or dry kissing.

Low-to-moderate risk behaviors include fellatio without climax, cunnilingus or anilingus, and vaginal or anal intercourse with condoms.

High-risk behaviors include anal or vaginal intercourse without a condom, sharing sex toys, fisting, or any sexual behavior that may damage mucosal linings or draw blood.

Pamphlets with information about safe sexual practices should be openly available in the primary physician's office. Patients should not have to request them; they should be able to pick them up discreetly.

34. Why is sex such a crucial issue for physicians to know about and deal with?

Physicians are consulted when organs are not functioning properly—eyes, lungs, kidneys, bowels. Patients should feel just as comfortable in talking with a physician when their genitals do not function properly; they should be able to get help and support from physicians when their sex life is not satisfactory.

Problems with sexuality not infrequently lead to divorce. Certainly they cause tremendous psychological pain and distress. There simply are not many people to whom patients can talk about sexual concerns. Physicians should make clear that they will listen and be interested in the patient's sexual concerns and offer information, suggestions, support, and, when needed, referral for solution.

BIBLIOGRAPHY

1. Anderson WB: Use of a "permission giving" patient checklist in identification of social and sexual problems. Henry Ford Hosp Med J 34:267–269, 1986.
2. Barbach L: For Yourself: The Fulfillment of Female Sexuality. New York, Doubleday, 1976.
3. Barbach L: For Each Other: Sharing Sexual Intimacy. New York, Doubleday, 1982.
4. Feldman HA, et al: Impotence and its medical and psychosocial correlates: Results of the Massachusetts Male Aging Study. J Urol 151:54–61, 1994.
5. Goldstein, et al: Oral sildenafil in the treatment of erectile dysfunction. New Engl J Med 338:1397–1404, 1998.
6. Krane et al: Impotence. N Engl J Med 1648–1649, 1989.
7. Lauman, Paik, Rosen: Sexual dysfunction in the United States: Prevalence and predictors. JAMA 281:537–544, 1999.
8. Levine S: Sexual Life: A Clinician's Guide. New York, Plenum Press, 1992.
9. Padma-Nathan, et al: Treatment of men with erectile dysfunction with transurethral Alprostadil. New Engl J Med 336:1–7, 1997.
10. Rendell: Sildenafil for treatment of erectile dysfunction in men with diabetes. JAMA 281:421–426, 1999.
11. Rosenthal S: Sex Over 40. New York, St. Martin's Press, 1987.
12. Russell: Sex and couples therapy: A method of treatment to enhance physical and emotional intimacy. Journal Sex & Marital Therapy 16:111, 1990.
13. Schiavi et al: Healthy aging and male sexual function. Am J Psychiatry 147:766–771, 1990.

28. EATING DISORDERS

Andrew W. Brotman, M.D.

1. What are the criteria for the diagnosis of anorexia nervosa?
- Inability to maintain body weight at or above minimally normal weight for age and height (within 85% of expected)
- Intense fear of becoming fat
- Disturbed body image
- In post-menarcheal females, the presence of amenorrhea

The DSM-IV includes two subtypes of anorexia nervosa (AN): the restricting type, and the binge eating/purging type. Restricters do not binge eat or purge. The other type of anorectic alternates binge eating and purging with food restriction.

2. What are the clinical and demographic characteristics of patients with anorexia nervosa?
The prevalence of AN is approximately 0.5% of the female population; 90% of anorectics are female. The age of onset seems to be bimodal, occurring in the prepubertal period or in the late teens, generally between 12 and 30 years of age. Patients with AN are by definition cachectic, and the percentage who meet criteria for major depression may exceed 50%. Although suicide attempts and substance abuse are relatively rare in this condition, the mortality rate can approach 10%, usually because of an arrhythmia secondary to hypokalemia and low weight. Exercise can be common and ritualistic in AN, and the course of illness may be chronic. At 5–10 year followup, the remission rate is 40%. An additional 35% of patients may achieve 85% of their ideal weight but still have an abnormal relationship with food, and 25% have chronic anorexia nervosa.

3. What are the physical findings and medical complications of anorexia nervosa?

Signs and symptoms of AN typically include lanugo, dry skin, emaciation, cold intolerance, hair loss, sunken eyes, bradycardia, hypotension, edema, and hypothermia. Other changes are listed below.

Medical Complications of Anorexia Nervosa

Cardiovascular	Renal
• EKG (low voltage, ST depression, T-wave inversions)	• Elevated blood urea nitrogen levels
• Bradycardia, arrhythmia	• Partial diabetes insipidus
• Hypotension	• Stones
• Congestive heart failure (secondary to refeeding)	Skeletal—osteoporosis
• Mitral valve prolapse	Endocrine
Hematologic—mild pancytopenia	• Decreased T_3
Gastrointestinal	• Increased reverse T_3
• Decreased motility	
• Elevated liver function tests and amylase	
• Acute vascular compression of the duodenum	

4. What are the clinical criteria for hospitalization of these patients?

Studies do not address this issue, and therefore the decision to hospitalize remains arbitrary. Nonetheless, particularly low or unstable vital signs, severe metabolic abnormalities, persistent weight loss despite adequate outpatient treatment, cardiac arrhythmias, severe depression, severe suicide risk, unremitting comorbid substance abuse, and general treatment resistance are sufficient reasons for hospitalization. The threshold for hospitalizing still-growing younger people is somewhat lower than for older individuals whose growth will not be permanently affected.

The goals of hospitalization include nutritional rehabilitation; biologic, social, and psychological therapy; family evaluation; and multidisciplinary assessment and treatment. In AN, the main goal of treatment is weight restoration; in bulimia nervosa, it is control of binging and purging. A variety of protocols are in use, but outcome studies do not convince that one type of therapy is clearly better.

5. What is it like to talk to patient with anorexia nervosa?

The anorectic can be alert and cheerful or sad and withdrawn, depending on the stage of the illness. Patients with AN sometimes are hyperactive, but toward the end of the illness they *can* become hypoactive. They can have substantial mood swings, demonstrate rigidity of thinking, and be controlling and manipulative. Major defense mechanisms include denial of their illness and intellectualization. Their thinking can be black-and-white or good-versus-bad without the capacity to integrate the two. Anorectics frequently are mistrustful of others, strive for perfection, have obsessive-compulsive personalities and a constricted affect, and are socially isolated. They are, by and large, hyposexual.

6. Describe pharmacologic strategies for treating anorexia nervosa.

Unfortunately, no medication has consistently outperformed placebo for the treatment of AN. Controlled trials of medication have had modestly positive results with the serotonin antagonist cyproheptadine and with the antidepressant amitriptyline. However, results for both in other studies have been either equivocal or clinically insignificant. Controlled trials of clomipramine, lithium, thiothixene, pimozide, sulpride, THC, and naloxone also have not achieved clinically positive results.

Several pharmacologic strategies may be a useful *adjunct* to psychotherapy. Antianxiety agents can in some cases be used before meals to help the anorectic carry out a behavioral plan that includes a certain caloric intake. This is generally a time-limited strategy. Antidepressants, particularly the serotonin reuptake inhibitors (SRIs) and certain tricyclics, can be useful, particularly in the anorectic with depression, prominent neurovegetative signs, severe anxiety, or obsessive-compulsive disorder (OCD) or who is otherwise resisting treatment. The desired effects are weight gain, increased interest in eating, decreased anxiety and depression, decreased obsessional thoughts, and increased willingness for treatment. Antipsychotics are not commonly used in AN unless comorbid psychosis is present. Antipsychotic drugs are sometimes used for the anorectic with extraordinary anxiety and inability to eat, when antianxiety drugs are ineffective. There have been several case reports on the use of electroconvulsive therapy, but the evidence is anecdotal.

7. What are the criteria for the diagnosis of bulimia nervosa?

The diagnosis of bulimia nervosa (BN) requires recurrent episodes of binge eating defined as the rapid consumption of a large amount of food in a reasonably short period of time, usually less than 2 hours. One of the hallmarks of the disorder is a fear of not being able to stop eating when the binge is in progress. Individuals regularly engage in some sort of **compensatory behavior**, such as self-induced vomiting, laxative abuse, severe dieting, or fasting, to counteract the binge. The binge-eating episodes need to occur at least twice weekly for 3 months, and there must be an accompanying over-concern with body shape and weight.

8. Are there other types of eating disorder?

Certainly. Patients can meet criteria for both AN and BN. Some eating disorders are "not otherwise specified." For example, some individuals can eat normal meals but self-induce vomiting afterward to control weight. In this case, they do not binge, so they do meet the criteria for BN, and they are of normal weight, so they do not meet criteria for AN. However, they do engage in unusual eating behaviors.

9. What are the clinical characteristics for bulimia nervosa?

The prevalence rate for BN is approximately 0.6–0.8% in women, with a lifetime prevalence up to 8%. As with AN, BN is predominantly a disorder of women (9:1). Onset tends to be in the late teens, with ages ranging from 12 to 40. Weight is usually normal but individuals can engage in ritualistic exercise, fasting, or purging behaviors, including self-induced vomiting, laxative abuse, and the use of ipecac and diuretics. Unlike AN, **suicide attempts** are relatively common, as is **substance abuse**, particularly of stimulant drugs such as cocaine and amphetamines. BN tends to be chronic and is characterized by multiple relapses, with a 10-year followup remission rate of 50%.

10. What are the physical findings and medical complications of bulimia nervosa?

Signs and symptoms of BN include: dizziness, hypotension, parotidomegaly, dental problems, and abrasions of knuckles caused by biting down on them during self-induced vomiting.

Medical complications include: fluid and electrolyte imbalances (K decreased, CL decreased, dehydration, alkalosis); gastrointestinal disorders (sore throat, esophagitis, Mallory-Weiss tears, parotidomegaly, cathartic colon, constipation); dental problems (caries, enamel loss). Most of these complications are secondary to chronic vomiting or laxative abuse.

11. What is it like to talk to a patient with bulimia nervosa?

Outward signs of an eating disorder may be few. Bulimics can be superficially sociable and perceived by others as strong and giving. Unfortunately, they frequently have low self-esteem and conflicts with intimacy, feel misunderstood, and have difficulty managing anger. They may suffer from mood swings and by definition are preoccupied with control over eating. Ask about other impulsive behaviors, including stealing, substance abuse, and suicide attempts.

12. Describe the pharmacotherapy for bulimia nervosa.

The predominant treatment for BN is antidepressants. Controlled studies have shown several to be superior to placebo for the treatment of binge eating and purging: imipramine, phenelzine, amitriptyline, desipramine, isocarboxazid, trazodone, and fluoxetine. A trial of bupropion also was positive, but it is not approved for the treatment of BN because of associated seizures.

Comorbid depression is not necessary for the use of an antidepressant. Medications are generally given in a manner and dose similar to treating someone for depression. However, the SSRIs may be given in higher doses, similar to the treatment of OCD. Abstinence is not usually the outcome of a trial of antidepressants, but a significant diminution in binge eating and purging is common. Pharmacotherapy should be given in the context of an overall psychotherapeutic relationship with the eating disorder patient.

13. What is binge-eating disorder?

Binge-eating disorder is a new diagnostic category that is essentially a subtype of obesity. Most individuals with this disorder are obese, but have recurrent episodes of binge eating without any compensatory behavior. They have significant distress about this and struggle against it. The binges occur at least twice a week for a 6-month period, but the criteria for BN are not met. Most binge eaters have dieted repeatedly, and tend to have more disruption in their lives than other obese individuals of the same weight. The prevalence of the disorder in weight loss clinic samples is about 30%; in nonpatient samples, it is less than 5%. Unlike AN and BN, which occur predominantly in women, the female to male ratio for binge-eating disorder is 1.5:1.

14. Should treatment for obese individuals with binge-eating disorder be any different than for other obese individuals?

It is unclear whether obese persons who eat in binges have a different response to treatment. Some early indications suggest that cognitive behavioral therapy directed toward the binge and, possibly, antidepressants (particularly the SSRIs) may result in improved outcome. The diagnosis of binge-eating disorder and implications for treatment await validation.

15. What is the essential medical work-up for anorexia, bulimia, and/or binge-eating disorder?

Generally these disorders do not require a "million dollar work-up." They usually are apparent on clinical exam and psychiatric interview. AN is an inherently public disorder on the basis of obvious cachexia. BN can be difficult to diagnose if the patient is secretive about it, and no definitive medical tests exist to make the diagnosis, although amylase levels may be increased, and potassium levels are decreased with chronic vomiting. Individuals with binge-eating disorder tend to be obese and are generally forthright about their behavior. Routine laboratory work, including CBC, electrolytes, liver function, fasting blood sugar, and thyroid function tests, is useful. Other tests should be individualized depending on the patient's presenting complaint.

The formal differential diagnosis for AN and BN can include a variety of conditions such as colitis, enteritis, thyroid diseases, diabetes, ulcers, hypothalamic tumors, and seizure disorders. Psychiatric comorbidity can include depression, OCD, anxiety, substance abuse, bipolar disorder, and psychotic disorders.

16. What is the etiology of eating disorders?

No definitive etiology has been documented, but theories abound. The most prominent are:

Sociocultural theory suggests that the pressure to be thin as promoted by the media and societal values can lead to AN and BN. In these societies, patients with eating disorders usually have a weight phobia, which may be a way to avoid post-pubertal conflicts.

Cognitive behavioral practitioners believe that distorted cognitions and learned behaviors lead to eating disorders.

Psychodynamic theorists suggest that there may be a "developmental arrest" leading to eating disorders, and significant comorbidity of personality disorders.

Biochemical theories are numerous. (1) A line of evidence revolves around the comorbidity of major depressive disorder with eating disorders. Approximately 50% of all anorectics and more than 50% of bulimics have concurrent major depressive disorder. In many cases, onset of depression precedes onset of the eating disorder, suggesting a similar etiology between the two. (2) Some clinicians view eating disorders as addictive behaviors, and treat them as they would alcoholism or substance abuse. (3) An alteration of neurotransmitters may be present in eating disorders, although definitive proof is lacking. (4) Some evidence exists that decreased cerebrospinal fluid norepinephrine and decreased methoxyhydroxyphenylglycol may be associated with AN. (5) Decreased brain serotonin and impaired secretion of cholecystokinin in response to a meal may be associated with BN. (6) Other researchers believe that hypothalamic dysfunction may be a cause of or perhaps a result of eating disorders.

Familial disturbances have been widely cited as a potential etiology for both AN and BN. A familial aggregation seems to exist in AN, but it is unclear whether it is hereditary or environmental.

Feminist psychology theorists believe that the pressure to be a "super woman," particularly in Western industrialized society, predisposes women to eating disorders.

Dietary factors—including excessive dieting—predispose to AN and BN, as does a past history of obesity or a family history of obesity.

Other etiologic factors, including childhood sexual abuse, comorbid diabetes mellitus, participation in weight-restrictive sports, and participation in high-achieving occupations, have been researched with various results. *Note that no explanations for the preponderance of women suffering from these disorders are as potent as the feminist and sociocultural views.*

This author's view is that eating disorders are a heterogeneous group of conditions, some of which, in a minority of cases, are subsets of other psychiatric disorders such as depression, anxiety, or OCD. In most patients the eating disorder begins as a diet, as an attempt to match a culturally defined physical shape, or as a means of control, but soon it takes on a life of its own. It becomes almost addictive in quality, and is then employed as a response to all types of emotions.

17. Describe the treatments available for eating disorders.

Many approaches have been tried. Most of the evidence focuses on shorter-term, more easily measured treatments such as cognitive behavioral, interpersonal, and pharmacologic interventions. **Cognitive behavioral** treatments have been a useful intervention for both AN and BN. Patients unlearn distorted thinking, normalize eating habits, and eliminate purging through a structured treatment whose goal is unequivocally symptom control. Manuals have been written on the use of this treatment for eating disorders. **Interpersonal psychotherapy** is also a short-term treatment that has been codified in a manual. It focuses on here-and-now relationships and has demonstrated success with people with depression and eating disorders. **Psychodynamic treatment** is probably the most common approach, resolving underlying conflicts to reduce the symptoms of eating disorders. **Family therapy** is particularly successful with young anorectics who continue to live with their families and do not have chronic illness. **Nutritional counseling** is geared toward education and advice about calories and food groups. **Pharmacotherapy** has been found particularly useful in treating BN, and may have a role in AN as well. **Ongoing medical care** and more intensive programs such as day hospital programs, intensive outpatient programs, evening programs, and halfway houses are selectively employed.

This author begins with a treatment contract and a cognitive-behavioral approach. Adjunct medication is frequently helpful, and psychodynamic treatment may be indicated after eating behavior stabilizes to some degree.

18. Is it useful to have a "treatment contract" with an eating disorder patient?

This is somewhat controversial. Some practitioners continue to see an eating disorder patient on an outpatient basis irrespective of the patient's clinical condition, whereas others set up strict treatment parameters. Many practitioners find it useful to have parameters beyond which outpatient treatment is no longer possible and hospitalization or some other intervention becomes necessary. Targets include reaching minimally acceptable weight levels on an outpatient basis, maintaining potassium levels, reducing levels of laxative abuse, continuing proper use of medication, determining the status of medical conditions, and lowering the level of suicidality. The agreement between the patient and the clinician, negotiated explicitly at the beginning of treatment, is that if these levels are not maintained, hospitalization will occur. A review of this plan with patients and potentially their families can decrease later conflict and help to minimize the dilemma of whether or not to hospitalize.

19. Has managed care had an impact on the treatment of eating disorder patients?

Yes! The goal of hospitalization for a patient with AN traditionally has been weight restoration. The time it takes to get to within 90% of ideal body weight can be substantial. Generally, a maximum of 3 or 4 pounds a week are gained; if a patient needs to gain 30 pounds, the process can take 10 weeks. Hospitalizations of this length almost invariably are denied by insurance companies. Thus, the clinician frequently is asked to discharge patients when they are medically and psychologically stable but have not yet reached ideal body weight.

Alternatives to hospitalization, including intensive outpatient programs and day hospitals, have been initiated to deal with this problem. In a treatment contract, hospitalization may not be the alternative to a violation of the contract, and these other interventions may be necessary.

Finally, managed care pushes shorter-term treatments, which may be inadequate for some patients afflicted with chronic illness.

BIBLIOGRAPHY

1. Agras WS, Rossiter EM, Arnow B, et al: Pharmacologic and cognitive-behavioral treatment for bulimia nervosa: A controlled comparison. Am J Psychiatry 149:82–87, 1992.
2. Brotman AW, Rigotti NA, Herzog DB: Medical complications of eating disorders. Comp Psychiatry 26(3):258–272, 1985.
3. Fairburn CG, Jones R, Peveler RC, et al: Three psychological treatments for bulimia nervosa: A comparative trial. Arch Gen Psychiatry 48(5):463–469, 1991.
4. Garner DM, Garfinkel PE (eds): Handbook of Psychotherapy for Anorexia Nervosa and Bulimia. New York, Guilford Press, 1985.
5. Herzog DB, Keller MB, Lavori PW: Outcome in anorexia nervosa and bulimia nervosa: A review of the literature. J Nerv Ment Dis 176:131–143, 1988.
6. Hudsen JI, McElroy SL, Raymond CN, et al: Fluvoxamine in the treatment of binge-eating disorder. Am J Psychiatry 155(12):1756–1762, 1998.
7. Jimmerson DC, Herzog DB, Brotman AW: Pharmacologic approaches in the treatment of eating disorders. Harvard Rev Psychiatry 1(2):82–93, 1993.
8. Keel PK, Mirchul JE, Miller KB: Long-term outcome of bulimia nervosa. Arch Gen Psychiatry 56:63–69, 1999.
9. Mitchell JE: Subtyping of bulimia nervosa. Int J Eating Disorders 11(4):327–332, 1992.
10. Spitzer RL, Devlin M, Walsh TB, Hasin D, Wing R, et al: Binge eating disorder: A multi-site field trial of the diagnostic criteria. Int J Eating Disorders 11(3):191–203, 1992.
11. Steiner-Adair C: The body politic: Normal female adolescent development and the development of eating disorders. J Am Acad Psychoanalysis 14(1): 1986.
12. Walsh BT, Hadigan CM, Devlin MJ, Gladis M, Roose SP: Longterm outcome of antidepressant treatment for bulimia nervosa. Am J Psychiatry 148:1206–1212, 1991.
13. Walsh BT: Diagnostic criteria for eating disorders in DSM-IV: Work in progress. Int J Eating Disorders 11(4):301–304, 1992.

29. SLEEP DISORDERS IN PSYCHIATRIC PRACTICE

Martin Reite, M.D.

1. What are sleep disorders? How does the practitioner determine whether a sleep disorder is present?

Sleep disorders initially are indicated by the presence of sleep complaints, which generally are grouped into the following three categories:

• "I can't sleep." This complaint most often indicates the presence of an insomnia disorder—**insufficient sleep** to permit the patient to feel refreshed and awake during the day. Insomnia, of course, is a complaint and not a disease; it has multiple causes. An accurate differential diagnosis is important to determine specific appropriate treatment.

• "I'm too sleepy (or I fall asleep) during the day." This complaint usually indicates the presence of one of the disorders of **excessive sleep**. In about 80% of patients the cause is a sleep-related breathing disorder (such as sleep apnea) or narcolepsy. The symptom of excessive sleepiness demands careful work-up and often an all-night sleep study (polysomnogram) for accurate diagnosis. These disorders can be medically serious or result in serious accident or injury (for example, the patient may fall asleep while driving).

• "Strange things happen while I'm asleep." This complaint often indicates a **parasomnia disorder**, which constitutes a series of behaviors that would be normal while awake (e.g., walking, talking) but are not normal during sleep. Patients with parasomnia may arise from any sleep stage. The behaviors usually are not remembered because the patient is asleep while they occur, but they are complained about by bedpartners (or parents, in the case of children).

2. What is "normal sleep"?

Normal adults usually first enter slow-wave or non-REM sleep, which has four stages, depending on the nature of scalp-recorded EEG activity. **Stage 1** is characterized by 5–6 Hz theta activity; **stage 2**, by 12–14 Hz spindles and sharp, high-voltage K complexes; **stage 3**, by 20–50% high-voltage (over 75 μv amplitude) delta activity; and **stage 4**, by over 50% delta activity. After about 90 minutes, the EEG changes to a pattern of low-voltage, fast activity; the eyes move beneath the closed lids; and subjects report dreaming if awakened. This stage of sleep is termed rapid eye movement (REM) sleep, or dreaming sleep. This pattern of slow-wave stages followed by REM sleep is called a sleep cycle; a normal night's sleep is characterized by several such sleep cycles in sequence. Sleep cycles change as the night progresses. Stages 3 and 4 usually are confined to the first part of the night; REM periods become longer as the night progresses.

No hard and fast rule defines how much sleep is "enough"; individual variability is high. Most people need about 7½ hours of sleep at night to feel rested and alert the following day. "Short sleepers" may get along with as little as 4 hours, whereas "long sleepers" may need up to 10 hours.

3. How does one approach the differential diagnosis of chronic insomnia?

Again, insomnia is a complaint, not a disorder. Thus, accurate diagnosis requires the systematic evaluation and exclusion of the several etiologic factors that individually or together may result in chronic insomnia. **Comorbidity is the rule** in insomnia. The identification of one potential etiologic factor does not mean that the diagnostic work-up is complete. All possible contributing factors must be considered individually.

4. List some common causes of insomnia.

Medications	Central sleep apnea
Medical disorders	Delayed sleep-phase syndrome
Psychiatric disorders	Psychophysiologic insomnia
Sedative-hypnotic abuse	
Periodic limb movements	

5. Which medical disorders are especially associated with insomnia?

Medical disorders involving chronic pain, endocrine dysfunction, or chronic fatigue-like syndromes often produce insomnia. In addition, many common medications used in the treatment of medical disorder result in side effects of insomnia. Such factors should be systematically excluded.

6. Which psychiatric disorders often feature insomnia?

Anxiety and depression are associated with insomnia. The complaint may include difficulty in getting to sleep (common in anxiety), difficulty in staying asleep, or early-morning awakening (common in depression).

7. Elaborate on the relation of sedative-hypnotic abuse to insomnia.

Chronic sedative-hypnotic abuse, especially involving older sedative-hypnotic agents or alcohol, may result in chronic insomnia in susceptible patients. Examples are medications started for transient (several days) or short-term (up to 3 weeks) insomnia but not stopped, and patients self-medicating with alcohol because of difficulties in getting to sleep.

8. What are periodic limb movements of sleep?

Periodic limb movements of sleep (PLMS; formerly called nocturnal myoclonus) may cause insomnia in some patients. Short (one-half to several second) bursts of muscle activity in the anterior tibialis muscles, accompanied by a leg jerk or kicking movement, occur about every 30 seconds in bouts during the night. Such movements frequently are seen in normal people with no sleep complaints, but if the leg jerks cause a transient EEG arousal several hundred times a night, the result is fragmented sleep and a complaint of insomnia (or excessive daytime sleepiness). Bedpartners usually complain that patients kick during sleep; if patients sleep alone, they may kick the bedclothes onto the floor during the night.

A polysomnogram usually is necessary to establish the diagnosis. The important question is not only the number of jerks, but perhaps even more important, how many are accompanied by transient arousals?

9. How does central sleep apnea interrupt rest?

Central sleep apnea is a rare condition. Central apneas usually are short (about 20 seconds in duration) with little in the way of direct hemodynamic consequences, but they frequently are accompanied by arousals when breathing resumes. Several hundred short central apneas during the night, each accompanied by arousal, seriously fragment sleep and result in the complaint of insomnia. Patients usually are not aware of central apneas; bedpartners, however, say that the patient stops breathing for short periods during the night. Snoring may or may not be present, and the typical accompaniments of obstructive apnea (recent weight gain, mild hypertension, excessive daytime sleepiness) need not be present. A high index of suspicion is necessary, and a polysomnogram is required for accurate diagnosis.

10. What is delayed sleep-phase syndrome?

Circadian rhythm disorders, such as delayed sleep-phase syndrome, may masquerade as an insomnia disorder. In delayed sleep-phase syndrome the sleepy phase of the circadian sleep/wake rhythm is characteristically delayed about 6 hours, so that the patient is not ready to go to sleep until about 4 AM. If allowed to sleep until 10 or 11 AM, they have no sleep complaint and feel well rested; but if they have to get up early for work or school, they are fatigued and sleepy, perform poorly, and complain of insomnia. Such disorders frequently are familial, and many patients compensate by adopting a work schedule compatible with their phase delay. A careful history is most important in diagnosis; polysomnography usually is not necessary.

11. What is conditioned arousal?

Conditioned arousal, often termed psychophysiologic insomnia, is one of the most frequent causes of chronic insomnia and often complicates or is comorbid with other causes listed above. In such cases, a stress-related insomnia results, after several nights, in patients worrying about going to bed (and therefore becoming aroused) because they fear that once again they will not be able to sleep. In a short while, susceptible individuals are conditioned to arouse at the mere thought of going to bed or by going into the bedroom and getting ready for bed. This condition occurs most frequently in people with a history of fragile sleep (sleep easily disrupted by mild stress). Such cases of insomnia may become quite ingrained and persist for many years. When properly diagnosed (and other causes are excluded), patients frequently respond well to a combination of pharmacologic and behavioral therapies.

12. Are the causes listed in Question 4 the only ones of real concern?

There also is primary insomnia, not related to the aforementioned causes, which persists for over 1 month and causes clinically significant distress or impairment in social, occupational, or other important areas of function. (See Question 19.)

13. What is the difference between a nightmare and a night terror?

Nightmares are basically **anxiety-filled dreams**. They occur during REM sleep and may be quite frightening. Vivid dream content is the rule, but because REM sleep is associated with descending skeletal muscle inhibition, there is little motor activity during nightmares. Nightmares are most common in children but generally rare in adults except at times of stress. Most adults may expect to experience 1–2 nightmares per year. Nightmare content usually is remembered clearly on awakening.

Night terrors are **parasomnias**—that is, disturbances in arousal from slow-wave, usually stage 3 or 4 non-REM sleep. They may be accompanied by a feeling of terror or dread, but as a rule are not associated with vivid dream activity. Autonomic arousal may accompany night terrors (rapid breathing, fast pulse), and some patients may exhibit considerable motor activity, such as sitting up in bed, striking out, or flailing about. Patients may injure themselves or others during parasomnia events.

Patients usually do not remember parasomnia events clearly when they awaken. More complex parasomnias include somnambulism (sleep walking), a state that may include quite complex behaviors.

14. When is polysomnography necessary in the evaluation of a sleep disorder?

It is rarely necessary for complaints of insomnia. Most causes can be identified by careful medical and sleep evaluation, and appropriate treatment may be instituted on the basis of the office evaluation. Two exceptions are insomnia related to central sleep apnea and PLMS, for which a sleep study is necessary to establish the diagnosis.

Polysomnography usually is necessary for excessive daytime sleepiness (EDS) complaints. Most EDS complaints are associated with sleep-related breathing disorders or narcolepsy; polysomnography and sometimes multiple sleep latency tests establish the diagnosis.

Polysomnography generally is not warranted for parasomnia disorders. In most cases, a careful sleep evaluation will be strongly suggestive. In addition, it often is quite difficult to capture a parasomnia disorder during an all-night sleep study, because they rarely occur with sufficient frequency. However, if a parasomnia event occurs during a sleep study, the diagnosis is unequivocal.

15. Are all-night sleep studies useful in psychiatric disorders?

Probably not, at least on a routine basis. Certain changes in sleep are seen in affective disorders (depression and mania), including shorter than normal REM latency (minutes from sleep onset until the onset of the first REM period), increased REM density (number of REMS per minute of REM sleep), and decreases in slow-wave amplitude. Such changes, however, are not thought to be sufficiently specific to merit the cost of a sleep study. Sleep changes in other psychiatric disorders tend to be nonspecific and are unlikely to be of sufficient diagnostic utility to merit the cost and inconvenience.

16. Can patients commit violent or aggressive acts during parasomnia episodes?

Yes. Sleepwalkers often strike out if awakened forcibly, and patients may strike out and hit a bedpartner during other types of parasomnias. Patients also may injure themselves during parasomnia events. They may strike out at hard objects or walls and injure their hands, turn on the hot water and step into the bathtub, walk into traffic, or jump through a closed window. Violent acts such as killing other people have been reported during parasomnia events, but are rare. Such cases have not been considered murder, because the intent to kill was not present.

Patients usually are not aware of parasomnia events, nor do they remember them in the morning. Bedpartners (or parents), however, are aware of such unusual behaviors.

17. Is it possible to screen for a sleep disorder during a routine medical evaluation without taking a detailed and time-consuming sleep history?

Yes. The following three questions may be incorporated into a routine medical history to pick up the majority of significant sleep disorders:

1. Are you satisfied with your sleep? (insomnia disorders)
2. Are you excessively sleepy during the day? (EDS disorders and severe insomnias that cause EDS)
3. Does your bedpartner (or parent, in the case of children) complain about your sleep? (parasomnia disorders)

A positive answer to any of these three questions should be followed by a more detailed sleep history. If all three are answered negatively, a significant sleep disorder is unlikely.

18. If the three screening questions suggest the need for a more complete sleep evaluation, what does that consist of?

First and foremost is a careful sleep history. What is the nature of the complaint, how long has it been present, and how does it vary with time? Is it cyclic or periodic? Does it co-vary with stress or other symptoms or complaints? Is there a family history of similar sleep problems? A screen for medical, psychiatric, and other conditions known to be associated with sleep complaints or conditions is indicated. It may be helpful to have patients keep a sleep diary or detailed account of daily sleep patterns and symptoms to help determine periodicity, relationship to stressful events, and related issues.

Keep in mind the differential diagnoses of the major sleep complaints (insomnia, excessive day-time sleepiness, parasomnias)and include questions relevant to each.

19. How do you treat chronic insomnia?

Start with an accurate diagnosis. Find the (usually several) causes, and target treatments specific to the causes. Treat medical and psychiatric causes as indicated. Use specific treatment for PLMS, central apnea insomnia, or circadian rhythm disorders, as appropriate. In addition, consider a **combined approach** for the remaining primary insomnia or conditioned psychophysiological insomnia component. A combined approach incorporates a hypnotic agent for rapid and reliable response, and behavioral strategies to induce more long-lasting, sleep-promoting behavioral changes.

Approved Hypnotic Agents

DRUG CLASS	GENERIC NAME	BRAND NAME	DURATION OF ACTION	DOSE (MG)	APPROXIMATE HALF-LIFE (HRS)
Benzodiazepine	Flurazepam	Dalmane	Long	15–30	20–100
Benzodiazepine	Quazepam	Doral	Long	7.5–15	40–75
Benzodiazepine	Estazolam	ProSom	Medium	1–2	10–20
Benzodiazepine	Temazepam	Restoral	Medium	15–30	4–18
Benzodiazepine	Triazolam	Halcion	Short	0.125–0.25	1.5–5
Imidazopyridine	Zolpidem	Ambien	Short	5–10	1.4–4.5
Pyrazolopyrimidine	Zaleplon	Sonata	Very short	10	1–1.5

Use the lowest effective dose for the shortest time period possible. Use intermittent dosing (3–4 weeks) when possible. Underscore to the patient that, as a rule, hypnotic agents do not "cure" insomnia, but rather treat the symptom.

Behavioral treatments should include sleep hygiene education, and might include EMG or EEG biofeedback, meditation training, formal relaxation training, sleep restriction (for those patients spending 10 hours in bed to get 6 hours sleep), as well as other specific cognitive strategies that have been shown to be helpful in controlled studies.

20. Episodic outbursts of violent behavior are noted during the night in an elderly man. What is the differential diagnosis?

Rule out a **parasomnia disorder** (careful history, bedpartner interview, possibly a sleep study) or seizure disorder (EEG). Another problem not infrequently encountered in older men (rarely women) is **REM behavior disorder**, which is characterized by a failure of descending muscle inhibition normally seen during REM sleep; such patients act out their dream—not infrequently injuring themselves or others. Such violent behavioral outbursts usually are accompanied by vivid dream material, whereas parasomnia events typically are not accompanied by dreamlike mentation. A polysomnogram generally is required for accurate diagnosis.

21. Does melatonin have a role in the treatment of sleep disorders?

Melatonin is a natural hormone produced in the pineal gland. It has been shown to be important in the regulation of circadian rhythms. Melatonin levels are low during the day, but increase during sleep. In preliminary studies, low doses of melatonin have been found to improve sleep in neurologically disabled children, to facilitate phase advance in adolescents with delayed sleep-phase syndrome, and to decrease sleep latency and increase total sleep time in normal adults. Definitive well-controlled studies have yet to be reported, and the FDA has not yet approved melatonin for medical use. Thus the answer to the question remains uncertain.

22. How is bright light used in the treatment of sleep disorders?

Bright light acts on the superchiasmatic nucleus of the hypothalamus via the retinohypothalamic tract to alter the phase or timing of the circadian system. Bright light exposure in the evening at the beginning of the sleep cycle serves to *delay* the circadian system; light exposure in the early morning or at the end of the dark cycle serves to *advance* the circadian system. Thus exposure to a 10,000 lux bright light unit for 30–45 minutes in the early morning may be an effective treatment for delayed sleep phase syndrome. Similarly, bright light in the evening may help some patients with early morning awakening.

23. How do I approach and manage sleep complaints in elderly patients?

Elderly individuals have more frequent sleep complaints and tend to be more sleepy during the day, for several reasons.

First, **physiological** changes accompanying the aging process may adversely impact sleep. Sleep patterns change with age, including greater sleep fragmentation and less stage 3–4 sleep. Circadian rhythms tend to be lower amplitude, somewhat phase-advanced (earlier bedtimes), and less adaptable to change (greater vulnerability to jet lag/shiftwork problems). Melatonin production may diminish with increasing age.

Second, **medical and psychiatric disorders** associated with impaired sleep increase in frequency with age. The incidence of PLMS and sleep apnea increases with age. Depression is more common in the elderly. Illness and associated decreases in activity may adversely influence sleep.

The management of sleep complaints is not different in the elderly than in younger patients. It starts with a careful diagnostic evaluation, with treatment targeted to all (medical, psychiatric, behavioral) pathologies interfering with sleep. The use of hypnotics should emphasize shorter acting agents to minimize daytime sedation and impaired psychomotor performance. Melatonin supplementation may be helpful in some cases. Emphasis on good sleep hygiene and institution of of an aerobic conditioning program should be part of most interventions.

24. Do herbal remedies play in role in the treatment of insomnia?

Herbal remedies have been widely used for insomnia complaints, especially by individuals uncomfortable with prescription agents. Herbs reputed to have sedative and hypnotic properties are **German chamomile, ambient lavender oil, hops, lemon balm, passion flower, kava, and valerian**. Double-blind controlled studies of the effects of herbal remedies on insomnia are sparse, however.

Some evidence suggests the kavalactones may bind with benzodiazepine or GABA receptors and possibly act in a similar fashion as some anxiolytic drugs. These agents may be beneficial for treatment of insomnia connected with anxiety and tension of nonpsychotic origin. Therapeutic dosage can range anywhere from 50–200 mg of kavalactones daily in divided doses, or a single dose at bedtime. However, note that long-term, heavy usage may cause a scaly skin rash called kava dermopathy, and kava may potentiate barbiturates and alprazolam.

Valerian root is a mild sedative, but there is no evidence to suggest that it is superior to existing drug treatments for insomnia. Sleep-promoting effects have been described when taken with lemon balm. Dosage should be 2 to 3 g of dried root taken at bedtime. Caution should be exercised with any herbal remedy because of possible potentiating effects on other medications.

BIBLIOGRAPHY

1. Dijk DJ, Duffy JF: Circadian regulation of human sleep and age-related changes in its timing, consolidation, and EEG characteristics. Ann Med 31:130–140, 1999.
2. Kryger MH, Roth T, Dement WC: Principles and Practice of Sleep Medicine, 2nd ed. Philadelphia, W.B. Saunders, 1994.
3. Moldofsky H, Gilbert R, Lue FA, MacLean AW: Sleep-related violence. Sleep 18:731–739, 1995.
4. Morin CM, Culbert JP, Schwartz SM: Nonpharmacological interventions for insomnia: A meta-analysis of treatment efficacy. Am J Psychiatry 151:1172–1180, 1994.
5. Regestein QR, Monk TH: Delayed sleep phase syndrome: A review of its clinical aspects. Am J Psychiatry 152:602–608, 1995.
6. Reite M: Sleep disorders presenting as psychiatric disorders. Psychiatr Clin North Am 21:591–607, 1998.
7. Reite M: Treatment of insomnia. In Shatzberg AF, Nemeroff MD (eds): The American Psychiatric Press Textbook of Psychopharmacology, 2nd ed. Washington, DC, American Psychiatric Press, 1998, pp 997–1014.

8. Reite M, Buyesse D, Reynolds C, Mendelson W: The use of polysomnography in the evaluation of insomnia. Sleep 18:58–70, 1995.
9. Reite M, Nagel K, Ruddy JA: A Concise Guide to the Evaluation and Treatment of Sleep Disorders, 2nd ed. Washington, DC, American Psychiatric Press, 1997.
10. Wong AH, Smith M, Boon HS: Herbal remedies in psychiatric practice. Arch Gen Psychiatry 55:1033–1044, 1998.

30. IMPULSE-CONTROL DISORDERS

Michael H. Gendel, M.D.

1. Which disorders are classified as impulse-control disorders?

Intermittent explosive disorder, pyromania, kleptomania, trichotillomania (compulsive pulling of a patient's own hair), and compulsive gambling.

Disorders that involve the failure to resist impulses to use alcohol or drugs, eat abnormally (including purging and food restriction), or perform certain sexual behaviors are not classified in this group.

2. What fundamental features do impulse-control disorders have in common?

No one knows. Presumably they are grouped together because they are **disorders of behavior** resulting from the failure to resist a subjective impulse to perform that behavior. However, these irresistible impulses are very different in nature (e.g., violence and hair pulling), in frequency (rare violent outbursts, hair pulling throughout the day), and resulting behavior (e.g., gambling and fire-setting).

Many clinicians regard them as **disorders of tension regulation**. Feelings of excitement, tension, or arousal *before* acting; pleasure, euphoria, or relief *during* acting; and dysphoria or guilt *after* acting are more or less present in this cluster. Some empathic imagining of what this condition might be like should be attempted, if for no other reason than to help distinguish these illnesses from more ordinary experiences. For instance, in trichotillomania, one might become very agitated during any concerted attempt to stop hair pulling, such that focus on any other activity is impossible. Minutes to hours of hair removal provide only temporary relief of tension. Bitter depression and emptiness may envelop the sufferer as the day ends and he or she imagines the next day as little more than the same struggle repeated.

The propensity to act rather than express feelings is another common characteristic of this group. Many afflicted individuals are not aware of their feelings and cannot name or use them (alexithymia).

3. Are these disorders biologically similar?

The biologic substrate is not yet elucidated. Considerable evidence is mounting that abnormal serotonin metabolism is present, particularly low serotonin turnover with decreased CSF 5-HIAA, in some of these disorders. Intermittent explosive disorder (IED) is most clearly associated with these changes, though kleptomania, pyromania, and trichotillomania are implicated in some studies. The role of serotonin receptor subtypes also may be important. In various types of aggressive behavior, agonists of the 5-HT1A receptor and antagonists of the 5-HT2 receptor appear to reduce symptoms. It is not yet clear whether all of these disorders share a common neurobiologic basis.

4. What is an impulse?

An impulse is a feeling to which an action is connected. It is an urge to act.

The issue of time course or urgency is very confusing. Commonly used expressions such as "impulsive decision" and "electrical impulse" suggest *urgent action* or immediate discharge. Some of these disorders conform clinically to these images, such as the sudden violence in IED. In pyromania, however, a fire might be intricately planned and executed, implying either that the concept of the firesetting impulse is not easily approached through common language paradigms or that tension relief begins with the *internal act of planning* the fire.

5. How does one resist or fail to resist an impulse?

In traditional psychiatry, impulses fail to result in actions because of **adequate defenses**. Defenses are ego functions, which themselves may be healthy (i.e., lead to better organismic adaptation) or less healthy (i.e., lead to problems of their own). Defenses also may be effective in preventing expression of unwanted impulses. They are unconscious operations that serve to reduce internal tension. You might imagine that people with good defensive structures do not "leak" unwanted behaviors, and those with poorer ones do. Unfortunately, such is not the case. Impulse-control disorders involve, by definition, truly overwhelming internal states that sometimes coexist with sound psychological defensive structures which simply do not help with these behaviors. These problems occur in a variety of people. In fact, most of these diagnoses can be made only in the absence of a primary axis I or II illness, which suggests that there is no pervasive or typical deficiency in defenses. Treatments based on creating healthier defense structures have a poor track record in these disorders, as they do with substance abuse and sexual disorders.

Another framework from which to approach this question is that of the **ability to defer** an impulse-connected action. To what extent can a violent feeling be contained as just a feeling, and the urge to act on it be delayed, put off, or even permanently put aside? Here, we can examine the effect of conscious behavior-controlling schemes (such as using the knowledge that an act may be unlawful, dangerous, or unacceptable). Other such operations might include remembering a previous bad outcome, distracting oneself with other thoughts or actions, or calling a friend for support. The extent to which a patient has attempted to use such methods might help a clinician understand the extent to which a person wanted to control an impulse.

It may ultimately prove more useful to examine the **biology of the expression** of specific behaviors, when such information becomes available. This will allow understanding of the neurochemical regulation of impulses and actions in normal and pathologic states.

6. How is Einstein connected to this discussion?

General relativity teaches us to stop thinking about gravity as a force operating on an object. It suggests other metaphors. Gravity can be conceptualized as a property of mass that alters the shape of space in the vicinity of the mass, such that the motion of neighboring massful objects is changed. The earth thus alters nearby space such that the moon (which might otherwise travel in a different trajectory) orbits it; it does not "hold" the moon by force of gravity.

"Impulse," too, is an old concept that may profit from newer conceptualizations or metaphors. Perhaps acting on impulse is experiencing a particular internal mental state that is less separable from behavior: the "shape" of our being would be altered by a feeling of this type. An impulse-control disorder might then be conceptualized as a condition of having more behavior-shaping feelings in which thoughts, fears, and concerns have less relevance. Although the underlying neurochemistry of such a condition is unclear, it is possible that the impulse-control-disordered phenomenon may be "wired" differently than ordinary feelings. If so, then gambling for the normal person may not be the same activity as gambling for the pathologic gambler.

7. What role do clinician attitudes play in impulse-control disorders?

One of the difficulties of working with patients with these sorts of problems is the negative feelings we have toward the behaviors themselves. Further, the problems tend to be repetitive and difficult to treat, leading to feelings of helplessness and powerlessness in the physician. Under these conditions we are likely to view such patients in moralistic and oversimplified ways. Anything we can do to generate intellectual interest, conceptualize the issues differently, or otherwise tilt the problem on its end will aid us in the effort to approach these disorders and the afflicted patients with scientific and humane interest.

8. What diagnostic problems are associated with impulse-control disorders?

As a group, these disorders are less well studied than most psychiatric conditions. When knowledge is sparse, diagnostic difficulty is inherent. Earlier versions of the DSM emphasized neurologic abnormalities in IED. In the current diagnostic schema, if a clearly diagnosable general medical condition is causing the explosive outbursts, you should diagnose "Personality Change Due to a General Medical Condition" rather than IED. However, soft neurologic signs and nonspecific EEG abnormalities do not constitute a diagnosable medical disorder and do not exclude the diagnosis of IED. Patients with IED demonstrate a greater frequency of EEG abnormalities when compared to various control samples.

Certain of these diagnoses cannot be made if the behavior is better accounted for by another condition, yet in reality it may rarely be seen in the absence of another serious disorder. For instance, IED should not be the diagnosis if antisocial or borderline disorders, in which explosiveness and poor temper regulation are common, better account for the behavior. However, many cases that conform well to the picture of the clinical entity of IED occur in the context of these serious character pathologies.

DSM-IV adds the "better accounted for" exception to the diagnostic criteria of all disorders in this group. For trichotillomania the accompanying condition is most likely dermatologic. For pathologic gambling, the other condition is specifically manic.

A patient's history is the most important diagnostic aid when two disorders may be present. If compulsive gambling clearly precedes the onset of identifiable manic symptoms, or is present in a euthymic period, both diagnoses may be appropriate. Many patients with an impulse-control disorder suffer major depression. Such depression often results from the damage created by the disorder, and historically follows the disorder's onset. If the impulse disorder occurs only in the context of an affective episode, excluding or at least deferring the impulse disorder diagnosis is quite sensible.

In this chapter, characterizations of the diagnostic entities are based on DSM-IV.

9. How to you differentiate intermittent explosive disorder and a bad temper?

A bad temper is not an illness; nor is explosive behavior. In IED, there are several episodes of aggression that result in serious destruction or assault and are not better accounted for by other psychiatric disorders, including substance abuse, or a medical condition. Some people known to have bad tempers may suffer from IED; most IED sufferers have bad tempers.

10. What is the difference between kleptomania and other forms of stealing?

The defining feature of kleptomania is that the sufferer steals in the absence of need for the stolen object or its monetary value. Kleptomaniacs tend to experience the impulse to steal as foreign and unwanted (ego dystonic). They steal on the spur of the moment despite the more constant pressure of the urge to steal. Any item may be stolen. The article may be kept, hoarded, thrown away, or even returned. The individual may worry about getting caught, but fail to plan the crime with such a consequence in mind. Kleptomaniacs generally are not antisocial. They steal alone, without accomplices. They are more often female than male.

Other stealing behavior has many forms. Shoplifters typically are seeking the item stolen, even if it is low in value. Many individuals steal for profit, gain, or revenge. The stealing may be planned, and the thief may carefully consider the dangers and consequences of apprehension. These motives and thought patterns are not typical of kleptomania and if present should lead to doubt about such a diagnosis, as should a more general pattern of antisocial behavior. The cycle of tension building before the theft, pleasure or relief during its commission, and depression afterward usually is not present in criminal stealing, though sensation-seeking may be a factor. Accomplices are more common in other forms of stealing.

11. How do you distinguish between trichotillomania and other causes of hair loss?

Trichotillomania consists of the pulling out of one's hair, resulting in noticeable hair loss, coupled with the cycle of tension preceding the act, gratification of doing so, and sometimes dysphoria afterward. A patient with trichotillomania may be quite ashamed of the condition and may not report the true source of the hair loss. Hair may be pulled from any area of the body: most often from the head (eyelashes, eyebrows, scalp), and also from the axilla, pubic, or perirectal areas.

Other conditions with hair loss include alopecia areata, male-pattern baldness, chronic discoid lupus erythematosus, lichen planopilaris, folliculitis decalvans, pseudopelade, and alopecia mucinosa. Skin inflammation generally does not occur in trichotillomania, in contrast to alopecia areata.

Biopsy in trichotillomania shows short and broken hairs, with normal and damaged follicles in the same vicinity. Follicles often show trauma, or may be empty. More catagen hairs (those hairs in the short phase between growth and resting, or between anagen and telogen phases) are seen. Also look for evidence of nail biting and scratching behaviors. This condition may present with gastrointestinal symptoms caused by bezoars, generated by trichophagia (eating hairs).

12. What pharmacologic treatment(s) are useful in these disorders?

Medicines used to treat IED include anticonvulsants (especially carbamazepine, valproate, and phenytoin), serotonergic antidepressants, buspirone, beta blockers, lithium, neuroleptics, and calcium-channel blockers. Of these, anticonvulsants and beta blockers show promise.

Antidepressants, especially SSRIs, have been found useful in trichotillomania. Some suspect trichotillomania to be related to obsessive-compulsive disorder.

Anecdotally, kleptomania, pyromania, and pathologic gambling have responded to a variety of medicines, usually antidepressants, buspirone, or thymoleptics (mood stabilizers such as lithium, carbamazepine, or valproate).

13. If you suspect the diagnosis of pyromania, should steps be taken to ensure safety?

Anyone who sets fire is dangerous, whether or not they meet the criteria for pyromania. The proportion of mentally disordered arsonists diagnosed with pyromania is low, suggesting that other firesetters also represent a dangerous population. Systematically evaluate potentially dangerous behavior; suicide and homicide risk assessments are models. Query pyromaniacs about past fires, including scope, damage, and associated injuries or deaths. This information-gathering is not for the purpose of reporting to authorities, but to measure the potential for danger. Evaluate current fantasies and plans for firesetting, including specific sites and individuals who may be involved. Even a general fantasy or plan involving no definite place or person should be noted—particularly if the patient believes there is a likelihood of action.

Such patients may meet criteria for involuntary commitment. Be aware of the standards for civil commitment in each state. Mental health professionals have been found liable for failure to warn possible victims of firesetting (*Peck v. Counseling Service of Addison Country*, 146 Vt. 61, 499 A.2d 422 [1985]). The duties to warn and protect are clearly defined in some jurisdictions because of state law or case law, and you should be familiar with the applicable standards in your geographic area of practice. Depending on the jurisdiction, such duties may be carried out by warning the individual endangered, calling the police or other authorities, detaining the dangerous person, or other measures. Issues of confidentiality (and privilege, if court actions ultimately ensue) are raised if warnings are given without the patient's consent.

14. Is pathologic gambling an addiction?

This question is controversial in psychiatry and among addiction experts. It should not be construed to suggest that impulse-control disorders are hard to distinguish from addictive disorders. Clinically, pathologic gambling has such similarity to addictive behavior that it has been called a "process addiction." This resemblance is much closer than to the other impulse-control disorders (which are so different from each other that their main commonality is that they are classified together). Below are arguments against and for this question.

Against

- Too many problems already are miscast as addictions. The word and concept are trivialized by such usage.
- Such diagnosis lends an aura of respectability to behavior which is better thought of as simply impulse-ridden.
- Addiction is a term that should be reserved for activities in which an exogenous chemical is introduced into the body, not for any other repetitive behavior.
- Many conceptual models of pathologic gambling exist. No single model explains all such behavior. Any model may prove useful in a given case. Some cases might be best understood from a psychoanalytic or behaviorist perspective, as a habit disorder, or as a condition comorbid with other psychiatric illness or directly related to other psychiatric illness (especially manic state, depression, and obsessive-compulsive disorder).
- Diagnosis implies treatment. One may too narrowly prescribe addiction-modeled treatment for a disorder with other available approaches.

For

- Loss of control over a compulsively repeated behavior (with resulting adverse consequences) is the hallmark of addiction. Pathologic gambling fits this model.
- DSM-IV diagnostic criteria for pathologic gambling are strikingly similar to the criteria for addictive illness (see table). This reflects the similarity in conditions.
- Some studies of compulsive gamblers document that upon cessation of gambling, physical withdrawal symptoms occur similar to those of opioid and central nervous system depressant withdrawal symptoms.
- Gamblers Anonymous, a 12-step program modeled on Alcoholics Anonymous, has proved helpful to many pathologic gamblers, and may be the most effective intervention currently available. Gamblers have been successfully treated in programs with other addicts.
- Addiction itself has many conceptual models. The notion of addiction should not impede thinking conceptually or diagnostically.
- Medicine is eclectic and empiric. Any treatment that helps, does not pose excessive risk of harm, and is ethical should be considered.

This author sides with the arguments for calling gambling an addiction. It may not be conceptually neat, but practically speaking, pathologic gambling behaves like an addiction, including its response to treatment and 12-step support programs. More knowledge or more effective treatment may lead to a reconsideration of this conclusion.

DSM-IV Diagnostic Criteria

SUBSTANCE DEPENDENCE	PATHOLOGIC GAMBLING
Tolerance: need for more substance to achieve desired effect or diminished effect with same amount of substance (1)	Need to gamble with increasing amounts of money in order to achieve the desired excitement. (2)
Withdrawal: characteristic withdrawal syndrome or substance taken to relieve withdrawal symptoms. (2)	Is restless or irritable when attempting to cut down or stop gambling. (4)
Substance taken in larger amounts or longer than intended. (3)	After losing money gambling, often returns another day to get even ("chasing" losses). (6)
Persistent desire or unsuccessful attempts to cut down or control use. (4)	Has repeated unsuccessful efforts to control, cut back, or stop gambling. (3)
Much time spent in obtaining, using, or recovering from substance use. (5)	Is preoccupied with gambling (e.g., preoccupied with reliving past gambling experiences, handicapping or planning the next venture, or thinking of ways to get money with which to gamble). (1)
Important social, occupational, or recreational activities are given up or reduced because of substance use. (6)	Has jeopardized or lost a significant relationship, job, or educational or career opportunity because of gambling. (9)
	Lies to family members, therapist, or others to conceal the extent of involvement with gambling. (7)
Substance use continues despite knowledge of a physical or psychological problem likely caused or exacerbated by the substance. (7)	Gambles as a way of escaping from problems or relieving a dysphoric mood. (5)
	Has committed illegal acts such as forgery, fraud, theft, or embezzlement to finance gambling. (8)
	Relies on others to provide money to relieve a desperate financial situation caused by gambling. (10)

Numbers in parentheses correspond to numbered diagnostic criteria in DSM-IV. Grouping of criteria is for the purpose of comparison and is *not* part of DSM-IV, and some material has been paraphrased or shortened.

15. True or false: The expression of an impulse disorder is more likely to occur under the influence of substances of abuse.

True. Further, these disorders have considerable comorbidity with substance use disorders, as well as with mood disorders and personality disorders.

BIBLIOGRAPHY

1. American Psychiatric Association: Diagnostic and Statistical Manual of Mental Disorders, 4th ed. Washington, DC, American Psychiatric Association, 1994.
2. DeCaria CM, Hollander E, Grossman R, et al: Diagnosis, neurobiology, and treatment of pathologic gambling. J Clin Psychiatry 57(suppl 8):S80–S84, 1996.
3. Drake ME, Hietter SA, Pakalnis A: EEG and evoked potentials in episodic-dyscontrol syndrome. Neuropsychobiology 26:125, 1992.
4. Gerner RH: Pharmacological treatment of violent behaviors. In Rosner R (ed): Principles and Practice of Forensic Psychiatry. New York, Chapman and Hall, 1994, pp 444–450.
5. Kavoussi R, Armstead P, Coccaro E: The neurobiology of impulsive aggression. Psychiatr Clin North Am 20(2):395–403, 1997.
6. Marohn RC, Custer R, Linden RD, et al: Impulse control disorders not elsewhere classified. In American Psychiatric Association: Treatments of Psychiatric Disorders: A Task Force Report of the American Psychiatric Association. Washington, DC, American Psychiatric Association, 1989, pp 2457–2496.
7. McElroy SL, Hudson JI, Pope HG, et al: The DSM-III-R impulse control disorders not elsewhere classified: Clinical characteristics and relationship to other psychiatric disorders. Am J Psychiatry 149:318, 1992.
8. McElroy SL, Soutullo CA, Beckman DA, et al: DSM-IV intermittent explosive disorder: A report of 27 cases. J Clin Psychiatry 59:203–210, 1998.
9. Murray JB: Review of research on pathological gambling. Psychol Rep 72:791, 1993.
10. Schalling D: Neurochemical correlates of personality, impulsivity, and disinhibitory suicidality. In Hodgins S (ed): Mental Disorder and Crime. Newbury Park, CA, Sage, 1993, pp 208–226.
11. Stein DJ, Hollander E, Liebowitz MR: Neurobiology of impulsivity and impulse control disorders. J Neuropsychiatry and Clin Neurosci 5:9, 1993.
12. Virkkunen M, Linnoila M: Serotonin in personality disorder with habitual violence and impulsivity. In Hodgins S (ed): Mental Disorder and Crime. Newbury Park, CA, Sage, 1993, pp 227–243.

31. MEDICALLY UNEXPLAINED SYMPTOMS

Alan M. Jacobson, M.D.

1. Define the term "medically unexplained symptoms."

Patients commonly present to their primary physicians with medical symptoms that cannot be fully explained by specific somatic illnesses. Such unexplained symptoms may vary considerably in duration and severity; often they are transient and mild, resolving without specific intervention. Simple explanation and reassurance, supported by physician assessment (history, physical exam, and office-based laboratory tests), may significantly reduce others.

The severity, intensity, and persistence of the symptoms dictate consideration of in-depth diagnostic evaluation, which may include more extensive medical and psychiatric work-ups. Even with detailed assessment, a clear somatic explanation may remain elusive, and the symptoms may persist. Four groups of psychiatric disorders comprise the more severe and/or persistent presentations of medically unexplained symptoms: **somatoform disorders, factitious disorders, other psychiatric disorders** (e.g., anxiety and depression), and **malingering**. When assessing patients with medically unexplained symptoms that are more than mild or transient, consider etiologies in all four spheres.

2. Do all severe and/or persistent unexplained presentations have psychiatric causes?

No. Some unexplained symptoms are due to biomedical syndromes that are not yet diagnosable. Indeed, in the course of ongoing somatoform and other psychiatric disorders, patients may develop medical problems that require treatment. This scenario can be especially demanding when somatization occurs in the context of chronic medical illness. Thus the clinician must maintain a balance: helping the patient with underlying psychiatric problems while remaining attuned to unfolding medical conditions. Careful psychiatric assessment helps to identify classic patterns of psychopathology, which may guide the evaluator to consider the possibility of unrecognized medical conditions.

3. What are the common characteristics of somatoform disorders?

Somatoform disorders present with physical symptoms that are not fully explained by clear medical disorder, the effects of substance abuse, or other psychiatric syndromes. The physical symptoms are *not intentional* and not under voluntary control. There are five general categories:

Somatoform Disorders

CATEGORY	KEY CHARACTERISTICS
Somatization disorder	Multiple symptoms—pain, gastrointestinal, sexual dysfunction Symptoms vary over time Chronic condition—often with extensive treatment history Not intentional
Conversion disorder	Symptoms affect voluntary motor or sensory system Symptoms do not conform to neuroanatomic structures May reflect, symbolically, past or current stressor Patient may not be upset by the symptoms Not intentional
Hypochondriasis	Chronic preoccupation with having a serious disease Patient misattributes symptom or test results Preoccupation not solely due to affective status
Body dysmorphic disorder	Preoccupation with an imagined defect in physical appearance May exaggerate mild anomaly
Chronic pain syndrome	Pain is the central feature May begin after specific injury Can lead to serious functional impairment and medication overuse

4. Describe somatization disorder.

Previously somatization disorder was referred to as hysteria or Briquet's syndrome. It is a chronic fluctuating condition that usually begins after the age of 30 and extends over many years. The patient presents with multiple symptoms, including pain, gastrointestinal symptomatology, neurologic symptoms, and sexual dysfunction, which may vary considerably over time. He or she may have a long history of past extensive treatment, including surgery. Typically, the patient seeks out multiple providers because of dissatisfaction with prior treatment, and may end up on complex combinations of medications because of frustration on the part of both patient and physician. Significant impairments in work and social functioning are common.

As described in the *Diagnostic and Statistical Manual–IV*, patients should have a history of pain in at least four different sites: two different gastrointestinal symptoms other than pain, at least one sexual symptom, and one neurologic symptom. Symptoms vary in type and frequency across cultures and countries, and between genders. In North America, somatization disorder is more commonly found in women; up to 2% of women and less than 0.2% of men have a lifetime prevalence of this disorder.

5. What is revealed in the work-up of a patient with somatization disorder?

The work-up of the patient with somatization disorder usually reveals a positive history of multiple medical and surgical treatments, current symptoms without abnormal laboratory test results, and a physical exam that fails to identify objective findings that explain subjective complaints. As with other patients with unexplained medical symptoms, past treatment may give rise to new symptoms, as well as clear physical findings. For example, the patient may have had an exploratory laparotomy, and as a result he or she now is experiencing persistent symptomatic cramping pain due to adhesions.

6. Describe conversion disorder.

Conversion disorder presents with deficits of the voluntary motor or sensory neurologic system, and often mimics recognized neurologic or other medical conditions. As with somatization disorder, the symptoms are not intentionally produced; rather, underlying psychological factors are expressed in physical symptoms. Common presentations include loss of sensation in a single limb or part of a limb, double vision, blindness, deafness, difficulty with swallowing, and paralysis.

On careful exam, the symptoms typically do not conform to recognized anatomic pathways. For example, a classic sensory loss due to conversion disorder may conform to a glove or stocking distribution. Recognize, however, that unusual distributions of sensory and motor loss can occur in some neurologic disorders, such as multiple sclerosis.

7. How are underlying psychological factors expressed physically in conversion disorders?

Historically, conversion reactions have been thought to symbolize unresolved conflict. For example, the patient who feels guilt-ridden because he or she stole something loses all ability to move the hand that grabbed the object. Such conversion symptoms may occur in patients with a history of physical and emotional abuse or borderline personality disorder.

Conversions disorders are likely to be associated closely in time with an acute stressor. However, the stressor itself may be mild and important only as a symbolic representation of past psychological trauma or conflict. For example, a patient who suffered oral rape may develop trouble with swallowing (sometimes called globus hystericus) on viewing a movie that depicts sexual violence. Most patients (but not all) do not concurrently remember the earlier event; gagging is felt without an accompanying memory of trauma or conflict.

8. Are these patients seeking pity and sympathy?

While reinforcing social responses may occur, the conversion disorder is thought to derive primarily from inner psychic gain. In the previous example (Question 7), the muffled ability to speak may represent the individual's earlier sense of suffocation and gagging as an abused child. The inner conflict also may have been caused by the authority figure's threat to kill the patient if he or she told anyone and/or by the patient's inner shame or guilt.

Because the early event commonly is forgotten or poorly remembered and only the symbolic physical symptom is experienced, the patient with a conversion disorder may present with minimal upset. This reaction has been termed "la belle indifference." In other instances, the patient may be confused and even terrified by the new symptom, even while having no anxiety about the actual trauma.

9. Describe hypochondriasis.

Hypochondriasis refers to a **chronic preoccupation** with and fear of having a serious disease. It typically is based on the individual's continual misperception of bodily symptoms and/or test results, and may occur in the context of a well-recognized and diagnosed illness, such as diabetes, or in the absence of known illness. The preoccupation persists despite all reasonable medical testing and reassurance; it may cover a wide range of body functions and systems over time as various evaluations demonstrate healthy functioning. Although the preoccupation cannot be attributed solely to the presence of comorbid anxiety, depression, obsessive-compulsive disorder, or psychotic disorder, it may be associated with these conditions.

Hypochondriasis may occur at any age. The course is usually chronic, with waxing and waning symptoms and presentations. It seems to be equally common in men and women and may be made worse by the diagnosis of new medical problems.

10. What should the physician guard against in treating a hypochondriac?

Hypochondriacs frequently "doctor shop" when dissatisfied by the responsivity of their current physician. "Doctor shopping" may occur in response to failure to diagnose a condition, but more commonly occurs when a physician unwittingly becomes irritated by the patient's persistent complaints. Such irritation may manifest as avoidance behavior—failure to return phone calls, abrupt referral to a psychiatrist without careful preparation, or unwillingness to reassure the patient for the "umpteenth" time that the dark urine does not represent kidney failure.

11. What is the treatment for hypochondriasis?

Treatment of the hypochondriac should include careful assessment and reassessment for comorbid psychiatric disorders. Particularly important is aggressive treatment of symptomatic anxiety, depression, and frank delusions, which may worsen hypochondriacal complaints and/or occur in response to the chronic fear of disease. Although hypochondriasis and chronic somatization disorder should be considered as separate entities and are differentiated by the hypochondriac's intense preoccupation, in practice they exist on a continuum.

12. How does hypochondriasis differ from body dysmorphic disorder?

Hypochondriasis does not focus on a specific, circumscribed concern about appearance (see Question 13).

13. Describe body dysmorphic disorder.

Body dysmorphic disorder refers to preoccupation with an **imagined defect** in physical appearance. The sense of defect may occur in response to a mild physical anomaly or with no identifiable trace of abnormality. A common example is the person obsessed with the ugliness of his or her nose because of a small bump. Distress frequently leads to a search for cures through techniques such as plastic surgery or dental treatment. The patient frequently is tormented with feelings of inadequacy and may go to extreme lengths to resolve them; make-up, exercise, and diet may be part of important rituals.

Clearly, the intense focus of western culture on physical beauty provides a setting for a continuum of concern about bodily perfection. Body dysmorphic disorder represents an extreme of this continuum. In **anorexia nervosa** the focus is on being too fat; thus, the patient uses diet-related methods rather than surgery to cure the problem.

14. Describe pain disorders.

Pain disorders are characterized by a specific, predominant focus on pain as the presenting symptom. The pain usually does not follow established anatomic patterns. However, it may be impossible to differentiate from established medical conditions such as lumbar disc disease. Although work-ups typically are negative, prior invasive treatment may lead to physical findings that completely muddy the diagnosis (see Question 5). Indeed, pain disorders may develop after prior injury or treatment, which provides some pathophysiologic explanation for the symptoms.

Pain disorders may occur throughout the lifespan and are more common in women than men. The course may be persistent and lead to severe functional impairment and extensive use of pain medication.

15. How are pain disorders assessed and treated?

Pay careful attention to the presence of comorbid depression, which may present with pain symptoms. Psychotic and anxiety disorders also may feature pain, as one of an array of symptoms.

The management of chronic pain syndromes is described at length in Chapter 69. Rehabilitation programs combining behavioral and physical therapies may be helpful in some patients. External gains (e.g., social, financial) may affect the success of treatment, but as with somatization disorder, the primary cause is inner psychic gain.

16. Describe malingering.

The essential feature of malingering is an *intentional* causing or faking of physical or psychological symptoms motivated by external incentives. Such incentives may be monetary or related to avoidance of work, prosecution, or military service; they also may involve the goal of obtaining drugs.

Several factors are suggestive of underlying malingering. Most commonly, the symptom is complex and/or vague, and the patient is involved in a law suit because of an injury or accident. The discrepancy between the symptomatic presentation and the apparent physical findings may be marked. Lack of cooperation in the evaluation process and poor compliance with recommended treatment are also common. Finally, the presence of an antisocial personality disorder may suggest malingering in a patient presenting with unexplained symptoms associated with possible external rewards or motivations. Thus malingering, unlike somatoform disorders, is motivated primarily by **external gain**.

17. Describe factitious disorder.

In factitious disorder, external factors may be present, but they play a minor role in providing support or reinforcement for symptoms. The motivation for a factitious disorder appears to derive from assuming the role of a sick person. Factitious disorders may involve fabrication of subjective complaints, such as headache; self-inflicted injury; and/or exaggeration of pre-existing medical conditions.

Patients with factitious disorder usually engage in some form of **lying**. They may present with vague, inconsistent histories, often with a dramatic flair. Patients often have prior experience with medical routines and are knowledgeable about medical terminology. They eagerly await work-up results, and their complaints may change with normal or negative findings. They even ask for multiple invasive procedures. Patients usually deny any suggestion that symptoms are self-induced or exaggerated and upon confrontation usually discharge themselves, only to appear in another emergency department or clinic.

The onset of factitious disorder is usually in adolescence or early adulthood. Although it may involve only a few episodes, chronic patterns often develop; in some instances, the patient travels to multiple cities—even countries—seeking hospitalization.

18. What is Münchausen's syndrome?

An extreme form of chronic, recurrent factitious disorder that typically involves wandering from place to place and taking on a lifestyle that centers on repeated evaluation, treatment, and hospitalization. The extensive wandering and search for different treatments may result from confrontations by angry hospital staff. However, it is not entirely clear whether the wandering and the accompanying disorder can be prevented by alternative treatment approaches.

Severe factitious disorders also have been described in children. The parent reports symptoms in the child in the manner described in adults. Termed **Münchausen's by proxy** (see Chapter 81), this syndrome should be considered as a possible instance of child abuse and reported to appropriate authorities under the guidance of state and local laws.

19. How are malingering and factitious disorder distinguished from somatoform disorders?

Malingering
Motivated by external gain (e.g,. winning a lawsuit)
Symptoms intentionally caused or feigned
Poor cooperation in evaluation and treatment
May be accompanied by antisocial personality disorder

Factitious Disorder
Motivated by assumption of the sick role
Symptoms fabricated and/or injury self-inflicted
History vague and confusing
Often chronic
Patients may go from hospital to hospital seeking care

Somatoform Disorders
Motivated by inner, psychic gain
Unintentional, involuntary
May be result of past or current, traumatic stressor

20. Describe a general approach to the patient with unexplained medical symptoms.

The management of unexplained medical symptoms is a series of recurring steps.

• **In the acute presentation**, careful assessment of the medical symptoms, physical findings, and associated psychological responses may be followed by thoughtful, nonjudgmental reassurance when the symptoms are relatively mild, circumscribed, and of recent origin. The psychoeducational approach (information, reassurance, and explanation of probable cause) is often sufficient, and the symptoms remit. For example, a child may present with headaches before school is to begin. Exploration of the stress may help the parents and child to find methods of reassurance that alleviate the source of the anxiety-based symptoms.

Such an approach can be used in combination with more in-depth medical assessment. For example, a patient hospitalized for treatment of a compound fracture of the left leg spontaneously developed paresis in the good leg. The paresis appeared to have no anatomic basis. Assessment by a consulting neurologist confirmed the initial evaluation by the primary physician. The consultant's suggestion that the symptoms would improve gradually over time was sufficient; over the following several days of recuperation the symptoms completely remitted.

• **When symptoms are persistent and/or severe**, further steps are warranted, including more medical evaluation and detailed psychosocial assessment to identify psychological factors and social triggers. The laboratory and physical findings should be presented unambiguously and in a nonjudgmental manner. The treatment plan may require negotiation with the patient to set limits on the nature of investigations, specialty referrals, and unwarranted treatment.

Avoid simplistic dual models in which the diagnosis is either physical or mental. Present, as part of the medical evaluation, a psychological explanatory model of the symptom process using words that are both understandable and safe. The model can indicate that the symptoms may be stress-related.

21. Won't the patient balk at any suggestion that symptoms are stress-related?

Sometimes; but the approach recommended can improve patient acceptance. As one part of this approach, underline that stress-related symptoms are just as real as symptoms produced by a clear medical illness. For example, the patient fearing cancer needs to understand that the presenting symptom, if it is said to be stress-related, is just as important to you as if it were caused by cancer. Furthermore, emphasize that the suggested treatments for somatoform disorders are just as real as treatments for feared medical conditions, though they differ.

Careful assessment also should include evaluation for comorbid psychiatric conditions such as depression, anxiety, personality disorders, and psychosis. It is helpful to have a single medical doctor or team approach in treating the chronic somatisizing patient. The team may include a physician and a mental health professional who work either in the same institution or in close collaboration. Be open and honest at all steps of the treatment. "Sneaking in" a psychiatric referral leads only to greater mistrust and resistance to treatment recommendations.

22. How can the physician facilitate the process?

Consistency and flexibility are both important. Avoid unnecessary, new medical assessments. Offer a clear, sensible, and consistent pronouncement of your findings and recommendations. Patients often need to hear repeatedly what the doctor thinks, why he or she thinks it, and why a specific treatment is or is not recommended.

At times of increased anxiety, flexibility may be required. For example, the patient who is chronically worried about renal failure may require periodic (and superficially unnecessary) simple kidney function tests to demonstrate kidney health. Letting the patient's concerns help to dictate evaluation and treatment decisions provides a sense of control. Continual renegotiation with the patient is essential. Flexibility also is warranted because in the course of chronic somatisizing problems other psychiatric disorders commonly develop (e.g., the hypochondriac may require antidepressant treatment). Likewise, inflexibility may lead to missing the diagnosis of newly emerging medical illness.

Finally, by maintaining a consistent, stable, nonjudgmental attitude the physician helps patients to feel understood, encouraging continuation of treatment and avoiding "doctor shopping."

23. Are specific treatment approaches applied differentially to the different forms of somatoform disorders?

There are more similarities than differences in treating patients with medically unexplained symptoms. As noted, the severity and chronicity of the complaint are important determinants of the initial approach. Additionally, certain therapeutic variations derive from the type of somatoform disorder.

• Patients with **body dysmorphic disorder** may benefit from a supportive therapeutic approach that helps the patient to understand possible sources of the distorted beliefs. Cognitive-behavioral therapy may be useful (see Chapter 41). Beliefs about body shape and deformity are so powerful, however, that short-term cognitive approaches are unlikely to lead to radical improvement. Thus, they should be considered in the context of chronic management that helps the patient to avoid recurrent, invasive treatment. The distorted perceptions can be so severe as to become delusional; such patients may respond to low doses of antipsychotic medication.

• A focused approach is less likely to be effective in **somatization disorder** and **hypochondriasis** because of the broad range of symptoms and complaints. In all instances the therapy for chronic conditions needs to be considered as long-term and supportive. Recognition of serious underlying psychological problems may not only guide therapy but also serve to allay the doctor's sense of being used and abused by the patient, thereby helping to maintain a positive therapeutic alliance. Especially in patients with **conversion disorder**, hypnotherapy and/or other methods for exploring sources of particular stress may bring out unresolved conflicts and concerns that were not previously identified. Uncovering such issues can be useful in treating conversion symptoms.

24. What is especially important to remember in caring for patients with medically unexplained symptoms?

The therapist and physician must recognize that these patients often produce intense emotional reactions in the caretaker. They may arouse anger by repeated complaints and disturbances as well as cause embarrassment with multiple visits to the emergency department, seeming to represent treatment failures in the eyes of the clinician and possibly his or her colleagues. Furthermore, chronic demands for pain medications and letters to housing boards and employers may lead the clinician to feel used by the patient. Remember that while external gain may be a secondary motivation for some symptoms in some patients, it is usually not the primary causal factor.

25. How do approaches to treatment differ for patients with factitious disorder or malingering?

In many ways the approaches to treatment are similar. The critical differential with the malingering patient is recognizing that the patient always has another, external goal; consistency and clarity are required so that the patient understands what the physician is recommending. Many such patients leave treatment because they do not obtain an external reward. The patient with factitious illness also may leave treatment if the drive for the sick role comes in conflict with the physician's unwillingness to perform more invasive tests.

26. How are medical symptoms associated with other psychiatric conditions differentiated from those associated with somatoform and factitious disorders and malingering?

Three psychiatric syndromes most commonly present with subtle and sometimes vague physical symptoms: depression, anxiety, and psychosis. Diagnosis depends on a careful history that explores for the symptoms of each psychiatric disorder. When the patient presents with symptoms suggestive of either anxiety or depression, such as headaches or other bodily pains, a trial of appropriate medication may be useful. Such therapeutic trials are also valuable because anxiety and depressive disorders may well coexist with somatoform conditions. Treatment of the comorbid psychiatric condition may lead to considerable improvement in the somatoform disorder. In addition, symptomatic treatment of depression, anxiety, and psychosis often is more effective than treatment of chronic somatizing conditions.

BIBLIOGRAPHY

1. Bass C, Benjamin S: The management of chronic somatisation. Br J Psychiatry 162:472–480, 1993.
2. Reference deleted.
3. Kellner R: Psychosomatic syndromes, somatization and somatoform disorders. Psychother Psychosom 61:4–24, 1994.
4. Kellner R: Somatization: Theories and research. J Nerv Mental Dis 178:150–160, 1990.
5. Lipowski ZJ: Somatization: The concept and its clinical application. Am J Psychiatry 145:1358–1368, 1988.
6. Margo KL, Margo GM: The problem of somatization in family practice. Am Fam Physician 1873–1879, 1994.
7. Mayou R: Somatization. Psychother Psychosom 59:69–83, 1993.
8. Somatoform disorders. Diagnostic and Statistical Manual–IV. Washington, DC, American Psychiatric Association, 1994.
9. Wise MG, Ford CV: Factitious disorders. Prim Care 26:315–326, 1999.

32. GRIEF AND MOURNING

Stephen R. Shuchter, M.D., and Sidney Zisook, M.D.

All psychiatrists encounter patients who have experienced the death of a loved one. Such losses often are quite traumatic and painful and can precipitate both psychological and medical sequelae which may require intervention. Appreciating the effects of death on survivors can be a crucial element in assessing the patient.

1. What is grief?

Grief comprises the myriad psychological, physiologic, and behavioral responses which accompany the human awareness of an irrevocable loss, such as a pending or actual loss of a close friend or relative. It is an extraordinarily powerful emotion.

Manifestations of Normal Grief

Psychological	Physiologic
Numbness or dissociation	Autonomic discharge: gastrointestinal,
Sense of loss	cardiovascular, respiratory, neuromuscular
Anguish	Insomnia
Yearning	Agitation
Anger	Anorexia
Guilt	
Apathy	
Anxiety and fear	
Intrusive images	
Cognitive disorganization	
Distractibility	
Hallucinatory experiences	
Regression	

2. What are the psychological aftereffects?

The psychological sequelae may include experiences of intense anguish and emotional pain accompanied by crying, feelings of loss, and yearning for the one who has died; feelings of anger or guilt; transient periods of numbness, shock, or disbelief, when the loss does not register emotionally; a sense of apathy or lack of direction; anxiety and fearfulness; intrusion of painful images and memories, especially if the nature or course of death was traumatic to the survivor; and cognitive disorganization. Behaviorally, survivors frequently search for evidence that their loved one is still alive. They may experience multiple sensory hallucinations of the deceased, most often in the form of sensing their presence but also including auditory, visual, haptic, and olfactory hallucinations.

Many grieving persons attempt to isolate themselves from social contacts, which are too painful because of the memories they evoke. They may avoid discussing their loss or even confronting mundane experiences of life or possessions of the deceased which can trigger their anguish. The aggregation of these powerful emotional and cognitive forces often leads to a **regression**: an emotional state in which the grieving person feels overwhelmed, out of control, helpless, and child-like in heightened dependency.

3. What forms of physiologic responses are common?

Physiologic responses occur frequently, often in reaction to reminders of the loss. They take the form of sudden autonomic discharge with acute symptoms reflecting the pangs of grief: chest pain ("heartache"), gastrointestinal distress ("a knife in the belly"), dyspnea, paresthesias, palpitations, dizziness, nausea, tremulousness, and others. Acutely grieving survivors may demonstrate hypercortisolism, sleep and appetite disturbances, and continuously heightened autonomic arousal.

4. Are all losses the same?

No. Although the word "grief" generally is reserved for the feelings and behavior associated with death (e.g., bereavement), the same sort of reaction is seen after any loss considered important by the individual. Examples are stillbirth and miscarriage, loss of a job, failing health, disability, amputation, loss of home, or divorce. Indeed, divorce, especially when dependent children are involved, can lead to some of the most tumultuous and persistent grief reactions. Sometimes a loss that seems trivial to the outside observer, such as the death of a pet or a favorite celebrity, or losing an object of sentimental value, is followed by a severe grief reaction because the loss has a disproportionate significance. The grief also can occur when the loss is intangible, such as after a stroke or cataract, when the loss is a *function* of a part of the body. In each of these examples, the individual loses someone or something that is emotionally or physically "part of themselves." The meaning of such losses, the intensity of the grief, and the way people ultimately cope with the changes in their lives vary from person to person.

5. What is mourning?

Mourning is an important aspect of the total grief reaction. It refers to a prescribed set of experiences—which may include a time-frame and a series of behaviors, rituals, and observances—that reflect a given culture's or religion's views about the meanings of life and death and the role of the individual survivor within this context. Mourning customs may be strictly defined: the widow should wear black and avoid pleasantries for a year; the funeral and memorial services should contain certain elements; prayers for the dead are said on particular occasions. Some grief experiences, such as hallucinations, may be more acceptable or even desirable in certain cultures.

In the United States, no standard traditions dictate the decisions and behavior of survivors. There are few tight-knit communities where widowed men and and women are scrutinized or monitored. Individuals' religious beliefs may dictate some traditions, but for the most part, mourning has evolved toward a more individualized and relatively unstructured experience.

6. What is pathologic grief?

Pathologic grief is a commonly used term with an elusive definition. It originally referred to those patients whose grief was absent or excessively intense or prolonged. It also referred to situations where grieving patients developed medical or psychiatric illnesses. Although clinicians will likely continue to encounter references to pathologic grief, it is not a useful concept. First, the spectrum of normative responses to loss is enormous. Some people's grief is brief and limited in terms of their emotional responses and sequelae; others grieve profoundly for a long time. Furthermore, particularly following the death of a spouse or a child, survivors are likely to continue to manifest elements of grief intermittently throughout their lives. Responses at both ends of this continuum are normal and not pathologic.

Second, some individuals are vulnerable to the development of medical and psychiatric illnesses in the context of grief. These illnesses also do not constitute pathologic grief, but idiosyncratic vulnerability (genetic and developmental), as expressed at a point of an enormous stressor.

7. How long does grief last?

There is great variability in the course of grief. The most important determinant of the length and intensity of grief is the closeness of the relationship between the deceased and survivor: how central that person was to the survivor's emotional life. In the closest of relationships, an acute period of grief may last from a few weeks to several months, and protracted grief may last for years. If you encounter such extended grief, or a persistent, intense grief a year or more after the death, consider the possibility of major depression.

8. Does grief end?

The most common and clinically normal forms of protracted grief occur on an intermittent basis for several years, or forever. A person who has lost a child may experience elements of acute grief every time he or she hears the name of the child, on special occasions (birthdays, holidays, anniversaries), or when seeing the child's picture. Such grief, often referred to as *anniversary reactions*, usually is short-lived and dissipates in minutes. Similarly, when a clinician makes an inquiry into the emotions of any patient's loss, it should be recognized that in such a regressively oriented exploration, elements of grief are likely to appear and are normal. It is a mistake to think that grief "resolves" in the sense that it disappears or goes away. In most people, grief is circumscribed and suppressed, only to re-emerge in response to familiar triggers.

9. What is the relationship between grief and depression?

Acute grief represents one of the most powerful paradigms for the stress-diathesis model of medical illness, including psychiatric illness (see figure). The death of a loved one is likely to be the most profound and intense stressor that most people will encounter. Studies repeatedly have demonstrated the association between grief and the development of numerous stress-related medical disorders, including heart disease, cancer, and the common cold. The bereaved are vulnerable, as well, to psychiatric syndromes, especially depression.

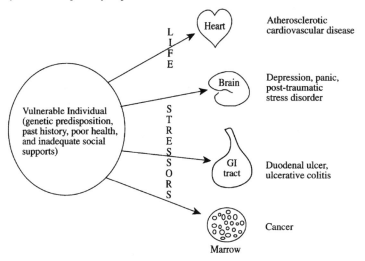

Stress-diathesis model of medical illness.

Historically, bereaved individuals, their families, and physicians have taken the position that grief is "depressing" and that "mourning" and "melancholia" are inseparable phenomena. No one is surprised when a survivor is depressed; it seems normal and natural. Consequently, the physician exhibits less zeal in treating a disorder that otherwise would be the object of aggressive therapy.

At some time during the first year after the death of a spouse, 30–50% of widows and widowers meet the criteria for a major depressive episode. Recognizing the ubiquity of depressive symptoms in grief, the DSM-III and DSM-III-R introduced the term *Uncomplicated Bereavement* to demarcate depressive syndromes occurring shortly after the death of a close friend or relative from a major depressive disorder. Because uncomplicated bereavement is not considered an illness, the clinical rule-of-thumb has been benign neglect rather than active treatment. Such depressions often are persistent, however, and may be associated with substantial morbidity. Therefore, the DSM-IV changed the term uncomplicated bereavement to *Bereavement*, suggesting that only mild depressive syndromes beginning and ending within 2 months of the death should be considered "normal."

10. Can grief and depression be distinguished?

Although manifestations of acute grief frequently mimic or overlap those of depression, they can be differentiated by the **intermittent** and **trigger-related quality** of grief symptoms and the autonomous quality of depressive symptoms. Once depression has a "life of its own," the intermittent periods of good functioning and relatively normal affects that punctuate the lives of the nondepressed grieving individual are less likely. Other differential points are: *several* symptoms of depression occur simultaneously most of the time, for at least 2 weeks; and relentless anhedonia is common in depression but less frequent in grief uncomplicated by major depression.

The DSM-IV lists several additional factors that should alert the clinician that a major depression may be present. These include: (1) guilt unassociated with the death; (2) preoccupation with death independent of the specific death of the loved one; (3) morbid preoccupation with worthlessness; (4) marked psychomotor retardation; (5) prolonged and marked functional impairment; and (6) hallucinations not involving the deceased.

Differentiation of Mourning and Melancholy

	NORMAL DEPRESSION OF BEREAVEMENT (DSM-IV)	MAJOR DEPRESSIVE EPISODE (MDE)
Onset	Within 2 months of death	Any time after death (or before death in response to prolonged dying)
Duration	Less than 2 months	Weeks to years; typically at least 6–9 months
Course	Circumscribed episode: symptoms associated with "triggers," then resolve	History of chronic, intermittent, or recurrent symptoms; current symptoms autonomous (i.e., independent of trigger)
Symptoms	Rarely include severe guilt, suicidal ideation, morbid worthlessness, psychomotor retardation, or psychosis	All symptoms of MDE, often including atypical, melancholic, or psychotic features
Impairment	Brief and mild to moderate	May be prolonged and marked
Self-perception	Normal	Disordered

11. Are grief and depression intrinsically connected?

Yes. Another complicating element in the relationship between grief and depression is that **depression recruits grief**; that is, depressive states have a tendency to exacerbate prior experiences of grief. Patients with a major depression whose focus is on some relationship that ended, or on the death of someone important in their lives, are not uncommon. Such losses may have occurred years before. This presentation often leads a clinician to believe that the depressive episode is a manifestation of "unresolved grief" and to begin to focus treatment on the grief. Remembering that grief does not resolve but only subsides, the correct assessment will reveal that the grief is a manifestation of depression; it will subside once the depression is treated. In this scenario, depression begets grief, rather than the converse.

12. Should grieving patients be treated with psychopharmacologic agents?

It depends. Grief itself is a normal response to loss. At times, people feel overwhelmed by the power of their emotions. They often try to "dose" themselves, by allowing exposure to stimuli that evokes anguish and then avoiding it when it becomes too much. People learn what is painful and what is not, which activities they can do safely and which are "dangerous" as triggers for their grief. For those who are experiencing this type of distress, there is no indication to medicate despite what may be a perceived need by the patient for relief. However, there are exceptions.

13. When should grieving patients be treated with psychopharmacologic agents?

When grief-related symptoms of anxiety are expressed so continuously that they interfere with cognitive and other **functions of living** in a substantial way, consider the use of a benzodiazepine. This medication also is an option in patients who have a higher risk of development or exacerbation of a major depression or anxiety disorder. Usually, benzodiazepines are used as needed for relatively brief periods.

When substantial **sleep disorders** develop, short-term intervention with pharmacology can be both humane and helpful. Agents include: (1) hypnotics, (2) short-acting anxiolytics, or (3) low doses of sedating antidepressants (e.g., trazodone, 50 mg). A persistent and continuous sleep disorder with features of early, middle, or late insomnia may indicate the onset of major depression, requiring closer monitoring and possible use of antidepressants in standard doses.

Depression is under-diagnosed and often under-treated even when diagnosed. Historically, physicians have been reluctant to treat the depression of bereavement aggressively, feeling that treating such depression interferes with normal grief and nature's restorative properties. However, depression is depression, regardless of the context in which it appears or the existential reasonableness of its presentation. Depression carries with it substantial morbidity, both medical and psychological. *Treat major depression aggressively, even if it appears in the context of bereavement!*

14. How can I counsel the bereaved to get past their loss or to put it behind them?

You cannot, and you ought not try. The death of one's spouse or child or sibling is forever, and elements of the survivor's grief also will last forever. Healthy people find many ways to cope with their losses and grief. One of the most "human" ways to deal with such loss is to mitigate against it by keeping the loved one alive. It is normal and healthy for survivors to maintain a relationship with the deceased.

Survivors frequently have a sense that their loved one is with them, watching over them, protecting them. It is not uncommon for a widow to carry on conversations with her dead husband or to ask for his advice. These and similar phenomena occur in healthy people with intact reality-testing whose sensory perceptions are highly directed toward keeping their loved ones alive. As time goes by, the actual sense of their loved one's presence evolves into an emotional feeling of the person's place in their heart. Qualities of the deceased may become incorporated into the identity of the survivor. Cherished possessions and memories keep the deceased alive for those who have physically lost them. Important emotional ties do not disappear when our loved ones die, and clinicians must learn to appreciate these connections, respect them, and even foster communication about them. For survivors, life will go on, and more comfortably once they have established an emotionally viable way of sustaining their relationship with the deceased.

Therefore, it is *not* helpful to convince a bereaved individual to "let go" or get on with life in a way that disregards the loved one. Instead, let such patients know you care. Listen when they feel like talking. Offer the perspective of someone who identifies with the painful and often protracted course of grief. Be ready to step in when, and if, a major depression or other medical or psychiatric complications develop.

15. What are the other common problems of the bereaved?

Frequently, problems develop because of the **reactions of others to grief**. Friends and family may be unable to tolerate grief and may avoid the bereaved or, when with them, discourage them from expressing what they feel. Grieving persons may feel isolated, at times because of their reluctance to inflict their own suffering on others. In time, they will find closeness and comfort with others who have felt such pain and with whom they feel a common bond. For this reason, involvement in a bereavement support group usually is helpful.

Of particular concern is the difficulty physicians and therapists can have in dealing with the bereaved, particularly those in the most acute throes of grief. Empathetic clinicians may find themselves experiencing much anguish and helplessness in the face of their patients' suffering. At times this may feel intolerable, and clinicians may become inclined to push their patients away or to divert them from their grief. Other therapists may fear being "swallowed up" by the intense need of the grieving person. The intense regression of grief is, however, a time-limited phenomenon, and the clinician's emotional availability is central to his or her ability to help the bereaved. The healthy clinician emerges from the suffering, often stronger for the experience.

BIBLIOGRAPHY

1. Burnell GM, Burnell AL (eds): Clinical Management of Bereavement: A Handbook for Healthcare Professionals. New York, Human Sciences Press, 1989.
2. Jacobs S (ed): Pathologic Grief: Maladaptation to Loss. Washington, DC, American Psychiatric Press, 1993.
3. Osterweis M, Solomon F, Green M (eds): Bereavement: Reactions, Consequences, and Care. Washington, DC, National Academy Press, 1984.
4. Prigerson HG, Reynolds CF, Jacobs SC, et al: Results of a consensus conference to refine diagnostic criteria for traumatic grief. Br J Psychiatry, In Press.
5. Raphael B (ed): The Anatomy of Bereavement. New York, Basic Books, 1983.
6. Reynolds CF, Miller MD, Pasternak RE, et al: Treatment of bereavement-related major depressive episodes in later life: A controlled study of acute and continuation treatment with nortriptyline and interpersonal psychotherapy. Am J Psychiatry 156:202–208, 1999.
7. Rynearson EK (ed): Bereavement. Psychiatric Annals (Special Issue) 16:268–318, 1986.
8. Rynearson EK (ed): Pathologic Bereavement. Psychiatric Annals (Special Issue) 20:294–348, 1990.
9. Shuchter SR (ed): Dimensions of Grief: Adjusting to the Death of a Spouse. San Francisco, Jossey-Bass, 1986.
10. Stroebe MS, Stroebe W, Hansson RO (eds): Handbook of Bereavement: Theory, Research and Intervention. Cambridge, Cambridge University Press, 1993.
11. Worden JW (ed): Grief Counseling and Grief Therapy: A Handbook for the Mental Health Practitioner. 2nd ed. New York, Springer, 1991.
12. Wortman CB, Silver RC: The myths of coping with loss. J Consult Clin Psychol 57:349–357, 1989.
13. Zisook S, Shuchter SR: Major depression associated with widowhood. Am Assoc Geriatr Psychiatry 1:316–326, 1993.
14. Zisook S (ed): Grief and Bereavement. Psychiatr Clin North Am 10:329–510, 1987.
15. Zisook S, Chentsova-Dutton Y, Shuchter SR: PSTD following bereavement. Ann Clin Psychiatry 10(4):157–163, 1999.
16. Zisook S, Shuchter SR: Psychotherapy of the depressions in spousal bereavement. Psychother Pract 2:31–45, 1996.
17. Zisook S, Schuchter SR, Pederelli P, et al: Bupropion: Treatment of bereavement. Am J Psychiatry, In Press.

IV. Dementia, Delirium, and Related Conditions

33. BEHAVIORAL PRESENTATIONS OF MEDICAL AND NEUROLOGIC DISORDERS

C. Alan Anderson, M.D., and Christopher M. Filley, M.D.

1. Why is the identification of an underlying medical or neurologic disorder important?

What initially seems to be a standard psychiatric illness on closer examination may prove to be a medical or neurologic disease. Patients with medical illness who present with behavioral or psychiatric symptoms as the major manifestation have been shown to have significant morbidity and mortality that worsens with delay in diagnosis and treatment. Illnesses as diverse as brain tumors and renal failure may present with behavioral syndromes, and for many of the conditions there are specific and effective therapies. Psychiatric treatment is unlikely to be effective and the condition may worsen unless the primary problem is addressed. Hence, the timely and expeditious identification of patients with secondary or induced behavior syndromes is crucial.

2. What are the typical behavioral presentations of medical and neurologic diseases?

Whereas nearly every symptom, syndrome, and psychiatric diagnostic category has been described, several presentations are particularly common. Confusional states, psychosis, depression, and personality changes are the most frequent, with anxiety, mania, and conversion disorder occurring less often. All varieties of presentation are seen. Affected patients may present with isolated symptoms or with multiple symptoms of sufficient duration and severity to meet DSM-IV criteria. The problem may be acute and progressive, or it may present as a chronic condition with little or no change over months to years. The bad news, therefore, is that we need to consider an underlying medical or neurologic problem in nearly every patient that we see. The good news, however, is that clinical clues help to identify patients at higher risk and assist in focusing the evaluation.

In general, the **absence of prior psychiatric problems**, **lack of family history of psychiatric illness**, and **onset of symptoms after age 40** should raise the suspicion of medical or neurologic illness. A thorough review of systems may uncover other problems that otherwise would be overlooked in the face of major behavioral disturbances. A history of headaches, syncope, seizures, head trauma, focal neurologic problems (i.e., visual disturbance, weakness, incoordination), cardiopulmonary complaints, incontinence, weight change, or fevers should prompt further investigation. Finally, presenting complaints that have a higher likelihood of representing medical illness include progressive intellectual deterioration, apathy or indifference, and visual hallucinations without accompanying auditory hallucinations.

3. What is confusion?

Because of its everyday use, confusion as a medical term has confused many clinicians. In clinical terms, confusion means the inability to maintain a coherent line of thought. Confusional states are exceedingly common, and most arise acutely because of a reversible toxic or metabolic disorder with prominent effects on the brain. The patient with an acute confusional state typically presents with impaired attention, disorientation, incoherent thinking, hallucinations, delusions, illusions, disturbed sleep-wake cycles, and variable alterations in level of consciousness. The cardinal feature is the disturbance of attention; other symptoms present in varying combinations and degrees.

Synonymous terms terms include delirium and metabolic or toxic encephalopathy, and each may be used to emphasize certain aspects of the syndrome. The term acute organic brain syndrome, however, is inadequate, both because it lacks specificity and because it promulgates the unlikely belief that some behavioral disorders do not result from brain dysfunction. This terminology has been deleted from the DSM-IV, and we suggest that it be dropped from common medical usage as well.

4. Which disorders may present with confusion?

Patients at higher risk for developing an acute confusional state include the elderly, patients with prior brain disease or injury, postoperative or burn patients, and patients with acquired immunodeficiency syndrome (AIDS). The list of causes for the acute confusional state is long but the more common disorders associated with confusion are listed below:

Common Causes of the Acute Confusional State

Intoxications—alcohol; prescription, over-the-counter, and street drugs; solvents; heavy metals; pesticides; carbon monoxide

Withdrawal states—alcohol, sedative-hypnotic drugs

Nutritional deficiencies—thiamine (Wernicke's encephalopathy), vitamin B_{12}, folate, niacin

Metabolic disorders—electrolyte and acid-base disturbances; hepatic, renal, pancreatic disease

Infections—pneumonia, urinary tract infection, sepsis, AIDS

Endocrinopathies—hypo- and hyperthyroidism, hypo- and hyperglycemia, hypo- and hyperadrenocorticism

Structural brain disease—traumatic brain injury, seizure disorders, stroke, subarachnoid or parenchymal hemorrhage, epidural or subdural hematoma, encephalitis, brain abscess

Postoperative states—anesthesia, electrolyte disturbances, fever, hypoxia, analgesics

5. Differentiate primary and secondary psychosis.

The essence of psychosis is loss of contact with reality. This breakdown in perception, thought content, and communications takes various forms, including hallucinations, delusions, motor disturbances, paranoia, and changes in affect. Although the typical constellation of symptoms and signs of schizophrenia has been described in medical and neurological illness, usually other clues suggest an underlying pathologic process.

Secondary or induced psychosis often has a more abrupt onset, more prominent alterations in level of consciousness, and more evidence of intellectual deterioration. The character of symptoms also may be different, with induced psychosis more likely to cause visual hallucinations without auditory hallucinations, and poorly defined delusions.

Primary psychosis, due entirely to psychiatric illness, more often manifests auditory hallucinations, preserved level of alertness and orientation, and more complex and stable delusions.

6. Which disorders may present with secondary psychosis?

Disorders Associated with Secondary Psychosis

Complex partial seizures	Traumatic brain injury
Alcohol withdrawal	Stroke
Drugs (prescription, over-the-counter, street; for example bromocriptine, levodopa, diet pills, amphetamines)	Brain infections
	Brain neoplasms
Metabolic disorders (hepatic, renal, thyroid disease; vitamin deficiencies)	Dementia (Alzheimer's disease, Pick's disease, Huntington's disease, Wilson's disease)
Multiple sclerosis	

7. Which disorders may present with depression?

The depressed patient presents with low mood, psychomotor retardation, apathy, and anhedonia, plus the vegetative signs of decreased appetite, diminished libido, and sleep disturbance. The more common concern is overlooking functional depression while searching for medical and neurologic illness, but the reverse situation also occurs. Systemic illnesses can present with a clinical picture typical of major depression in every respect. Clues to distinguishing these patients include the absence of previous psychiatric problems or family history, no precipitating event, older age at onset, and associated medical and neurological signs and symptoms.

Frequent Medical and Neurologic Causes of Depression

Drugs (oral contraceptives, beta-blockers, opiates, benzodiazepines, barbiturates, methyldopa)	Metabolic disorders (thyroid disorders, adrenal disorders, hepatic disease, hypoglycemia, pancreatic and gastrointestinal cancer)
Stroke	Dementia (Alzheimer's disease, Parkinson's disease, Huntington's disease)
Systemic lupus erythematosus	Neurosyphilis
Brain neoplasms	
Traumatic brain injury	
Multiple sclerosis	

8. Which disorders may present with mania?

Manic patients present with increased energy, flight of ideas, grandiosity, and impaired judgment against a background of an abnormally elevated or irritable mood. There may be delusions and hallucinations as well. Mania has been described as the presenting symptom of many medical disorders and also as a consequence of head trauma and seizure disorder. The diagnosis of secondary or induced mania is suggested by associated neurologic signs and symptoms and initial presentation after the age of 40.

Common Medical and Neurologic Causes of Mania

Drugs (e.g., excessive thyroid hormone, amphetamines, cocaine, monoamine oxidase inhibitors, steroids)	Multiple sclerosis
	Dementia (Huntington's disease, Wilson's disease, Pick's disease)
Hyperthyroidism	Herpes simplex encephalitis
Seizure disorders (especially complex-partial)	Neurosyphilis
Traumatic brain injury	Brain neoplasms
Stroke	

9. Which disorders may result in personality change?

Personality changes are like good art: they are hard to describe and categorize, but we know them when we see them. Subtle alterations in basic character and temperament often herald the onset of neurologic illness. Comportment, motivation, affect, judgment, and impulse control may change dramatically in the face of disease or injury of the brain. Whereas nearly any illness or injury may alter personality, the following lists provides a clinical guide.

Medical and Neurologic Causes of Personality Change

Traumatic brain injury	Complex partial seizure disorder
Dementia (Pick's disease, Alzheimer's disease, Huntington's disease, Wilson's disease, normal pressure hydrocephalus)	Drug and alcohol abuse
	Neurosyphilis
	Infection with human immunodeficiency virus (HIV)
Brain neoplasms	Hypo- and hyperthyroidism
Stroke	
Multiple sclerosis	

10. Which disorders may present with anxiety?

Patients with anxiety typically display apprehension, fear, hyperattentiveness, trembling, restlessness, dizziness, dry mouth, and palpitations. These are common autonomic responses to psychological stress but also may represent an undiagnosed medical or neurologic illness. As in the examples above, absence of related history, lack of precipitating event, and older age at onset suggest an underlying disorder. In large series of patients, endocrine diseases and cardiopulmonary conditions were most likely to present with anxiety.

Likely Disorders Associated with Anxiety

Hyperthyroidism	Pulmonary disease
Hypoglycemia	Drugs
Pheochromocytoma	Alcohol or sedative-hypnotic withdrawal
Hypoparathyroidism	Systemic lupus erythematosus
Cardiovascular disease	Wilson's disease

11. Why is it important to recognize conversion disorder?

Many patients present with symptoms and signs that suggest medical or neurologic illness, but are due to unconscious manifestations of emotional conflict. The clinician needs to be able to recognize this pattern, both for accurate diagnosis of psychiatric illness and for isolation of hysterical clinical features from those that may be due to medical or neurologic illness. An important point to remember is that signs and symptoms of conversion disorder are common in patients with known neurologic illness. For example, nonepileptic seizures may be encountered in patients with established seizure disorders. Such traditional signs of conversion disorder as give-way weakness, nonanatomic sensory changes, and la belle indifference may be seen in patients with multiple sclerosis and other neurologic disorders (see Chapter 31 for further discussion of conversion disorder). Disorders that frequently accompany hysteria include:

Multiple sclerosis	Complicated migraine
Systemic lupus erythematosus	Neurosyphilis
Seizure disorders	Endocrine disorders

12. What is an appropriate evaluation of patients presenting with behavioral syndromes?

As with all medical disciplines, it is wise to start with a detailed history, paying close attention to onset and course of symptoms, past and present medical and surgical history, and complete review of medications and drugs (prescription, over-the-counter, borrowed, stolen, or obtained on the street). The family history should be reviewed for both medical and psychiatric illness. A complete review of systems also is necessary. At this point, we suggest "going where the money is" and reviewing medications and drugs again.

A detailed general physical examination, including neurologic and mental status testing is next. Laboratory evaluations should include a complete blood count, urinalysis, thyroid function studies, and toxicology screen. For example, you may encounter delirium due to hypoglycemia, or psychosis related to hyperthyroidism. Pulse oximetry or arterial blood gas studies, lumbar puncture, syphilis serology, HIV testing, B12 and folate levels, vasculitis screening, and measurements of heavy metals, copper, ceruloplasmin, and porphyrins may be indicated. Consider these tests when signs and symptoms suggest particular organ system involvement or the presence of reversible disorders.

Additional tests include electroencephalography (EEG) and neuroimaging studies. EEG provides information about the physiology of the brain and is safe and readily available at modest cost. Another advantage is that it can be performed at bedside if necessary. The utility of EEG is best documented in seizure disorders, but it often is useful in the diagnosis of acute confusional states, dementia, and focal brain lesions.

Both computerized tomography (CT) and magnetic resonance imaging (MRI) generate detailed anatomic information, and MRI in particular shows elegant views of brain regions that may be implicated in the pathogenesis of behavioral and psychiatric disorders. Because of high cost, however, the indications for obtaining such scans have been controversial. Several behavioral presentations should generally prompt a neuroimaging scan, including acute confusional state or dementia of unknown cause, the initial episode of undiagnosed psychosis, and the first presentation of personality change after age 40. Other indications include focal neurologic findings, movement disorders, incontinence, or evidence of increased intracranial pressure such as headache, nausea, vomiting, and papilledema on funduscopic examination.

BIBLIOGRAPHY

1. Cummings JL: Organic delusions: Phenomenology, anatomical considerations, and review. Br J Psychiatry 146:184–197, 1985.
2. Cummings JL: Psychosis in neurologic disease: Neurobiology and pathogenesis. Neuropsychiatry Neuropsychol Behav Neurol 5:144–150, 1992.
3. Cummings JL, Miller BL: Visual hallucinations: Clinical occurrence and use in differential diagnosis. West J Med 146:46–51, 1987.
4. Gorman DG, Cummings JL: Organic delusional syndrome. Semin Neurol 10:229–238, 1990.
5. Gould R, Miller BL, Goldberg MA, Benson DF: The validity of hysterical signs and symptoms. J Nerv Ment Dis 174:593–597, 1986.
6. Larson EW: Organic causes of mania. Mayo Clin Proc 63:906–912, 1988.
7. Mackenzie TB, Popkin MK: Organic anxiety syndrome. Am J Psychiatry 140:342–344, 1983.
8. Skuster DZ, Digre KB, Corbett JJ: Neurologic conditions presenting as psychiatric disorders. Psychiatr Clin North Am 15:311–333, 1992.
9. Strub RL: Mental disorders in brain disease. In Frederiks JA (ed): Handbook of Clinical Neurology, Vol 2. Amsterdam, Elsevier, 1985, pp 413–441.
10. Taylor D, Lewis S: Delirium. J Neurol Neurosurg Psychiatry 56:742–751, 1993.
11. Filley CM, Kleinschmidt-DeMasters BK: Neurobehavioral presentations of brain neoplasms. West J Med 163:19–25, 1995.
12. Lyoo IK, Seol HY, Byun HS, Renshaw PF: Unsuspected multiple sclerosis in patients with psychiatric disorders: A magnetic resonance imaging study. J Neuropsychiatry Clin Neurosci 8:54–59, 1996.
13. Yudofsky SC, Hales RE (eds): Neuropsychiatry, 2nd ed. Washington, DC, American Psychiatric Press, 1992.

34. DEMENTIA

Roberta M. Richardson, M.D.

1. Define dementia.

Dementia is an impairment in intellectual functioning in at least two spheres. One of the spheres is memory; the second may be any other area of cognition.

Cognitive Functions That May Be Impaired in Dementia

Language	Ability to dress and do other semiautomatic tasks
Visuospatial ability	
Personality	Abstraction
Judgment	Calculation
Object recognition	Information synthesis
	Problem solving

In contrast to delirium, the deficits of dementia are **relatively stable** over at least a few months. In contrast to mental retardation, the deficits are **acquired**. Memory disturbance is an early feature. It may be evidenced by inability to learn new material or loss of ability to recall previously learned material.

The degree of interference in the patient's life should be taken into account, as should education and intelligence. For example, a highly educated man may "pass" a screening test but still have significant impairment in his usual complex occupation. Alternatively, a retired manual laborer may show some deficits on exam but have no problems in his daily life. Third-party informants are helpful. People who know the patient best can report changes in functioning from a previous level as well as notice signs or symptoms of which the patient is unaware. More extensive, formal neuropsychological testing may be helpful if the diagnosis is in doubt.

2. Why is dementia an increasingly important problem?

The population of the U.S. is aging. It is estimated that by the year 2010 about 15% of Americans will be 65 or older, and 25% will be 55 or older. Currently the fastest growing segment of the population is people over the age of 85. The incidence of dementia rises steadily with age. About 5% of people over 65 have severe dementia, and another 10–15% show mild-to-moderate symptoms. Of people over 80, one-fourth have severe dementia.

Dementia is presently the fourth leading cause of death in the U.S. Death occurs because so much of the nervous system has failed that the entire body is profoundly affected. Such patients are mute, unable to eat, incontinent, and immobile. The immediate cause of death may be pneumonia, dehydration, malnutrition, or sepsis.

3. What are the causes of dementia?

Alzheimer's disease is the most common cause of dementia, accounting for about 50% of cases. Multi-infarct dementia accounts for about 25%, and the remaining 25% are caused by a wide variety of other conditions or agents.

Causes of Dementia

Cortical dementias	Normal pressure hydrocephalus
Alzheimer's disease	Dementia syndrome of depression
Pick's disease (frontal lobe degeneration)	Chronic confusional states
Lewy body disease	Infections
Vascular dementias	Toxic-metabolic encephalopathies
Multiinfarct dementia	Trauma
Lacunar state	Neoplasms
Binswanger's disease	Demyelinating diseases
Movement disorders	
Parkinson's disease	
Huntington's disease	
Wilson's disease	
Progressive supranuclear palsy	
Spinocerebellar degeneration	

4. What are the differences between cortical and subcortical dementias?

Subcortical dementias are caused by disorders that affect mainly the basal ganglia, thalamus, and brainstem. Clinical characteristics contrast with those of the cortical dementias, which, as the name implies, affect mainly the cerebral cortex. Recognizing this distinction assists in differential diagnosis. Movement disorders exemplify the subcortical dementias. In addition to effects on the motor system, cognition and comprehension are slowed. The ability to synthesize and manipulate information for problem solving and decision making is impaired. Memory deficits are characterized by retrieval deficits. Clinically, patients with subcortical dementias may be helped by clues, structure, and prompting. Information registers, but it is difficult to retrieve from storage. Such strategies do not help patients with Alzheimer's disease, because the information was not learned.

Cortical dementias are characterized by language disturbances, agnosia and apraxia, visuospatial deficits, and impairment of judgment, abstraction, and calculation. Many deficits are characterized by problems with registering new information and, as the dementia progresses, with remote recall. For example, the patient with Alzheimer's disease has great difficulty recalling the three objects commonly requested during mental status screening. Clues do not help. The patient may not even remember that three objects were mentioned, because the information was not registered in the memory. The neurologic exam shows no abnormalities in motor function, gait, reflexes, or posture. Alzheimer's disease is the prototypic cortical dementia.

Mixed dementias have features of both cortical and subcortical type. Multi-infarct dementia and Lewy Body disease (LBD) are the most common examples. LBD differs from Alzheimer's disease in that it shows psychotic symptoms and parkinsonian features early in the course. Also, the course is more fluctuating. A tell-tale sign is extreme sensitivity to extrapyramidal side effects of antipsychotic medications. Cognitive deficit is more prominent than movement disorder, distinguishing it from Parkinson's disease.

5. What conditions are commonly mistaken for dementia?

Normal aging is associated with some alterations in mental functioning. Benign senescent forgetfulness refers to alterations in memory function with age; it is characterized by decreased retrieval of learned information rather than inability to learn. Word-finding difficulties, especially proper names, are common in the elderly. If cognitive decline does not interfere with social or occupational functioning, it is not considered to indicate dementia.

Delirium is an acute or subacute decline in mental functioning associated with a specific organic cause. Because patients with dementia are predisposed to delirium, the two conditions may be superimposed. Delirium is temporary and should remit when the underlying organic cause is treated. Medication effects are the most common, and most commonly missed, cause of delirium mistaken for dementia.

Focal brain syndromes, such as isolated amnesias or aphasias, may be mistakenly diagnosed as dementia. Dementia, however, involves disturbances of memory and at least one other area of cognition. The careful clinician is not fooled by the aphasic patient who at first glance seems to have memory deficits. Nor does the careful clinician assume that an amnestic patient has dementia. All areas of cognition must be considered and tested.

Major depression may cause reversible dementia, especially in the elderly. It may also cause symptoms that may be misdiagnosed as dementia: apathy, withdrawal, decrease in attention to personal grooming, personality changes, and loss of interest in activities. Such symptoms are prominent features of major depression as well as common symptoms of senile dementia. Because major depression may cause memory loss and actual decrease in cognitive abilities, it is considered a reversible cause of dementia. Careful attention to full mental status testing, including subtleties of mood and thought, is essential for proper diagnosis and treatment. Like delirium, depression also may coexist with dementia.

6. How is delirium distinguished from dementia?

It is important to distinguish delirium from dementia, but the distinction is especially difficult when delirium overlies preexisting dementia. The main distinguishing feature is **level of attention**, which is impaired in patients with delirium. When interviewed patients answer a question asked of the person in the next bed rather than the question just posed to them, impairment of attention is suggested.

An easy and accurate bedside test of attention is the so-called A test. The examiner recites a series of random letters at a steady rate of about one per second and asks the patient to indicate by a gesture every time he or she hears the letter A. The examiner should sometimes say the letter A two or three times in a row and also allow a long list of letters to pass by without an A. The patient should be able to perform this task for about a minute without error. Errors indicating impairment of attention include omissions and gesturing for the wrong letter. Perseverating after a series of letter As suggests frontal lobe dysfunction.

Other features that suggest delirium rather than dementia include:
  • **Acute or subacute onset**. Family and friends of the demented patient will have noticed problems for at least a few months.

- **Fluctuating course**. The delirious patient may be confused one hour, clear the next, and confused again a few hours later.
- **Clouding of consciousness**. The delirious patient may not be fully alert or aware of surroundings.
- **Florid hallucinations**, most often visual or tactile.
- **Illusions**, or misrepresentations of sensory stimuli, such as believing that the coat rack is a person or the stethoscope a snake.

7. How are depression and dementia related?

Both depression and dementia are common in the elderly. They may coexist, either in a causative manner or coincidentally, and at times they are difficult to distinguish.

Depressive pseudodementia describes what once were thought to be apparent but not real cognitive deficits associated with severe major depression. More recent research indicates that major depression is a cause of reversible dementia; that is, major depression may cause true cognitive deficits that resolve with successful treatment of depression. The term **depressive pseudodementia** should be replaced by the more precise term, **dementia syndrome of depression**.

If the clinician is uncertain whether major depression is a part of a presentation that includes dementia, it is best to treat depression empirically, not only for the emotional well-being of the patient, but also because cognition may improve. The classic clue to the diagnosis of dementia syndrome of depression is the occurrence of many "I don't know" answers. Patients with pure dementia are likely to try their best or even to invent answers when memory is poor. But severely depressed patients have a motivational deficit and negative attitude. They may even emphasize and complain about thinking problems in a catastrophic way, whereas patients with Alzheimer's disease are often poorly aware or in denial of cognitive difficulties. Rapid decline in functioning, inconsistency in the mental status exam, pervasively dysphoric mood, and suicidal ideation or expression of a wish to die are other important clues to major depression.

8. Describe the elements of the work-up for dementia.

There is no definitive work-up for dementia. The astute clinician takes a careful history, completes a careful examination, and orders further tests as indicated in each case. However, certain chronic confusional states are difficult or impossible to rule out by history and physical exam but common enough to warrant routine laboratory investigation. Others should be considered if the history, physical exam, or preliminary blood tests are suggestive.

Laboratory Tests for Work-up of Dementia

Routine	Supplementary
Complete blood count	Serum antibody for human immunodeficiency virus (HIV)
Syphilis serology	Electroencephalogram
Chemistry panel	Computed tomography scan of head
Thyroid function tests	Magnetic resonance imaging of head
Vitamin B12 and folate	Heavy metals screen
Sedimentation rate	Lumbar puncture
Urinalysis	Antinuclear antibody test
	Pulse oximetry
	Serum amylase

9. Describe the most common cause of nontraumatic dementia in young people.

HIV encephalopathy, also known as AIDS dementia complex (ADC), was first described in detail in 1986. Nearly all patients with AIDS develop HIV encephalopathy at some time during the course of the disease. In 20% of HIV-infected people, changes in mental status precede immunologic abnormalities, and in another 10% changes in mental status and immunologic abnormalities are recognized simultaneously. All persons with changes in mental status should be questioned about risk factors for HIV exposure; if any are present, serum testing should be performed.

HIV encephalopathy is the most common but by no means the only neurologic manifestation of HIV infection. Although a wide variety of infections and neoplastic brain diseases may occur, the dementia syndrome progresses in a fairly predictable fashion. Forgetfulness, poor concentration, and slowing of thought are early symptoms. Apathy and social withdrawal often appear early and become progressively severe. Psychomotor retardation occurs. Memory impairment and disturbances of higher cortical functioning become apparent as the disease progresses. Delusions, hallucinations, and agitation may occur. The terminal state is usually characterized by "quiet confusion."

10. Name the two behaviors of patients with dementia that most commonly lead to nursing home placement.

The two behaviors of demented individuals most commonly leading to nursing home placement are insomnia and aggression. Caregivers often feel helpless to deal with these problems, which are distressingly frequent and extremely difficult to tolerate.

11. Discuss the management of insomnia in patients with dementia.

Normal sleep patterns are disrupted in many patients with dementia. In addition to actual brain changes that can be demonstrated in sleep EEGs, changes in behavior and lifestyle may cause the demented patient to be awake and active at night. For example, disinterest and inability to participate in usual activities may lead to excessive napping during the day. Decreased sensory stimulation at night may foster hallucinations or confusion. Inability to recall structure and social norms may encourage arousal and activity at night.

Increasing structure and activity during the day should be the first approach to insomnia. Senior centers and day programs for patients with dementia are excellent resources. Exercise, especially in the late afternoon, encourages appropriate desire for rest at night. Routine bedtime and rising, with structure and ritual as cues, also may be helpful. The caretaker should react calmly if the person arises at night. Offering guidance to the bathroom or a drink of water or milk and then leading the individual back to bed often allows a return to sleep.

If such approaches are not enough, medication may be considered. Sedatives-hypnotics should be used sparingly in patients with dementia, because they may further impair memory, cause paradoxical excitement, and interfere with balance, leading to falls. *All over-the-counter sleep aids, including Benadryl and Tylenol PM, should be avoided*, because their anticholinergic properties frequently cause confusion in the demented patient. The sedating tricyclic antidepressants and antipsychotics are also highly anticholinergic and may cause significant orthostatic hypotension, increasing the risk of falls as well as cardiovascular complications. Sometimes a low dose of trazodone is effective. Trazodone is not sedating for all individuals but may be effective without the hazards of more traditional sleeping medications. A dose as low as 25 mg may be sufficient. Melatonin also has been found to be helpful for some.

12. How should aggression be approached in patients with dementia?

Aggression is a disturbing problem for caregivers and frequently brings the patient to the attention of a physician. The first response that comes to mind for many doctors and caregivers is sedating medication. However, medications involve significant risks and are usually only partially effective. It is best to attempt behavioral approaches first.

Caregivers should be instructed to note the circumstances that commonly precede outbursts of aggression. Usually, there is a period of increasing agitation in response to something that the patient has difficulty in understanding or handling. Often the responses of caregivers increase rather than resolve the agitation. For example, caregivers may argue, raise their voice, or use physical force to make patients do something that they are resisting. It is much more effective to stop immediately whatever is happening when the patient begins to show warning signs of aggression and to initiate more soothing and relaxing activity. If possible, the patient's underlying concern should be addressed. For example, if the patient is accusing someone of stealing, help the patient to find what has been lost. The Alzheimer's Association, a national organization with chapters in many cities, is an invaluable asset for educating caregivers in how to deal with these and other difficult behaviors associated with dementia. *The 36-hour Day*, by Nancy Mace and Peter Rabins, is an excellent reference to recommend to caregivers.

13. If pharmacologic treatment of aggression or agitation becomes necessary, how should it be managed?

First, consider the cause. Treating an underlying medical condition that is causing pain or discomfort may resolve the problem. The presence of depression, delirium, or psychosis will guide your choice of agent.

Controlled studies have shown a modest improvement in overall agitation in dementia with the use of conventional **antipsychotic agents**. The high-potency agents are preferred to the more anticholinergic ones. For most, a dosage equivalent to haloperidol 2 mg/d is necessary. However, many elderly develop debilitating extrapyramidal symptoms, particularly parkinsonism, with this treatment. The second-generation antipsychotics risperidone and olanzapine are being used with success, and fewer side effects. Even so, it is wise to reserve the antipsychotic agents for those with psychotic symptoms.

Benzodiazepines may be used carefully, in small doses, to treat agitation and aggression. Lorazepam or oxazepam are preferred; both are metabolized at the same rate regardless of patient age, and therefore do not accumulate in the aging body. Caution is needed because more than a small dose often causes postural instability, leading to falls. Consider starting a delayed-action agent such as buspirone or an antidepressant, with the intent to taper the benzodiazepine as soon as possible.

Divalproex was the third most commonly used medication to treat these symptoms in the elderly in 1997, according to a medication usage study,[9] following haloperidol and risperidone. Although controlled data on its effectiveness are lagging behind, the widespread use of this medication for this purpose most likely represents clinician experience, as well as its safety and relative lack of side effects. Effective dosages may be lower than those used to treat epilepsy or mania.

Buspirone also is widely used, and is most recommended for the long-term treatment of anxiety. It generally is well tolerated and safe. **Trazodone** is helpful in many cases, as well.

14. Are there any medications that can treat Alzheimer's disease directly, rather than just the behavioral symptoms?

At present, there is no way to cure or stop the progression of Alzheimer's disease. However, there are agents that can enhance cognition in some, in the early to middle stages of the disease, and slow the rate of decline.

The anticholinesterase inhibitors were developed in response to the finding of cholinergic cell loss in the brains of Alzheimer's disease patients. The first one available was **tacrine**. It has many side effects, including a fairly high rate of liver toxicity necessitating frequent blood monitoring, and a short half-life, requiring frequent dosing. **Donepezil** may be dosed once daily, and because it is more specific to brain tissue, the side effects are few. Use of these agents can produce measurable but quite modest improvement in cognition, and modest slowing of the decline.

There is now sufficient data to recommend supplemental **vitamin E** for those with Alzheimer's disease. **Selegiline** is about equally as effective but much more expensive. Many other substances are being studied but as yet data is insufficient to recommend them routinely.

BIBLIOGRAPHY

1. Alexopoulos GS, Silver JM, Kahn DA, et al (eds): Treatment of Agitation in Older Persons with Dementia. From The Expert Consensus Guideline Series. A Special Report of Postgraduate Medicine. April, 1998.
2. Cummings JL, Benson DF: Dementia: A Clinical Approach, 2nd ed. Boston, Butterworth-Heinemann, 1992.
3. Eberling JL, Jagust WJ: Neuroimaging and the diagnosis of dementia. Psychiatr Ann 24:178–185, 1994.
4. Horowitz GR: What is a complete work-up for dementia? Clin Geriatr Med 4:163–180, 1988.
5. Kim E, Rovner BW: Depression in dementia. Psychiatr Ann 24:173–177, 1994.
6. Mace NL, Rabins PV: The 36-Hour Day, rev. ed. Baltimore, Johns Hopkins University Press, 1991.
7. Mortimer JA: The dementia of Parkinson's disease. Clin Geriatr Med 4:785–797, 1988.
8. Moss RJ, Miles SH: AIDS dementia. Clin Geriatr Med 4:889–895, 1988.
9. Schneider L: Clues to psychotropic prescribing practices in geriatric medicine. Primary Psychiatry 5:23–26, 1998.
10. Strub RL, Black FW: Neurobehavioral Disorders: A Clinical Approach. Philadelphia, F.A. Davis, 1988, p 58.
11. Webster J: Recognition and treatment of dementing disorders in the elderly. Clinical Geriatrics 7:61–69, 1999.

35. DELIRIUM

J.S. *Kobayashi*, M.D.

1. Why should the psychiatrist be concerned about the recognition of delirium?

Delirium is frequently misdiagnosed by physicians, is common among the medically ill, and often is either iatrogenic or the initial presentation of a major medical disorder. Although rarely treated as such, *delirium is a medical emergency*, and patients with delirium have greater morbidity and mortality than other patients. The delirious patient typically is referred to a psychiatrist because of presenting psychiatric symptomatology, but misdiagnosis may result in delay of appropriate medical intervention.

2. Give an example of a situation in which delirium was detected.

A 58-year-old man was brought to the emergency department because of the sudden onset of irritable, labile mood, paranoia, agitation, and auditory hallucinations. The prominence of psychiatric symptoms led to a request for a psychiatric consultation. The psychiatrist also noted tachypnea, diaphoresis, and disorientation to place and date. A call to the patient's daughter revealed no prior history of psychiatric disorder, no recent change in mental functioning, and no history of substance abuse. Medical history of recent evaluation for breathing difficulties also was obtained from the family. An arterial blood gas showed severe hypoxemia. A diagnosis of delirium due to severe respiratory compromise was made, and treatment of his respiratory condition was initiated.

3. What common presenting clinical symptoms are immediate clues that a patient may be delirious?

- Intermittent disorientation to time or place
- Easy distractibility by irrelevant stimuli
- Mumbling or muttering (dysarthric speech)
- Hyper- or hypoactivity (agitation or hypersomnolence)
- "Sundowning" (increased confusion in the early evening), or a subjective feeling of confusion
- Illusions and misperceptions or a predominance of visual hallucinations
- Extreme emotional lability
- Sudden inability to remember the events of the previous day
- Transient difficulties in word-finding, or disorganized speech

4. How can these clinical phenomena be easily differentiated from other psychiatric symptoms?

- The disorientation and confusion of delirium fluctuates over the day.
- Manic flight of ideas usually has some thread of coherence, in contrast to simple distractibility.
- Neologisms (newly created words) or idiosyncratic speech (new meanings or usage) are not simply mispronounced or poorly articulated words, as in dysarthric speech.
- Manic hyperactivity rarely, if ever, suddenly lapses into somnolence as a delirium can; and a depressive stupor is more stable than a lapsing consciousness.
- Illusions are misperceptions or misinterpretations of a real stimulus (such as thinking a loud noise is gunfire), whereas hallucinations are devoid of a reality-based stimulus.
- Histrionic emotionality usually demonstrates less frequent and less acute switches in mood (e.g., from laughing to crying).
- Acute problems with memory or word-finding are not the profound deficits of expressive aphasia or global amnesia.

5. How is the clinical presentation of the psychotic patient different from the delirious patient?

Chronically psychotic individuals are rarely disoriented; do not customarily identify themselves as confused; may demonstrate nonsensical speech rather than incoherence; hallucinate more than misperceive; and tend to substitute **the unfamiliar for the familiar** (such as thinking the nurse is a relative) **rather than the familiar for the unfamiliar** (as in Capgras syndrome, believing someone else has taken on the identity of a family member).

6. What are the formal criteria for diagnosing delirium?

There are four primary elements in the diagnosis of a delirium: **time course, disturbance of consciousness, change of cognition**, and **evidence of medical cause**. Change in mental status usually occurs over a period of hours to days, and tends to fluctuate during the day. Disturbance in consciousness (i.e., reduced clarity or awareness of the environment) is a core dysfunction, along with reduced ability to focus, sustain, or shift attention. Changes in cognition (e.g., memory deficit, disorientation, language disturbance), disorganized thought process, or perceptual disturbance should not be attributable solely to dementia, and the history, physical examination, or laboratory findings should provide evidence that symptoms are caused by the direct physiologic consequences of a general medical condition.

Presumptive causes are among the changes in the DSM-IV categorization of delirium. Substance-induced delirium, for example, includes intoxication and withdrawal syndromes from substances of abuse, as well as medication toxicity.

7. What factors predispose a patient to delirium?

Patients with dementia, head injury, cerebrovascular or other disorders of the central nervous system tend to be more easily precipitated into a delirious state. Other risk factors include age over 65 years, with or without prior psychiatric history; history of significant substance abuse; and major medical illness or recent major surgery.

8. What are important elements in a good history for the evaluation of a possible delirium?

In addition to identifying predisposing risk factors, the history should include: exposure to medications, substances, or toxins; premorbid level of function; psychiatric and medical history; time course, including acuity of onset and fluctuating symptoms; recent medical procedures or treatments (such as fluid or electrolyte changes); current medical symptomatology.

9. Which medications can cause delirium?

Any psychoactive medication can cause delirium, particularly in high-risk patients, even at therapeutic levels. Toxic levels can cause delirium in any patient. Medications that are well tolerated orally may cause delirium on intravenous administration, and vice versa.

Common Pharmacologic Causes of Delirium

Narcotics	Beta blockers
Barbiturates	Cimetidine
Benzodiazepines	Clonidine
Anticholinergics	Digitalis
Medications with anticholinergic side effects	Pressors (lidocaine)
(e.g., amitriptyline, thioridazine, some anti-	Theophylline derivatives
histamines)	Bromides
Steroids	Antibiotics (cephalosporins, aminoglycosides)
Sympathomimetics	(less common)
Anticonvulsants	Antifungals (amphotericin B) (less common)
Antihypertensives	Over-the-counter agents (e.g., antitussives and
Antiarrhythmics	sedatives)
Antidepressants	
Antineoplastics (e.g., 5-fluorouracil)	

10. What common medical disorders may be associated with delirium?

In addition to causation by medications, substances, and toxins (e.g., heavy metals), delirium can be caused by infection, hypoxia or hypoglycemia, metabolic or fluid and electrolyte disturbance, trauma, vitamin deficiencies, endocrinopathies, cerebrovascular events (strokes, hemorrhage), seizures, and other CNS pathology (e.g., tumors, infections or abscesses, cerebritis, acute hypertensive crisis, hydrocephalus). Finally, a summation effect, in which subclinical factors combine to cause delirium may occur, particularly in predisposed patients. For example, such factors as sleep deprivation, dehydration, anemia, or stress may precipitate delirium in conjunction with a clinical condition, such as a low-grade infection in an elderly patient.

11. What is the differential diagnosis of delirium in psychiatric patients?

Substance intoxication or substance withdrawal are differentiated from substance intoxication delirium and substance withdrawal delirium "if the symptoms of the delirium are in excess of those usually associated with the intoxication or withdrawal syndrome and are sufficiently severe to warrant independent clinical attention" (DSM-IV). If hallucinations and/or delusions are present, consider all psychotic disorders, including brief psychotic disorder, schizophrenia, schizoaffective disorder, and mood disorders with psychotic features. Dementia may predispose the elderly individual to delirium, or may confound the diagnosis.

12. How can the psychiatrist differentiate delirium from other psychiatric diagnoses?

Systematic review of risk factors, history, acuity of onset, course, associated symptoms, and possible medical etiologies may determine the diagnosis. Serial mental status examinations can be useful in demonstrating a fluctuating course. Careful clinical observation facilitates the differentiation of illusions from hallucinations, cognitive distractibility from manic flight of ideas, dysarthric from idiosyncratic speech, word-finding difficulties from expressive aphasia, and emotional lability from mood disorder.

In **schizophrenia**, age of onset is rarely after the fifth decade, auditory hallucinations are more common than visual, memory is fundamentally intact, speech is not dysarthric, disorientation is rare, and symptoms do not tend to worsen or fluctuate significantly over the course of the day. The deterioration of ability to function is more gradual and prolonged, and there are more prominent deficit symptoms, such as marked social isolation or withdrawal.

Mood disorders with psychotic symptoms manifest a persistent rather than labile disorder of mood, with gradual onset, sometimes with prior similar episodes. Although there may be a "manic delirium" in a very agitated state, cognitive performance is not routinely impaired (and sometimes it is heightened); flight of ideas may be differentiated from cognitive distractibility by a thread of coherence; and disorientation is unusual. The "pseudodementia" of depression rarely fluctuates over the day, and patients experience more anhedonia than confusion.

A **brief reactive psychosis** is associated with an acute major emotional precipitant. Patients usually are not disoriented, and memory is intact. There may be emotional lability and some fluctuation of symptoms.

Patients with **dementia** are susceptible to a comorbid delirium but usually experience a gradual decline in memory and other higher cortical functions such as abstract reasoning, judgment, or language prior to manifesting paranoid delusions or hallucinations. In late stages or with significant deterioration, there may be overlapping symptoms such as dysarthric speech, emotional lability, and disorientation. In the past, delirium sometimes was contrasted with dementia as being "reversible," but the "secondary dementias" associated with various medical conditions such as hypothyroidism, B12 deficiency, porphyria, and nutritional deficiencies are reversible.

13. In which medical conditions may mood disturbances—instead of or in conjunction with cognitive dysfunction—be a prominent manifestation of delirium?

Steroid toxicity, hypocalcemia and hypercalcemia, exacerbations of thyroid disease, and tertiary syphilis may result in prominent disturbance of mood.

14. Why should the diagnostic category of delirium replace terms such as: toxic psychosis, ICU psychosis, acute confusional state, organic psychosis, organic mental syndrome, organic brain syndrome, encephalopathy?

The formal DSM-IV diagnosis of delirium should replace these historic terms because they are simply descriptive or reflective of the presumed causes of the confusional state. Psychoses caused by identifiable biologic factors were historically termed "organic" to differentiate them from the "functional" psychoses such as schizophrenia, but this distinction is no longer useful. The term organic may be useful as a descriptive term encompassing a variety of biologic etiologies (physiologic, metabolic, structural) causing changes in mental status, but is less precise than the diagnoses of delirium and dementia.

15. What is the pathophysiology of delirium?

There are many differing hypotheses, based primarily on animal research. They involve neurotransmitter abnormalities; inflammatory response with increased cytokines; intraneuronal signal transduction or chemical messenger systems; increased activity of the hypothalamic-pituitary-adrenal axis; or changes in blood-brain barrier permeability.

16. What treatment and clinical management should be provided for the delirious patient?

First, identify and treat the underlying disorder. When this is not possible, or there is not a rapid reversal of symptoms, environmental or pharmacologic treatments may be useful.

Environmental interventions should make the immediate environment, such as the hospital room, seem more familiar. Methods include having friends and relatives visit frequently, placing familiar objects like photographs nearby, and maintaining a routine. Orientation can be enhanced by the use of calendars, nightlights, and clocks, and by making an effort to orient the patient with each encounter. Confusion can be minimized by structuring activities; maintaining a daily schedule in the same location; keeping directions and discussions simple and brief; minimizing changes in personnel and procedures; and writing down instructions. Rarely, behavioral restraints may be required for the safety of the individual in an acutely agitated state.

Pharmacologic agents that are useful in decreasing psychotic symptoms, confusion, and agitation include: (1) Low-dose high-potency antipsychotic medication in divided doses, such as haloperidol (0.5 mg–4 mg/day), trifluoperazine (1–4 mg/day), or possibly risperidone (0.5–4 mg/day); antipsychotics of the butyrophenone class usually are recommended as superior. (2) Benzodiazepines such as lorazepam (0.5–6 mg/day) alone or in combination with antipsychotic medication may be useful for physical agitation or sleep disturbance, as well as for alcohol and sedative withdrawal, but there is risk of further confusion. (3) Psychostimulants (methylphenidate 2.5 mg–20 mg) may be useful in patients with dementia and chronic delirium for increasing ability to focus attention.

During treatment, remember that the family of the patient also requires support, and education about the delirium can be helpful to them.

17. What psychotherapeutic issues should be considered in delirious patients?

As with any patient, the clinician must be aware of specific countertransference to delirious patients, who may range from passive and unresponsive to agitated and alarming. It also is helpful (but often not done) for a clinician to process the experience of the delirious episode with the patient for four reasons:

1. Delirious states, known to the Greeks as the "waking dream," often produce material that may be helpful for a patient to understand with a clearer consciousness at a later time.

2. It helps to allay patients' fears, which otherwise may remain unaddressed, that they are going crazy or losing their minds.

3. The experience may be followed by posttraumatic sequelae, and patient education as well as support and monitoring may be useful, particularly if the causes are iatrogenic.

4. If factors predispose to another episode of delirium, intervention or patient education may be appropriate as soon as the initial episode has resolved.

BIBLIOGRAPHY

1. Flacker JM, Marcantonio ER: Delirium in the elderly. Drugs and Aging 12(2):119–130, 1998.
2. Inouye SK: Delirium in hospitalized older patients. Clin in Geriatric Med 14(4):745–764, 1998.
3. Jacobson SA: Delirium in the elderly. Psych Clin North Am 20(1):91–110, 1997.
4. Jacobson S, Schreibman B: Behavioral and pharmacologic treatment of delirium. Am Fam Phys 56(8):2005–2012, 1997.
5. Mcartnery JR, Boland RJ: Anxiety and delirium in the intensive care unit. Crit Care Clin 10:673–680, 1994.
6. Trzepaca PT: Delirium. Advances in diagnosis, pathophysiology, and treatment. Psych Clin North Am 19(3):429–448, 1996.
7. van der Mast RC: Pathophysiology of delirium. Jnl Geriatric Psych & Neuro 11(3):138–145, 1998.
8. Wise MJ: Delirium. In Hales RE, Yudofsky SC (eds): Textbook of Neuropsychiatry, 2nd ed. Washington, DC, American Psychiatric Press, 1992.
9. Diagnostic and Statistical Manual of Mental Disorders, 4th ed. Washington, DC, American Psychiatric Association, 1994.

36. PSYCHOSIS WITH NEUROLOGIC/SYSTEMIC DISORDERS

C. Munro Cullum, Ph.D., and Myron F. Weiner, M.D.

1. What is psychosis?

Psychosis is an impairment of reality testing manifested by delusions, hallucinations, and/or disordered thought processes. Psychotic symptoms define mental illnesses such as schizophrenia and delusional disorder, but also occur in neurologic disease or CNS dysfunction due to systemic disorders. It is important to differentiate between the mental illnesses and other forms of CNS dysfunction that cause psychotic symptoms because of the differences in treatment and prognosis, but in the acute phase, schizophrenia or mania may be indistinguishable from psychosis secondary to neurologic/systemic disease (see Question 3).

2. What are some of the more common symptoms of psychosis?

- Delusions (false ideas, e.g., paranoid, bizarre, grandiose, somatic)
- Hallucinations (false perceptions)
- Aberrant, bizarre, and disorganized thinking
- Incoherent speech (as occurs with extreme, pressured speech in mania)
- Neologistic speech (coining new words)
- Bizarre, disorganized behavior

Psychotic symptoms, much like fever, are not diagnostic of a particular condition but are indicative of an underlying disorder. The development of psychotic symptoms de novo in a previously normal person clearly requires prompt attention, because it may be related to any of numerous neuromedical factors. Metabolic, medication, and illicit drug effects must be considered early in the diagnostic process so that appropriate (and possibly life-saving) interventions can be instituted.

3. Give the differential diagnosis of conditions associated with psychosis.

Psychotic symptoms associated with neurologic or systemic disease often differ from symptoms of primary psychiatric disorders.

Differences in Psychotic Symptoms in Psychiatric and Neurologic/Systemic Disease

SYMPTOM	PSYCHIATRIC DISORDER	NEUROLOGIC/SYSTEMIC DISORDER
Delusions	Fixed, with more stable themes and elaborate contents, bizarre	Transient, less systematized, "homely"
Hallucinations		
Auditory	Prominent in *psychiatric* disorders. Accusatory in schizophrenia, mood-congruent in bipolar disorder or depression	*Less common in* neurologic/systemic disorders Often ill-developed
Visual	Less common: typically related to delusional themes, usually frightening	Common in Alzheimer's disease, Parkinson's treated with dopamine agonists. Often not frightening. Usually associated with delusions.
Tactile	Rare	A hallmark of delirium
Olfactory	Uncommon	More common in temporal lobe disorders
Incoherent or neologistic speech	Meanings of neologisms tend to be consistent and context-specific	"Word salad" more generalized and inconsistent, characteristic aphasic symptoms per syndrome
Bizarre behavior	May be related to delusional themes and tend to be stereotyped	Little organization or purpose; often sporadic

As with any set of symptoms, the clinical history is critical, including an assessment of the initial onset, frequency, changes over time, and context in which they occur. Psychotic symptoms may have vastly different etiologies and prognosis. For example, an adolescent who begins to withdraw socially and who slowly develops the delusion that he is being persecuted by classmates because he has special powers differs greatly in treatment and prognosis from another adolescent who experiences the sudden onset of persecutory delusions, visual hallucinations, and violent behavior during a time when he and friends are using illicit drugs. The frightening hallucinations of mental illness are of persecutors, while the "homely" hallucinations in persons with neurologic/systemic disorders often include friends and relatives. Benign hallucinations include the imaginary companions of young children and unformed or vague hallucinations that may occur on going to sleep and awakening.

A thorough medical work-up is indicated in any patient with new-onset psychotic symptoms, but the worsening of psychotic symptoms in mentally ill persons must also be investigated; persons with schizophrenia or other psychiatric disorders may develop neurologic or systemic disease that may present initially as an increase in psychosis.

4. What is the frequency of psychotic symptoms in neurologic disorders?

Psychotic symptoms may arise in association with a host of disorders affecting the CNS. Chronic metabolic disturbances or drug effects are common causes, although given the overlap between some psychiatric and neurological symptoms, it is not surprising that many neurologic conditions result in at least transient psychotic symptoms.

Neurologic/Systemic Conditions Associated with Psychotic Symptoms

Seizure disorders	Brain tumor, abscess
Head injury	Systemic lupus erythematosus
Dementing illnesses	Chronic metabolic disturbances
Alzheimer's disease	Hypo-, hyperthyroidism
Parkinson's disease	Cushing's disease
Huntington's disease	Porphyria

Table continued on following page

Neurologic/Systemic Conditions Associated with Psychotic Symptoms (Continued)

Pick's disease	Pernicious anemia
Stroke	Obstructive or normal-pressure hydrocephalus
Korsakoff's syndrome	
Subdural hematoma	
Chronic encephalitis/meningitis	
Neurosyphilis	
AIDS and opportunistic CNS infections	
Acute or chronic substance abuse	

This list represents only a handful of the conditions in which psychotic symptoms have been reported. Specific estimates of the frequency of psychotic symptoms or full-blown psychosis in any of these diagnostic categories are not easily derived from the existing literature. Some reliable data exist for Alzheimer's disease: up to 20% of patients have been reported to demonstrate hallucinations, and up to 50% experience delusions at some point during their illness. Similar estimates of psychotic symptoms in general are as high as 50% among persons with various types of epilepsy.

5. How can psychotic symptoms of mental illness be distinguished from those of neurological/systemic conditions?

Obtain a detailed history from the patient and a knowledgeable informant. Review all available medical and psychological records. Perform physical, neurological, and mental status examinations. Depending on the patient and symptoms, many of the following studies may be useful in the differential diagnosis.

Diagnostic Procedures to Be Considered in the Evaluation of the Patient with Psychosis

- History
- Physical examination
- Mental status examination
- Neurologic examination
- Laboratory studies (e.g., CBC, B_{12}, TSH, liver enzymes, BUN, electrolytes, VDRL test for syphilis, urine toxicology screen, HIV)
- Neuropsychological evaluation
- Neuroimaging (MRI, CT, functional imaging)
- Electrophysiological studies (e.g., EEG, evoked potentials)

Good premorbid adjustment is seen more often in patients with psychosis due to neurologic/systemic disorders, whereas poorer adjustment is more common in patients with mental illness. Baseline behavior also is a useful discriminant. Persons with schizophrenia, for example, often demonstrate evidence of disturbed thinking between psychotic episodes. Likewise, interpersonal relationship and work histories tend to be more disrupted in patients with primary psychiatric disease. Thus, a variety of background information and historical data can be useful in helping to delineate the nature of psychotic symptoms.

Various neurodiagnostic procedures (see above) are useful in estimating the likelihood of neurologic disease in patients with major psychiatric illnesses, although this task is challenging and sometimes impossible. Neurobehavioral examination, including formal neuropsychological studies, may be helpful, particularly when emphasis is placed on qualitative as well as quantitative aspects of test performance. Establishment of a patient's intellectual status and assessment of relative cognitive strengths and weaknesses across cognitive domains (e.g., memory, attention/concentration, language, visuospatial function) also are also useful in evaluating medication effects and planning treatment.

6. Discuss the treatment of psychotic symptoms.

Treatment of psychotic symptoms varies, depending on the underlying causative factors. Resolution of the causative neuromedical condition often results in the amelioration of psychotic symptoms without additional interventions. In chronic neurologic/systemic disorders, antipsychotic medications may be indicated to control more severe symptoms. In general, high-potency antipsychotic medications are preferable to low-potency antipsychotics in psychoses due to medical conditions because of their more benign side-effect profile. Low-potency antipsychotic agents can cause delirium through their anticholinergic effects. Atypical antipsychotic drugs are the drugs of choice in psychosis associated with Parkinson's disease because they do not aggravate extrapyramidal symptoms by adding to dopaminergic blockade.

Psychological and environmental interventions also may be effective in reducing psychotic symptoms, regardless of their etiology. These include simple reassurance and simplifying and/or routinizing environmental demands, but may extend to more intensive behavioral treatment programs.

BIBLIOGRAPHY

1. Burns A, Jacoby R, Levy R: Psychiatric phenomena in Alzheimer's disease. Br J Psychiatry 157:72–94, 1990.
2. Naugle R, Cullum CM, Bigler ED: Introduction to Clinical Neuropsychology: A Casebook. Austin, TX, Pro-ed, 1998.
3. Rabins PV, Starkstein SE, Robinson RG: Risk factors for developing atypical (schizophreniform) psychosis following stroke. J Neuropsychiatry Clin Neurosci 3:6–9, 1999.
4. Strub RL, Black FW: Neurobehavioral Disorders. Philadelphia, F.A. Davis, 1988.
5. Weiner MF: Hallucinations in children. Arch Gen Psychiatry 5:54–63, 1961.
6. Weiner MF (ed): The Dementias: Diagnosis, Management, and Research. Washington, DC, American Psychiatric Press, 1996.
7. Yudofsky SC, Hales RE (eds): The American Psychiatric Press Textbook of Neuropsychiatry. Washington, DC, American Psychiatric Press, 1997.

V. Personality Disorders

37. PERSONALITY AND PERSONALITY DISORDERS

Alexis A. Giese, M.D.

1. What is the difference between a personality trait and a personality disorder?

Everyone has a distinct *personality style*, including typical ways of perceiving the self and the world, preferred coping mechanisms in response to stress, and values derived from cultural, familial, and individual experiences. Although personality development continues throughout life, most characteristic traits are formed by early adulthood.

Personality disorders, on the other hand, are distinguished by persistently inadequate adaptive capacities affecting several realms of functioning, such as social relationships or occupational performance. People with personality disorders have chronic problems dealing with responsibilities, roles, and stressors; they also have difficulty understanding the causes of their problems or changing their behavior patterns.

2. Give an example of each.

A person with dependent personality traits may be somewhat overreliant on others, but generally functions fairly well. During a crisis (such as an acute medical illness), he or she may exhibit exaggerated neediness in the healthcare setting or increase demands on family and friends to make decisions and provide care. However, when the illness is over, previous patterns of relating and functioning return. By contrast, someone with dependent personality disorder has trouble making even routine decisions without extensive support and advice, is underfunctioning socially and occupationally because of the inability to initiate things independently, and is submissive, clinging, and fearful of loss of nurturance, even in everyday situations.

3. What is the natural history of personality disorders?

Early manifestations of personality disorders generally are evident in adolescence or even childhood. By young adulthood, maladaptive traits cause major problems in social or occupational functioning or significant distress to the individual. Developmental tasks common to late adolescence or early adulthood, such as completing an education, emancipation from the family of origin, obtaining employment, and pursuit of romantic relationships, often are mishandled or delayed. Impairment from a personality disorder (especially antisocial and borderline personality disorders) is usually most pronounced during the third and fourth decades and decreases thereafter. However, some personality disorders, such as obsessive-compulsive and schizotypal, are less likely to remit with age and may become more problematic in later life.

4. Give examples of age-related manifestations.

Borderline personality disorder may present first in the middle or late teens with onset of self-mutilatory behaviors, eating disorder symptoms, depression, or suicide attempts. The twenties and thirties can be tumultuous, with frequent crises and hospitalizations. By 40 years of age, however, the features of borderline personality disorder typically have attenuated, with decreased impulsive behaviors, but with residual feelings of emptiness and identity disturbance. Crises that occur in mid-life (e.g., loss of employment) may precipitate a recurrence of some borderline symptoms such as self-mutilatory behavior, but such symptoms tend to be more limited than earlier because of some degree of social stability and coping skills.

Older adults may manifest previously quiescent personality disorders, especially dependent and obsessive-compulsive, when faced with late-life stressors such as illness or loss of partner.

5. Describe the clinical features that help distinguish an axis I disorder from an axis II disorder.

Axis I disorders (clinical syndromes) are primarily focal disturbances affecting one mental dimension, such as thought (as in psychotic disorders) or mood (as in mania). Axis I disorders may be episodic, chronic, or progressive, but in general they represent a distinct departure from premorbid functioning. Many axis I disorders are highly amenable to specific pharmacotherapeutic and psychotherapeutic interventions.

Axis II (personality) disorders represent an impairment in baseline functioning, in which the person generally functions below the level expected for his or her intelligence, education, and resources. The impairment is most evident in self-perceptions and interpersonal relationships. By definition the personality impairment has an early onset and affects several realms of functioning.

Clinical tip-offs to an axis II problem include **atypical presentations** that do not fit readily into the usual axis I categories. For example, a patient who complains of mood swings and depression that are of insufficient severity and duration to meet criteria for bipolar disorder or cyclothymia may have histrionic or borderline personality disorder. Another clue is the presence of **multiple, conflicting psychiatric diagnoses**. For example, a patient seen in several clinics and diagnosed variably with schizophrenia, chronic depression, and social phobia may have schizotypal personality disorder. A high degree of **chaos** and **emotional response** is sometimes a tip-off to personality disorder, especially the cluster B group (see Question 6). In addition, failure to respond to appropriately aggressive treatment of an axis I disorder may suggest an underlying axis II problem.

The distinction between axis I and axis II symptoms often is made only after extensive longitudinal data are obtained. A thorough diagnostic evaluation for axis I disorders must precede or accompany consideration of a personality disorder diagnosis.

6. Name the three clusters of personality disorders in DSM-IV.

Cluster A is the odd or eccentric group, which includes paranoid, schizoid, and schizotypal personality disorders. **Cluster B** is the dramatic, overly emotional, or erratic group, including antisocial, borderline, histrionic, and narcissistic personality disorders. **Cluster C** is the anxious or fearful group, including avoidant, dependent, and obsessive-compulsive personality disorders.

7. Describe the general characteristics of cluster A.

This group is characterized by a general **distrust** of others, **misinterpretation of others' actions**, **odd or idiosyncratic beliefs**, and a tendency toward **social isolation**. The assessment that beliefs and behaviors are abnormal must take into account the patient's cultural and religious background. Some religious and ethnic traditions may appear bizarre on the surface (e.g., voodoo, dietary restrictions) but are pervasive in certain cultures. The distinction that the finding is pathologic is strengthened by evidence that the belief or behavior puts the patient at odds with his or her society and interferes with social or occupational functioning.

The initial presentation of cluster A personality disorders often is **hostility** or **conflict with others**; the underlying mistrust and unusual ideas become apparent over time. Only rarely do people with cluster A disorders self refer for mental health treatment. Referral for psychiatric evaluation may be prompted by primary medical providers when depression or frank psychotic symptoms develop or when the odd beliefs interfere with treatment of a general medical condition. Occasionally, such persons come to psychiatric attention through the legal system when idiosyncratic behaviors conflict with social convention or laws. For example, a person with schizotypal personality disorder may live an isolated lifestyle with dozens of cats, ignoring hygiene and health codes; he or she may refuse to leave the home when it is condemned by authorities and ultimately be brought to mental health care by the police.

DSM-IV Personality Disorder Clusters

CLUSTER	DESCRIPTION	PERSONALITY DISORDERS
A	Odd/eccentric	Paranoid Schizoid Schizotypal
B	Dramatic/erratic	Antisocial Borderline Histrionic Narcissistic
C	Anxious/fearful	Avoidant Dependent Obsessive-compulsive

Reprinted with permission from the Diagnostic and Statistical Manual of Mental Disorders, 4th ed. Copyright 1994 American Psychiatric Association.

8. Describe individuals in cluster B.

Such people often are characterized as **labile, unpredictable, unlikable**, and **impulsive**. The initial presentation typically is crisis-related and chaotic, often involving severe symptoms (that may decrease after the crisis has passed), substance abuse, and conflicts with family members, employers, or the healthcare system. Persons with cluster B disorders have difficulty establishing and maintaining interpersonal relationships (e.g., with medical providers) and often have a history of discharge against medical advice, doctor shopping, or failure to follow recommended treatment.

9. What are the characteristics of patients in cluster C?

Patients often are anxious, timid, perfectionistic, and conflict-avoidant; presentation frequently is triggered by depression or somatic complaints. Although sometimes reluctant to engage in general medical or psychiatric treatment, they may become highly attached because they have few other important relationships and have difficulty disengaging at the appropriate time.

10. How frequently do personality disorders occur in the general and psychiatric populations?

Standardized, structured diagnostic interviews estimate the lifetime prevalence of personality disorders in the general population at 10–13%. Schizotypal personality disorder is the most common cluster A disorder in the general population, borderline personality disorder the most common in cluster B, and dependent personality disorder the most common in cluster C.

The prevalence of personality disorders in clinical psychiatric populations is, of course, much higher than in the general population. Psychiatric inpatients have prevalence rates of personality disorders ranging from 30–60%. In most studies, borderline personality disorder is the most frequently found axis II disorder in hospitalized psychiatric patients (20–30%). In outpatient psychiatric clinics prevalence rates of personality disorder fall between those for the general population and inpatients, ranging from 20–40% in some estimates. Avoidant, dependent, and borderline personality disorders have been reported most frequently in psychiatric outpatient clinics.

Many individuals meet criteria for more than one personality disorder. Multiple diagnoses of axis II disorders are allowed in DSM-IV, and the clinician should list all disorders in order of clinical importance.

11. Describe common comorbid psychiatric disorders in persons with personality disorders.

Mood disturbances, such as depression, anger, and anxiety, are frequent findings in people with personality disorders. Major depressive episodes and suicide attempts are more common in persons with a personality disorder than in those without. Anxiety disorders such as social phobia are frequent comorbid diagnoses in the cluster C group, particularly avoidant personality disorder. Posttraumatic symptoms (e.g., intrusive memories and flashbacks of traumatic events) are common in borderline personality disorder, although only a minority of cases meet full criteria for posttraumatic stress disorder.

Substance abuse is a frequent comorbid diagnosis with personality disorders, especially in cluster B. Substance intoxication or withdrawal may contribute to some of the presenting symptoms, and may explain why some of the symptoms are severe at presentation yet remit fairly quickly.

Transient psychotic symptoms may lead to treatment, especially in the cluster A group and borderline personality disorder.

People with personality disorders often present to primary medical providers with physical complaints, rather than seek mental health services. A personality disorder may complicate or prolong medical treatment and result in higher service utilization and costs if unidentified.

12. What types of psychiatric treatment approaches are useful for treating personality disorders?

By definition, personality disorders are chronic and relatively fixed and thus are not easily "cured." In short-term treatments, **adaptational approaches** that help the patient to cope with the current crisis and solve problems more effectively are most helpful. Commonly used treatment modalities include crisis intervention, supportive psychotherapy, environmental manipulation (such as change in living situation), and treatment for substance abuse. Behavioral therapies (such as assertiveness training or systematic desensitization) may be helpful for avoidant and obsessive-compulsive personality disorders. Careful consideration of comorbid axis I disorders may lead to a diagnosis with specific treatment implications, including medications.

Certain patients with personality disorders may benefit from long-term psychotherapy that attempts to restructure faulty coping mechanisms. Because of the intensity and complexity of the therapeutic relationship, such treatment is best undertaken by professionals with specific expertise (such as a psychiatrist, psychologist, or psychiatric social worker with psychodynamic training). This type of treatment is not without its risks and should be recommended only to patients who are not in crisis, who have some degree of stability in their lives, and who have resolved substance abuse problems.

13. What personality changes commonly are seen when underlying organic brain disease is present?

Personality changes are a feature of many organic brain diseases, sometimes presenting as the earliest signs of illness or even its major manifestation. Dementias due to Alzheimer's disease and other neurodegenerative disorders often begin with subtle personality changes that are typically recognized in retrospect after other findings, such as memory deficits, are evident. Structural damage to the brain may result from tumors, trauma, or infarcts and cause significant, permanent personality changes—especially if the frontal and/or temporal lobes are involved. The abrupt and/or late onset of personality changes should not be attributed to a personality disorder until a thorough diagnostic investigation (e.g., premorbid functioning, neurologic history, review of systems, physical exam) has been conducted.

Disorder	Common personality changes
Dementias (e.g., Alzheimer's)	Early: apathy, narrowing of interests, loss of humor, poor social judgment, impulsivity, immaturity
	Late: irritability, oppositionality, aggressive outbursts, suspiciousness
Frontal lobe damage	Apathy, indifference
	Depression
	Disinhibition, excitement
Temporal lobe epilepsy	Heightened emotional tone
	Rigidity, hypermoralism
	Circumstantiality, loquaciousness
	Dissociative symptoms
	Temper outbursts
Acquired immunodeficiency syndrome (AIDS)	Early: social withdrawal, apathy, agitation
	Late: progressive dementia, paranoia, manic symptoms
Head trauma	Impulsivity, aggression, affective lability

14. Are personality disorders caused by environmental or constitutional factors?

The DSM-IV avoids the question by taking an empirical, atheoretical approach; the disorders are defined by descriptive criteria emphasizing observable behaviors. In the past, personality was traditionally viewed as a product of upbringing, whereas the major mental illnesses were thought to be related to biologic vulnerabilities. These issues are now understood to be much more complex, and a substantial body of evidence suggests that both biologic and environmental variables play important interacting roles in personality development and disorders.

A familial relationship may exist between schizophrenia and cluster A personality disorders, especially schizotypal personality disorder. Family studies also have suggested a hereditary component to antisocial personality disorder. Borderline personality disorder clusters in families, although this is not clearly genetically determined. Some axis I illnesses such as depression are present at elevated rates in families of personality disordered probands, suggesting that in some cases personality disorder symptoms may be inherited subsyndromal forms of axis I problems.

Data supporting the role of environmental factors are strongest in the cluster B group, including high rates of childhood sexual and physical abuse as well as elevated rates of childhood stressors such as divorce, parental loss, inadequate parenting, frequent moves, and institutional placements. Although the association between borderline personality disorder and childhood abuse is the most strongly established (70–80% prevalence in most studies), other personality disorders have been estimated to have childhood abuse prevalence rates of approximately 50% compared with estimates of 20–40% in mixed psychiatric populations and 10–15% in the general population.

15. Are psychotropic drugs useful in treating personality disorders?

Most clinicians agree that psychotropic drugs have at least limited usefulness. If an axis I disorder that usually responds to pharmacologic intervention is present, such as a major depression, treatment should be not be withheld because a personality disorder is suspected. Some of the apparent personality disorder symptoms may remit with adequate treatment of depression and anxiety.

Even in the absence of a formal axis I diagnosis, medications are sometimes moderately effective for certain target symptoms in personality disorders. For example, the perceptual distortions and brief psychotic symptoms in paranoid or schizotypal personality disorders may respond to low doses of antipsychotics. Severe behavioral dyscontrol (as sometimes seen in antisocial and borderline personality disorders) may respond to carbamazepine or beta blockers at high doses.

16. Can psychotropic drugs be the mainstay of treatment?

A treatment plan that focuses largely or exclusively on medications probably will not meet the needs of a patient with a personality disorder. Many such patients desperately want amelioration of distress, and seek pharmacologic intervention as a panacea. Multidrug regimens carry the risk of combined toxicity and provide a ready means of suicide and drug dependence, particularly if substance abuse is a comorbid diagnosis. The definitive resolution of many problems faced by personality disordered patients requires the development of new coping mechanisms and better social skills; even with aggressive pharmacotherapy, such goals are usually best reached through **psychotherapeutic processes**.

BIBLIOGRAPHY

1. American Psychiatric Association: Diagnostic and Statistical Manual of Mental Disorders, 4th ed. Washington, DC, American Psychiatric Association, 1994.
2. Andreasen NC, Black DW (eds): Introductory Textbook of Psychiatry. Washington, DC, American Psychiatric Press, 1991.
3. Gorton G, Akhtar S: The literature on personality disorders, 1985–88: Trends, issues, and controversies. Hosp Community Psychiatry 41:39–51, 1990.
4. Hori A: Pharmacotherapy for personality disorders. [Review] Psychiatry Clin Neurosci 52:13–19, 1998.
5. Oldham JM: Personality disorders: Current perspectives. JAMA 272:1770–1776, 1994.
6. Oldham JM, Skodol AE: Personality disorders and mood disorders. In Tasman A, Riba MB (eds): Review of Psychiatry, vol 11. Washington, American Psychiatric Press, 1992, pp 418–435.
7. Perry JC, Banon E, Ianni F: Effectiveness of psychotherapy for personality disorders. [Review] Am J Psychiatry 156:1312–1321, 1999.
8. Shea MT, Pilkonis PA, Beckham E, et al: Personality disorders and treatment outcome in the NIMH treatment of depression collaborative research program. Am J Psychiatry 147:711–718, 1990.

9. Siever LJ, Davis KL: A psychobiological perspective on the personality disorders. Am J Psychiatry 148: 1657–1658, 1991.
10. Turkat ID: The Personality Disorders: A Psychological Approach to Clinical Management. Elmsford, NY, Pergamon Press, 1990.
11. Tyrer P: Personality Disorders. Management and Course. London, Butterworth, 1988.

38. BORDERLINE PERSONALITY DISORDER

Robin A. McCann, Ph.D., and Elissa M. Ball, M.D.

1. What is borderline personality disorder?

The key to recognizing borderline personality disorder (BPD) is instability—**instability in affect, interpersonal relationships, and self-identity**. The emotional instability of patients with BPD is characterized by vulnerability, intensity, and poor regulation. Emotions are quickly and easily aroused and more intense than those of others; patients often experience difficulty soothing themselves and returning to a stable emotional baseline. They are particularly vulnerable to perceived or actual abandonment and often react with rage, panic, and despair.

As people with BPD have difficulty in soothing themselves, they may attempt to block the experience of pain by experiencing, if not inducing, changes in consciousness, including feelings of derealization, depersonalization, and brief psychotic reactions with delusions and hallucinations. Substance use, gambling, overspending, eating binges, and/or self-mutilation, including suicidal threats, gestures, and attempts, are often used to escape intensely painful affect. People with BPD frequently engage in self-injurious acts, ranging from minor scratches or self-inflicted cigarette burns to overdoses or other acts requiring ICU admissions; such nonfatal, intentionally self-harmful acts are referred to as **parasuicidal behaviors.**

2. What are the diagnostic criteria for BPD?

The criteria for BPD were developed by consensus rather than empirical study and were first published in 1980 in DSM III. Specific DSM IV diagnostic criteria[1] for BPD are as follows:

A pervasive pattern of instability of interpersonal relationships, self-image, and affects, and marked impulsivity beginning by early adulthood and present in a variety of contexts, as indicated by five (or more) of the following:

1. Frantic efforts to avoid real or imagined abandonment. Note: Do not include suicidal or self-mutilating behavior covered in Criterion 5.

2. A pattern of unstable and intense interpersonal relationships characterized by alternating between extremes of idealization and devaluation.

3. Identity disturbance: markedly and persistently unstable self image or sense of self.

4. Impulsivity in at least two areas that are potentially self-damaging (e.g., spending, sex, substance abuse, reckless driving, binge eating). Note: Do not include suicidal or self-mutilating behavior covered in Criterion 5.

5. Recurrent suicidal behavior, gestures, or threats, or self-mutilating behavior.

6. Affective instability due to a marked reactivity of mood (e.g., intense episodic dysphoria, irritability or anxiety usually lasting a few hours and only rarely more than a few days).

7. Chronic feelings of emptiness.

8. Inappropriate, intense anger or difficulty controlling anger (e.g., frequent displays of temper, constant anger, recurrent physical fights).

9. Transient, stress-related paranoid ideation or severe dissociative symptoms.

3. How is emotional lability evidenced in the BPD patient?

Emotional lability is often associated with a cognitive style characterized by all-or-nothing, either-or thinking. Patients vacillate suddenly between rigidly held, yet contradictory points of view and find it extremely difficult to formulate compromise positions. This cognitive style contributes to an unstable self-concept and unstable interpersonal relationships. For example, the belief that Dr. X is totally trustworthy leads to worship or idealization of Dr. X. When Dr. X inevitably disappoints the patient, perhaps by saying no to a particular request, the patient predictably decides that Dr. X is as totally untrustworthy individual who deserves punishment and denigration; Dr. X's reasons for denying the request are not considered. Thus, relationships between patients with BPD and their significant others, including spouses, children, and treatment providers, often begin on a highly positive note (idealization), but deteriorate quickly into a chronically irritating and often emotionally and physically abusive interchange (devaluation).

Unstable self-concept and emotional lability predict difficulty in maintaining commitment to long-term goals. Commitment to school, occupation, friends, mores, and treatment plans is erratic. Behavior is impulsive and unpredictable and further contributes to unstable relationships. People with BPD often frantically seek the company and attention of others to avoid feeling lonely, empty, and worthless. Examples of such characters in literature and film include Alex in *Fatal Attraction* and Natalya Fillipovna in Dostoyevsky's *The Idiot*.

4. How common is BPD?

BPD is commonly diagnosed, particularly among women. Approximately 10% of psychiatric outpatients and 20% of psychiatric inpatients meet criteria for BPD. Approximately 75% of patients diagnosed with BPD are women.

5. Explain the origin of the term borderline.

The term *borderline* has both historical and colloquial uses extending beyond the DSM IV criteria. Historically, the term described individuals with both neurotic and psychotic symptoms who were believed to be on the borderline or continuum between psychosis and neurosis. Some patients diagnosed with schizophrenia before 1980 (when DSM III criteria for schizophrenia were constricted and refined) probably would be diagnosed with BPD today. Historically, the term also described a pathologic level of personality organization, subsuming some but not all of the characteristics of the current DSM IV criteria, including instability of self-concept and poor differentiation between self and others. Colloquially, the term sometimes has been used pejoratively to describe patients who evoke anger or hate in treatment providers.

6. What causes BPD?

The many proposed etiologies reflect a variety of theoretical paradigms. From a **psychodynamic paradigm**, BPD is the result of poor mothering. Because the mother-child relationship serves as a template for later relationships, it is important that it is "good enough." A "good-enough" mother adequately responds to her child's needs and fosters an adequate balance between dependence and independence. Without a mother who is adequately reflective and responding, the child who later develops BPD is unable to develop a sense of self that is strong, cohesive, and good. Without a strong sense of self, the child is unable to separate and differentiate self from mother. Thus, without a sufficiently cohesive sense of self, the child is unable to differentiate self from others. To an excessive degree, the child seeks self-definition and safety through others.

A **biologic paradigm** suggests that BPD is the result of an innate inability to modulate or tolerate emotion. Regulation of emotion is complex and involves multiple areas of the brain. Research to date does not suggest any single neurologic or genetic factor common to all borderline patients. Abnormalities in limbic system reactivity have been suggested as causal factors of emotion dysregulation. Limbic abnormalities may result from genetic influences, intrauterine events, or negative effects on brain development of early childhood environments. Some researchers have suggested that chronic sexual abuse and other severe, recurrent traumas (more common in patients with BPD than in those without BPD or normative samples) may physiologically alter the limbic system and thereby cause permanent adverse effects on emotional arousal, sensitivity, and modulation. Some studies have suggested additional biologic vulnerability; first-degree relatives of borderline patients were found to have a higher prevalence of mood disorders than relatives of control groups.

Biologic and psychodynamic paradigms have been incorporated into a variety of interactional, diathesis-stress, and transactional models. An example of a **transactional model** is the biosocial model described by Linehan, who attributes BPD to a transaction between biologic vulnerability to intense and unmodulated emotions (the diathesis) and an invalidating, unpredictably punishing environment. In invalidating environments, an individual's perception of personal experience is trivialized, punished, disregarded, or dismissed. An example is a sexually or physically abusive environment. Such an environment transacts with the child in that it causes the child to become even more emotionally vulnerable and unmodulated. Such an emotionally vulnerable and unmodulated child may then transact with the environment, in other words change his or her interpersonal milieu so that it becomes even more invalidating. For example, due to overwhelming emotions, a child may not consistently report her experience of sexual abuse to adults who could potentially help her, thus increasing the probability of disbelief, dismissal, disregard, or even punishment.

7. Why is BPD more frequently diagnosed among women?

Some theorists argue that, at best, the paradigms described above miss the point, and at worst (particularly the psychodynamic paradigm) are "women-blaming." Such theorists argue that the cause of BPD—a disorder so overwhelmingly diagnosed among women—is a society that disempowers and victimizes women.

Extensive research has confirmed differences in the interpersonal relationship styles of men and women. Studies suggest that **socialization**, beginning in infancy, may render women generally more affectively connected and interpersonally perceptive than men. By age 6, girls and boys already communicate and socialize in significantly different ways. Girls are more likely to play in intimate, confiding dyads; boys are more likely to play in rough-and-tumble, competitive groups. Studies have shown that rough-and-tumble play is aversive to some girls. Thus, when girls play with boys, they become relatively passive, allowing the boys to monopolize or control the game. This pattern may be reinforced by adults, who consciously or unconsciously encourage aggression in boys yet discourage identical behavior in girls.

Perhaps as a result of such socialization, emotional health and sense of well-being among women is highly correlated with the degree of social support and intimacy. This socialization leaves women especially vulnerable to the needs, whims, and vicissitudes of others. Given a pathologic, invalidating environment, this vulnerability may lead to the instability of self, affect, and relationships of BPD. Such gender role socialization also may be related to the increased sexual victimization experienced by girls compared with boys. Although most theorists focus on the effects of early invalidating experiences, similar effects may result from later spouse abuse, especially if such experiences are cumulative.

In addition, the high frequency of diagnosis among women may reflect **clinician bias**. It has been suggested that clinicians attribute specific symptoms to women to BPD yet attribute the same symptoms in men to antisocial or narcissistic personality disorder.

8. Is BPD caused by sexual and/or physical abuse?

Possibly. Data suggest that the risk of sexual abuse is 2–3 times greater for girls than boys. Physical abuse rates are not significantly different for boys and girls, yet rates of physical abuse for patients with BPD are reported to be as high as 76% vs. 38% for patients with BPD. Eighty-six percent of inpatients with BPD report a history of sexual abuse compared with 34% of inpatients without BPD; 70% of outpatients with BPD compared with 26% of outpatients without BPD report such a history. Studies also have suggested a relationship between both sexual and physical abuse in childhood and adult suicidal behavior. Although childhood victimization appears to be tragically common, data suggest a unique relationship among female gender, sexual abuse, perhaps physical abuse, and BPD.

9. List and discuss the differential diagnosis of BPD. What particular disorders are associated with BPD?

- Major depression
- Substance abuse or dependence
- Bipolar disorder
- Posttraumatic stress disorder

Major depression and **bipolar disorder** are commonly considered in the differential diagnosis. Up to 50% of individuals diagnosed with BPD also may have concomitant diagnoses of either major depression or bipolar disorder. BPD can be described as marked *instability* of self, mood, interpersonal relationships, and symptoms. In contrast, a diagnosis of major depression requires *stability* of affective symptoms, notably a period of at least 2 weeks in which the patient experiences depression or anhedonia every day. The marked changes in mood in BPD generally occur within hours or days rather than within weeks or months as in bipolar disorder.

Substance abuse frequently results in impulsive, emotionally labile behavior and unstable interpersonal relationships. The impulsivity associated with BPD often results in substance abuse or dependence. Studies suggest that 10–50% of hospitalized chemical abusers meet criteria for BPD.

The high prevalence of physical and sexual trauma among patients with BPD suggests a differential diagnosis of **posttraumatic stress disorder** (PTSD). However, whereas rates of abuse and BPD in the general population are high, baseline rates for PTSD in the general population are low (1%). Whereas patients with either PTSD or BPD may have histories of abuse and experience intense emotional arousal, patients with PTSD avoid the feared stimuli and yet reexperience the trauma through dreams, flashbacks, or intrusive thoughts. For example, a rape victim with PTSD may avoid all men and experience nightmares of the rape. If a patient with BPD has a recent history of trauma but does not actively avoid similar stimuli or reexperience the trauma, a concomitant diagnosis of adjustment disorder may be more appropriate.

10. Describe the main risks involved in the treatment of BPD. How significant is the risk of suicide in such patients? How are the risks assessed?

Symptoms of BPD such as impulsivity, anxiety, anger, and concomitant affective and substance abuse disorders result in a high risk of suicide. Between 70–75% of patients with BPD have histories of at least one self-injurious act. Rates of completed suicides are about 9% for patients with BPD vs. 1% in the general population. In one longitudinal study in which psychiatric inpatients were followed for 10–23 years after discharge, patients who met all 8 of the DSM III criteria for BPD had a suicide rate of 36% vs. 7% for patients who met 5–7 of the criteria.

Suicidal threats should be taken seriously and warrant psychiatric consultation. You cannot easily tell if a patient is really suicidal or "just manipulating." **Imminent risk factors include:**

- Current suicidal ideation
- Current or recent suicide threats
- Current or completed suicide planning
- Suicide attempt in the last year
- Indirect references to own death
- Recent disruption or loss of a relationship
- Recent medical care
- Severe anxiety or panic
- Hopelessness

Long-term risk factors include:

- Incarceration
- Family history of suicide
- Childhood sexual abuse history
- Diagnosis of borderline personality disorder
- Substance abuse diagnosis
- White male over age 45
- Poor physical health
- Unemployment

11. What feelings are commonly generated in professionals by patients with BPD?

Patients with BPD often live in a state of chaos. Their moods shift rapidly and without apparent cause. They often appear to have normal cognitive abilities and yet demonstrate extremely poor judgment. They repeatedly present to emergency departments for treatment of self-inflicted injuries or overdoses. They overdramatize or give inconsistent reports of symptom history. One minute they appear to have a good relationship with their doctor and the next minute they are angry, hostile, and critical. They report an understanding of the risks and benefits of recommended treatment, but then are noncompliant. They miss scheduled follow-up appointments, yet demand immediate attention or call at all hours to discuss new symptoms.

Such behaviors not surprisingly engender feelings of anger, irritation, confusion, helplessness, and hopelessness in providers. These feelings may lead providers to engage in treatment-destructive behaviors, including:

- Blaming the patient for lack of improvement
- Believing that the patient would be better off dead
- Failing to return phone calls
- Failure to carefully assess ongoing risk of prescribing medications
- Labeling the patient's motivation as cause of treatment failure
- Overzealous use of potentially addictive medications
- Arguing with patient
- Arguing with other professional staff regarding the patient

Borderline patients also may induce intensely positive feelings in treatment providers. Such feelings may lead providers to engage in other treatment-destructive behaviors, such as:

- Omnipotent beliefs and behaviors
- Rescue fantasies and behaviors: "Only I can rescue this patient."
- Romantic and sexual fantasies or behaviors
- Keeping secrets
- Making housecalls
- Violations of usual boundaries: having coffee, talking about provider's personal problems

12. When are providers especially vulnerable to experiencing these reactions? Can this experience be helpful?

All of these reactions are especially likely to arise when care providers are particularly stressed (e.g., sleep deprivation during internship or in marital discord). Recognize that many such feelings are engendered simply by contact with the borderline patient. Borderline patients experience a broad range of emotions, which all humans are familiar with to some degree. Borderline patients simply experience emotions and defenses with less ability to modulate reactions and to maintain or regain a balanced perspective.

When care providers become involved, they also may experience some loss of their normal ability to maintain balance. This emotional experience can be a highly useful tool to help professionals recognize what a patient suffers from BPD. The cognitive and behavioral techniques that the professional uses to reestablish balance also provide useful clues to treatment and management of the patient.

Thus, a physician's acknowledgment of his or her own feelings, obtaining consultation or peer supervision, and possibly limiting clinical contact may be useful strategies.

13. What are some clues that the doctor-patient relationship is in trouble?

- Rescue fantasies ("Only I can treat this patient")
- Defensive posture with colleagues, family, or other staff; concern expressed by clinic or hospital staff about the physician's involvement with the patient.
- "Special" behaviors or deviation from routine behaviors or procedures, including keeping secrets from supervisors, staff, or consultants; making house calls; giving out personal information; talking to the patient about personal stress in an intimate way; agreeing "just to have coffee"; feeling sexual tension when the patient is present; or feeling guilty about time spent with the patient, or thoughts or feelings about the patient.

These become clues to problems within the doctor-patient relationship when they become the pattern rather than the unusual event. The common denominator for each is *loss of equilibrium and objectivity in the professional's thinking, feelings, or behavior* in regard to the specific patient. The key to reestablishing the necessary objectivity is recognition that something within the relationship is out of balance and must be rectified to provide competent treatment. Formal or informal consultation with a colleague often is helpful.

14. Are there guidelines for successful management of BPD patient behavior when the physician's primary goal is medical stability and compliance with treatment?
   Management of emotional dyscontrol:
   • Provide structure. Patients with BPD experience intense, poorly understood emotions, and their thinking becomes diffuse and disorganized. They have difficulty consistently providing order to internal experience. At times, self-destructive behaviors are their best, although primitive, attempt at "grounding" their emotional state. Borderline patients experience significantly less turmoil and engage in fewer negative behaviors if the environment around them is clearly structured. They need clear expectations and clear role definition.
   • Be matter-of-fact. Patients with BPD become overwhelmed by emotions and are reassured by a professional who calmly addresses affect-laden issues. Avoid expression of extreme emotions.
   • Help patients to validate their own experience by acknowledging their feelings while also clearly stating the expectation of behavior control. Many (perhaps most) patients with BPD were raised in traumatic and abusive environments. The child's feelings and needs were ignored. Such children grow into adults who, on the one hand, overvalue the importance of their emotions and, on the other hand, are profoundly confused and distrustful of their emotional experience.
   • Consider frequent, brief, scheduled contacts for needy, demanding, or somaticizing patients with BPD. Gently encourage the patient to consider the relationship between psychological stressors and emotional stress and somatic symptoms.
   • Be alert to the risk of suicide. Discuss this risk openly with the patient. Weigh potential overdose potential when deciding to prescribe medication, amount to be dispensed, and number of refills.
   • Have a low threshold for seeking psychiatric or psychological consultation. Consider a referral for psychotherapy. Take care to make this referral in a nonrejecting manner, clearly defining the roles of medical and psychotherapy professionals.
   Management of interpersonal boundaries:
   • Interact in a genuine manner, balancing appropriate warmth and concern with appropriate professional boundaries. Avoid interactions conveying either unresponsiveness or overinvolvement.
   • Convey a demeanor of professional competence, yet also openly and matter-of-factly acknowledge minor errors. Presentation of oneself as infallible or omnipotent plays into the borderline patient's idealization. Idealization invariably leads to devaluation and rage; no one can live up to the fantasy of perfection. Model comfort with nonperfection to decrease the intensity of expressed anger in response to expected disappointments.
   • Perform physical examinations with a chaperone present, regardless of gender of doctor or patient. Patients with BPD have significant boundary problems and may misinterpret the meaning of physical exams or other procedures. When angry, patients also may consciously or unconsciously distort their recall of physical contact.
   Additional general guidelines:
   • Be aware of the high risk of comorbid substance abuse and major depression. Avoid prescription of addictive medications. Consider providing treatment or referring the patient for treatment of these conditions.
   • Confront noncompliance in a direct, calm, nonjudgmental manner; consider use of written contracts.
   • Avoid global, black-white, all-or-none statements and thinking. Present the patient with choices. Think compromise.
   • Set limits in a calm, nonhostile, nonjudgmental manner.

• Think balance. Continually ask, "Am I over- or underreacting to the patient's complaints?" Aim for the middle ground.

15. Are patients with BPD competent to make medical decisions?

Generally, yes. Patients with BPD are prone to brief psychotic episodes and to distortions in thinking, especially under stress; this at times may interfere with competency. Providing information about risks and benefits in a calm, structured manner often is sufficient to reestablish their capacity to participate in medical decisions. When in doubt, consult a mental health professional.

CONTROVERSY

16. Patients with BPD just need to try harder and be more motivated to act in a mature, adult manner. Psychotropic medications have no place in treatment.

For

1. Although studies support biologic, genetic, and environmental contributions to the development of BPD, studies support no pharmacologic "treatment of choice." Effects of all classes of medication studied are modest at best.

2. Patients with BPD have inadequate coping skills; medication does not replace the need to learn new coping skills.

3. Evidence suggests that the behavioral dyscontrol exhibited by patients with BPD is within their control. For example, when limits are set firmly, behavior improves. All medications have associated risks, which are not justified if control can be attained through behavioral interventions.

4. Patients with BPD cannot be trusted. They will use the medications in an attempt to kill themselves, will self-medicate their unstable moods and become addicted psychologically or physiologically, or will simply comply with prescribed medication in such an erratic manner that treatment trials are inadequate and inconclusive.

Against

1. Having BPD does not provide protection from the typical medication-responsive axis I disorders. In fact, mood disorders, substance use disorders, anxiety disorders, gender identity disorders, eating disorders, and other personality disorders often coexist with BPD. BPD has the greatest overlap with other personality disorders; comorbidity with mood disorders (particularly dysthymia and major depression) and substance use disorders is extensive. At times, comorbidity may be due to overlap in diagnostic criteria, but studies suggest that, at least for some patients, borderline symptoms represent a characterologic variant within the affective spectrum. Clinicians must consider additional syndromes that may warrant separate treatment approaches. Withholding effective medications for coexisting psychiatric conditions cannot be justified.

2. Psychopharmacologic interventions reduce specific target symptoms (anxiety, behavioral dyscontrol, acute or chronic perceptual disturbances, and emotional lability). Symptom reduction may increase the patient's ability to benefit from other psychosocial interventions.

3. Low-dose neuroleptics have been shown to decrease cognitive symptoms such as magical thinking, illusions, ideas of reference, tangentiality, and circumstantiality. Studies have shown superiority over placebo in measures of global functioning, hostility, anger, impulsivity, and subjective feelings of depression. Most patients, however, show only modest improvement and continue to meet criteria for BPD. Other patients show no improvement and/or cannot tolerate side effects. Because of the risk of tardive dyskinesia, antipsychotics are used more frequently during periods of acute stress or decompensation rather than for long-term maintenance.

4. Controlled pharmacologic trials and clinical experience suggest that some patients with BPD symptoms experience a decrease in emotional lability and impulsivity with use of carbamazepine, lithium, and monoamine oxidase inhibitors.

5. The minor tranquilizers generally should be avoided in patients with BPD because of their potential for abuse and disinhibition of impulses. Despite this relative contraindication, some patients benefit from cautious, controlled use.

6. Although the risk of suicide must be weighed in the decision to use any medication, overdose is commonly an interpersonal event and patients provide extensive opportunity for "rescue." Many physicians find that when this issue is addressed in a serious, matter-of-fact manner, patients with BPD consciously and consistently avoid overdose of physician-prescribed psychotropic medications.

17. Is BPD treatable? How is it treated?

By definition, a personality disorder is a disorder with an enduring pattern. Hence, some theorists suggest that BPD is not treatable and that therapy, particularly analytic therapy, may have a worsening effect. More recent theorists (particularly brief dynamic and cognitive-behavioral theorists) have suggested that the symptoms of BPD can be significantly ameliorated and perhaps resolved.

Linehan[6] successfully taught patients with BPD to monitor, recognize, and regulate painful affect; to inhibit inappropriate behaviors associated with affect; and to refocus attention on nondistressing stimuli. This technique ameliorates the negative effects of intense affect on interpersonal relationships. In clinical practice, to manage angry feelings, patients may be taught first to recognize the anger, to analyze its causes, to soothe themselves and then consciously to initiate a behavior that is the opposite of anger. For example, after recognizing anger related to her husband's interest in a friend's art work, the patient may gently avoid discussion of the work and instead ask about her husband's work day, thereby resisting the impulse to attack. The success of this approach has been validated with controlled empirical data.

Compared with controls, patients with BPD who were treated with DBT were less likely to engage in parasuicidal acts and to receive inpatient hospitalizations and more likely to remain in treatment and to rate themselves higher on measures of occupational and other role performance. A study of an adaptation of DBT for substance-using BPD patients found that patients assigned to DBT had greater reduction in illicit substance abuse (as measured by urinalysis) both during treatment and at followup, and greater improvements in global functioning and social adjustment at followup.

BIBLIOGRAPHY

1. American Psychiatric Association: Diagnostic and Statistical Manual of Mental Disorders, 4th ed. Washington, DC, American Psychiatric Association, 1994.
2. Beck AT, Freeman A: Cognitive Therapy of Personality Disorders. New York, Guilford Press, 1990.
3. Cowdry RW: Psychopharmacology of borderline personality disorder: A review. J Clin Psychiatry 48:15–22, 1987.
4. Dimeff LA, McDavid J, Linehan MM: Pharmacotherapy for borderline personality disorder: A review of the literature and recommendations for treatment. Clin Psychol Med Sett, In Press.
5. Kreisman JJ, Straus H: I Hate You—Don't Leave Me: Understanding the Borderline Personality. New York, Avon, 1989.
6. Linehan MM, Schmidt H, Kanter JW, et al: Dialectical behavior therapy for patients with borderline personality disorder and drug-dependence. Arch Gen Psychiatry, Submitted.
7. Paris J: The treatment of borderline personality disorder in light of the research on its long term outcome. Can J Psychiatry 38:S28–S34, 1993.
8. Sansone RA, Sansone LA: Borderline personality disorder: Office diagnosis and management. Am Fam Physician 44:194–198, 1991.
9. Sedright HR: Borderline personality disorder: Diagnosis and management in primary care. J Fam Pract 34:605–612, 1992.
10. Tasman A, Hales RE, Frances AJ (eds): American Psychiatric Press Review of Psychiatry, vol. 8. Washington, DC, American Psychiatric Press, 1989.

39. ANTISOCIAL PERSONALITY DISORDER

Elissa M. Ball, M.D., and Robin A. McCann, Ph.D.

1. What is antisocial personality disorder?

Clues to a diagnosis of antisocial personality disorder include (1) a high frequency of behaviors that violate rules or the rights of others and (2) a cognitive style characterized by lack of motivation to understand the world from any point of view except one's own. To meet criteria for the diagnosis of antisocial personality disorder, such behaviors must begin in childhood (before age 15 years) and persist through adulthood. Childhood behaviors that violate rules or the rights of others include frequent lying, stealing, and physical fights; fire setting and other destruction of property; and cruelty to people or animals. For adults such behaviors include impulsivity, consistent failure to follow through with occupational and family commitments, frequent lying, and lack of remorse. Examples of such characters in literature and film include Fagin in Dickens' *Oliver Twist*, the Benefactor in Dickens' *David Copperfield*, and the title characters in *Bonnie and Clyde*. The specific criteria for the DSM IV[1] diagnosis are presented below:

A. There is a pervasive pattern of disregard for and violation of the rights of others occurring since age 15, as indicated by 3 or more of the following:
   1. failure to conform to social norms with respect to lawful behaviors as indicated by repeatedly performing acts that are grounds for arrest.
   2. deceitfulness, as indicated by repeated lying, use of aliases, or conning others for personal profit or pleasure.
   3. impulsivity or failure to plan ahead.
   4. irritability and aggressiveness, as indicated by repeated physical fights or assaults.
   5. reckless disregard for safety of self or others.
   6. consistent irresponsibility, as indicated by repeated failure to sustain consistent work behavior or honor financial obligations.
   7. lack of remorse, as indicated by being indifferent to or rationalizing having hurt, mistreated, or stolen from another.
B. The individual is at least 18 years.
C. There is evidence of conduct disorder with onset before age 15 years.
D. Occurrence of antisocial behavior is not exclusively during the course of schizophrenia or a manic episode.

From American Psychiatric Association: Diagnostic and Statistical Manual of Mental Disorders, Fourth Edition. Washington, DC, American Psychiatric Association, 1994, with permission.

Antisocial personality disorder, as currently conceptualized in DSM IV, is a quantitative (behaviorally anchored) rather than qualitative (trait- or predisposition-based) diagnosis. However, it is important to recognize the difference between specific antisocial acts and the chronic maladaptive pattern of antisocial behavior that characterizes the patient with antisocial personality disorder. For example, most adolescents have committed the following illegal activities at least once: driving a car without a license, skipping school, fist fighting, stealing, drinking alcohol, or using marijuana. Similarly, many adults have committed some of the following illegal or hurtful behaviors: lying, use of marijuana and other illegal drugs, extramarital affairs, failure to provide child support, and spouse and child abuse. In a randomly sampled survey, 25% of married individuals reported that their spouse had physically abused them in the past year. Despite a few behaviors that particularly distinguish the antisocial individual (vagrancy, the use of aliases, impulsivity, and a poor marital history), the differentiation between antisocial personality disorder and normative legal and social violations is largely quantitative. Individuals with antisocial personality disorder, beginning in childhood, consistently and inflexibly commit a higher frequency of antisocial behaviors resulting in maladaptive social or occupational functioning.

The credo of the individual with antisocial personality disorder can be summarized as "I believe; therefore, it is so." Such individuals are 100% certain of the veracity of their viewpoint, 100% certain that because they want something, they should receive it. They are 100% certain that because they believe that a particular rule is silly, they need not follow it. Because they believe that they can avoid negative consequences, they are 100% certain that they will not happen. Because they believe that another is not worthy of respect, they feel 100% justified in denigrating the person. The high frequency of antisocial behaviors may be maintained by this egocentric cognitive style, notable for a lack of motivation to understand events from any other point of view. Such individuals do not think about how others perceive them and are not concerned about the effect of their behavior on others. Qualities such as empathy, remorse, reliability, and sincerity depend on understanding events from the vantage of others. The antisocial individual's low motivation to understand another's point of view may account for his or her limited ability to demonstrate empathy, remorse, sincerity, or reliability.

2. List clues for the general practitioner that he or she is treating a patient with antisocial personality disorder.

Such clues include physical, historical, and interpersonal characteristics of the patient and the practitioner's response to the patient. **Physical characteristics** of the patient include (1) multiple tattoos, especially "jail-house" tattoos, which generally are of poor quality and completed by nonprofessional tattoo artists or the patient; and (2) "biker" or otherwise nonconformist appearance modeled after groups known to approve or sanction violence or disregard for the rights of others. **Historical characteristics** include (1) multiple injuries or scars not explained by occupation or involvement in sports and (2) unstable lifestyle. **Interpersonal characteristics** include an ingratiating interaction style, (2) entitled attitude with frequent demands, (3) superficial charm with overall functioning and level of success well below the level anticipated on the basis of perceived level of intelligence, (4) references in the interview to prison time or use of prison slang (e.g., "the man," "snitches," "hooch," "the joint"), (5) unsolicited statements that "I'm telling you the truth, doc!" and (6) statements suggesting a pattern of projecting blame onto others. Examples of such statements include, 'Yeah, doc, those doctors in the pen, they're not like you, they don't know what they're doing. They never told me I shouldn't drink . . . smoke . . ." or "yeah, they really screwed up" or "yeah, those fast food restaurants, they really ought to be sued by somebody . . . it is their *fault* we all got this cholesterol problem."

The **practitioner's responses** often include:

1. A perception that the patient's complaints or requests are manipulative, including an uncomfortable feeling that the patient is seeking drugs. Suggestive evidence includes an unusual degree of knowledge about pain medication, a request for *specific* addictive medication, vague responses to questions about prior treatment providers, or subjective complaints justifying addictive medication without supportive physical findings.

2. Suspicion that the patient is not being truthful about the medical history. This suspicion may be based on inconsistencies in the patient's report, vague answers to many questions, or an irritable, defensive response to detailed questioning.

None of these clues are pathognomonic for the diagnosis of antisocial personality disorder. They are sufficiently suggestive to warrant particular notice and consideration of more detailed questioning, special precautions, or external validation of history before implementing treatment.

3. How common is antisocial personality disorder?

Antisocial personality disorder is the only personality disorder studied in recent large-scale U.S. surveys: the Epidemiologic Catchment Area (ECA) study, and the National Comorbidity Survey (NCS). The prevalence of antisocial personality disorder in these studies was 2.4% and 3.5%, respectively. In the National Comorbidity Study, 5.8% of men and 1.2% of women met criteria for antisocial personality disorder.

4. What is a psychopath? What is a sociopath? Are these terms synonymous with antisocial personality disorder? What is the diagnostic reliability of antisocial personality disorder?

Often, the terms psychopath, sociopath, and antisocial personality disorder are loosely used synonymously. This is unfortunate as it fosters poor communication and poor diagnostic reliability. Historically, the terms psychopath and sociopath referred to persons who not only exhibited bad behavior, but suffered from a disorder characterized by deficits in empathy and an inability to manage interpersonal relationships. Factor-analytic studies suggest two separate elements in psychopathy: criminality and pathologic interpersonal/affective behavior. Hare's Psychopathy Checklist measures both elements. When both elements are considered, only 10-25% of criminals meet diagnostic criteria for psychopathy. In comparison, between two-thirds and three-quarters of male prison populations meet the definition of antisocial personality disorder when DSM IV criteria are used. In other words, psychopaths are probably a more pathologic subset of the broader category of those with antisocial personality disorder.

The Cleckley and Hare term psychopath involves a trait-based description of personality. The traits of psychopathy include: superficial charm, irresponsibility, insincerity, lack of remorse, impulsiveness, egocentricity, shallow affect, and a failure to learn from experience. Criteria based on traits are generally less diagnostically reliable. A trait approach requires the diagnostician to determine absolutely the presence or absence of qualities such as irresponsibility and insincerity in an all or none fashion. In actuality, such traits reflect a continuum of behaviors rather than a dichotomy. Psychopathy, as measured by the Hare Psychopathy Checklist-Revised can be reliably assessed, though such reliability requires extensive training, and the test is time consuming. In contrast, the DSM IV criteria are behaviorally anchored, resulting in considerably greater ease in attaining diagnostic reliability. Though it may be difficult to reach agreement on whether a given patient is irresponsible, it is relatively easy to determine whether a person has or has not failed to honor financial obligations or provide child support. Although clinicians can diagnose reliably the presence or absence of a personality disorder, they are not able to distinguish reliably between the different personality disorders. Because of its behavioral anchors, however, the diagnosis of antisocial personality disorder has the highest diagnostic reliability of all personality disorders.

5. Discuss the differential diagnosis of antisocial personality disorder.

Antisocial personality disorder must be differentiated from antisocial behavior. Antisocial behavior may be committed intermittently by many people without mental disorders or may be a symptom of another disorder. To differentiate between antisocial behavior and antisocial personality disorder it is necessary to consider whether the patient meets criteria for a personality disorder. Patients must demonstrate a pervasive, enduring, and inflexible antisocial pattern of perceiving, relating to, and thinking about themselves, others, and their environment.

Although antisocial personality disorder, not unexpectedly, is represented disproportionately in prison populations, a pattern of criminal behavior (beginning before or after age 15) is insufficient to make the diagnosis. Studies of prison populations have reported prevalence rates of antisocial personality disorder as low as 40% and as high as 75%. Prisoners without antisocial personality disorder may include "professional criminals," those involved in organized crime, and one-time offenders. Many such persons clearly disregard the rights of others and may have no remorse for their harmful effects. However, if they are neither aggressive nor impulsive, they probably do not meet criteria for antisocial personality disorder.

Criminal or antisocial behavior is commonly associated with substance use disorders. Correlations between the diagnoses of antisocial personality disorder and alcohol or other substance abuse or dependence are statistically significant. The presence of one of the three diagnoses increases the probability of the presence of the others. Despite this association, the diagnosis of antisocial personality disorder should not be given if criminal behavior and other antisocial behavior occur only in the context of addiction.

Specific symptoms of antisocial personality disorder are associated with many psychiatric disorders. Patients with schizophrenia, mania, sexual perversions, mental retardation, organic brain syndromes, and other personality disorders (including narcissistic personality disorder) may demonstrate some but not all features of antisocial personality disorder. For example, patients with schizophrenia, mental retardation, and organic brain syndromes are likely to demonstrate impaired occupational and parental functioning. All of these disorders are sometimes associated with impulsive acts, including repeated unlawful behavior. Sometimes, such impulsive acts may be associated with lack of remorse. For example, sex offenders may not experience remorse with regard to their sexual victims because of false beliefs that their behavior is not harmful or in fact is desired by the victim. At times, only the absence of symptoms of a conduct disorder as a child clarifies that the patient does not have antisocial personality disorder.

6. What is the cause of antisocial personality disorder?

Antisocial personality disorder is likely the result of an interaction among multiple factors, including individual vulnerabilities, particular developmental learning histories, and environmental stressors. Individual vulnerabilities include genetic factors. Twin studies have demonstrated that there is significant heritability involved in criminal behavior. EEG studies have found a high frequency of abnormalities in sociopaths. There are studies which suggest those who develop antisocial personality are born with an "uninhibited temperament," lack of normal fearfulness, and a constitutionally based failure to learn from negative experiences. Another biologic factor in psychopathy is possible comorbidity with attention-deficit hyperactivity disorder. About one-third of children with attention-deficit hyperactivity disorder later demonstrate adult criminal behavior.

Patterson and others have proposed a developmental theory of antisocial behavior which is empirically anchored. This theory has generated interventions, primarily prevention, with demonstrated success. Patterson proposes the following learning history: First, parents teach their children antisocial behavior through inappropriate and inconsistent parenting. Inappropriate parenting may occur when the parent positively reinforces the child for antisocial acts. For example, the parent may laugh or praise the child when the child hits another. Inconsistent parenting may occur when the parent negatively reinforces the child. For example, a mother asks her son to clean his room. Like most children, he does not comply immediately, so the mother asks again. The child throws a tantrum. The mother experiences the tantrum as aversive and stops asking him to clean his room. Thus the child is negatively reinforced for his tantrum; in other words, when he throws a tantrum, the mother stops asking him to be responsible. The mother also learns that if she does not ask her child to be responsible, he will not throw a tantrum. The child learns to use aversive behavior to avoid responsibility.

The second step in the development of antisocial behavior occurs when the child begins school. The child's aversive behavior leads to a predictable social outcome: the child is rejected. He or she does not follow instructions, is unable to complete a task on time, and does not cooperate with others. The child lacks the skills to do well academically and thus may fail to learn to read or compute math. Such failures have dire consequences for occupational and social future. Step three of the inexorable sequence occurs when after being rejected, the child gravitates toward deviant peer groups. Such peers are likely to provide positive feedback for antisocial behaviors and punishment for prosocial behaviors.

Epidemiologic studies have identified clear environmental and social factors which correlate with antisocial personality disorder. Social structures affect the prevalence of personality disorders by lowering or raising the threshold at which other risks influence their development.[6] Though there are no differences in prevalence of antisocial personality disorder among U.S. racial groups, there are important cross-cultural differences in its prevalence. In east Asian cultures with low comorbid alcoholism, antisocial personality disorder has an unexpectedly low prevalence (0.03–0.14% vs. 2–4% in the U.S.). This difference has been attributed to strong vs. weak family structures. The importance of social factors is further supported by the fact that the prevalence of antisocial personality disorder is increasing dramatically in North America. Both the ECA and NCS studies found that the lifetime prevalence of antisocial personality disorder nearly doubled among young people in 15 years. Such rapid increases in such a short time period can be accounted for by changes in the social environment.

7. What is the prognosis for the patient with antisocial personality disorder?

Impairment is the rule, although it may range from mild to severe. Not uncommonly, professionals or laypersons refer to various prominent persons, such as politicians, as "sociopaths." Sociopathic qualities such as disregard for the truth and lack of remorse are perhaps present in many individuals drawn to positions of national recognition or power. However, economic or political success is unlikely if a person truly meets criteria for antisocial personality disorder. Characteristics of antisocial personality disorder such as early onset, related impairment in educational achievement, impulsivity, and aggression generally preclude success.

Impairment due to the disorder is frequently severe. Typically, such individuals fail to become independent, experiencing years of institutionalization, usually penal rather than medical. Although estimates vary, such individuals appear significantly more likely to die prematurely as a result of suicide, homicide, or complications of drug or alcohol abuse.

Although people who meet criteria for antisocial personality disorder are at risk of early death, the prognosis for those who live to middle-age is somewhat encouraging. Spontaneous improvement with age appears to be the rule rather than the exception. In the ECA study, there was a striking decrease in the prevalence after age 44. In a large follow-up study, fewer than 10% met criteria for antisocial personality disorder 29 years after initial hospitalization. The vast majority has ongoing impairments, particularly in interpersonal relationships. The most consistent improvements are in criminal behavior. The prognosis for the psychopathic subset of antisocial personality disorders appears more grim. The psychopaths are significantly more likely to recidivate than non-psychopathic antisocials.

8. What kind of difficulties do professionals have with patients diagnosed with antisocial personality disorder?

Health care professionals frequently experience the following problems with patients diagnosed with antisocial personality disorder: (1) difficulty in collecting reliable history, (2) difficulty in managing the patient, (3) conflict between responsibility to the patient and responsibility to society, and (4) because of the conflict, negative feelings such as anger, boredom, and hopelessness.

The dishonesty of patients with antisocial personality disorder makes it difficult to collect reliable history. Inconsistency or vagueness is a clue that the patient may be lying. Nonverbal cues include stammering, short answers, hesitations, excessive blinking, dilated pupils, and excessive touching of clothing. The patient is likely to blame the clinician who questions inconsistencies (e.g., "aren't you listening?" "you heard that wrong," "I didn't say that," or "use your head, doc"). In such situations, straightforward delineation of the costs and benefits of presenting an accurate history is useful. Patients with antisocial personality disorder respond best to an approach based on self-interest. Fortunately, they typically have the capacity and motivation to discuss honestly their physical history (in contrast to social or occupational history).

Keys to the second difficulty, difficulty in management, include the following:

1. It is the patient's responsibility to deal with the consequences of antisocial behavior.
2. The clinician must set clear expectations regarding acceptable behavior.
3. The clinician must take a nonjudgmental stance and objectively help the patient to consider the costs and benefits of his or her behavior to self.

For example, the patient may wish to consider whether the benefits of denigrating nursing staff (reduction in tension) outweigh the costs (probable reduction in care). Given the patient's difficulty appreciating any point of view other than his or her own, it is more effective to emphasize the effects on self than on others.

The health care provider also may experience conflict between responsibility to the patient and responsibility to the patient's dependents or society. Informing the patient of the limits of confidentiality at the onset of treatment helps to ameliorate such problems. For example, the patient should be informed that the clinician will be unable to maintain confidentiality if the patient threatens to harm self or others, or reveals plans to commit a crime. Similarly, the patient should be informed that the clinician is unable to maintain confidentiality if the patient reports physical abuse or neglect of a child or, in some states, an elderly person. Before breaking confidentiality, the clinician is well advised to consult. Consultation not only provides information but also enables the clinician to wear one rather than multiple hats. For example, in the case of mandated reporting of child abuse, by consulting with specialists in psychiatry and social work the clinician avoids the potentially conflicting roles of investigator, therapist, and physician. Data indicating that hospital personnel report less than 50% of child abuse cases suggest a conflict between medical and social responsibilities.

The above difficulties may result in the fourth difficulty: the health professional may experience negative feelings such as anger, boredom, hopelessness, and hatred toward the patient. Whereas it is the patient's responsibility to deal with the consequences of his or her behavior, the provider must deal appropriately with her or his own feelings. The clinician's perusal of police reports may result in anger, fear, or horror. Some clinicians avoid reading police reports for fear that such feelings may prevent them from providing adequate care. As a result of the marked tendency of patients with antisocial personality disorder to project blame and responsibility, the clinician may experience guilt, impotence, and hopelessness. It is important, particularly for the introspective health care provider, to study the patient's behavior, not his or her own. Finally, it is important to recognize that feelings of apathy or boredom may shield more intense feelings. Signs that clinicians may be acting out their feelings inappropriately include forgetting appointments and other commitments, colluding with staff in denigrating the patient, colluding with the patient in denigrating staff, giving the patient special consideration, or giving the patient less than appropriate consideration.

9. What are the guidelines for management of medical conditions in patients with antisocial personality disorder?

1. Err on the side of caution. If anyone (clinician, spouse, colleague, or support personnel) expresses concern about personal safety, whether based on clearcut logic or "gut" feeling, evaluate the patient with a chaperone present.

2. The clinician at times will be required to evaluate patients in restraints or chains. The patient should be evaluated as thoroughly as possible with restraints in place. If adequate assessment is not possible, adequate security personnel should be obtained before removal of restraints and completion of physical examination. The clinician should defer security assessment decisions to security personnel. The clinician must not try to be a hero.

3. The clinician should consider a diagnosis of malingering (exaggeration or complete fabrication of symptoms for secondary gain). For example, the patient may wish to avoid work, military conscription, or prison time or to obtain financial gain, disability payments, or drugs. Clinicians should ask themselves, "Why is this patient in my office right now?" "What does this patient really want?"

4. The clinician should be cautious in prescribing medication and avoid prescription of addictive medications when possible. When such medications are prescribed, the clinician must be explicit and write out exactly how much is to be dispensed—e.g., "dispense 4 (four)." The clinician must think, "Is this written in such a way that the patient could alter what the pharmacy dispenses?" "No refills" should be specified. If the clinician follows a patient with antisocial personality disorder or antisocial symptoms, precise amounts should be prescribed from visit to visit. The patient should be notified that the clinician will not provide extra prescriptions if they are "lost," "stolen," or "accidentally flushed down the toilet."

CONTROVERSY

10. Is antisocial personality disorder a treatable condition?
Against:

1. Prior comprehensive, costly programs in which offenders were diverted to secure treatment facilities rather than prison demonstrated no sufficient improvement or decrease in recidivism to warrant the cost to society. In fact, in one study (Rice, et al.) a psychopathic subset actually demonstrated increased violent recidivism after receiving treatment, in contrast to the non-psychopathic antisocial individuals who demonstrated a decrease in violent recidivism.

2. Psychiatric or psychological treatment of individuals with antisocial personality disorder is a poor allocation of financial and social resources.

3. Psychiatric or psychological treatment of incarcerated individuals is coercive, unethical, and unconstitutional.

For:

1. Previous treatment outcome studies of patients with antisocial personality disorder involve significant methodologic problems: (1) Few outcome studies identified subjects by DSM-III or

DSM-III-R criteria; (2) no studies in which diagnostic criteria were well-defined employed non-treated control group; and (3) although expert opinion supporting the lack of benefit of individual psychodynamic treatment is pervasive, no information in the literature addresses outcome for patients with antisocial personality disorder treated with other modalities for an extended time in a forensic setting. Schizophrenia does not respond to psychodynamic psychotherapy but is generally agreed to be a treatable condition. Depression does not generally improve with psychoanalysis but often responds to cognitive therapy, antidepressant medication, or a combination of the two.

Studies of treatment outcome with conduct-disordered children, who may potentially become adults with antisocial personality disorder, suggest that antisocial personality disorder can be prevented. Parent-management training, cognitive therapy, and court-diversion appear to be promising approaches. In summary, conclusions about the treatability of antisocial personality disorder are premature; it is as scientifically valid to say that such patients are treatable as it is to say that they are not.

2. Patients with antisocial personality disorder have a significant risk of early death but also a good chance of spontaneous remission (or at least substantial improvement) if they live till age 30 or 35. At a minimum, this observation supports crisis intervention strategies aimed at decreasing the risk of early death and minimizing negative effects of antisocial behaviors on both the patient and others.

3. For unclear reasons, the standard for psychiatric medical conditions appears to equate "treatment" with "cure." Diabetes mellitus, coronary artery disease, and chronic obstructive pulmonary disease are only three of the many medical disease that are "treatable" (i.e., morbidity and mortality can be reduced by medical interventions) but not currently "curable."Accurate assessment of treatability of antisocial personality disorder requires clear definition of the target symptoms to be reduced or relieved. Target symptoms may include prevention or treatment of violent death, aggression, substance abuse, impulsivity, or concomitant major mental disorders. Individuals with antisocial personality disorder have a 5–50-fold increased risk of experiencing concurrent mania, schizophrenia, and alcohol or drug abuse. Prognosis is improved by treatment of concurrent anxiety and depression. Treatment of such disorders may prolong life and decrease personal and societal damage while awaiting possible spontaneous remission.

BIBLIOGRAPHY

1. American Psychiatric Association: Diagnostic and Statistical Manual of Mental Disorders, 4th ed. Washington, DC, American Psychiatric Association, 1994.
2. Beck AT, Freeman A: Cognitive Therapy of Personality Disorders. New York, Guilford Press, 1990.
3. Cleckley H: The Mask of Sanity, 5th ed. St. Louis, Mosby, 1976.
4. Frances AJ, Hales RE (eds): American Psychiatric Association Annual Review, vol. 5. Washington, DC, American Psychiatric Press, 1986.
5. Hare RD: Psychopathy: A clinical construct whose time has come. Criminal Justice Behavior 23:25–54, 1996.
6. Kessler CR, McGonagle KA, Zhao S, et al: Lifetime and 12-month prevalence of DSM-IIIR psychiatric disorders in the United States. Arch Gen Psychiatry 51:8–19, 1994.
7. Paris J: A biopsychosocial model of psychopathy (227–287). In Millon, et al (eds): Psychopathy. New York, Guilford Press, 1998.
8. Patterson GR, DeBaryshe BD, Ramsey E: A developmental perspective on antisocial behavior. Am Psychol 44:329–335, 1989.
9. Rice ME, Harris GT, Cormier CA: An evaluation of a maximum security therapeutic community for psychopaths and other mentally disordered offenders. Law Hum Behav 16:399–412, 1992.
10. Schubert DS, Wolf AW, Patterson MB, et al: A statistical evaluation of the literature regarding the associations among alcoholism, drug abuse, and antisocial personality disorder. Int J Addict 23:797–808, 1988.
11. Treatment outlines for antisocial personality disorder. The Quality Assurance Project. Aust N Z J Psychiatry 25:541–547, 1991.
12. Widiger TA, Corbitt EM, Millon TM: Antisocial personality disorder. APA Rev Psychiatry 11:63–79, 1992.

VI. *Therapeutic Approaches in Psychiatry*

40. PSYCHOANALYTICALLY ORIENTED PSYCHOTHERAPIES

James L. Jacobson, M.D., and Alan M. Jacobson, M.D.

1. Describe psychoanalytically oriented psychotherapy.

Psychoanalytically oriented psychotherapy (sometimes called psychodynamic psychotherapy) encompasses a group of psychotherapeutic approaches founded on the discoveries of Sigmund Freud and later refined and expanded by a number of other researchers, clinicians, and theoreticians. This group of approaches is based on the belief that current behavior, emotions, capacities for functioning, and patterns of relationship are deeply influenced by one's experiences early in life.

2. How might early life experiences affect the present?

Psychoanalytically oriented therapists believe that early developmental experiences influence later behavior and that such influences often are outside of normal awareness. The early experiences are retained in the unconscious mind as expectations about relationships, beliefs about ourselves and the world around us, and mechanisms to control uncomfortable feelings and thoughts and prevent them from coming into the conscious mind. These unconscious processes determine present feelings and actions. Thus, the past shapes the present through forces that are sometimes known and sometimes unknown.

For example, a person may maintain a haughty, aloof attitude toward others that results in a painful lack of emotional closeness. In the course of therapy, it is discovered that this way of relating was developed to protect the person earlier in life against a hostile relationship with a demeaning caregiver. Hence, the person developed false superiority to protect from internal feelings of inadequacy, and aloofness to maintain distance from relationships that may be perceived as threatening to self-esteem.

3. How is psychoanalytic therapy conducted?

Psychoanalytic therapy comprises verbal interaction between patient and therapist in an effort to elucidate unconscious past forces that affect current emotions and actions. Intensive therapy often is paced at 1–2 sessions per week over several weeks to years. In **psychoanalysis**, the most involving approach based on psychodynamic principles, the course of treatment often is longer, with more frequent meetings (up to 4–5 times per week). This process allows the patient to reexperience with the analyst, in a deeply felt way, earlier emotional involvements. The bringing forward of past experiences and reexperiencing them in the present is called **transference**. Most people are unaware of transference, although it frequently shapes the way in which they relate to other people.

Such unawareness is maintained by unconscious mental processes known as **defense mechanisms**. Although defense mechanisms vary widely (e.g., repression of memory, denial, disconnection of emotion from event [isolation], externalization of blame, internalization, sublimation), their common purpose is to keep potentially anxiety-provoking events and feelings out of awareness. In psychoanalysis and in some forms of psychodynamic therapy, the therapist or analyst interprets (i.e., comments on) defensive maneuvers to gradually uncover their origins by expanding the patient's awareness of current events (defensive maneuvers) and historical events (origins). This process stirs uncomfortable feelings and seemingly unacceptable thoughts, and defense mechanisms may be activated in the relationship with the therapist. They may present as apparent resistances, such as reactions to the therapist that lead to breaks in the free flow of discussion. In such cases, the therapist offers further commentary on the nature of the resistance, which may lead to further understanding of the difficulties in the interpersonal relationship.

4. What are the benefits to the patient?

Through repeated, successive interpretation and intense experience of the connection between current personal involvement (with both the therapist and other people) and past events, the patient learns about the forces directing his or her own behavior. As unconscious sources of difficulty gradually emerge in the therapeutic relationship, the therapist or analyst explains them to the patient over and over again in an effort to expand understanding.

Unconscious forces are demonstrated in daily life, in work, in dreams, and in every human endeavor. The patient, in an intimate, evolving relationship with the therapist or analyst, experiences increasingly deep emotional and intellectual understanding of these forces and how they shape attitudes and relationships. Moreover, he or she can compare previously unconscious perceptions to current experiences with the therapist. This comparison provides an opportunity to gain control over the previously unknown impulses and defensive reactions, leading to changed feelings about self and improved relationships with others. The result is greater freedom to make choices in work and in establishing loving relationships. Often, new developmental processes or the reestablishment of normal development ensues.

5. Define transference and countertransference.

In its broadest form, *transference* is bringing into a current life experience, such as a relationship, the beliefs, expectations, and perceptions from previous relationships. In analytic therapy transference often refers to relationships from particular stages of development. For example, a patient may experience his wife in the same way that he experienced one of his parents in childhood. Although there may be some similarity to the way his wife behaves, the total perception is colored by the early experience; hence, this is a transference relationship.

Countertransference is a specific reaction of the therapist to the patient's transference. Examples include feelings, thoughts, and attitudes that are reactions to specific events in therapy. The therapist may experience such a reaction or feeling as being unlike him- or herself; this is often a hint to the presence of a countertransference reaction. For example, the therapist may be unusually silent, angry, or affectionate.

Both transference and countertransference can be elucidated to increase understanding of behavior and to assist in the progress of therapy. If not addressed and discussed, such reactions may stall the therapeutic endeavor or lead to negative reactions and cessation of treatment.

6. How are dreams used in psychodynamic psychotherapy and analysis?

Dreams were initially seen by Freud as "the royal road to the unconscious." They were thought to contain a direct view into the unconscious life of the individual. Thus, dream interpretation was once considered the central method for understanding unconscious phenomena.

Dream elements are **symbolic representations** of current life events as well as earlier life experiences and conflicts. Although dreams still play an important role in psychodynamic psychotherapy, they now are seen as one of many sources of information about hidden wishes and fears that are relevant to both current and past functioning. The therapist or analyst may focus on current concerns manifested by the content of the dream or on representations of the past. He or she may ask a patient to associate (i.e., let the mind wander and freely react to different thoughts and feelings) to the dream as a whole or the different elements of the dream to unmask and elaborate what the symbols in the dream represent. Such associations are termed the **latent content**.

Current analytic thought places equal (or perhaps more) emphasis on transference as the royal road to the unconscious. Other phenomena that help to elucidate unconscious processes include slips of the tongue (known as parapraxis), fantasies, daydreams, resistance, and virtually any recurrent way of relating in life.

7. What are defense mechanisms?

Defense mechanisms are the methods by which individuals seek to regulate basic instincts. Instincts may be thought of primarily as aggressive and sexual. Defense mechanisms are conceptualized as part of a process called the ego or the "I." Freud's initial theory of personality highlighted a conflict between the desire for gratification of basic instincts and the need to control unwanted or dangerous pressure for gratification. He conceptualized repression as the ego's central mechanism of defense, but various defense mechanisms are now recognized.

Repression refers to the mechanism by which internal urges, thoughts, and feelings and memory of events are "forgotten." They are contained in unconscious (or repressed) memory. The repressed is not recognized, but the effects of what has been repressed tend to remain. For example, a person may "forget" or repress a traumatic event, yet retain an emotion that he or she cannot connect to a particular situation. Inexplicable sadness unattached to a memory, but present in response to certain interpersonal cues, likely results from repression.

Other mechanisms of defense include **denial, altruism, intellectualization, projection, internalization**, and **sublimation**. Each mechanism represents a somewhat different method of dealing with unacceptable thoughts, feelings, wishes, or events. Although such defensive operations occur largely outside the individual's awareness, they become manifest as types of behavior in all relationships, including the therapeutic relationship. The therapist helps the patient to understand defensive maneuvers and become more aware of their influence on everyday functioning. With the therapist's help, the patient can change behavioral patterns.

8. Who is treatable with psychoanalysis or psychoanalytic psychotherapy?

The clinician must assess the patient's relative strengths and capabilities as well as relative weaknesses and difficulties. Psychoanalysis and psychoanalytic psychotherapy are not specifically indicated or contraindicated by particular disorders. The individual who is likely to benefit from psychoanalytic psychotherapy suffers long-standing symptoms such as depressed mood, anxiety, and repetitive patterns of behavior that result in a sense of limited choices and enjoyment. The person's capacities may be thwarted by his or her own actions; there may be a sense of falling short or disappointment with the outcome of behavior and ways of relating. The person may have difficulty being spontaneous or feeling close to others. There also may be a sense of inordinate suffering.

Concurrently, there must be adequate psychological and emotional strength to endure the explorations of psychoanalytically oriented therapy. For example, the person must have demonstrated some capacity to achieve, such as a history of satisfaction in relationships with friends or work. The capacities to form relationships, self-observe, and contain strong feelings adequately also are strengths that may aid in the psychotherapeutic process.

The psychoanalyst or therapist assesses specific patterns of defensive functioning and the nature of relationships to evaluate to the required sturdiness and motivation. Exploratory and exposing approaches demand considerable patient resilience—as well as support from the clinician.

9. Are risks associated with exploratory psychoanalytic psychotherapy or analysis?

Yes. As with any treatment, risks are involved. Dynamic analytic therapy often is anxiety-provoking because of its attempt to pierce the comforting defensive operations used by the patient to cope with **unwanted feelings**. Ideally, these unwanted feelings gradually emerge into awareness. The therapist must first determine whether the patient is prone to impulsive actions, which may be dangerous if anxiety-provoking feelings and instincts become more accessible (sometimes called "acting out"). The therapist must assist in managing the expression of such impulses. The goal is a balance between uncovering unconscious elements and maintaining current emotional stability.

Psychoanalytically oriented psychotherapy is designed to promote a transitory **regression** in which the patient experiences earlier ways of relating to people. Regression by definition means returning to a former state. Earlier states of development can be painful to experience and lead to behavior that is no longer appropriate. The result may be transient functioning that is less adaptive. For example, a patient may reexperience the full force of a humiliating experience with his or her father and hence be left more vulnerable. A criticism from a supervisor at work may feel humiliating, and an over-reaction can lead to an angry response or even quitting the job. Furthermore, such regression may persist and lead to chronic over-dependence on the therapist.

10. Differentiate exploratory and ego-supportive approaches.

The psychodynamic framework includes exploratory therapies that *uncover* unconscious motives and experiences, thereby weakening defenses. The use of psychoanalytic understanding to *strengthen* rather than diminish defenses is called ego-supportive psychotherapy. Some of the techniques of supportive psychotherapy are similar to those used in cognitive and behavioral therapies (see chapters 41 and 42). One particularly well-defined method, based in part on psychodynamic principles and developed by Klerman and Weissman, has been termed interpersonal psychotherapy. It is a commonly used short-term, dynamic psychotherapy that contains supportive therapy principles.

11. Describe interpersonal psychotherapy.

Interpersonal psychotherapy was designed as a short-term treatment model for patients with depression. It has been empirically evaluated in a series of studies. A manual describes the methods and techniques for therapeutic intervention in a consistent, reproducible fashion. Interpersonal therapy focuses primarily on the **social roles** and **interpersonal interactions** in the patient's past and current life experiences. Although the entire life-span is covered, the interpersonal therapist places a clear emphasis on current factors, especially a patient's disappointment in personal role expectations as well as disputes and problems in relationships. The interpersonal therapist directs the patient to one or two problem areas in current functioning, which then become the primary focus of the therapy. Examples include grief over a loss; disputes in marriage, family, and work; role transitions such as retirement or job demotion; and loss through divorce.

Although the interpersonal therapist recognizes the importance of defense mechanisms, he or she does not attempt to address internal conflict as a source of current problems. Instead, behaviors and emotions are examined as they relate to current interpersonal problems.

12. Differentiate interpersonal psychotherapy and "uncovering" approaches.

Interpersonal therapy, as a supportive approach, helps to *build on* current capacities to function rather than uncover inner conflict. The primary focus is not enduring personality and character problems or earlier life experiences, although they may play a role in depression. The twin goals are: (1) relieve symptoms through reduction of grief, and (2) help the patient develop better strategies for dealing with current problems associated with the onset of depressive symptoms.

Interpersonal Psychotherapy	*"Uncovering" Analytic Psychotherapies*
What has contributed to the patient's current depression?	Why did the patient become what he or she is and/or where is the patient going?
What are the current stresses?	What was the patient's childhood like?
Who are the key persons involved in the current stress? What are the current disputes and disappointments?	What is the patient's character?
Is the patient learning how to cope with the problem?	Is the patient cured?
What are the patient's assets?	What are the patient's defenses?
How can I help the patient to ventilate painful emotions and talk about situations that evoke guilt, shame, resentment?	How can I find out why this patient feels guilty, ashamed, or resentful?
How can I help the patient clarify his or her wishes and have more satisfying relationships with others?	How can I understand the patient's fantasy life and help him or her to gain insight into the origins of present behavior?
How can I correct misinformation and suggest alternatives?	How can I help the patient discover false or incorrect ideas?

Adapted from Klerman G, Weissman M, Rovsanville B, Cherron E: Interpersonal Psychotherapy of Depression. New York, Basic Books, 1984.

13. How long do psychoanalytically oriented therapies take?

Therapeutic approaches range from short-term, well-defined therapies with specific focus, which may require only 2–8 sessions, to psychoanalysis, which may require 4 or 5 sessions per week for many years. Brief forms of treatment focus on specific current problems that result in an outbreak of particular symptoms, such as anxiety or depressed mood. The long-term forms address the source of current difficulty, but also attempt to understand and change basic, long-held patterns of relating to others as well as feelings about self that have developed over a lifetime. Hence, *the goals of each particular form of therapy are directly related to the length of treatment.*

The longer forms of treatment involve the development of an **intense interpersonal relationship**, the elucidation of of multiple aspects of that relationship, and the development of the personal strength and ability to move beyond it. This relationship may be viewed similarly to other important interpersonal relationships that enhance development, such as with a parent, sibling, friend, grandparent, or mentor. The length of treatment is influenced, therefore, by the goals of therapy and the degree to which the primary focus is on the relationship between patient and therapist.

Supportive psychotherapies also vary greatly in duration. Support can last through a **specific life event** (job change, divorce, grief over the death of a parent), or it may be a long-standing therapeutic relationship that helps *fragile* patients sufficiently to allow them to function at work and avoid suicide attempts and costly hospitalizations.

14. Differentiate dynamic analytic and behavior therapies.

In simple terms, behavior therapies attempt to modify observable behavior through various **reinforcement strategies**. For example, if an individual is afraid of snakes, behavioral therapy may desensitize the patient to this fear by having him or her learn a specific method of attaining a relaxed state, and then, during relaxation, introducing the idea of a common earthworm. Subsequently, a picture of an earthworm is introduced, followed by the idea of a common, nonthreatening snake. After a picture of a snake, gradual steps may lead to viewing a snake in a contained environment such as a zoo. There is no focus on the origin or symbolic representation of the fear.

In psychodynamic psychotherapy, the therapist focuses on both the origin and the object of the fear. Behavior therapy offers a strategy of *managing* a symptom without the necessity of understanding its meaning or origin. In psychodynamic psychotherapy, management strategies are developed secondarily.

15. Are there uses of psychoanalytic principles other than for psychotherapy?

The psychoanalytic method in which the patient says everything that comes to mind in the context of an interpersonal relationship is both a method of psychotherapy and a tool for learning about human mental functioning. Based on such information, various theories of human mental functioning and normal development from infancy to old age have evolved. Hence, these principles also provide a tool for investigating inner life, a theoretical framework for human development, and a mechanism of viewing the functioning of the human mind.

From a more practical viewpoint, psychoanalytic principles can be used to understand patients reactions to medical illness, compliance and adherence problems in outpatient medical and psychiatric practice, and the complexities of human behavior as manifest in any form of clinical practice. It may well be that the psychodynamic perspective has its broadest application in understanding doctor-patient interchange rather than as a specific method for therapy. Indeed, clinicians using psychopharmacologic, behavioral, and other techniques can use this approach to enrich their understanding of the patient.

BIBLIOGRAPHY

1. Balint M, Balint E: Psychotherapeutic Techniques in Medicine. London, J.B. Lippincott, 1961.
2. Binder JL: Research findings on short-term psychodynamic therapy techniques. In The Hatherleigh Guides Series. New York, Hatherleigh Press, 1996, pp 79–97,
3. Greenson RR: The Technique and Practice of Psychoanalysis, vol. 1. New York, International University Press, 1967.

4. Jacobson AM, Parmelee DX: Psychoanalysis: Critical Explorations in Contemporary Theory and Practice. New York, Brunner/Mazel, 1982.
5. Klerman G, Weissman M, Rovsanville B, Chevron E: Interpersonal Psychotherapy of Depression. New York, Basic Books, 1984.
6. Luborsky L: Theories of cure in psychoanalytic psychotherapies and the evidence for them. Psychoanalytic Inquiry 16(2):257–264, 1996.
7. Mann J: Time-Limited Psychotherapy. Cambridge, MA, Harvard University Press, 1973.
8. Sloane RB, Staples FR, Cristol AH, et al: Psychotherapy Versus Behavior Therapy. Cambridge, MA, Harvard University Press, 1975.
9. Wachtel PL: Psychoanalysis and Behavior Therapy. New York, Basic Books, 1977.
10. Stern DN: The Interpersonal World of the Infant. New York, Basic Books, 1985.
11. Rothstein A: Models of the Mind. New York, International Universities Press, 1985.
12. Vaillant GE (ed): Ego Mechanisms of Defense: A Guide for Clinicians and Researchers. Washington, DC, American Psychiatric Press, 1992.

41. COGNITIVE-BEHAVIORAL THERAPY

Jacqueline A. Samson, Ph.D.

1. What is cognitive-behavioral therapy?

Cognitive-behavioral therapy (CBT) combines treatment approaches of both cognitive and behavioral therapy. The principles were first outlined in a treatment manual specifically targeted to depression by Beck et al.[3]

The basis of **cognitive therapy** is the observation that negative feelings result from faulty cognitive processing. Incoming information is selectively filtered so that perceptions are distorted toward negative conclusions. Faulty processing is identified by examining a patient's spontaneous thoughts occurring throughout the day or after specific events. These "automatic" thoughts are key to understanding a patient's core system of assumptions and beliefs about the self and the world. CBT treatments first help a patient become aware of automatic thoughts and underlying assumptions and beliefs. The patient is then encouraged to seek evidence by which to support or refute the assumptions, and to modify beliefs based on a more balanced view of all available information.

Behavioral techniques are integrated throughout CBT treatment to facilitate change. Specific exercises for thought stopping, relaxation, and impulse control may be combined with monitoring and adjusting daily activities to increase mastery and pleasure experiences. Graded task assignments and systematic graded exposures also may be used.

2. Give an example of cognitive distortion.

A depressed patient reported to her cognitive therapist that she felt sad over the weekend. In reconstructing the events of the weekend, she noted that the sadness began during a telephone call on Saturday morning from an old friend. The therapist then encouraged her to remember the conversation and the point at which she first felt sadness. She remembered that her friend Sarah was discussing her plans to take a vacation but did not invite the patient to come along. Her first "automatic" thought was: "Sarah doesn't want me along because I'm no fun." Her next thought was, "Nobody wants to be with me. I have no friends." She then thought, "I will be alone for the rest of my life." Gloomy thoughts indeed!

The patient's faulty processing began with her first reaction to the news of Sarah's vacation. When the therapist asked the patient to examine the evidence for her assumption that Sarah did not want to be in her company, she had to say that there was no evidence; the fact that Sarah called indicated that Sarah enjoyed her company. Once the distortion in the automatic thought was worked through, the patient felt more hopeful about the future and was able to say that she might ask Sarah if they could plan to do something together soon.

3. What is the cognitive triad?

The cognitive triad refers to negative biases that are characteristic of depressed patients. The patient tends to: (1) view him- or herself in a negative light and assume excessive responsibility for failures or negative experiences; (2) view the world in a negative light and as presenting obstacles that cannot be overcome; (3) view the future negatively, consisting only of more failure and insurmountable obstacles.

4. What are the main cognitive processing errors that contribute to maintaining negative biases?

In general, cognitive errors involve: (1) making predictions about the future or how others will behave without sufficient evidence; (2) selectively focusing only on information that is consistent with one's expectations and ignoring information that runs counter to expectations; (3) assuming too much responsibility for negative events without acknowledging the contributions made by others or the situation; and (4) seeing situations as all-or-nothing and failing to acknowledge partial success or progress.

Cognitive Processing Errors

Emotional reasoning: A conclusion or inference based on an emotional state; e.g., "I feel this way; therefore, I *am* this way."

Overgeneralization: Evidence drawn from one experience or a small set of experiences to reach an unwarranted conclusion with far-reaching implications.

Catastrophic thinking: An extreme example of overgeneralization, in which the impact of a clearly negative event or experience is amplified to extreme proportions; e.g., "If I have a panic attack I will lose *all* control and go crazy (or die)."

All-or-nothing (black-or-white; absolutistic) thinking: An unnecessary division of complex or continuous outcomes into polarized extremes; e.g., "Either I'm a success at this, or I'm a total failure."

Shoulds and musts: Imperative statements about self that dictate rigid standards or reflect an unrealistic degree of presumed control over external events.

Negative predictions: Use of pessimism or earlier experiences of failure to prematurely or inappropriately predict failure in a new situation; also known as "fortune telling."

Mind reading: Negatively toned inferences about the thoughts, intentions, or motives of another person.

Labeling: An undesirable characteristic of a person or event is made definitive of that person or event; e.g., "Because I *failed* to be selected for ballet, I am a *failure*."

Personalization: Interpretation of an event, situation, or behavior as salient or personally indicative of a negative aspect of self.

Selective negative focus (selective abstraction): Focusing on undesirable or negative events, memories, or implications at the expense of recalling or identifying other, more neutral or positive information. In fact, positive information may be ignored or disqualified as irrelevant, atypical, or trivial.

Cognitive avoidance: Unpleasant thoughts, feelings, or events are misperceived as overwhelming and/or insurmountable and are actively suppressed or avoided.

Somatic (mis) focus: The predisposition to interpret internal stimuli (e.g., heart rate, palpitations, shortness of breath, dizziness, or tingling) as definite indications of impending catastrophic events (heart attack, suffocation, collapse).

Adapted from Thase ME, Beck AT: Overview of cognition therapy. In Wright JG, Thase ME, Beck AT, Ludgate JW (eds): Cognitive Therapy with Inpatients. New York, Guilford, 1993, pp 3–34.

5. How do patients learn to correct cognitive processing errors?

By working with a therapist who questions their logic. The therapist may use the socratic method and encourage the patient to identify errors in rational thinking by asking questions such as: "What is the evidence that this is true? What is the evidence that this is not true? Is there another way of looking at this?" Once alternative explanations have been generated, the therapist may collaborate with the patient to design a mini-experiment in which the patient gathers information to confirm, refute, or modify the assumption.

6. How does correction of cognitive errors result in mood change?

Although the exact mechanisms involved in clinical change are not known, it is hypothesized that the tendency to filter incoming information through a negative lens systematically excludes the positive information needed to maintain a **balanced perspective**. The process of change involves completing homework assignments. This is a critical step because it requires that the patient take concrete action to gather data (i.e., fill out daily activity monitoring forms). Patients are more likely to follow through on such assignments when they understand the rationale of the treatment, and evidence of its usefulness has been demonstrated in the initial therapy sessions (see Question 2). This behavioral component increases the patient's activity level and, usually, sense of self-efficacy. Once the patient becomes more active and is feeling somewhat empowered, opportunities for positive feedback from others increase. Mood improves as the negative cognitive biases are refuted by experience or evidence, and the patient begins to see more options.

7. How is the role of the cognitive-behavioral therapist different from more psychodynamically oriented therapists?

The cognitive-behavorial therapist takes an **active**, **problem-oriented**, and **directive** stance in the therapy relationship. Early in the relationship, the therapist assumes a direct teaching role and conveys the basic principles of cognitive therapy to the patient. In later sessions, the therapist assumes the role of coach, as the patient takes on more responsibility. Sessions are structured: the therapist and patient (1) jointly set an agenda, (2) briefly review the previous session, (3) review homework completed since the last session, (4) work on additional topics spurred by the homework or events of the week, (5) set up homework for the following week, and (6) end with a summary of the key points from the session. Throughout the session the therapist actively summarizes and highlights points as they occur and selectively pursues issues for further work.

Structure of a Typical CBT Session

---

1. Mood check
   • Examination of symptom severity score (e.g., Beck Depression Inventory)

2. Set the agenda

3. Weekly items
   • Review of events since last session
   • Feedback on reactions to previous session and review of key points
   • Homework review

4. Today's major topic

5. Set homework for next week

6. Summarize key points of today's session

7. Feedback on reactions to today's session

---

8. How many sessions typically are involved?

Protocols for CBT of depression and anxiety disorders are relatively brief (typically 12–20 sessions). The patient is expected to gradually master the skills of this method so that he or she may continue to monitor automatic thoughts and test assumptions independently after therapy termination. For patients with multiple diagnoses or comorbid personality disorders, more sessions may be needed to address target problems.

9. To what degree is early developmental experience examined in CBT?

In general, cognitive-behavioral therapists are oriented toward the present and encourage patients to examine how *present thoughts* affect specific behaviors. Examination of a number of automatic thoughts may reveal recurring themes. Such themes can then be examined in more detail to understand core beliefs or "schemas" about oneself or the world that may be driving the thoughts. Although core beliefs are likely to have developed as a result of early experience, it is not necessary to spend a great deal of therapy time exploring such experiences. Rather, the patient may be encouraged to write a brief autobiography outside the session from which likely links between schemas and early experiences can be drawn with the therapist in the next session. The therapist can help the patient to trace how the core belief may have evolved from painful early experiences and to see how they are understandable in that light. However, the emphasis is primarily on examining the ways in which old beliefs distort present thinking and behaviors and on developing an action plan for change.

10. Is there research evidence that CBT works?

Yes. A growing number of well-designed studies demonstrate that CBT is effective for patients with depression or anxiety disorders. Studies also show CBT to be as effective as antidepressant medication in mildly to moderately depressed patients; in patients with severe depression, this evidence is mixed. For both disorders, there is no clear evidence that a combination of CBT and medication is superior to either alone, or that the combination is less effective than either alone.

Studies comparing CBT to psychodynamically oriented therapies have not been conclusive, partly because of differences in the length of the treatments and difficulties in establishing standardized treatment protocols.

11. How do relapse rates for CBT and pharmacotherapy compare?

Follow-up studies find that 70–80% of depressed patients treated with CBT alone continue to be well 2 years later. These rates are significantly higher than the maintenance rates in patients who are withdrawn from antidepressant medication after a comparable initial trial, and equal to the rate in patients who continue on antidepressant medications.

12. Which disorders are responsive to CBT?

Efforts to apply CBT techniques to various types of patients have expanded rapidly in the past decade. Included among the disorders shown to be responsive to CBT are panic disorder, generalized anxiety disorder, social phobia, and bulimia nervosa. Preliminary studies show some promise applying CBT techniques to post-traumatic stress disorder, obsessive compulsive disorder, and dysthymia. There are guidelines for applying CBT techniques to personality disorders, but efficacy has not been established across all diagnostic groups. Such application may require more extensive (longer) treatment, and may explain why some depressed and anxious patients with comorbid personality disorder do not show complete response to a brief trial of CBT. Cluster C personality disorders are likely to be most responsive.

13. Are there patients for whom CBT does not work?

Studies predicting outcome based on patient characteristics are only now being completed. A strong predictor of positive outcome is whether a patient completes **homework assignments** between sessions. Preliminary work suggests that patients who have borderline personality disorder or a great deal of **difficulty forming a work alliance** with the therapist are likely to show a poor response to a brief trial of cognitive therapy. However, these patients also are likely to show poor response to other forms of brief therapy. Historically, patients with bipolar depression or psychotic features have been excluded from research trials and assumed to be less responsive to intervention with CBT alone. CBT recently has had some success in relapse prevention in bipolar patients; it also has decreased the conviction of psychotic beliefs in patients with delusional features.

BIBLIOGRAPHY

1. Beck AT: Depression, Causes and Treatment. Philadelphia, University of Pennsylvania Press, 1967.
2. Beck AT, Emery G: Anxiety Disorders and Phobias: A Cognitive Perspective. New York, Basic Books, 1985.
3. Beck AT, Rush AJ, Shaw BF, Emery G: Cognitive Therapy of Depression. New York, Guilford Press, 1979.
4. Beck JS: Cognitive Therapy: Basics and Beyond. New York, Guilford Press, 1995.

5. Beutler LE, Engle D, Mohr D, et al: Predictors of differential response to cognitive, experiential and self-directed psychotherapeutic procedures. J Consult Clin Psychol 59:333–340, 1991.
6. Dobson K: A meta-analysis of the efficacy of cognitive therapy for depression. J Consult Clin Psychol 57:414–419, 1989.
7. Elkins I, Shea T, Watkins J, et al: National Institute of Mental Health Treatment of Depression Collaborative Research Program. Arch Gen Psychiatry 46:971–982, 1989.
8. Evans M, Hollon SD, DeRubeis RJ, et al: Differential relapse following cognitive therapy and pharmacotherapy for depression. Arch Gen Psychiatry 49:774–781, 1992.
9. Fennell MJ: Depression. In Hawton K, Salkovskis PM, Kirk J, Clark DM (eds): Cognitive Behavior Therapy for Psychiatric Problems. A Practical Guide. New York, Oxford University Press, 1989, pp 169–234.
10. Hollon SD, Beck AT: Cognitive and cognitive-behavioral therapies. In Bergin AE, Garfield SL (eds): Handbook of Psychotherapy and Behavior Change, 4th ed. New York, John Wiley & Sons, 1994, pp 428–466.
11. Hollon SD, DeRubeis RJ, Evans MD, et al: Cognitive therapy and pharmacotherapy for depression: Singly and in combination. Arch Gen Psychiatry 49:774–781, 1992.
12. Hollon SD, Shelton RC, Loosen PT: Cognitive therapy and pharmacotherapy for depression. J Consult Clin Psychol 59:88–99, 1991.
13. Thase ME, Beck AT: Overview of cognitive therapy. In Wright JG, Thase ME, Beck AT, Ludgate JW (eds): Cognitive Therapy with Inpatients. New York, Guilford, 1993, pp 3–34.

42. BEHAVIOR THERAPY

Garry Welch, Ph.D., and Jacqueline A. Samson, Ph.D.

1. What is behavior therapy?

Behavior therapy is a scientifically based approach to the understanding and treatment of human problems. It arose from laboratory experiments of animal behavior conducted in the early 1900s and has developed since from a large body of clinical research and experience. The goals of behavior therapy are:

- Improve daily functioning
- Reduce emotional distress
- Enhance relationships
- Maximize human potential

Behavior therapy first came into common use in the 1960s and is now applied to a wide range of human problems. Originally the emphasis was on overt, **measurable behavior** and the application of classical and operant conditioning principles. However, since the 1980s it has been expanded to include **cognitive aspects** that emphasize the role of inner mental processes and emotional states. In addition, a new consideration of the broader **social context** of behavior has developed. The current focus of behavior therapy is not only what we overtly do, but also what we think and feel; all of these elements are influenced by the fundamental principles of learning.

2. Which patients are most likely to benefit from behavior therapy?

Behavior therapy has been proven effective for the treatment of specific health problems requiring behavior change, such as smoking cessation, weight loss, stress, and pain management. In addition, treatment protocols for anxiety disorders and phobias such as obsessive-compulsive disorder (OCD), agoraphobia, and panic disorder show success equivalent to or exceeding medication alone. Behavior therapy and token economy systems (see Question 15) have been used with good outcome in patients with developmental disabilities and severely disturbed psychotic patients. It is the treatment of choice for severely ill patients who cannot participate in standard insight-oriented or cognitive therapies.

3. How do operant and classical conditioning differ?

Behavior therapy draws heavily on principles derived from classical (or pavlovian) and operant (or instrumental) conditioning. Both forms of conditioning are important influences in daily life because they permit a rapid behavioral response and adaptation to inner changes and external events. Learning may occur through personal experience or the experience of others (i.e., through vicarious learning and modeling). Classically conditioned reflexes generally function to maintain *internal* bodily processes, and the conditioned responses that arise from this conditioning are stereotypic. Operant behaviors, on the other hand, are typically instrumental in managing the *external* environment. They involve skeletal muscles under voluntary control and the ongoing learning of a changing repertoire of new and varied behaviors.

4. Describe classical conditioning.

Classical conditioning involves the acquisition of **new cues** (or triggers) to "wired-in" physiologic reflexes. These reflexes, which function naturally to protect us and to maintain our inner physiologic state, are principally linked to the autonomic nervous system. They are found in many internal bodily systems and are triggered by specific, unconditioned stimuli. For example, a nausea-vomiting reflex typically occurs in response to the eating of overly rich, diseased, or poisonous food. This reflex helps to protect us from sickness.

Classical conditioning occurs when a neutral stimulus that normally does not evoke a given reflex is paired repeatedly with the unconditioned stimulus that naturally provokes the reflex. Under such conditions, the neutral stimulus takes on the ability to evoke the reflex. For example, the nausea reflex in response to eating rich or poisonous food can become linked to the sight or smell of the food (or even just the thought of it). Cancer patients, who experience nausea and sickness as side effects of chemotherapy treatment, may develop anticipatory nausea on entering the hospital for treatment. Both responses to a previously neutral stimuli result from classical conditioning.

5. Give examples of classically conditionable reflexes.

Many potential reflexes in the reproductive, muscular, respiratory, and circulatory systems can be classically conditioned. Note that the emotional components of reflexes (e.g., fear, pleasure, anxiety) can be conditioned as well as the physical components. In daily life, classical conditioning can be **adaptive** (e.g., it helps us learn quickly to avoid danger or unpleasantness) or **maladaptive**. For example, the normal adult response of sexual arousal and pleasant feelings with genital stimulation can become classically conditioned to inappropriate cues such as children (as in pedophilia) or nonanimate objects (as in fetishism).

Examples of Internal Reflexes and Conditioned Stimuli

Digestive system
   Vomiting and nausea in response to food poisoning (e.g., nausea on sight or smell of target food)
Reproductive system
   Sexual arousal and pleasurable feelings in response to genital stimulation (e.g., arousal on viewing erotic books or videos)
Respiratory system
   Asthma attack in response to allergens (e.g., an asthma patient feels the beginning of an attack on seeing an allergy-producing cat enter the room)
Circulatory system
   Pounding heartbeat and anxiety produced by involvement in an auto accident on the freeway (subsequent fear and anxiety when driving in similar circumstances)
Muscular system
   Relaxation response to ingestion of alcohol (relaxation felt on pouring the first drink at home at the end of a tense day)

---

6. Describe important principles of classical conditioning that are used in behavior therapy.

• **Extinguishing** occurs when the conditioned stimulus is not subsequently paired with the original unconditioned stimulus; the classically conditioned response weakens and becomes less frequent.

• **Generalization** occurs when similar stimuli evoke a similar conditioned response. For example, a child frightened by the barking of a large dog may develop an anxious, fearful response to all dogs.

• **Discrimination** occurs when the individual learns to respond differently to two similar or related stimuli. For example, the child frightened of dogs may subsequently learn that large dogs that bark aggressively are more dangerous than small, quiet dogs.

• **Counter-conditioning** occurs when a conditioned stimulus is paired with a new stimulus that produces an incompatible or opposite response. The original, problematic conditioned response is extinguished by this technique, and new, healthy conditioning is introduced simultaneously. For example, a patient with a spider phobia can be taught relaxation techniques and then in therapy be asked to recreate the relaxed feeling during simultaneous exposure to the anxiety-provoking spider stimulus. Under such conditions, the old conditioned anxiety response to spiders weakens.

• **Aversive counter-conditioning** is used to reduce problematic behaviors that are pleasurable. For example, an alcoholic patient may be given disulfiram (Antabuse) so that drinking alcohol becomes associated with nausea and unpleasantness, thereby helping to reduce the frequency of later drinking.

• **Covert conditioning** is classical conditioning that occurs through imagery techniques rather than actual (in vivo) experience.

7. Describe operant conditioning and its important principles.

• **Consequences** shape and modify behavior in operant conditioning (also known as trial-and-error learning). Behavior that produces good effects becomes more frequent (positive reinforcement occurs), whereas behavior that produces bad effects becomes less frequent (negative reinforcement occurs). Learning occurs when the consequences are **contingent** (interpreted to be causally linked) on the operant behavior.

• **Situational, antecedent cues** influence behavior in operant conditioning; any given operant behavior may produce good effects in one situation but bad effects in another. Thus we learn to discriminate between situations in which behavior may be rewarded or punished. For example, stepping on the gas pedal when driving a car produces good effects when traffic lights are green (the driver can proceed quickly with the intended journey) but bad effects when they are red (the driver may receive a speeding ticket or have a serious accident).

• **Shaping** occurs when new, complex behaviors are learned through reinforcement of successive approximations of the desired goal behavior.

• **Discrimination** occurs when an individual learns to respond differently to two similar predictive cues through differential reinforcement (i.e., one predicts reinforcement and the other does not, or one predicts more reinforcement than the other). For example, a shopper may drive to store A rather store B because he or she has learned that store A has better bargains.

• **Generalization** occurs when stimuli that resemble a predictive cue become cues to the operant behavior. For example, a child who learns to bang in a nail with a hammer may then enjoy hammering many objects that look like a nail.

Understanding important situational cues and the negative or positive consequences of behavior are the two keys to understanding how operant behavior arises and is subsequently maintained, shaped, or extinguished.

8. Describe systematic desensitization.

Systematic desensitization, which is used principally in the treatment of phobias and OCD, combines **counter-conditioning** with **extinction**. It can be carried out through patient imagination or (more effectively) in vivo. This approach reduces the conditioned anxiety response by pairing incompatible, positive feelings (e.g., relaxation, calm) with the original anxiety-provoking, conditioned stimulus.

The patient first learns relaxation techniques. Then a hierarchy of anxiety-provoking situations is identified by the therapist and patient to guide treatment planning. The patient is taught to rate the conditioned anxiety he or she feels on a scale from 0 (e.g., no fear or anxiety) to 10 (e.g., extreme fear, panic) to provide immediate feedback during each treatment exercise. Then, in therapy and in homework, the patient is systematically exposed to graded levels of conditioned anxiety through imagination or in vivo. At each anxiety-provoking level, the patient pairs relaxed feelings and thoughts with the conditioned stimulus and endures the conditioned stimulus until the anxiety subsides to a low level.

For example, a patient with a fear of flying may work through a hierarchy of fears by going through airport procedures before a flight, sitting in a plane, taking off, and then finally flying and landing. This process often is preceded by practice sessions in the office in which each phase is imagined along with a paired relaxation exercise. The aim of treatment is for the patient to feel little anxiety in the most difficult flying-related situations.

Research has shown that the relaxation component of systematic desensitization is not always necessary for successful treatment.

9. Describe the use of exposure with response prevention in the treatment of simple phobias.

In this method, the conditioned anxiety reaction is extinguished through enduring exposure to the feared phobic object. This strategy is combined with prevention of usual escape (avoidance) behaviors that provided reinforcement in the past through negative reward (i.e., relief from phobic anxiety). For example, if a patient with a spider phobia is exposed to pictures or thoughts of spiders without escape or avoidance, he or she will experience a gradual reduction of anxiety and fear as the presence of the unconditioned stimulus (the spider) persists. In therapy, patients are taught the rationale behind the treatment, receive specific exposure with response prevention treatments, practice homework assignments at fixed times, discuss homework with the therapist, receive new assignments, and carry out maintenance exercises in follow-ups if needed.

For simple phobias, exposure in vivo is generally preferred to exposure through imagination of the phobic object. Exposure and cognitive restructuring approaches (used to overcome irrational fears and negative thoughts) have become the psychosocial treatments of choice for panic, agoraphobia, and social phobia (see Chapters 14 and 15).

10. Name the essential elements of behavior therapy for obsessive-compulsive disorder.

• Behavioral assessment identifies the nature of obsessional thoughts and compulsive rituals as well as related fear and anxiety responses.

• Gradual exposure in vivo to the problematic conditioned stimuli (e.g., exposure to dirty objects for patients with fears of dirt and contamination) is based on a hierarchy drawn up by the patient and therapist. This exposure allows extinction of the conditioned anxiety response.

• Response prevention is applied to obsessive rituals (e.g., compulsive hand-washing behaviors) used by the patient to alleviate anxiety after exposure to the feared situation.

• Faulty patient cognitions (self-talk) are identified.

• Ongoing structured homework includes further exposure and response prevention assignments and correction of maladaptive self-talk.

11. Describe flooding.

In flooding, patients are exposed in vivo or through imagination to their conditioned object of fear at the most anxiety-provoking level possible until the fear and anxiety responses have been extinguished. Flooding differs from systematic desensitization, in which graded levels of exposure are introduced. Furthermore, in flooding the therapist controls the exposure, whereas in systematic desensitization the patient determines progression through the hierarchy of conditioned fears. Flooding may be poorly tolerated by some patients because of the high level of unpleasant feelings. In vivo flooding generally is considered more effective than flooding through imagination.

12. What is the Premack principle?

If, as a precondition made in therapy, the patient must complete desired low-frequency behavior before high-frequency behavior can be carried out, the desired behavior will increase in frequency. For example, if an obese patient in behavior therapy for weight control contracts to complete a 20-minute walk each evening before sitting down to watch a favorite television show (something the patient does often), regular walking will increase in frequency and weight loss and health gains will be more likely to occur. The high-frequency behavior typically is pleasurable and provides positive reinforcement for the low-frequency behaviors. This principle is applied in many forms of behavior therapy.

13. What is the role of cognitive factors in behavior therapy?

An understanding of the role of cognitive factors in the development and maintenance of problem behaviors enables the therapist to identify cognitive distortions (negative self-talk and beliefs) arising from false assumptions or interpretations of life experiences and fear-inducing self-instructions. Cognitive interventions aim to teach the patient to recognize distortions of thinking and to replace them with more realistic, positive thoughts. They are particularly helpful in the treatment of anticipatory anxiety, demoralization, avoidance behaviors, and low self-esteem (see Chapter 41).

14. What is assertiveness training?

Assertiveness training uses principles of operant reinforcement to improve social skills through **shaping, modeling** of appropriate social behaviors by the therapist, **role rehearsal** of new skills in therapy sessions, and patient homework assignments. Typical problems include poor refusal skills; difficulties with self-disclosure, expression of negative emotions, and giving or receiving criticism; and opening, maintaining, and closing conversations. Such deficits can be incorporated into a broader treatment plan for the presenting clinical problem.

Treatment begins with a careful recording of the problematic social situations and the circumstances under which problem behaviors and thoughts arise. Patients are taught new social responses for each specific problematic social situation. Problem solving is used in reviews of patient homework exercises, and new goals are set as the patient progresses to more challenging social situations based on a previously agreed hierarchy of social difficulty. Mastery of problem situations may combine with newfound enjoyment of social activities to reinforce new behaviors through positive reward.

15. Describe token economies and their use.

Token economies are based on the operant conditioning principle that positive reward of a desired behavior increases its frequency. They often involve the use of behavior shaping (i.e., the selective reinforcement of successive approximations to the target behavior). All token economies have in common a clear definition of the appropriate behavior that the therapist wishes to promote and a contract with the patient that details the explicit rewards for carrying out desirable behaviors. Target behaviors may range from simple tasks related to feeding, personal hygiene, or politeness to complex social interaction behaviors that are the end result of a systematic behavior-shaping schedule.

Token economies may be based on the use of **primary reinforcers** (e.g., food, drink) or **secondary (acquired) reinforcers** (e.g., tokens, points, praise, smiles). Tokens or points are accumulated by the patient and exchanged for tangibles such as television time, toys, or privileges. Points or tokens also may be taken away for inappropriate behavior (negative punishment). Note that some primary reinforcers, such as food (e.g., candy), may be problematic as they can reach levels of satiation, whereas secondary rewards (e.g., tokens) cannot.

Token economies have been used to promote adaptive, normal, or healthy behaviors in classrooms, adult day hospitals, sheltered workshops, and patient psychiatric settings; to help family functioning; and to promote individual self-development.

16. What is stimulus control?

Large numbers of stimuli from the environment and from within our bodies influence behavioral responses in any given situation at a given point in time. Depending on past learning, significant stimuli may be (1) unconditioned or conditioned stimuli that produce classical responses, (2) discriminant stimuli that predict operant responses, or (3) stimuli that operate in both capacities. Treatment approaches based on stimulus control involve the identification of this array of antecedent stimuli through a careful behavioral assessment and implementation of strategies to limit their influence. Stimulus control approaches have been used notably in the management of obesity and smoking cessation.

For example, obese patients are taught to recognize conditioned stimuli (from previous classical learning) and predictive stimuli (from previous operant learning) that may promote eating when the patient is not hungry. A patient who eats when depressed, bored, or angry is taught to recognize these cues and is instructed to carry out healthier, incompatible behavior instead (e.g., go for a walk, phone a friend). Food can be hidden from view outside of mealtimes, and eating can be restricted to the dining table only (instead of while watching television or reading). The patient may be given specific exercises to slow down the rate of eating and to increase awareness of consumption. A slower eating speed with improved awareness of the pleasurable, hedonic value of food may reduce overall calorie intake. In addition, slower eating is thought to give the brain sufficient time to respond appropriately to rising blood glucose levels that provide feedback signals of satiety.

17. How does biofeedback work?

Biofeedback involves the use of specific machines that provide information (feedback) about variations in one or more of the patient's physiologic processes that are not ordinarily perceived (i.e., brain wave activity, muscle tension, blood pressure). Feedback over a period of time may help the patient to learn to control certain target physiologic processes (i.e., anxiety, muscle tension responses) through operant conditioning. For example, awareness of alpha wave patterns through a graphic representation of wave activity on a biofeedback monitor may help the patient to elicit a relaxation response (see Chapter 46).

18. How is behavior therapy structured?

The foundation of behavior therapy is the **initial behavior analysis**, a process of careful documentation and recording of the specific conditions under which presenting problem behaviors arose and are maintained. Based on the behavioral analysis, a specific series of **treatment tasks** devised by the therapist and patient are implemented in therapy sessions and in regular patient homework. Because behavior therapy is highly goal-oriented, **treatment goals** are clearly spelled out for the patient, progress is assessed and discussed, and new goals are set for the next stage of treatment. Treatment gains are maintained with follow-up sessions and ongoing homework assignments. Through this process, behavior therapy reshapes the problem behavior in a more desirable direction.

The treatment plan may include a microanalysis that focuses on the conditions surrounding the presenting clinical problem and a macroanalysis that relates the presenting problem to other broader problem areas (e.g., social skill deficits, marital problems).

19. What differentiates behavior therapy from psychodynamic therapy?

	Behavior Therapy	*Psychodynamic Therapy*
FOCUS	Conditions surrounding current problematic behavior and past circumstances that may highlight maladaptive learning relevant to the current problems	Historical and early life experiences, parenting dynamics, enduring personality traits; links between these and current life experiences and problematic emotions and behaviors
GOAL	Improve problematic behaviors, cognitions, and emotions directly, through application of principles of classical and operant learning theory and cognitive therapy	Reshape the intrapsychic structure of the patient to produce favorable symptom change based on specific theories about the nature of early childhood nurturance experiences and parenting dynamics
STRUCTURE	Highly structured and goal- and outcome-oriented	Unstructured approach facilitates unexpected associations and derives new information and insights into the causes of current problems

Although behavioral and psychodynamic therapies differ markedly in theoretical basis and treatment approach, elements of each may be found in the other. Information gathering is important in both, as part of the continual exploration for new ideas and connections. Repeated discussion of anxiety-producing concerns in the comfortable environment of psychodynamic therapy sessions may lead to extinction of a conditioned anxiety response (as in systematic desensitization). In behavior therapy, open-minded questions and chance discussions in unstructured parts of a treatment session may lead to important insights into the broader psychosocial context of specific problematic behaviors (e.g., the presence of marital or work difficulties that exacerbate problem behaviors).

BIBLIOGRAPHY

1. Baldwin JD, Baldwin J: Behavior Principles in Everyday Life. Englewood Cliffs, NJ, Prentice-Hall, 1981.
2. Emmelkamp PMG: Behavior therapy with adults. In Bergin AE, Garfield SL (eds): Handbook of Psychotherapy and Behavior Change, 4th ed. New York, John Wiley and Sons, 1994, pp 377–427.
3. Emmelkamp PMG, Bourman TK, Scholing A: Anxiety Disorders. A Practitioner's Guide. Chichester, John Wiley & Sons, 1992.
4. Griest JH: Behavior therapy for obsessive compulsive disorders. J Clin Psychol 55:60–68, 1994.
5. Noyes R: Treatments of choice for anxiety disorders. In Coryell W, Winokur G (eds): The Clinical Management of Anxiety Disorders. New York, Oxford University Press, 1991.
6. Sloane R, Staples F, Cristol A, et al: Psychotherapy Versus Behavior Therapy. Cambridge, MA, Harvard University Press, 1975.
7. Wachtel P: Psychoanalysis and Behavior Therapy. New York, Basic Books, 1977.

43. PLANNED BRIEF PSYCHOTHERAPY

Mark A. Blais, Psy.D.

1. What is the "natural" course of psychotherapy?

Despite the common perception that psychotherapy is a long-term, even timeless, enterprise, most of the existing data indicate that psychotherapy as it is practiced in the real world is a time-limited process. National outpatient psychotherapy utilization data from 1987 (obtained before the nationwide impact of managed care) reveals that 70% of psychotherapy users received 10 or fewer sessions, and only 15% received 21 or more sessions.[18] These data are highly consistent with findings from other utilizations studies. Clearly, most patients have a time-limited or brief psychotherapy experience.

This chapter will help you deliver psychotherapy in an organized, planned, and thoughtful manner that more closely matches the "natural" course of psychotherapy.

2. How did brief psychotherapy develop?

Freud was one of the first practitioners of brief psychotherapy. A review of his early cases reveals that he treated many patients in a span of weeks to months rather than years. Over time, as psychoanalytic theory became more complex, the goals of psychoanalysis became more ambitious, and the length of treatment increased greatly. As early as 1925 this trend had become a concern to some.

Alexander and French can be considered the true fathers of brief psychotherapy. Their book *Psychoanalytic Psychotherapy* outlined the first systematic attempt to develop a shorter and more efficient form of psychotherapy. Although not generally accepted in its time, this work laid the foundation for both psychoanalytic psychotherapy and modern brief psychotherapy.

The modern era of brief treatment began with the work of Malan and of Sifneos. At present, brief psychoanalytic psychotherapies are supplemented by several other time-limited treatments, such as Beck's cognitive therapy, Mann's "existential" psychotherapy, and Klerman's interpersonal treatment of depression.

3. How does brief psychotherapy differ from long-term psychotherapy?

Four dimensions, considered common to all brief therapies, differentiate short-term from the more traditional long-term therapies: (1) the setting of a fixed time limit for the treatment, (2) holding to specific patient selection criteria, (3) using a treatment focus to limit the scope of the therapy, and (4) requiring increased activity by the therapist.

Summary of Selected Planned Brief Psychotherapies

THERAPY SCHOOL	NUMBER OF SESSIONS	TYPE OF FOCUS	PATIENT SELECTION
Analytic			
Sifneos			
Anxiety suppressing	4–10	Crisis and coping	Fairly open, less healthy
Anxiety provoking	12–20	Very narrow, Oedipal conflict and grief	Very selective, top 2–10% outpatients
Malan	20–30	Very narrow, similar to Sifneos	Responds to trial interpretation
Davanloo	1–40	Resistance and suppressed anger	Less healthy, top 30% outpatients
Existential			
Mann	12 exactly	Central issue and termination	Broad patient selection (passive-dependent)
Cognitive			
Beck	1–14	Automatic thoughts	Very broad, not psychotic
Interpersonal			
Klerman	12–16	Patient's interpersonal experience	Depressed patient, any level of health
Eclectic			
Budman	20–40	Interpersonal, developmental, and existential	Broad range
Leibovich	36–52	One borderline trait	Borderline outpatients

Adapted from Groves J: The short-term dynamic psychotherapies: An overview. In Ritan S (ed): Psychotherapy for the 90s. New York, Guilford Press, 1992.

Comparison of Brief and Long-Term Therapy

BRIEF	LONG-TERM
Specific focused goals	Broad goals: "insight and character change"
Specific time frame	Time unlimited
Emphasizes patient selection	Down-plays patient selection
Here and now focus	Inner life, historical focus
Attempts to restore psychologic functioning quickly	Techniques can cause increased psychological distress and temporary dysfunction
The therapist is active and directive	Therapist is nondirective; therapy unfolds
Uses between-session homework	Is mostly limited to treatment hour

4. What is the best attitude for learning brief therapy?

There must be a willing suspension of disbelief and cynicism about brief treatment. Trainees are frequently taught that quick improvement is suspect and likely represents a transient "flight into health." This can be a hard lesson to unlearn. Remember, brief therapy is not a fad, but rather a form of treatment developed and refined over many years, based upon clinical experience and treatment outcome studies.

• It must be recognized from the outset that therapy will end after a set number of sessions (or in some cases on a planned date). This can be difficult, particularly for therapists trained in long-term therapy, because this mindset has ramifications for all treatment decisions and requires a clinician to reconsider every intervention during the treatment.

• The brief therapist should accept (and expect) that patients will return to therapy periodically across their life span. This perspective allows a brief therapist to focus on the patient's current difficulties rather than attempting a "total" lifelong cure.

5. For which patients is brief therapy appropriate?

Patient selection is an important (and distinguishing) part of brief therapy. Basically, patient selection is the art of finding the right patient with the right problem for brief psychotherapy. A two-session format is recommended to alleviate time pressure and allow the clinician to conduct a complete psychiatric evaluation while also assessing the appropriateness of the patient for brief psychotherapy.

6. Name some useful criteria for excluding or including a patient for brief psychotherapy.

Exclusion criteria are best seen as *categories* (either the condition is present or absent); if any is present, the patient should be considered a poor candidate for brief treatment. Inclusion criteria are best viewed as *dimensions*, and as such they are likely present to a varying degree in every patient. The more of these qualities a patient has, the better the candidate for brief psychotherapy.

Patient Selection Criteria for Brief Therapy

Exclusion Criteria	**Inclusion Criteria**
Actively psychotic	Moderate emotional distress
Abusing substances	Seeking relief from pain
At significant risk for self harm	Able to articulate or accept specific cause or circumscribed problem as focus of treatment
	History of at least one positive mutual interpersonal relationship
	Functioning in at least one area of life
	Ability to commit to treatment contract

7. How does the brief therapist focus the treatment?

Developing a treatment focus is probably the most misunderstood aspect of brief therapy. Many clinicians write about "the focus" in a mysterious and circular manner. It often appears as if the whole success of the treatment rests on finding the *one* correct focus. Rather, what is needed for a successful brief treatment is the establishment of a **functional focus**; that is, a focus on which both the therapist and patient can agree to work.

8. How is a functional focus established?

One powerful, straightforward technique is the "Why now?" question used by Budman and Gurman. It is applied by repeatedly asking the patient: "Why did you come for treatment now?" "Why are you here now?" Attention is directed to the current problem, rather than last week's or tomorrow's. (Try this simple technique a few times to see how effective it can be.)

For example, a male patient (Pt) presents with significant depressive symptoms to a therapist (Th) at a walk-in clinic.

Th: "I hear from what you say that you are depressed and are feeling terrible, but I wonder what made you come in today?"

Pt: "I can't take it any more. I know I need help."

Th: "You can't take it. What makes it impossible to take it now?"

Pt: "It's getting too bad. I just can't take it any more."

Th: "It sounds like something happened recently that made you realize how bad things were. What made you realize that you had to get help now?"

Pt: "I just felt so bad I couldn't go to work yesterday. I stayed home in bed all day. I never miss work. I must be falling apart."

This line of questioning led to establishing the patient's physical inactivity as a functional focus for treatment. As a result, his depression was successfully treated by increasing his physical activity.

9. Describe some typical functional foci.

Budman and Gurman describe five common treatment foci:

• Losses past, present, or pending

• Development dyssynchronies; being out of step with expected developmental stages (Therapists should be able to identify with this because years of extended schooling and training usually keep life events such as marriage and children on hold.)

• Interpersonal conflicts (usually repeated disappointments in important relationships)
• Symptomatic presentations and desire for symptom reduction
• Severe personality impairment (In brief therapy, one aspect of personality impairment can be selected as the focus of therapy.)

Beginning brief therapists should use these five common foci to help organize their patient's complaints and problems. The most important thing to remember is that you are not finding *the* focus, only *a* focus for the therapy.

10. How does the therapist complete the evaluation?

Brief therapy is demanding for the therapist and patient. In addition to doing a full psychiatric interview, by the completion of the second evaluation session you need to have (1) determined whether the patient is suitable for brief treatment; (2) developed a functional focus; and (3) articulated a clear treatment contract.

The patient and therapist must agree on a **treatment contract**. The contract identifies the treatment focus and spells out details, such as the number of sessions, procedure for missed appointments, and guidelines for post-termination contact. Brief therapy typically lasts 10–24 sessions, but may include as many as 50 sessions. (A 15-session treatment, not including the evaluation sessions, is a good length for a beginning brief therapist to start with). A flexible approach to missed appointments is recommended, and if the patient has a valid reason, the therapist should try to reschedule. if a session is missed without a valid reason, the missed session should be counted and the patient's motivation should be explored, because this is resistance to treatment.

11. What is another advantage (besides the extra time) of a two-session evaluation?

It allows an assessment of how the patient responds to the therapy (and therapist), providing important additional information about the appropriateness of brief treatment. Some form of **intervention** at the end of the first evaluation session is helpful in this regard. This initial intervention can be as simple as summarizing the patient's problem and offering a tentative treatment focus or as complex as requiring the patient to fill out a psychological questionnaire. At the start of the second session, inquire about the intervention. If the patient responds positively (e.g., found it helpful to think of the problem in this new light; is interested in the psychological test results) and/or is feeling better, it is a sign that brief therapy may work. If the patient has not followed up on the intervention (e.g., did not think about the potential focus) or reacted angrily to it, it is a negative sign.

12. Can the functional focus change?

No. Once a functional focus has been established, the therapist must maintain it. One way is by working consistently from within one style or orientation, of which there are basically three: (1) psychodynamic, (2) interpersonal, or (3) cognitive-behavioral. The one you use depends on your preference and, to some extent, your patient's problem.

13. Describe the three approaches used in brief therapy.

Most **psychodynamic** treatments are limited in their range of application and are appropriate for only a small percentage of clinic patients, typically those suffering from reactive or neurotic forms of depression (such as failure to grieve, fear of success and competition, and triangular, conflicted love relationships). These are demanding treatments for the therapist to undertake and require that the patient be able to tolerate considerable affective arousal.

Brief **interpersonal** psychotherapy (IPT) was developed by Klerman and colleagues specifically to treat depression. It is a highly formalized (manualized) treatment often used in research studies. It can be considered a mix of psychoeducation and supportive therapy. In IPT, the patient's symptoms are explained (psychoeducation) and interpersonal interactions, expectations, and experiences are explored. IPT seeks to clarify what the patient wants to receive from relationships and helps patients develop necessary social-interpersonal skills. No effort is made to understand the deeper unconscious meaning of the patients' social interactions or desires.

The **cognitive-behavioral** therapies, like Beck's, are more broadly applicable, both in the percentage of patients who can benefit and the range of problems that can be treated. These therapies aim at bringing the patient's "autonomic" (pre-conscious) thoughts into awareness and demonstrating how these thoughts maintain negative behaviors and feelings.

14. Are all three approaches employed simultaneously?

No. A minimal, thoughtful amount of mixing of techniques from different therapy styles is acceptable. Therapeutic flexibility is necessary in brief treatment. It is important, however, to conceptualize and work predominantly from within one orientation to keep treatment focused and clear. Especially avoid uncritical wholesale mixing of styles and orientations, because such "wild" treatment confuses and disappoints both the therapist and patient.

15. What does it mean to be an active therapist?

Completing a psychotherapy in 12–15 sessions requires sustained activity on the part of the therapist to maintain treatment focus and move the therapy process forward. The brief therapist works to structure every session, thereby increasing productivity.

The Active Therapist

Structure each session	Use confrontation and clarification
Give homework assignments	Quickly address negative and overly positive transference
Develop and use the working alliance	Limit regression
Limit silences and vagueness	Use supervision

16. Discuss important factors for the active therapist in structuring sessions.

Starting each session with a **summary** of important material from the last session and restating the treatment focus organizes therapy and keeps the treatment on track. Giving homework to the patient to be completed between sessions helps increase the impact of therapy on the patient's current life and situation and monitor the patient's motivation for change. If the patient does not complete the homework, the motivation for change must be explored.

The **working alliance** between therapist and patient must be developed quickly. It is frequently invoked to return the patient to the treatment focus. Patients may attempt to escape the anxiety inherent in brief therapy by bringing up interesting but diverting material. The therapist should meet such tactics with reminders of the agreed-upon focus (thus invoking the working alliance) and queries about how the new material relates to it. Prolonged silences (by either the therapist or patient) are considered unproductive in brief therapy and also are quickly confronted as resistance.

The brief therapist must know how to **limit regression**. Two useful techniques are (1) organizing interpretations about events in the "here and now," using either the therapy relationship or the patient's current life situation, rather than around early developmental traumas; and (2) moving the patient away from feelings and into thoughts—"What are you thinking" rather than "What are you feeling?" Regressions within sessions are permitted and even encouraged in some short-term work. For example, it is quite common, when employing a treatment modeled after that of Sifneos, to keep a patient focused on an anxiety-provoking conflict despite mild confusion or panic.

17. What are two valuable tools in brief therapy?

The brief therapist makes heavy use of **confrontation** and **clarification**. Confrontation helps the patient recognize when he or she is avoiding or resisting the treatment focus, usually as a result of anxiety. Clarification techniques are used whenever the patient is communicating in a vague or incomplete manner. Usually the therapist asks for specific examples of unclear situations or feelings.

18. How does transference manifest in brief therapy?

Regardless of the style of therapy you employ (psychodynamic, cognitive, or interpersonal) patients inevitably react to some of your interventions based on their past experiences. When such reactions are negative ("You always criticize me") or excessively positive ("You know me better than anyone on earth"), they must be explored and interpreted quickly. Rapid attention can help keep the patient's transference under control and reduce the likelihood of it becoming a major resistance to treatment.

19. Is supervision unnecessary due to the short-term nature of this type of treatment?

As in all psychotherapy, supervision is important in both learning and practicing brief psychotherapy. Supervision by an experienced colleague provides an excellent vehicle for beginning therapists. More advanced practitioners find that some form of ongoing supervision, either formal or informal, helps maintain the treatment focus and aids in identifying subtle, but often important, changes in the patient's manner. Such subtle changes can represent the first signs of transference.

20. What are the phases of brief therapy?

The **initial phase** includes evaluating and assessing patient appropriateness for brief therapy, selecting a treatment focus, and establishing the main treatment orientation. For the patient this phase is usually accompanied by slight symptom reduction and mildly positive transference. Both of these factors help with the quick development of a working alliance.

In the **middle phase**, the work gets more difficult. Typically the patient becomes concerned about the time limit and, in addition to the treatment focus, issues of dependency become important. The patient often feels worse, and the therapist's faith in the treatment process is tested. The early middle phase of brief therapy can be particularly hard for the therapist, who must be active in sustaining treatment focus, keeping the patient working, and countering patient skepticism while projecting optimism. Good supervision is invaluable during this phase for the beginning brief therapist.

In the **termination** phase, therapy tends to settle down. The patient accepts that treatment will end as planned and that symptoms will decrease. Now, in addition to the treatment focus, post-therapy plans and the patient's feelings about termination are explored. Among the most common termination problems is the introduction of new material by the patient. The therapist may be tempted to explore the new information and extend the therapy. This is usually a mistake, because the patient likely is attempting to avoid the treatment focus, and in most cases the treatment should end as planned.

21. How do I handle post-treatment contact with the patient?

This difficult question must be answered individually by each therapist. During training, the beginning therapist should have the experience of handling the intense feelings (both his or her own *and* the the patient's) that accompany the termination of a treatment in which there will be no post-therapy contact. This teaches the therapist how to deal openly with these powerful and important feelings. In ongoing practice, however, it is important to encourage patients to return for treatment when new difficulties develop, and to foster the understanding that help is available if needed. Patient care should be guided by the understanding that "Therapy is for living and not vice versa." The brief psychotherapist practices as a primary care physician, available to help patients with (psychological) troubles or crises that develop.

22. How does brief psychotherapy relate to managed care?

In a managed care environment, payors are encouraging the use of shorter treatments such as planned brief psychotherapy. However, managed mental health care and brief psychotherapy are not identical. Managed health care is primarily concerned with controlling cost. Planned brief psychotherapy represents a clinically proven procedure for helping some patients in need of psychiatric services. To be administered properly, brief psychotherapy must be based on clinical, not financial, considerations. Although many patients covered by managed care contracts benefit from brief psychotherapy, not all patients are appropriate. Many variables are involved in selecting patients for brief psychotherapy—but mental health insurance coverage is not one of them. Finally, therapy that is considered brief for clinical work (i.e., 15–20 sessions) may be considered too long by managed care companies, who often suggest 6–8 sessions.

BIBLIOGRAPHY

1. Alexander F, French T: Psychoanalytic Psychotherapy. New York, The Ronald Press, 1946.
1a. Beck AT: Cognitive therapy for depression and panic disorder. Western J Med 151:9–89, 1989.
2. Beck S, Greenberg R: Brief cognitive therapies. Psychiatr Clin North Am 2:11–22, 1979.
2a. Book HE: How to Practice Brief Psychodynamic Psychotherapy: The Core Conflictual Relationship Theme Method. Washington, DC, American Psychological Association Press, 1998.
3. Budman S, Gurman A: Theory and Practice of Brief Therapy. New York, The Guilford Press, 1988.
4. Burk J, White H, Havens L: Which short-term therapy? Arch Gen Psychiatry 36:177–186, 1989.
5. Davanloo H: Short-Term Dynamic Psychotherapy. New York, Jason Aronson, 1980.
6. Ferenczi S, Rank O: The Development of Psychoanalysis. New York, Nervous and Mental Disease Publishing Company, 1925.
7. Flegenheimer W: History of brief psychotherapy. In Horner A (ed): Treating the Neurotic Patient in Brief Psychotherapy. New Jersey, Jason Aronson, 1985, pp 7–24.
8. Goldin V: Problems of technique: In Horner A (ed): Treating the Neurotic Patient in Brief Psychotherapy. New Jersey, Jason Aronson, 1985, pp 56–74.
9. Groves J: Essential Papers on Short-Term Dynamic Therapy. New York, New York University Press, 1996.
10. Groves J: The short-term dynamic psychotherapies: An overview. In Rutan S (ed): Psychotherapy for the 90's. New York, Guilford Press, 1992.
11. Hall M, Arnold W, Crosby R: Back to basics: The importance of focus selection. Psychotherapy 4:578–584, 1990.
12. Horner A: Principles for the therapist. In Horner A (ed): Treating the Neurotic Patient in Brief Psychotherapy. New Jersey, Jason Aronson, 1985, pp 76–85.
13. Horath A, Luborsky L: The role of the therapeutic alliance in psychotherapy. J Consult Clin Psychol 61:561–573, 1993.
14. Klerman G, Weissman M, Rounsaville B, Chevron E: Interpersonal Psychotherapy of Depression. New York, Basic Books, 1984.
15. Leibovich M: Short-term psychotherapy for the borderline personality disorder. Psychother Psychosom 35:257–264, 1981.
16. Malan D: The Frontier of Brief Psychotherapy. New York, Plenum Medical Book Company, 1976.
17. Mann J: Time-Limited Psychotherapy. Cambridge, Harvard University Press, 1973.
18. Olfson M, Pincus HA: Outpatient psychotherapy in the United States. II: Patterns of utilization. Am J Psychiatry 151:1289–1294, 1994.
19. Sifneos P: Short-Term Anxiety Provoking Psychotherapy: A Treatment Manual. New York, Basic Books, 1992.

44. MARITAL AND FAMILY THERAPIES

Margaret Roath, M.S.W., LCSW

1. What are marital and family therapies?

Marital and family therapies are therapeutic modalities whose focus of assessment and treatment is on the relationship, not on the individual. Assessment includes gathering data related to the following areas:

- History of the relationship
- Goals of the individuals in the relationship
- Coping mechanisms which have been unsuccessful
- Precipitant for seeking therapy—"why now?" or "what changed?"
- Communication patterns, both constructive and destructive
- Description of the strengths of the relationship
- Unmet needs of the individuals in the relationship

Assessment of the precipitant for seeking marital or family therapy is especially important in determining the **relationship equilibrium**—which may have worked previously for all members of the relationship, but is now out of balance. The precipitant might be a change in external circumstances or a change within an individual that is affecting the relationship.

Marital and family therapies identify these changes and then examine patterns of communication, behavior, and coping mechanisms which may have been destructive, not constructive, in responding to the identified changes. The goal of therapy is to provide the marriage and the family with new ways of responding that are helpful and constructive to the relationships. Sometimes, there is no acute precipitant to the request for marital or family therapy, but instead there are long-standing destructive patterns of communication that have been identified, and the married couple or the family are interested in changing those patterns.

2. What are the indicators for marital and family therapies?

Statements or complaints expressed by individuals that reflect concerns about the relationship and also show the inability to resolve those concerns. Indications might include internal and external changes within individuals in the relationship or changes within the relationship itself.

Internal and External Indicators for Marital and Family Therapy

INTERNAL CHANGES	EXTERNAL CHANGES
A person, through individual therapy or through life experience, is making a decision about whether to remain in the relationship	Recently diagnosed illness of one of the marital or family members—the illness may mean death or adjustment to changing abilities
A person, through experience or therapy, realizes that he or she is of a different sexual orientation than originally believed	Change in financial status through loss of a job or a decrease in pay
A person may be experiencing an internal crisis, such as a mid-life crisis, and desires to change or maybe end the relationship	Addition of members to the marriage or family: the birth of a child, an in-law or children of a previous marriage joining the family
Normal developmental changes of children, such as adolescence	Children leaving home, which may exacerbate unresolved relationship issues for the marriage
Developmental changes of adults, such as the wife desiring to return to a career after being a homemaker	A decision to divorce which causes all relationships to be renegotiated

3. What treatment models are used for marital and family therapies?

In the *most common model for marital therapy*, both partners of the marriage are seen together by one therapist. Sometimes one or both partners will also be in individual therapy. In preparation for the marital sessions, the individuals may be working on issues pertinent only to themselves or developing a better understanding of their needs as partners in a marriage. It is usually optimal for the individual's therapist not to be the couple's therapist because the therapist may learn secrets which would compromise the marital therapy. However, when it is not possible or deemed optimal for separate therapists for each treatment modality (e.g., in rural areas), the therapist and the patients must establish clear boundaries regarding the content discussed in each treatment modality. When several therapists are involved, communication among them can be helpful to clarify that they are working together and not at cross-purposes. Confidentiality needs to be addressed by each therapist with their respective patient or patients.

In the *most common model for family therapy*, all members of the immediate family are seen together. Concurrent individual therapy should be handled as noted above for marital therapy.

Group therapy is another possible modality for both marital and family therapy. It affords the possibility of learning from others in similar situations and also the benefit of feeling less alone with the issues being addressed. Couples and families often can listen and integrate advice from others in similar situations better than they can integrate advice from therapists. A disadvantage is that each couple's or family's specific issues may take longer to address because time is spent on developing relationships among couples or families. The therapist's role is to facilitate interaction among participants.

4. What is the role of the therapist in marital and family therapies?

Typically quite active. The therapist assists marriage and family members in **defining the problem** and **determining goals to address it**. The therapist may need to stop certain behaviors and encourage others within therapy—for example, stopping one person from doing all of the talking and encouraging another to talk more. He or she also may have to direct marriage and family members to stop certain behaviors outside of the treatment session, such as marathon discussions which might escalate into arguments or physical actions. The therapist might suggest a time limit for all discussions which have not resolved an issue, and also set very specific rules prohibiting physical violence, both in and out of therapy. When individuals in a marriage or family cannot stop physical violence, a separation with strict guidelines for being together may be suggested.

The therapist also **reframes problems** or feelings among marriage and family members by removing labels of good and bad and making statements about differences among the members. He or she may suggest problem-solving with the directive that if the solution is not effective, it only means that the participants, including the therapist, did not have all of the information necessary to develop a better solution. The therapist may give homework to the marriage and family members so that the therapy does not just take place in the office, but also becomes a part of daily home life. The therapist may serve as **coach**, **educator**, or **mentor** to the marriage and the family when destructive communication is observed, by giving specific examples of what to say or by participating in role-playing. The therapist joins with the marriage partners and the family to develop new coping mechanisms, communication skills, and negotiation skills to address the identified problems.

5. What assessment and treatment techniques are used by the therapist?

The techniques of marital and family therapy focus on the relationships and relationship issues.

Assessment Techniques

- Ask each individual to describe their sense of the problem and its history
- Ask each individual the same question that has been asked of another
- Identify nonverbal communication
- Ask each individual's reaction to what another has said
- Identify themes common to the relationship and individuals within that relationship

Treatment Techniques

- Ask individuals to speak with "I" phrases, not "you" phrases, which sound accusatory
- Ask that each expressed need be accompanied by a proposed solution
- Assign homework or tasks that respond to the assessed problem
- Clarify—repeat what the other said and ask if the repeated statement was heard as intended

Many other techniques exist. Their common goal is strengthening the marriage or the family's bond even when the individuals feel polarized, disappointed, and angered at the time of therapy.

6. How long does marital or family therapy take?

It is not possible to say specifically. However, it is possible to establish specific goals and assess at the end of each session or after an agreed-upon number of sessions whether the goals have been met and what will need to happen for any remaining goals to be met. The length of time needed depends on how much blame is present, how much desire or ability there is for the participants to move from blame to identification and problem solving, and how much empathy all members have for other marriage and family members. The more blaming, the less problem-solving behavior, and the less empathy, the longer the therapy will take. The more willing each individual is to examine his or her behavior and develop solutions for changing it, the less time therapy is likely to take.

7. Are there any patients with specific psychiatric diagnoses who should not be referred to marital or family therapy?

Yes. If one member of a marriage or family is psychotic or so severely depressed that he or she is unable to focus cognitively on marriage and family issues, then such therapy is not recommended.

Once treatment for psychosis or depression has occurred, however, there can be a referral for marriage or family therapy if the issues identified indicate the need for it. Otherwise, because marriage and family therapies focus on changes in behavior, coping mechanisms, and problem-solving, they have the potential to be successful if the members are motivated to pursue those changes, irrespective of the members' DSM-IV diagnoses. Some research shows that marital and family problems may increase vulnerability to mood disorders, and those same problems may slow recovery or cause exacerbations of additional episodes of severe illness. Treatment to promote marital and family harmony may prevent recurrences of the illness.

Family therapy may be very helpful in reducing severity or relapses for persons with schizophrenia. Family members often respond positively to information about mental illness and coping strategies and feel less alone when professionals are interested in working with them in management and caretaking. Partners and families of schizophrenics usually identify relapses earlier than the patient does; if they are working collaboratively with professionals, they can provide data that increase services being provided. Also, partners and families who have a positive relationship with professionals and are able to express their feelings and worries in marital and family therapy sessions are less likely to be intrusive or hovering, possibly causing the patient to express hostility and anger, which could precipitate a relapse. The intrusive or hovering behavior is referred to as **expressed-emotion behavior**. The greater the level of this behavior, the more likely a relapse by the patient; the lower the level, the less likely.

8. Can marital and family therapies be effective if one of the members is resistant?

If one of the members displays resistance by not attending meetings, the issues in the marriage and the family may still be addressable, but with the understanding that the only ones who can change behavior are those willing to attend meetings. *The focus cannot be on the person not present.* If the resistant person attends the meetings, it may be possible to lessen the resistance by having everyone listen to and understand the reasons for the resistance. If an individual maintains resistance, a decision can be made for that person not to attend, and therapy can proceed for those members who are motivated.

9. Are marital and family therapies different for different cultures, races, ages, and sexual orientations?

No. The assessment process remains the same, as does the treatment process. In other words, assessment and treatment always focuses on needs, expectations, complementarity of roles, communication, and behavior patterns. However, cultural differences between individuals in a marriage or a family may lead to different goals or expectations, and those differences need to be elucidated and clarified by the therapist.

10. Does there have to be a match with the therapist in the areas of culture, race, age, and sexual orientation?

No, although couples and families do request it. Accommodating that request may facilitate the beginning process of therapy. However, it is not necessary because a competent therapist addresses the lack of complementarity in the beginning, which creates **alliance-building**. The alliance encourages the members of a marriage or family to express feelings, either negative or positive, about the lack of complementarity and allows the therapist to empathize with those feelings. The therapist also may encourage the couple or family to share information about culture, history, traditions, or lifestyle as a way to bridge the gap between those differences.

11. Are marriage and family therapies always successful in keeping marriage and family together and improving the relationships?

No. Approximately 50% of the marriages that enter marital therapy end in separation or divorce. Some couples come to marital therapy when anger has created too great a distance and one, if not both, partners have already decided on separation or divorce. The therapy can be a forum through which to accomplish this goal. Sometimes one partner is hoping the other will connect with the **therapist as a source of support** in order to feel less guilty or fearful about abandoning the partner.

Marital and family therapies are sometimes unable to promote change because the desire to change and enter into the unknown is weaker than the comfort of the known. The therapist shares that observation with a marriage and family in a nonjudgmental way, encouraging them to return should the situation change. Some marriages and families experience several attempts at therapy before they decide to make changes and risk the unknown. Part of the process in marital and family therapy is learning whether the members of a marriage or family can meet the needs expressed. If, through therapy, it is learned that needs cannot be met, decisions may be required to meet those needs other than through the marriage or family.

12. What are some of the controversial issues?

The biggest issue today is "**Who are the family members?**" when the therapist is making decisions such as who to invite to family therapy sessions. The divorce rate has altered the composition of family systems and relationships. There may be parents, step-parents, children, step-children, half-siblings, grandparents, and step-grandparents. There also are gay and lesbian couples who may have ex-spouses by previous marriages. Children of those marriages will most likely be sharing time with both their homosexual and heterosexual parents. Another recent social phenomenon is the choice being made by both men and women to have children outside of marriage. Children of such relationships may be living with both biologic parents, a single parent, or one biologic parent and a significant other of that biologic parent.

Another controversial issue is whether couples and families dealing with **domestic violence** should be treated with marital or family therapy. Some professionals say "Never," because they believe that marital and family therapies support blaming the victim. Those professionals say that only the perpetrator needs to be in therapy; however, the basic tenet of couples' therapy is that both people contribute to destructive behavior. Other professionals argue that the domestic violence occurred in the context of a relationship and that the most helpful treatment program is individual help for the perpetrator in addition to therapy that addresses marital or family relationships. It may be that the decision should not be viewed as "either-or," but rather as a *clinical* decision that depends on whether or not the goal is to reunite the couple or family.

BIBLIOGRAPHY

1. Balcom D, Lee R, Tager J: The systemic treatment of shame in couples. J Marital Family Ther 21:55–65, 1995.
2. Beck RL: Redirecting the blaming in marital psychotherapy. Clin Soc Work J 15:148–158, 1987.
3. Berg KI, Jaya A: Different and same: Family therapy with Asian-American families. J Marital Family Ther 19:31–38, 1993.
4. Carter B, McGoldrick M: The Changing Family Life Cycle, A Framework for Family Therapy. New York, Gardner Press, 1988.
5. Cordova J, Jacobson N, Christensen A: Acceptance versus change interventions in behavioral couple therapy: Impact on couples' in-session communication. J Marital Family Therapy 24:437–455, 1998.
6. Dattilio F, Padesky C: Cognitive Therapy with Couples. Sarasota, FL, Professional Resource Exchange, 1990.
7. Gottman J, Notarius C, Gonso J, Markman H: A Couple's Guide to Communication. Champaign, IL, Research Press, 1976.
8. Greenspan R: Marital therapy with couples whose lack of self-sustaining function threatens the marriage. Clin Soc Work J 21:395–404, 1993.
9. Guerin PP, Fayu L, Burden S, Kautto G: The Evaluation and Treatment of Marital Conflict. New York, Basic Books, 1987.
10. Gurman A, Kriskern D: Handbook of Family Therapy. New York, Brunner/Mazel, 1981.
11. Hugen B: The effectiveness of a psychoeducational support service to families of persons with a chronic mental illness. Res Soc Work Pract 3:137–154, 1993.
12. Marley J: Content and context: Working with mentally ill people in family therapy. Soc Work 37:412–417, 1992.
13. Moltz D: Bipolar disorder and the family: An integrative model. Family Process 32:409–423, 1993.

45. GROUP THERAPY

John F. Zrebiec, M.S.W.

1. What is group psychotherapy?

It often has been defined in the broadest terms, encompassing many kinds of groups with goals that range from behavioral change to educational exchange. Group psychotherapy is considered here as a field of clinical practice and a specific approach within the realm of psychotherapy. All group therapy is aimed at alleviating illness or distress with the help of a trained leader. What distinguishes group treatment from other methods is the use of **group interaction** as the agent for change.

2. How did group therapy begin?

In 1905, Dr. Joseph Pratt, a Boston physician, brought his tuberculosis patients together for weekly discussion groups and found that these meetings seemed to improve mutual support, alleviate depression, and decrease isolation. Moreno, who is best known for developing psychodrama, first used the term "group therapy" in the 1920s. Group treatment largely was considered ineffective until World War II. The many neuropsychiatric casualties returning from the war compelled the governments of the United States and England to find ways to treat these veterans more efficiently and economically. Since then, the group therapy field has mushroomed and is now applied in many different clinical settings for many different types of problems.

3. What are the advantages of group therapy?

• The patient recreates characteristic difficulties in the group. Interactions in the group quickly expose patterns of behavior.

• The "hall of mirrors" concept refers to the group's ability to confront an individual with behavior he or she had been unable to recognize. Individual members are more likely to accept feedback about their behavior if it comes from multiple observers.

• Multiple supporters who empathize with the patient's struggle can make confrontation more tolerable and dealing with intense affect more possible.

• The revelation of shameful secrets can lead to immense relief.

• Group interactions pull for socially acceptable responses and interchanges.

• The group offers alternative models for behavior.

• Group therapy often is experienced as less regressive than individual therapy.

4. What are the disadvantages?

• Patients get less exclusive time and attention than in individual therapy.

• Groups can create a feeling of being lost in the crowd, and of not being appreciated for one's uniqueness.

• Confidentiality has limitations. The group leader cannot guarantee that members will maintain confidences.

• Termination is more complicated (less flexible, more final) than in individual therapy.

5. Are there different theoretical viewpoints?

Originally, most group therapy was established on psychodynamic principles; now most group therapists use a combination of theories. For example, a common blend of models is psychodynamic (focused on individual group members), interpersonal (focused on interactions between members), and group as a whole (focused on the group processes). This chapter blends those models into some general principles that are broadly applicable to a wide variety of groups, of any length and type, in any clinical setting.

6. What do I need to do first?

A successful group requires thoughtful planning:

Clarify your own values about why group treatment is valuable.

Assess the institution in which you work and whether it values group treatment. Will the institution and your colleagues be friend or foe in your attempts to start a group? Who values or devalues groups? Who has the authority to help you start a group? What kinds of groups are already in existence? What kinds of patients need a group? How will you get your group members? How much competition is there between professionals for these patients?

Consider the type of group you are offering. Groups range from discussion and theme-centered or supportive/educational to process-oriented therapy. It is essential to be clear about the type of group so that you can explain the purpose of the group to potential patients and referral sources and define your role as leader. For example, in a social skills training group, the leader's primary role is teacher, whereas in a psychodynamic group, the leader's role is interpreter of unconscious phenomena.

7. How do I select patients for groups?

Many different criteria have been proposed for selecting patients. In general, most patients can work effectively in some type of group therapy. If patients are willing to listen to others and talk about themselves, then they are group therapy candidates. Exclusionary criteria are: refusal to enter a group or abide by group agreements and serious problems with interpersonal relatedness. Contrary to popular opinion, people who do not do well in groups are *not* the prime candidates for groups. Caution also needs to be exercised in including patients who are highly impulsive, acutely suicidal, homicidal, or psychotic.

8. Which group for which patient?

Groups are not random collections of strangers thrown together because a clinic has too few therapists and too many patients. It is important not only to select patients who will benefit from group therapy, but to place them in a group that is particularly appropriate. Beginning groups traditionally comprise members who are similar in terms of ego development but different in terms of interpersonal style. For example, the ability to establish trust or capacity for concern is similar, but degrees of shyness or submissiveness are different. Most important is that no members see themselves as one of a kind in the group because they will be at high risk to drop out. To use a broad example, the only elderly, widowed man in a group with young, new mothers is going to find little common ground with other members and is likely to quickly leave the group.

There are **three reasons why patients drop out** of groups:
• The right group at the wrong time (the patient is not ready for group).
• The wrong group at the right time (e.g., the elder widower with the young mothers).
• The patient is not suited for group treatment.

9. Should I conduct a screening interview?

Ideally, there should be at least one individual interview before a patient is accepted into a group. Some patients may require more if they are unfamiliar with therapy or ambivalent about joining the group. Assessment of a patient, for group therapy in general and for your group in particular, requires face-to-face contact. The interview also helps form an alliance between leader and member, establish goals, provide education about the role of the leader and the members, review the group agreements, answer questions, and address potential problems. Finally, it gives the patient an opportunity to make an informed decision about joining the group.

The Screening Interview: Common Questions

What do you want to get out of this group?

Why do you want to joint this group at this time?

What is your experience in groups (prior treatment, but also including family, school, job, social groups)?

Table continued on following page

What do you imagine this group will be like?
What do you think you will contribute to this group?
What will be the most difficult aspect of this group for you?
May we review group agreements?

10. Should I have a group agreement?

Yes. All groups need some operational guidelines that provide structure and a baseline for addressing any future behavior that jeopardizes the group. The following guidelines traditionally have been used by psychodynamic group therapists. They can be modified for time-limited groups, and for groups with a variety of patients in different settings. Members agree to:

- Attend each meeting, be on time, and remain for the entire meeting.
- Work on the problems which brought them to the group.
- Realize that communication is verbal and not physical.
- Protect the names and identities of other group members.
- Use relationships therapeutically and not socially.
- Remain in the group until the problems which brought them to the group are resolved.
- Give appropriate time to themselves and to the group to understand the reasons for leaving, should they decide to leave, and to say good-bye.
- Give the leader permission to speak with their individual therapist (if they have one) at any time that the leader feels it is in their best interests.
- Be responsible about payment.

11. What are the basics in terms of time, size, and place?

Most groups meet weekly, although some groups meet twice weekly, and others meet twice monthly. The important point for therapeutic benefit is that patients do not lose contact with the affect and process of the previous meeting. The usual time period is 90 minutes, with the range 75–120 minutes. Less than 75 minutes is not enough time for members to get their fair share, and meetings longer than 120 minutes can be exhausting for members and leaders.

Group size is four to ten members. Fewer than four members provides a temptation to focus on individuals, not group processes; more than ten seems to become unmanageable and less productive. Most group experts recommend seven as the ideal number with higher-functioning patients, and starting with at least that many patients to compensate for potential early drop-outs.

It is the group leader's responsibility to arrange for a comfortable, private room with enough chairs for everyone. Most group leaders prefer chairs in a circle so that members are not physically hidden from one another by tables or other furniture.

12. What is the role of the leader?

To help the group members understand themselves by understanding their behavior in the group. The leader, then, has the challenge of deciding how the group can best be helped. Several decisions are involved:

- What to say, how much to say, and when to say it.
- How much attention to give to the present experience versus past events or future hopes.
- How much attention to give to individuals while still observing interactions between members.
- How much value to give to feelings and emotional experience without ignoring reason and intellectual understanding.
- How to integrate dialogue about group members with discussions about people outside the group.
- How to blend understanding of the content (obvious meaning) with the process (symbolic meaning)
- How much to respond to group demands or wishes.
- How much personal information to share.

All of these leadership decisions are influenced by theoretical orientation, personality, and context of the group. Moreover, all are a matter of degree, not all or nothing, and each has consequences for the group.

10 Useful Rules for the Group Therapist

1. Each meeting is in a context (time, place, purpose).
2. Each group member has a context. Try to keep in mind their history and presenting problems.
3. Pay attention to what is happening in the group at that very moment . . . the "here and now" focus. Ask yourself: What is happening? Why is it happening now?
4. Remember everything that happens in the group has something to do with the group.
5. Each group meeting has a theme or connecting thread.
6. Pay special attention to the beginning words and behaviors that might predict the theme.
7. Think in terms of metaphors or analogies as a clue to the theme of the group.
8. Pay attention to your own emotional response to the group as a barometer of what is happening in the meeting.
9. Do not panic if you do not always know what is happening in the group. This is a common experience. Remember the above points and try to formulate hypotheses that can help you make an educated guess about the theme.
10. Prepare a summary statement whether you actually state it or not, as a way of organizing the group theme.

13. Are there advantages to co-leadership?

Co-therapy is a frequently used model, primarily for training. The most important and time-consuming aspect is the need for the co-therapists to maintain their communication and attend to their relationship.

Advantages

For Patients
Enhances continuity in case of leader absence
May provide a constructive relationship model for imitation
Replicates a two-parent family
Provides more limit-setting capability

For Leaders
Provides mutual support and co-supervision
Offers two vantage points on group
Allows leaders to share or change roles from verbal to observational and focus from whole group to individual
Helps in dealing with crises and concrete tasks

Disadvantages

Increased cost
Destructive competition
Lack of communication
Serious disagreement based on each leader's different professional, clinical, or administrative role
Distancing from the emotional impact of the experience
One leader overshadowed by more experienced other

14. Are there stages in group development?

It is valuable for the group leader to have a developmental framework for understanding group themes and the myriad interactions of group process. Yalom proposes a useful framework for thinking about these four developmental stages.

Stage 1 ("in or out")—searching for purpose, getting to know other members, finding similarities, and learning the ground rules. Members are primarily concerned with acceptance and nonacceptance. Do the others like me? Are we similar? Communication in this stage often is superficial, polite, focused on giving or seeking advice, and gaining approval from the leader. The leader's primary role is to promote trust and safety, and to help members find common ground.

Stage 2 ("top or bottom")—jockeying for positions of control, dominance, and power among members, but above all, between members and the leader. The honeymoon comes to an end as safety and trust are established. Now, members want to know how they are different, how much autonomy the group leader will permit, and how much they can challenge one another and the leader. How can they batter, bend, and break group guidelines? Who are the strong ones? Whereas in the first stage members were primarily concerned with being seen as the same, now they are primarily concerned with being accepted as different. Criticism of one another, hostility toward the leader, and disenchantment with the group are typical. The group has great expectations of the leader so it should come as no surprise that they are disappointed in the leader's failure to fulfill their dreams. It is essential that the group leader tolerate their disappointment, encourage their confrontation, and not respond punitively. Remember that this rebellious, emotionally stormy phase is a sign that the group is moving ahead.

Stage 3 ("near or far")—the chief concern of the group is intimacy and closeness. How close to get to others? How many secrets to share? Following the previous stage of conflict there is more trust, cooperation, openness in communication, and group spirit. The leader sets the stage for progress by making sure that the group does not suppress all negative affect for the sake of group cohesiveness. The group is now ready to become a mature working group, with focus, flexibility, compassion, a greater tolerance for affect, a realistic appraisal of the leader, and a recognition of the value of other members.

Stage 4—termination. It is the leader's job to draw the attention of the group members to the loss. Ordinarily, termination resurrects feelings around three themes: mortality and death, separation, and hope.

These stages are present in all groups, but the depth and breadth of expression differ depending on the goals, time, and leadership style. There is overlap, with no clear boundaries between stages or consistency between groups. Groups never ultimately resolve these developmental issues, but periodically cycle through them at progressively deeper levels as stresses and conflicts emerge.

15. How do I handle difficult patients?

The difficult patient, often self-centered or demanding, can create a difficult group and a scapegoated group member. Volumes have been written about managing difficult patients, but it is worth mentioning one particularly constructive approach in groups. It is based on the premise that the difficult patient plays an important role for the group and represents aspects of everyone else in the group. The most therapeutic response is to focus on the reaction of other group members rather than on the pathology of the individual patient. This approach avoids further attack on the individual patient and encourages others to take responsibility for their share of the interaction.

16. What about combining group therapy with pharmacotherapy or individual therapy?

Psychotropic medications are common in groups and essential for psychotic patients. Attitudes about and reasons for medication typically become a topic for group discussion.

Many patients receive concurrent individual and group therapy, which can be a powerful combination. There are two variations: combined therapy, in which the same therapist sees the patient in both individual and group therapy, and conjoint therapy, in which the patient is seen in individual and group therapy by two different therapists. Group therapy often is added to individual treatment, but patients can be referred for individual treatment from group, as well. Note that neither mode of treatment should be viewed as better than the other. When considering combined or conjoint therapy, be sure to review repercussions for communication, confidentiality, and countertransference.

17. How do I decide when to terminate?

Time-limited groups come to a preordained ending. Other groups end because of the leader's decision to terminate. Patients leave groups because they have successfully completed treatment or leave prematurely for a variety of personal, group, and circumstantial reasons. The leave-taking process is more complicated than in individual therapy because it affects a number of people, not just the therapist. The leader should attempt to prevent premature termination and should draw attention to the feelings surrounding termination. Two helpful questions are: (1) Has the patient leaving gained the most possible from the group? (2) Why is the patient leaving at this particular time? The decision also can be examined on the basis of whether the original goal for joining the group has been accomplished. Interestingly, groups often assess the constructive changes and continuing conflicts exhibited by the terminating member.

18. Is there a place for brief group therapy?

Time-limited treatment is becoming more common because of cost-limited care. Time-limited groups often are formed around specific symptoms, crises, or common issues (for example, medical illness, divorce, or adolescence) with limited goals of symptom relief, crisis management, or support and psychoeducation. Brief-treatment groups also are designed for more aggressive interpersonal intervention and more ambitious therapeutic change. They have in common a careful selection of patients, explicit goals, a well-defined working focus, rapid application of learning, active leaders, the use of interpersonal resources, and the use of time limits to accelerate behavior change. Unlike longer-term groups, patients can return for several courses of treatment; in both, success is predicated on careful pregroup preparation.

Time-limited groups also can be conceptualized as having developmental stages (see Question 14). Progression through stages may be intensified because of the time limit.

19. Can the leader guarantee confidentiality?

The legal and ethical responsibility to protect the patients' privacy and confidentiality is uncompromised and uncomplicated for the therapist doing individual treatment. However, although the same standard applies for the group therapist, group therapy poses special problems because patients are expected to respect the identities and protect the information shared by other group members. In actuality, group therapy places limits on confidentiality (when one group member violates the confidentiality of another) because neither the leader nor the other group members have any legal means of enforcement.

BIBLIOGRAPHY

1. Agazarian YM: System-Centered Therapy for Groups. New York, Guilford Press, 1997.
2. Alonso A, Swiller HI (eds): Group Therapy in Clinical Practice. Washington, DC, American Psychiatric Association Press, 1993.
3. Bernard HS, MacKenzie KR (eds): Basics of Group Psychotherapy. New York, Guilford Press, 1994..
4. Dies RR: Models of group psychotherapy: Sifting through the confusion. Int J Group Psychother 42:1–17, 1992.
5. Kaplan HI, Sadock BJ (eds): Comprehensive Group Psychotherapy. Baltimore, Williams &Wilkins, 1993.
6. Klein RH, Bernard HS, Singer DL (eds): Handbook of Contemporary Group Psychotherapy: Contributions From Object Relations, Self-Psychology, and Social Systems Theories. Madison, CT, International Universities Press, 1992.
7. Roth BE, Stone WN, Kibel HD (eds): The Difficult Patient in Group. Madison, CT, International Universities Press, 1990.
8. Rutan JS, Stone WN: Psychodynamic Group Psychotherapy. New York, Guilford Press, 1993.
9. Scheidlinger S: Group dynamics and group psychotherapy revisited: Four decades later. Int J Group Psychother 47:141–159, 1997.
10. Steenbarger BN, Budman SH: Group psychotherapy and managed behavioral health care: Current trends and future challenges. Int J Group Psychother 46:297–309, 1996.
11. Yalom ID: The Theory and Practice of Group Psychotherapy. New York, Basic Books, 1995.

46. RELAXATION TRAINING

William H. Polonsky, Ph.D.

1. What are the major forms of relaxation training?

Meditation	Self-guided, passive attention to single object of focus
Progressive muscle relaxation	Systematic contraction and relaxation of major muscle groups
Hypnosis	Verbal and repetitive suggestions, often involving mental imagery, to relax mind and body
Autogenic training	Structured series of formalized suggestions directed toward promoting body sensations associated with relaxation

Biofeedback	Machine-based detection and amplification of tension-related physiological signals; signals are fed back to patient, who learns to sense and modify signal

2. Describe meditation.

Abbreviated (i.e., nonreligious) versions of meditational systems, usually of the *concentrative* form, have become increasingly popular in the West. In concentrative meditation, the patient is taught to attend passively to a single object of focus that is unchanging or repetitive (e.g., a visual image, a repeated word or mantra, or a body sensation such as breathing). The emphasis is on present-centered, effortless attention, often without any directive guidance that relaxation or any other psychophysiological change should occur. *Nonconcentrative* forms are similar, though usually more difficult, with the attention directed in a more expansive or "mindful" manner towards the ever-changing flow of mental activity.

3. Describe progressive muscle relaxation.

The patient is guided in the tensing and relaxing of 16 major muscle groups, one group at a time. Of the major relaxation forms, progressive muscle relaxation may be the most simple, straightforward, and teachable. Voluntary muscle contraction allows the patient to sense the difference between tension and relaxation in each of the muscle groups and enables subsequent muscle relaxation. Recent research, however, suggests that the tensing component may not be necessary; abbreviated techniques involving awareness of each muscle group followed by suggestions for relaxation may be just as effective. As the progressive muscle relaxation skill is developed, patients are encouraged to combine muscle groups, until relaxation is achievable through simple recall.

4. How is hypnosis relaxing?

Hypnosis and self-hypnosis both focus on formalized suggestion, often involving mental imagery. Hypnotic suggestion may be applied toward a variety of different ends, of which the most well known is relaxation. With a rhythmic and calming voice, repetitive suggestions are used to guide the patient toward somatic relaxation (e.g., "the muscles of your body are relaxing more and more") and cognitive relaxation (e.g., "slowly let go of the day's worries"). Of all the hypnotic suggestions, relaxation is one of the easiest to attain, though there is considerable evidence that individuals differ greatly in their ability to respond to hypnotic suggestion.

5. Is autogenic training a form of hypnosis?

Yes. It involves a series of six self-suggestions referring to specific body sensations. In the course of treatment, patients are slowly guided in the promotion of each group of sensations (e.g., "the heart is beating quietly and strongly," "the forehead is cool") in a step-by-step manner, which is believed to promote relaxation. Strong emphasis on passive concentration encourages the patient to allow, rather than force, changes in body sensations. As in progressive muscle relaxation, after autogenic skills are acquired, abbreviated forms are introduced so that the patient can more reliably and rapidly achieve states of deep relaxation.

6. In biofeedback, it's hard to see the benefit of relying on a machine for relaxation.

The biofeedback system simply relays information, via visual and/or auditory signals, back to the patient. The patient then learns to modify the signals, thereby modifying the associated physiological system in the desired direction. Biofeedback interventions can promote states of deep relaxation through directed reductions in, for example, electrodermal activity, heart rate, and muscle tension. Ideally, the patient is slowly weaned from the biofeedback system.

7. Does biofeedback have other uses?

Biofeedback is a multidimensional tool in that it can be used to promote a number of potentially valuable physiological changes that are not necessarily associated with relaxation. For example, electromyographic biofeedback training is used in neuromuscular rehabilitation to assist patients in re-learning to perceive, activate, and/or relax specific muscles, followed by the regaining of patterned muscle movement. The complexity and specificity of such training is clearly distinct from relaxation training (RT). Biofeedback training has been proven useful in a variety of other syndromes, including Raynaud's disease and encopresis.

8. What is the "relaxation response"?

Benson suggested that all types of RT are remarkably similar. Almost all types involve verbal repetition and a passive attitude toward external stimuli, and all lead to the same, generic result—the relaxation response. This response is characterized by muscle relaxation, diminished heart rate, reduced blood pressure, and other psychopathological changes indicative of a broad reduction in sympathetic arousal.

9. True or false: All types of relaxation training produce the same result.

True *and* false. This is a point of considerable controversy. In contrast with the relaxation response model, some researchers argue for a "specific effects" model, suggesting that somatic and cognitive forms of relaxation may be more effective when matched with the appropriate form of anxiety (e.g., complaints of chronic muscle tension versus "racing thoughts"). The evidence to date suggests that a compromise is warranted: each form of RT has been shown to promote general, stress-reducing effects as well as specific effects. For example, progressive muscle relaxation and biofeedback (somatic) have more powerful effects than meditation (cognitive) on body-oriented anxiety, such as a rapid heart rate. Meditation appears to impact more strongly when the anxiety is primarily psychological, such as excessive worrying. (For a more comprehensive discussion, see Lehrer, et al., 1994.)

10. Which psychiatric problems have been helped by relaxation training?

Generalized anxiety disorder, social phobia, depression, chronic substance abuse, and other disorders in which anxiety is a central factor.

While RT is widely viewed as an effective panacea, as a solitary intervention it is unlikely to be sufficient for most conditions. Powerful and effective stress management treatment *packages* have been developed, especially for anxiety-related diagnoses. For example, cognitive intervention and therapist-directed exposure have been remarkably effective in promoting long-term symptom reduction in agoraphobia and panic disorder (Craske and Barlow, 1993). RT usually is part of a comprehensive treatment program, and as such it generally adds to treatment efficacy (especially when focused on "breathing retraining"—slow, paced diaphragmatic breathing), but it is clearly a **second-tier treatment**. Cognitive therapy interventions usually are central, and relaxation techniques are directed towards "situation-specific" practice (e.g., learning to relax before and during difficult social situations.)

11. How are stress management programs different from relaxation training?

Stress management programs commonly involve a broad range of techniques, usually including RT, directed towards the amelioration of stress-mediated conditions. In contrast to RT, these programs tend to be multifaceted. One well-known program is **anxiety management training** (Suinn, 1990), which packages a number of cognitive therapy techniques along with progressive muscle relaxation. The goal is applied relaxation, and patients are trained to: repeatedly imagine anxiety-provoking scenes and use their relaxation skills to reduce the anxiety; recognize and treat the early signs of stress; and practice their relaxation skills during anxious moments. Other programs are more directly focused on specific psychiatric conditions. For example, Barlow and colleagues have developed a program for panic disorder that features relaxation techniques, cognitive restructuring (to identify the common cognitive errors that contribute to panic), and graded exposure to fearful body sensations (to promote desensitization).

Again, stress management programs tend to be more effective than simple RT for most psychiatric conditions.

12. Should patients be discouraged from the broad usage of relaxation techniques?

Not at all! In addition to its role as a potentially valuable component in the treatment of anxiety and other psychiatric disorders, RT can be a potent means for relieving daily stress and attenuating psychophysiological stress responses (i.e., chronically exaggerated reactions to stressful stimuli in any of a variety of organ systems). It can be rewarding and effective in the alleviation of subclinical anxiety disorders, as an alternative coping response to self-destructive behaviors, as an adjunct to psychotherapy, and/or as a preventative to the accumulation of daily stress. In addition, data suggests that RT may be useful in the treatment of certain physical illnesses.

13. Relaxation training has been shown to be valuable in the treatment of which medical conditions?

RT has been applied to a variety of medical conditions, with both positive and negative results (Gatchel and Blanchard, 1993; Murphy, 1996). The strongest and most positive effects are apparent in **headache disorders**. Both progressive muscle relaxation and electromyographic biofeedback are effective in promoting a clinically significant reduction in tension headache symptoms (50% reduction in self-reported symptoms) in approximately 40–50% of sufferers. However, cognitive therapy (identifying situations where headaches occur, improving recognition of the early warning signs of headache, and learning to practice relaxation skills immediately prior to headache onset) appears to be even more effective. Evidence suggests that cognitive therapy in combination with RT is more effective in reducing symptoms than amitriptyline. RT, especially autonomic-directed approaches (temperature biofeedback and autogenic training) also can alleviate migraine, though the effects generally are not as great in tension headaches. Nevertheless, temperature biofeedback in combination with autogenic training has been found to be as effective in promoting long-term reductions in migraine frequency as many pharmacologic approaches.

RT may be of some benefit in low back pain and other **chronic pain** conditions (hypnotic interventions have been popular) and in reducing **chronic insomnia**. Again, however, more comprehensive, cognitive-behavioral programs are clearly the treatment of choice, and RT is best regarded as one component.

Stress management programs promote significant and long-term clinical improvement in **irritable bowel syndrome**, but the degree to which the relaxation component contributes to these effects is not clear. In **hypertension**, **bronchial asthma**, and **diabetes**, research findings generally have been disappointing. Antihypertensive medications consistently produce more powerful results than RT. In asthma, RT improves pulmonary function, but the effects are small. In patients with Type 1 diabetes, RT does not lead to consistent, direct effects on blood glucose levels. (Effects in Type 2 diabetes are more equivocal.) Note, however, that RT in *small subgroups of patients* (e.g., highly anxious patients) with these types of illnesses may lead to significant clinical improvement.

Efficacy of Relaxation Training

MEDICAL CONDITION	DEGREE OF BENEFIT	PREFERRED METHOD
Tension headache	**	Progressive muscle relaxation EMG biofeedback
Migraine headache	*	Autogenic training Temperature biofeedback
Chronic pain	*	Hypnosis Meditation EMG biofeedback
Chronic insomnia	*	Progressive muscle relaxation Meditation
Irritable bowel syndrome	*	Progressive muscle relaxation Temperature biofeedback
Hypertension, bronchial asthma, diabetes	—	

—   Small, often transitory improvements, but not clinically significant
*   Clinically significant, small effects
**   Clinically significant, moderate effects
***   Clinically significant, large effects

14. Which is the most effective type of relaxation training?

None of the forms can be considered "most" effective. Meditation is increasingly popular in hospital-based programs around the country, and indeed, for the management of *cognitive* anxiety, it often is an excellent choice (Kabat-Zinn, et al., 1992). However, in many patients *somatic* anxiety is paramount (e.g., chronic muscle tension). These patients typically do not respond well to the relatively unstructured directions for meditation (possibly experiencing relaxation-induced anxiety, see Question 19), and symptom-specific training is necessary (e.g. breath retraining). Progressive muscle relaxation—an easy and nonthreatening technique with concrete directions—is an excellent introduction to RT. It is especially useful in patients for whom somatic anxiety is central, helping to sensitize them to their own patterns of muscle tension. Biofeedback can be particularly effective as a reinforcer for further training. When immediate progress can be observed concretely (e.g., an on-screen display of a slowly increasing finger temperature), the skeptical patient may be more likely to appreciate the utility of relaxation.

15. Under what conditions are psychopharmacologic interventions a better choice than relaxation training?

Drug treatments and stress management approaches that include RT appear to have similarly potent, short-term effects in the treatment of anxiety. Long-term studies show that stress management training is somewhat more effective than psychopharmacologic intervention. In certain circumstances, however, medication is a better choice for *initial* treatment. For example, when anxiety is overwhelming, patients are unable to concentrate on RT tasks (or other stress management instructions). Psychopharmacologic agents may facilitate the introduction and use of RT at a later time. In addition, when time and/or finances are limited, referral for RT may not be practical.

However, given the high relapse rates for anxiety conditions following the discontinuation of drug therapy, practitioners should be wary of limiting their intervention to drug treatments, especially when the presenting problem does not appear to be a transient condition. At the very least, inclusion of stress management interventions expands the patient's range of coping strategies and significantly lowers the rate of long-term relapse.

16. Are relaxation tapes as clinically effective as live training?

No. Live training has been shown to be consistently more effective than taped instruction in providing patients with the skills to lower physiologic arousal. In live training, the patient has the opportunity to benefit from an individualization of training and ongoing feedback. Interpersonal factors, especially the therapist's involvement and warmth, also may be important contributors.

17. How important is home practice?

It is essential. However, few differences are observed between those who practice daily and those who practice only occasionally, and frequency of home practice typically does not correlate with degree of clinical improvement. Thus, while home practice is necessary, extensive and regular practice is not necessarily more advantageous than occasional practice.

18. What are the best methods for encouraging home practice?

Greater levels of self-efficacy (belief in personal success) and higher expectations of benefits are both associated with regular practice. Thus, the therapist may be most successful in promoting home practice by encouraging the patient to believe that RT is a worthwhile endeavor and that he or she can be successful at it. In addition, written prescriptions (detailing the specifics of practice duration, frequency, and timing) may effectively encourage home practice.

19. What is relaxation-induced anxiety?

While adverse effects are uncommon, a subset of patients experience paradoxical sensations of transient anxiety when beginning RT. On rare occasions, severe anxiety may develop (referred to as relaxation-induced panic). Anxiety responses appear to be more common with cognitive forms of relaxation (e.g., meditation) than with somatic forms (e.g., progressive muscle relaxation). The causes of relaxation-induced anxiety are not clear, but cognitive factors (e.g., fear of losing control) as well as somatic factors (e.g., subtle hyperventilation) are suspected.

In autogenic training, such responses (termed autogenic discharges) are not considered abnormal, and are thought to reflect the "unloading" of pent-up thoughts or muscular activity. A similar perspective is seen in many forms of meditation, where such anxiety is viewed as a too-rapid release, an "unstressing," of emotional tension.

Given the aversive nature of such responses, it is possible that relaxation-induced anxiety is a major contributor to the high dropout rate often seen in RT. However, in the hands of a skilled therapist, it may become a valuable part of ongoing training (as well as potentially useful in associated psychotherapy interventions) as the patient learns to relax and accept such experiences. Alternatively, the therapist can switch, at least initially, to a more structured form of relaxation (e.g., progressive muscle relaxation or biofeedback).

BIBLIOGRAPHY

1. Barlow DH: Cognitive-behavioral therapy for panic disorder. Current status. J Clin Psychiatry 58(Supplement 2):32–37, 1997.
2. Benson H: The Relaxation Response. New York, Morrow, 1975.
3. Borkovec TD, Mathews AM, Chambers A, et al: The effects of relaxation training with cognitive or nondirective therapy and the role of relaxation-induced anxiety in the treatment of generalized anxiety. J Consult Clin Psychol 55:883–888, 1987.
4. Craske MG, Barlow DH: Panic disorder and agoraphobia. In Barlow DH (ed): Clinical Handbook of Psychological Disorders, 2nd ed. New York, Guilford Press, 1993.
5. Gatchel RJ, Blanchard EB (eds): Psychophysiological Disorders: Research and Clinical Applications. Washington, DC, American Psychological Association, 1993.
6. Kabat-Zinn J, Maisson AO, Kristeller J, et al: Effectiveness of a meditation-based stress reduction program in the treatment of anxiety disorders. Am J Psychiatry 149:936–943, 1992.
7. Lehrer PM, Carr R, Sargunaraj D, Woolfolk RL: Stress management technqiues: Are they all equivalent, or do they have specific effects? Biofeedback and Self-Regulation 19:353–401, 1994.
8. Murphy LR: Stress management in work settings: A critical review of the health effects. Am J Health Promo 11:112–135, 1996.
9. Suinn RM: Anxiety Management Training: A Behavior Therapy. New York, Plenum Press, 1990.

47. MEDICAL TREATMENT OF DEPRESSION

Russell G. Vasile, M.D.

1. What symptoms are affected by antidepressant medications?

Antidepressant medications exert their effects on the psychological and neurovegetative physical symptoms of depressive illness. Psychological symptoms include feelings of sadness, hopelessness, helplessness, worthlessness, guilt, and suicidal ideation. Physical symptoms include lack of energy, trouble concentrating, insomnia or hypersomnia, appetite disturbance (with weight loss or, less commonly, weight gain), diminished interest and/or pleasure in daily activities, psychomotor agitation or retardation, diminished libido, increased anxiety and/or agitation, and impaired cognitive function.

2. What are the factors in clinical presentation that suggest prescription of an antidepressant medication?

The diagnosis of major depression—persistent presence of five or more of the above physical features together with psychological symptoms, for a period of 2 weeks—is a strong indication for prescribing antidepressant medications. Additionally, there is evidence that the persistent presence of psychological symptoms even in the absence of marked neurovegetative depressive features may be sufficient indication to prescribe antidepressant medications. Thus, patients with dysthymia also are candidates.

3. What do antidepressants accomplish?

Antidepressant medications reverse the neurovegetative and psychological symptoms of depression, restoring a sense of well-being and normal function, as existed prior to the onset of the depressive episode. Antidepressant medications typically take at least 2 weeks to begin exerting their therapeutic effects and may take up to 6 weeks at adequate dosage before full therapeutic effect occurs. They are not euphoriants and do not induce elevation of mood in the absence of a depressive disorder.

Before beginning antidepressant medication, the clinician should establish that there is no organic factor (such as anemia, frontal lobe tumor, or hypothyroidism), that is initiating and maintaining the depressive symptoms.

4. How do antidepressants work?

Current understanding suggests that they work by blocking the reuptake and degradation of important neurotransmitters including serotonin, norepinephrine, and epinephrine, enhancing their availability at the synaptic level. Thus, the transmission of neurochemical impulses in brain regions rich in noradrenergic and serotonergic neurons, which contribute to the regulation of neurovegetative and psychological function, is facilitated.

Recent theories postulate that antidepressant medications mediate various intracellular signaling mechanisms that operate to increase or decrease specific neurotrophic factors. These factors are necessary for the functional viability of neuronal systems involved in the regulation of mood.

5. Can antidepressants be used in conjunction with psychotherapy?

Yes, and they are commonly used in this manner. Psychotherapy exerts its primary effect on the psychosocial and interpersonal adaptation of the patient, but has little impact on the neurovegetative symptoms of depression and is not effective for the treatment of severe depressive symptoms. Once a diagnosis of major depression is established, initiate antidepressant medications to afford relief of major depressive symptoms and supportive psychotherapy to enable maintenance of hope and a realistic perspective. The psychotherapy should emphasize a psychoeducational approach, which includes teaching the patient how to marshal social support from family and others. Moreover, when the major symptoms of depression resolve, many patients find insight-oriented psychotherapy helpful in reducing stress by altering maladaptive patterns of behavior.

Several studies suggest that the combination of antidepressant medication and psychotherapy is the most comprehensive and effective approach for resolving an acute depressive episode.

6. What are the common antidepressant treatments?

• **Selective serotonin reuptake inhibitors (SSRIs):** fluoxetine (Prozac), sertraline (Zoloft), paroxetine (Paxil), citalopram (Celexa)

• **Cyclic antidepressants:** tricyclic antidepressants, such as imipramine (Tofranil) and amitriptyline (Elavil); heterocyclic or atypical antidepressants, such as amoxapine (Asendin), maprotiline (Ludiomil), bupropion (Wellbutrin), nefazodone (Serzone), trazodone (Desryl), mirtazapine (Remeron), venlafaxine (Effexor)

• **Monoamine oxidase (MAO) inhibitors:** phenelzine (Nardil), tranylcypromine (Parnate), isocarboxazid (Marplan)

A novel antidepressant with a unique chemical structure, venlafaxine (Effexor), has been introduced within the past year. In addition to effects on neurotransmitters (see Question 4), this antidepressant has dopamine-blocking properties.

7. Comment further on SSRIs.

SSRIs, developed in the mid-1980s, have become the most popular antidepressants in the world due to their relatively benign side-effect profile and relative safety in overdose. Citalopram (Celexa) is a useful alternative for the patient who has experienced intolerable side effects (see Question 11) on other SSRIs. Citalopram also exhibits limited medication interactions as it appears to have less effect than other SSRIs on the cytochrome P40 enzymes and, therefore, may be a useful choice for patients requiring pharmacologic treatment for medical conditions.

8. Describe the cyclic antidepressants.

The tricyclic antidepressants were first used in the early 1960s and subsequently were the standard in the field for many years. The heterocyclic antidepressants, reflecting a variation from the classic tricyclic molecular structure, have found a specific role in selected circumstances. They were introduced throughout the 1970s and 1980s. Each of these agents has specific clinical features that may be advantageous in specific circumstances:

• **Amoxapine** has significant dopamine blocking properties and may play a particular role in the treatment of psychotic depression.

• **Trazodone** has highly sedating properties and often is useful in the treatment of depressed patients with insomnia. It also is used in low dosage (25–50 mg in the evening) in conjunction with SSRI antidepressants, which usually are activating, to induce insomnia.

• **Bupropion** is a highly stimulating antidepressant, which may be of particular value in bipolar patients in the depressed phase of illness. Some clinical studies have suggested that it induces mania or hypomania less frequently than other antidepressants.

• **Nefazodone** is a less activating antidepressant with significant anxiolytic properties. It may be a useful choice in the anxious depressive who develops insomnia on standard SSRIs.

• **Mirtazapine** enhances central noradrenergic and $5-HT_1$ transmission while blocking $5HT_2$ and $5HT_3$ receptors. It may be helpful in underweight patients, as weight gain and increased appetite can be associated with this medication.

9. What is the relationship between MAO inhibitors and tyramine?

The MAO antidepressants also were discovered over 20 years ago but fell out of popularity for a time because of adverse reactions, often severe and occasionally (rarely) fatal, involving ingestion of tyramine-containing foods. Prevention of this adverse side effect requires a special tyramine-free diet.

10. What do the antidepressants have in common?

Similar rates of response to all antidepressant drugs have been documented. Antidepressant medications may not be fully effective before 6 weeks of administration at adequate dosage, although most treatment-responsive patients show a response 2–3 weeks into the treatment course. The choice of antidepressant is predicated on factors specific to the particular patient, such as tolerance to specific side effects, and previous history of response to a given antidepressant.

11. What are the common side effects of antidepressant treatment?

Pharmacology of Antidepressant Medications

DRUG	MOST COMMON SIDE EFFECTS
Tricyclics	
Amitriptyline	Anticholinergic side effects predominate: dry mouth, constipation,
Clomipramine	drowsiness, orthostatic hypotension, urinary hesitancy. Weight gain
Desipramine	excessive sweating, increased intraocular pressure may occur.
Doxepin	Side effects vary within group. Amitriptyline and clomipramine
Imipramine	are most anticholinergic; desipramine and nortriptyline are least
Nortriptyline	anticholinergic.
Heterocyclics	
Amoxapine	Amoxapine may induce mild parkinsonian symptoms. Bupropion
Bupropion	may be associated with agitation, insomnia, and seizures. Trazodone
Maprotiline	is highly sedating, and has been associated with priapism in males.
Trazodone	Maprotiline is sedating.
Nefazodone	

Table continued on following page

Pharmacology of Antidepressant Medications (Cont.)

DRUG	MOST COMMON SIDE EFFECTS
SSRIs	
Fluoxetine	Insomnia, agitation, headache, and GI upset, typically nausea and cramp-
Paroxetine	ing. Fluoxetine generally more activating (akethesia) than other SSRIs.
Sertraline	Sertraline may have more pronounced GI side effects. Paroxetine
Citalopram	has mild anticholinergic properties and may cause mild dry mouth.
Mixed reuptake blockers	
Venlafaxine (Effexor)	SSRI-like side effects include agitation, nausea, headache, and GI distress.
	Hypertension may occur over time; ongoing BP monitoring required.
Noradrenergic and specific	
serotonergic antidepressant	
Mirtazapine	Weight gain, sedation.
MAO inhibitors	
Isocarboxazid	Orthostatic hypotension, weight gain, adverse interactions with tyramine-
Phenelzine	containing foods. Adverse food interaction characterized by throbbing
Tranylcypromine	headache and BP elevation, with marked pressor response. Tranylcy-
	promine activating; may induce insomnia. Phenelzine sedating; has a
	greater effect on (lowers) blood pressure.

12. Discuss antidepressant effects on sexual function.

Cyclic antidepressants, SSRI antidepressants, and MAO inhibitors are not uncommonly associated with **sexual dysfunction**, including diminished libido, delayed ejaculation, and anorgasmia. These side effects are much less likely to occur with bupropion, and are probably less likely to occur with mirtazapine and nefazodone. Helpful strategies for countering sexual side effects include lowering doses of antidepressant if possible, considering drug suspension for 1–2 days prior to sexual activity, or adding counteracting medicines, typically stimulants, such as yohimbine 5.4 mg qd, or the serotonin antagonist cyproheptadine, which is taken 30 minutes before sexual activity.

13. How might these medications affect weight?

Weight gain may be encountered with cyclic antidepressants and MAO inhibitors, but is less likely with SSRIs. **Weight loss** has been reported with the use of SSRIs; thus, they should be used with caution in the treatment of anorectic or underweight patients.

14. What are possible neurologic side effects?

Neurologic side effects include an approximate 1% risk of induction of **seizures**. This risk is associated with elevated antidepressant blood levels, and is more commonly associated with tricyclic antidepressants (TCAs) and bupropion as compared to SSRIs and MAO inhibitors. Mild myoclonus and toxic confusional states, particularly in the elderly, also may be encountered, particularly with elevated blood levels of TCAs.

15. Describe potential cardiologic side effects.

Cardiovascular side effects of antidepressant medications include orthostatic hypotension, commonly seen with TCAs, MAO inhibitors, and trazodone. Among the TCAs, nortriptyline (Pamelor, Aventyl) and desipramine (Norpramin) induce less orthostatic hypotension. In patients with sinus node dysfunction, treatment with TCAs may on occasion induce bradyarrhythmias. Therapeutic concentrations of TCAs may lengthen the QT interval, which predisposes to the development of ventricular tachycardia.

Cardiovascular side effects are less commonly observed with the SSRI antidepressants, as well as mirtazapine, nefazodone, and venlafaxine. Venlafaxine may contribute to essential hypertension, particularly at high doses (greater than 225 mg/qd), and monitoring of blood pressure is required.

16. Which antidepressants have side effects especially worth noting?

Bupropion is quite activating and is associated with less sexual dysfunction than other antidepressants, but it has a tendency to induce insomnia and in high doses has caused a significant incidence of seizures in underweight patients. **Trazodone** has been associated with priapism in males, yet in low doses is often used adjunctively with SSRI antidepressants to facilitate sleep. **Mirtazapine** may be associated with weight gain in some patients, and at lower doses is often sedating.

17. What is important to remember about MAO inhibitors?

At least 2 weeks must elapse after discontinuation of other antidepressant medication prior to the initiation of treatment with MAO inhibitors. For long half-life SSRIs such as fluoxetine (Prozac), 6 medication-free weeks must elapse prior to initiating MAO inhibitor treatment.

18. What factors influence the choice of antidepressant medications?

Since all antidepressants are equally effective in clinical trials, factors specific to a given patient influence choice of antidepressant.

Depressive illness is heterogeneous in symptom expression, and individual patients exhibit different side effect patterns and treatment responses. If a patient has had an excellent response to a specific antidepressant in the past, it likely is the best choice for future administration. Similarly, if there is a history of a first-degree relative having had an excellent response to an antidepressant, the likelihood of the patient having a good response is enhanced.

In addition, antidepressant side effects are an important consideration. If a patient has insomnia, an antidepressant with sedative properties is advantageous. Conversely, if a patient is experiencing lethargy and hypersomnia, a more activating antidepressant is helpful. Antidepressants that induce orthostatic hypotension should be avoided in the management of patients at risk for falls, such as the elderly.

Another factor is safety in overdose. The SSRIs and nefazodone, venlafaxine, bupropion, and mirtazapine have a clear advantage in this regard as they are substantially safer in overdose than other antidepressants, especially TCAs. Ingestion of 2000 mg of a TCA (a 10-day supply of 200 mg/qd) can be fatal.

19. How might antidepressant medications be combined?

Combination with adjunctive medications, such as lithium carbonate 600–1200 mg qd, or triiodothyronine 25–50 mcg qd, can enhance efficacy. In some treatment-resistant patients, combinations of antidepressant medications such as low-dose Prozac 10–20 mg qd and low-dose desipramine 25–50 mg qd may be considered, provided that antidepressant blood levels are carefully monitored, as toxic levels of desipramine can result due to medication interactions. Clinicians often combine SSRI antidepressants with bupropion, mirtazapine, or mirtazapine plus bupropion. Busipirone (Buspar) also can be used synergistically with antidepressant medication.

20. Are there specific types of depression that respond more consistently to specific antidepressant treatments?

Yes. While all antidepressants are equally effective in general, specific subtypes of depressive disorder appear to respond preferentially to different antidepressant treatments. These subtypes include:

- Atypical depression
- Psychotic depression
- Manic-depressive illness
- Melancholia

Major Depressive Disorder Subgroups

SUBGROUP	ESSENTIAL FEATURES	DIAGNOSTIC ISSUES	TREATMENT ISSUES	PROGNOSTIC FEATURES
Psychotic	Delusions Hallucinations	More likely to be bipolar than non-psychotic types; may be misdiagnosed as schizophrenia	Antipsychotic plus antidepressant more effective treatment than antidepressant-alone ECT highly effective	Usually a recurrent illness Subsequent episodes usually psychotic Psychosis affect consonant in depressed patients Patients with mood incongruent features-have poorer prognosis

Table continued on following page

Major Depressive Disorder Subgroups (Cont.)

SUBGROUP	ESSENTIAL FEATURES	DIAGNOSTIC ISSUES	TREATMENT ISSUES	PROGNOSTIC FEATURES
Melancholic	Anhedonia Unreactive mood Severe vegetative depressive symptoms	Can be misdiagnosed as dementia; more common in elderly patients	Antidepressant medication essential ECT highly effective if medications fail to produce remission	Maintenance treatment should be considered if recurrent episodes occur
Atypical	Reactive mood Overeating and oversleeping Rejection sensitivity Waves of fatigue Prominent anxiety and irritability	Patients tend to be younger May be misdiagnosed as personality disorder	TCAs less effective than MAO inhibitors; SSRIs show promise as therapeutic agents	Unclear
Seasonal	Onset in low-light months	More frequent in nonequatorial latitudes	May respond to antidepressants Phototherapy is effective option	Recurs seasonally
Postpartum	Acute onset (<30 days) in postpartum period Severe, labile mood symptoms	Often heralds bipolar disorder	Hospital treatment required Medical treatment necessary	50% chance of recurrence in next postpartum period Associated with vulnerability to switch to mania and bipolar illness

ECT = electroconvulsive therapy.

21. Which antidepressants are best for atypical depression?

MAO-I antidepressants are more efficacious than classic TCAs for the treatment of atypical depression. Atypical depressions are characterized by overeating, oversleeping, prominent anxiety and phobic concerns, and worsening of depression in the evenings. Emotional lability, irritability, rejection sensitivity, and a dramatic, histrionic, yet dysthymic interpersonal style (sometimes termed hysteroid dysphoria) also may characterize these patients. Another atypical depressive symptom is the sensation of episodic waves of leaden fatigue.

Specifically, the MAO inhibitor phenelzine is distinctly superior to the TCA imipramine in the treatment of this subtype. SSRIs also are highly effective and unlike MAO inhibitors do not require attention to dietary concerns.

22. Panic/anxiety disorders respond more consistently to which medications?

The SSRI antidepressants paroxetine and sertraline are effective in the treatment of panic disorder, and now carry this indication. Imipramine also has distinct anti-panic properties, and may be a preferential choice for patients with comorbid panic and depressive illness who cannot tolerate SSRI antidepressants. Venlafaxine has been approved for treatment of generalized anxiety disorder. Nefazodone and mirtazapine also can reduce anxiety symptoms in depressed patients; they may have a dual efficacy. MAO inhibitors have demonstrated efficacy for the treatment of patients with panic and/or phobic symptoms, and warrant consideration in patients for whom SSRIs are ineffective or intolerable.

23. Which antidepressants are most effective for psychotic depression?

Depressive disorders associated with psychotic features respond to antidepressants when combined with antipsychotic medications. Psychotic depression also exhibits a high rate of response to electroconvulsive therapy. Some clinicians feel that amoxapine may have superior efficacy to other antidepressants in the treatment of psychotic depression. Increasingly, the novel neuroleptic, risperidone (Risperdal), 1–3 mg qd, is added. For patients with bipolar tendencies, consider olanzapine (Zyprexa) 5 mg qd, as it appears to have mood-stabilizing as well as anti-psychotic characteristics.

24. Which medications are best for manic-depressive illness?

Many clinicians feel that the antidepressant bupropion is a superior choice for the treatment of manic-depressive patients in the depressed phase of their illness, because it is less likely to induce mania than other antidepressants. Limited data suggests that paroxetine (Paxil) also is less likely to induce mania. Avoid TCAs because they are most likely to induce mania.

25. Which personality disorder traits respond best to which antidepressants?

Clinical trials currently underway suggest that SSRI antidepressants may have specific benefits in depressed patients with a proclivity towards inappropriate anger and impulsivity. Indeed, SSRIs reduce impulsivity and inappropriate anger in nondepressed patients with borderline or antisocial personality disorder.

26. True or false: In higher doses, SSRI antidepressants are highly effective for the treatment of OCD symptoms.

True. Fluvoxamine (Luvox) is specifically marketed in the U.S. with an OCD indication. The antidepressant clomipramine (Ananfranil) has specific beneficial effects on OC symptoms and may be a preferential choice for patients with depression and associated OCD or OC symptoms.

27. Is phototherapy helpful in depression?

In some patients who experience depression during low-light months, 30 minutes of bright, white artificial light in the morning and/or evening hours can reduce symptoms. Phototherapy-responsive patients also may respond to antidepressant medication, and the two can be used in combination. Phototherapy generally is not associated with side effects, but some patients report irritability, insomnia, or increased anxiety during the course of treatment, particularly if phototherapy is combined with antidepressant medication.

28. When should electroconvulsive therapy (ECT) be considered?

• When the patient has failed to respond to several antidepressant medication trials.

• When the patient is experiencing threatening acute symptoms such as intense suicidal pressure, food refusal, or catatonic stupor, which require a rapid antidepressant response. ECT can be effective within days (antidepressants commonly require 2–3 weeks).

• When the patient has agitation and/or psychotic symptoms, characterized by delusions or hallucination.

• When antidepressant medications are associated with unacceptable side effects.

• When the patient has a history of a positive response to previous ECT treatments.

• When the patient has a medical condition that precludes the use of antidepressants.

29. Is ECT an adjunct to antidepressants?

During the course of ECT, antidepressant medication treatment is suspended, although low-dose antianxiety medication may be used. High-dose antianxiety medications may interfere with the efficacy of ECT.

30. Is ECT effective?

ECT has shown a high rate of success in patients exhibiting marked neurovegetative symptoms, including marked agitation or psychomotor retardation, and in patients with psychotic depression. ECT has an excellent safety profile and rapid onset of action. There are no absolute contraindications. However, ECT causes a transient elevation in blood pressure, heart rate, cardiac workload, and blood-brain barrier permeability. Therefore, it should be considered with caution in patients with recent myocardial infarction, cardiac arrhythmias, and intracranial space–occupying lesions; consultation is advised.

31. Describe the side effects of ECT.

The most common side effects are a transient postictal confusional state and anterograde and retrograde periods of memory disturbance, which may take 2–3 weeks to resolve after completion of the course of ECT. Therapy usually consists of three treatments per week for up to 4 weeks. Recent advances in ECT instrumentation have reduced cognitive side effects and permitted some patients to be treated as out-patients, with careful day program and/or family monitoring.

32. Can electrode placement affect results?

Yes. There are two standard electrode placement positions, unilateral nondominant hemisphere placement and bilateral electrode placement, which utilizes a bitemporal positioning. Generally, bilateral electrode placement is reserved for patients who fail to respond optimally to unilateral treatment. A disadvantage of bilateral treatments is that they cause somewhat more confusion and transient memory impairment than unilateral treatments.

33. Are there any new approaches to treating depression somatically?

An experimental alternative to ECT, transcranial magnetic stimulation (TMS), currently is being evaluated in clinical research trials. This treatment involves highly topographically selective mild electrical stimulation of the left anterolateral prefrontal cortex. It does not require general anesthesia and has few side effects. TMS shows promise as an antidepressant treatment. It remains to be seen whether it will be a viable alternative to ECT.

34. How successful is pharmacologic treatment of depression?

Initial pharmacologic interventions are ineffective in 20–30% of patients with a major depressive disorder. The most common factors are inadequacy of dosage and treatment duration and failure to detect and treat a coexisting medical or psychiatric disorder. The duration of treatment required before a medication trial can be ruled a failure is 6 weeks. Blood levels of antidepressant medication can be assessed for adequacy of dosage, although appropriate levels are not precisely established for every antidepressant medication.

35. What steps should be taken if a medication fails?

If a patient does not respond to an antidepressant medication despite adequate dosage and sufficient duration, other interventions are required. Reassess possible medical factors contributing to treatment resistance. Rule out comorbid psychiatric conditions including anxiety disorders, alcohol or substance abuse, neuropsychiatric disorders, and personality disorders. Identify chronic psychosocial stressors as potential complicating factors. (See flow chart on facing page.)

Assuming none of the above issues is operative, possible modification of antidepressant treatment could include:
- Changing to an alternate class of antidepressant medication.
- Using adjunctive medications to boost antidepressant response.
- Using combinations of antidepressant medications.
- Considering the use of ECT as a treatment alternative.

36. What might changing to an alternate class of antidepressant involve?

Three options are: using an SSRI if a TCA has failed, switching to a mixed agent such as venlafaxine (Effexor), and considering an MAO inhibitor. Many clinicians combine a low dose of a TCA such as desipramine, 30 mg qd, with an SSRI medication such as sertraline (Zoloft), 100 mg qd. Take care to use low doses of TCAs for these purposes, as medication interactions with SSRI antidepressants drive up TCA blood levels. Alternative antidepressants including nefazodone and mirtazapine warrant consideration as options.

Note that serious adverse reactions can occur if SSRI and MAO inhibitor medications are combined; therefore, a waiting period of up to 6 weeks is required before beginning an MAO inhibitor following a trial of a long-half-life SSRI agent such as fluoxetine.

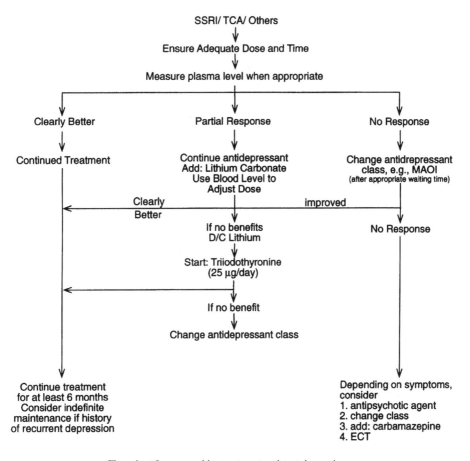

Flow chart for approaching treatment-resistant depression.

37. Which adjunctive medications can boost antidepressant response?

Commonly added are: lithium carbonate, in a standard dosage of 300 mg tid; Cytomel (T3), 25–50 mcg; or low doses of stimulants such as methylphenidate (Ritalin), 5–10 mg qd. Some clinicians add busipirone (Buspar), a serotonergic antianxiety medication, to an antidepressant regimen to enhance antidepressant response. Hormonal treatments, such as estrogen in women, are less well established as adjunctive agents.

38. Describe some antidepressant combinations that may be helpful.

Treatment-resistant patients may respond to a low-dose SSRI plus a low-dose TCA, typically fluoxetine, 10–20 mg qd, with desipramine, 10–20 mg qd. Also consider bupropion (Wellbutrin), nefazodone (Serzone), mirtazapine (Remeron), and venlafaxine (Effexor), all of which have slightly different biochemical properties from the SSRIs. Combinations of these agents, e.g., combining bupropion with nefazodone or mirtazapine, may be tried. In treatment-refractory cases, combinations such as bupropion and mirtazapine, or bupropion and nefazodone, can be helpful.

Note that it is less optimal to combine two simulating or two sedating antidepressants, and it is inadvisable to combine any antidepressant with an MAO inhibitor. A 2-week washout period is recommended before beginning an alternative antidepressant trial following a failed MAO inhibitor trial.

39. When is electroconvulsive therapy an alternative approach?

ECT is an option in treatment-resistant patients failing to respond to any of the interventions above. Approximately 50% of medication-resistant patients exhibit a positive response to ECT. The novel antidepressant venlafaxine, which acts on both noradrenergic and serotonergic neuronal systems, has shown promise in a subgroup of patients who have responded to other antidepressants. Venlafaxine generally is well tolerated, but has a spectrum of side effects (e.g., nausea, insomnia, and anxiety) similar to to the SSRIs.

40. Describe the phases of treatment with antidepressant medication.

Antidepressant treatment can be divided into three phases: acute treatment, which occurs in the initial stages of a depressive episode; continuation treatment, which covers the 6 months following the acute phase; and maintenance treatment, or chronic preventive treatment.

41. When is maintenance treatment appropriate?

Increasing evidence suggests that patients who have had three or more major depressive episodes, or histories of chronic low-grade depressive symptomatology are candidates for maintenance antidepressant medication. Note that adequate dosage is an important factor in effective prophylaxis of depression; thus, full dosage of medications should be administered for maintenance treatment. If a patient has had one initial depressive episode and does not exhibit any of the risk factors (see Questions 1 and 2), treatment should be continued for 6 months to 1 year prior to attempting a gradual tapering of antidepressant medication.

Decisions regarding precisely when to taper medication are best made collaboratively by the patient and doctor, with full consideration of the patient's life circumstances, including the likelihood of a recurrent episode of depression.

42. Why is tapering important?

Withdrawal symptoms may occur with the abrupt discontinuation of antidepressant medications. Withdrawal symptoms include feelings of malaise, agitation, lightheadedness, confusion, and increased dysphoria. The likelihood of withdrawal phenomena occurring is most pronounced with short-half-life antidepressants such as paroxetine (Paxil) as compared to long-half-life medications such as fluoxetine (Prozac). As a precaution, all antidepressants should be tapered over several days, if possible.

43. What are the risks of long-term treatment with antidepressants?

There are no well established long-term risks associated with chronic administration of antidepressant medications. Monitoring of cardiac status in the elderly by obtaining serial electrocardiograms and episodic assessment of liver function tests is recommended. Chronic administration of lithium carbonate requires periodic assessment (q 6–12 months unless symptomatic) of CBC with differential, thyroid tests, and measures of renal function including urine concentrating capacity following water restriction.

Since an increasing number of patients require maintenance antidepressant treatment, problems necessitating treatment modification may become more common simply due to the time factor. For example, the development of coronary vascular disease may lead to a risk of arrhythmia, and an alternative antidepressant with less cardiac toxicity, such as an SSRI, may be necessary.

44. What other psychiatric conditions commonly influence the medical treatment of depression?

It is crucial to have a high index of awareness of other psychiatric conditions that can influence and adversely affect the treatment of depressive disorder. These include:

• Substance abuse, particularly alcoholism
• Anxiety disorders, including panic disorder
• Personality disorders, most commonly borderline personality disorder
• Dementia superimposed on depression (The elderly are especially sensitive to the adverse cognitive side effects of antidepressant medication.)
• Temporal lobe epilepsy and neurologic conditions impacting the frontal lobes (particularly the left anterolateral prefrontal cortex)

45. What common medication interactions can influence antidepressant treatment?

Antidepressants can potentiate the sedative and central nervous system effects of a variety of medications, including antihistamines, barbiturates, and anticonvulsants. Do not use barbiturates with MAO inhibitors—this is a potentially fatal combination. TCA blood levels can be increased sharply with concomitant usage of SSRIs. MAO inhibitors and SSRI antidepressants should never be combined, as a potentially fatal "serotonergic syndrome" may occur. Many antidepressants can inhibit enzyme systems involved in the breakdown of common medications such as warfarin and digoxin. Citalopram (Celexa) appears to have less effect than other SSRIs on the P450 family of enzymes and thus may be favored in the medically complicated patient.

Carefully investigate medication interactions!

46. What are the treatment implications of concurrent general medical disorders?

Sympathomimetic agents, such as bronchodilators for **asthma**, must be avoided in patients on MAO inhibitors. Additionally, patients on MAO inhibitors should never be given meperidine, as fatal drug interaction may occur.

Patients with **cardiac disease**, including subclinical sinus node conduction disease or a history of ventricular arrhythmia, are best treated with bupropion, fluoxetine, sertraline, or ECT as opposed to TCAs.

Patients with **dementia**, given their vulnerability to adverse cognitive side effects of anticholinergic antidepressants, do well with low doses of antidepressants. If TCAs are to be used, low-dose desipramine or nortriptyline, which have minimal anticholinergic properties compared to other TCAs, are advised. Bupropion, fluoxetine, or trazodone with lower anticholinergic effects may be preferable.

Narrow angle glaucoma is a relative contraindication to anticholinergic antidepressants.

Obstructive uropathy usually secondary to prostatism mitigates against the use of highly antimuscarinic antidepressants. SSRI antidepressants, desipramine, or bupropion are advised in this circumstance.

Severe depression in **pregnancy** can be safely treated with ECT. The relative risk (particularly in the first trimester of pregnancy) of inducing birth defects, versus the benefits of antidepressant medication, should be reviewed on a case-by-case basis. Accumulating evidence supports the view that fluoxetine also is quite safe in pregnancy.

BIBLIOGRAPHY

1. Abramowicz M: Drugs for psychiatric disorders. Med Lett Drugs Ther 36(933):89–95, 1994.
2. Altshuler L, Post RM, Leverich GS, et al: Antidepressant-induced mania and cycle acceleration: A controversy revisited. Am J Psychiatry 152:1130–1138, 1995.
3. Ayd Jr F: Nefazadone: The latest FDA-approved antidepressant. International Drug Therapy Newsletter 30:4, April 1995.
4. Blacker D: Maintenance treatment of major depression: A review of the literature. Harv Rev Psychiatry 4:1–9, 1996.
5. Coccaro EF, Kavoussi RJ: Fluoxetine and impulsive aggressive behavior in personality-disordered subjects. Arch Gen Psychiatry 54:1081–1088, 1997.
6. Cohen LS, Altshuler LL: Pharmacologic management of psychiatric illness during pregnancy and the postpartum period. Psychiatr Clin North Am (Annual of Drug Therapy) 4:21–60, 1997.
7. Covey LS, Glassman AH, Stetner F: Major depression following smoking cessation. Am J Psychiatry 154:263–265, 1997.
8. Duman RS, Heninger GR, Nestler EJ: A molecular and cellular theory of depression. Arch Gen Psychiatry 54:597–606, 1997.
9. Ereshefsky L, Riesenman C, Francis Lam YW: Serotonin selective reuptake inhibitor drug interactions and the cytochrome P450 system. J Clin Psychiatry 57(supp 8):17–25, 1996.
10. Fawcett J, Marcus RN, Anton S, et al: Response of anxiety and agitation symptoms during nefazodone treatment of major depression. J Clin Psychiatry 56(supp 6):37–42, 1995.
11. Flint AJ, Rifat SL: Two-year outcome of psychotic depression in late life. Am J Psychiatry 155:178–183, 1998.
12. Frazer A: Antidepressants. J Clin Psychiatry 58(suppl 6):9–25, 1997.
13. Freeman MP, Stoll AL: Mood stabilizer combinations: A review of safety and efficacy. Am J Psychiatry 155:12–21, 1998.
14. Gatti F, Bellini L, Gasperini M, et al: Fluvoxamine alone in the treatment of delusional depression. Am J Psychiatry 153:414–416, 1996.

15. Gelenberg AJ: The P450 family. Biological Therapies in Psychiatry Newsletter. Vol. 18(8), August 1995.
16. Gershon S: Current therapeutic profile of lithium. Arch Gen Psychiatry 54, 1997.
17. Kupfer DJ, et al: Three year outcomes for maintenance therapies in recurrent depression. Arch Gen Psychiatry 47:1093–1099, 1990.
18. Leonard BE: New approaches to the treatment of depression. J Clin Psychiatry 57(suppl 4), 1996.
19. Nelson JC: Safety and tolerability of the new antidepressants. J Clin Psychiatry 58(suppl 6):26–31, 1997.
20. Nemeroff CB, Devane CL, Pollock BG, et al: Newer antidepressants and the cytochrome P450 system. Am J Psychiatry 153:311–320, 1996.
21. Nierenberg AA, Feighner JP, Rudolph R, et al: Venlafaxine for treatment-resistant unipolar depression. J Clin Psychopharmacol 14:419–423, 1994.
22. Quitkin FM, McGrath PJ, Stewart AW, et al: Atypical depression, panic attacks, and response to imipramine and phenelzine: A replication. Arch Gen Psychiatry 47:935–941, 1990.
23. Schatzberg AF: Fluoxetine in the treatment of comorbid anxiety and depression. J Clin Psychiatry 13:2–12, 1995.
24. Schatzberg AF, Cole JO, Debattista C: Manual of Clinical Psychopharmacology. 3rd ed. Washington, DC, American Psychiatric Press, 1997.
25. The Medical Letter: Citalopram for depression. 40(1041), December 4, 1998.
26. Wheatley DP, van Morraert M, Timmerman L, Kremer CME: Mirtazapine: Efficacy and tolerability in comparison with fluoxetine in patients with moderate to severe major depressive disorder. J Clin Psychiatry 59:306–312, 1998.
27. Wisner KL, Perel JM, Findling RL: Antidepressant treatment during breast feeding. Am J Psychiatry 153:1132–1137, 1996.

48. ANTIPSYCHOTIC MEDICATIONS

Herbert T. Nagamoto, M.D.

1. What are antipsychotic medications?

Antipsychotic medications are used to treat psychotic symptoms in patients with schizophrenia and other conditions. Symptoms may include hallucinations, delusions, paranoia, thought broadcasting, catatonia, bizarre behavior, and associated symptoms such as hypervigilance, agitation, and irritability. Typical antipsychotic medications also have neurologic side effects, leading to the alternate designation of neuroleptics ("of the neuron"). Antipsychotic medications are divided into **typical agents**, which are similar to haloperidol, and **atypical agents**, as exemplified by clozapine, which have different therapeutic and side-effect profiles and a different mechanism of action. This is a rapidly evolving area of psychopharmacology, and the newer atypical antipsychotic agents increasingly are used as first-line agents (see Question 21).

2. List the different typical antipsychotic medications by chemical class, specifying relative potency in chlorpromazine equivalents and usual range of daily oral dose.

Potency and Range of Oral Dose of Neuroleptics

ANTIPSYCHOTIC AGENT: GENERIC NAME (TRADE NAME)	APPROXIMATE AMOUNT (MG) OF DRUG NEEDED TO EQUAL 100 MG OF CHLORPROMAZINE	RANGE OF DAILY ORAL DOSE (MG)
Aliphatic		
Chlorpromazine (Thorazine)	100	25–2000
Piperazine		
Fluphenazine (Permitil, Prolixin)	2	1–40
Perphenazine (Trilafon)	10	4–64
Prochlorperazine (Compazine)	15	15–150
Trifluoperazine (Stelazine)	5	2–40

Table continued on following page

Potency and Range of Oral Dose of Neuroleptics (Cont.)

ANTIPSYCHOTIC AGENT: GENERIC NAME (TRADE NAME)	APPROXIMATE AMOUNT (MG) OF DRUG NEEDED TO EQUAL 100 MG OF CHLORPROMAZINE	RANGE OF DAILY ORAL DOSE (MG)
Piperidine		
Mesoridazine (Serentil)	50	75–400
Thioridazine (Mellaril)	100	75–800
Butyrophenone		
Haloperidol (Haldol)	2	1–100
Thioxanthene		
Chlorprothixene (Taractan)	100	30–60
Thiothixene (Navane)	4	6–60
Dihydroindolone		
Molindone (Moban)	10	15–225
Dibenzoxazepine		
Loxapine (Loxitane)	10	1–250

From Jenkins S, Gibbs T, Szymanski S: A Pocket Reference for Psychiatrists. Washington, DC, American Psychiatric Association, 1990, p 134, with permission.

3. What is the mechanism of action of typical antipsychotic medications?

The typical antipsychotic medications are believed to act via central blockade of dopamine receptors. This action in limbic areas leads to antipsychotic effects; in basal ganglia, to extrapyramidal side effects; in the brainstem chemoreceptor trigger zone, to antinausea and antiemetic effects; and in the hypothalamus (via blockade of dopamine inhibition of anterior pituitary prolactin release), to increased prolactin release.

4. Name several conditions that are indications for the use of antipsychotic medications.

Antipsychotic medications are used in a number of conditions to treat psychotic symptoms, including hallucinations, delusions, paranoia, combativeness, agitation and hostility, insomnia, catatonia, hyperactivity, and poor grooming and self-care.

Indications for Use of Antipsychotic Medication

- Acute and maintenance treatment of schizophrenia
- Psychosis associated with acute mania and major depression
- Psychosis from any number of medical causes (see chapters on schizophrenia, dementia, and delirium)
- As adjunctive treatment for agitation due to psychiatric conditions, delirium, delirium tremens, and dementia
- Tics due to neurologic conditions such as Huntington's chorea and Tourette's syndrome
- Flashbacks, nightmares, and agitation due to posttraumatic stress disorder
- Nausea and vomiting (prochlorperazine [Compazine], trimethobenzamide [Tigan], metoclopramide [Reglan])
- Gastroesophageal reflux and diabetic gastroparesis (metoclopramide [Reglan])
- Adjunctive use in anesthesia for medical and surgical procedures (droperidol [Inapsine])

5. List the general classes of side effects of typical antipsychotic medications.

Dopaminergic side effects

   *Pseudoparkinsonism

     Cogwheel rigidity

     Shuffling gait

     Parkinsonian tremor

     Masked facies

   *Acute dystonias, such as opisthotonus, torticollis, and †laryngospasm, which may cause acute airway obstruction

Increased prolactin secretion that may lead to galactorrhea
*Akathisia—subjective or observable restlessness ("thorazine shuffle")
Tardive dyskinesia, tardive dystonia (see question 12)
†Neuroleptic malignant syndrome (NMS)

Anticholinergic side effects
*Dry mouth
*Blurred vision (accommodation problems or frank blurred vision)
*Constipation that may lead to †adynamic ileus
*Urinary hesitancy or †obstruction
Memory and concentration difficulties, up to †frank delirium

Alpha-adrenergic blockade
*Hypotension
*Orthostatic hypotension

Antihistaminergic side effects
*Sedation, drowsiness
Weight gain

Others
†Agranulocytosis
ECG changes (prolonged QT interval)
Elevated liver function tests
Elevated creatine phosphokinase (in the absence of NMS)
Fetal toxicity
Photosensitivity
Pigmentary retinopathy (avoid doses of thioridazine > 800 mg/day)
Seizures (decreased seizure threshold)
*Sexual dysfunction (erectile problems, impotence, delayed, absent, or retrograde
  ejaculation, priapism)
Skin rashes

---

*Common side effects.
†Potentially dangerous side effects.

6. How is antipsychotic potency related to side effects?

In general, the lower-potency agents, such as chlorpromazine and thioridazine, tend to be high in sedation, orthostatic hypotension, and anticholinergic side effects, whereas the higher-potency agents, such as haloperidol and fluphenazine, tend to be high in pseudoparkinsonian, akathisia, and acute dystonic side effects.

7. Describe the treatment of common side effects of typical antipsychotic medications.

In general, decrease antipsychotic medications to the lowest effective dose whenever possible to minimize side effects and avoid polypharmacy.

Pseudoparkinsonism and acute dystonias are treated with antiparkinson agents. Benztropine (Cogentin, 1–2 mg up to 4 times/day), diphenhydramine (Benadryl, 25–50 mg up to 4 times/day), and trihexyphenidyl (Artane, 2–5 mg up to 15 mg/day in divided doses) are used for their anticholinergic effects to treat acute extrapyramidal side effects. Prophylactic treatment for approximately the first 10 days of treatment or after dosage increases may be considered for adolescents and other patients who (by history) are highly susceptible to pseudoparkinsonism and acute dystonias. Exercise care to avoid anticholinergic poisoning in combination with other anticholinergic agents, particularly in elderly or medically debilitated patients. The lowest effective doses are prudent, and they should be tapered and discontinued as soon as possible. Amantadine (Symmetrel), which is thought to potentiate dopaminergic neurotransmission, also may be used. In the case of laryngospasm, which may lead to acute airway obstruction, use Benadryl, 50 mg intravenously.

Akathisia usually responds well to dosage reduction, anticholinergic agents, or change to a different class of neuroleptics. Benzodiazepines and beta-adrenergic antagonists such as propranolol are also effective in treating akathisia. It is important to differentiate akathisia due to neuroleptic treatment from agitation due to psychosis. This differentiation may be difficult, but neuroleptic doses may be increased (which improves psychotic agitation but worsens akathisia) or decreased (which improves akathisia but worsens psychotic agitation). Some akathisia treatments (anticholinergics) are unlikely to affect psychotic agitation, whereas others may improve (benzodiazepines) or have differential effects (beta-adrenergic antagonists) on agitation due to psychosis.

Patients often develop tolerance to **anticholinergic side effects**, but they may persist. It is usually best to decrease dosage or switch to a more potent agent if anticholinergic side effects become intolerable. Alternatively, bethanechol (Urecholine, 5–10 mg up to 4 times/day; sometimes 25 mg up to 4 times/day) may be used to decrease dry mouth, blurred vision, constipation, and urinary hesitancy.

Hypotension and orthostatic hypotension are treated with oral hydration, careful instructions to the patient, dose reduction, or change to more potent agents. Occasionally, intravenous hydration is indicated. If a vasoactive agent is required, one should avoid agents with beta-adrenergic agonist properties (such as epinephrine), which may worsen hypotension via vasodilatation and peripheral pooling. In such cases, a selective alpha-adrenergic agonist such as metaraminol (Aramine) should be used.

8. What constitutes an adequate trial of typical antipsychotic medications?

Antipsychotic medications often induce sedation quickly, but their specific antipsychotic effects may take up to 6 weeks at therapeutic doses to develop fully. Conversely, when a stable schizophrenic patient decides to stop antipsychotic medication suddenly, it may take weeks for psychotic symptoms to return or for patients to decompensate. Therapeutic doses vary widely from patient to patient and within a given patient at various times. In general, maintenance doses range from approximately 100–700 mg/day, averaging 300 mg/day in chlorpromazine equivalents. Acutely ill patients may require higher doses, although the current trend is toward adjunctive use of benzodiazepines in acutely psychotic patients to avoid the side effects often associated with high-dose antipsychotic medications.

In an emergency situation, with a highly agitated or out-of-control patient, many antipsychotic medications can be given intramuscularly. In general, the lower-potency antipsychotics such as chlorpromazine or thioridazine are given in half the amount of oral doses. In some settings, particularly emergency departments, acutely psychotic, out-of-control patients are given intravenous haloperidol, often in very high doses. There is a small chance that intravenous haloperidol will induce the condition known as torsade de pointes, which may lead to ventricular fibrillation and sudden death. Intravenous haloperidol should be used with caution in women and patients with increased QT intervals on electrocardiogram, who are at increased risk for developing torsade de pointes.

9. Delineate an approach to patients who do not respond well to antipsychotic medications.

For patients who do not respond to treatment, **reassess the diagnosis**, particularly in the case of such illnesses as schizophrenia and bipolar affective disorder, which may be quite similar in the acute phases. When revisiting a patient's diagnosis: (1) rule out occult medical illness that may worsen symptoms or cause the illness under treatment; (2) rule out alcohol and substance abuse, which may mimic or worsen a number of psychiatric symptoms; and (3) ensure that the patient is receiving an adequate dosage of antipsychotic for an adequate length of time.

Typical antipsychotic medications may have a **therapeutic window**; thus patients out of the appropriate range may receive too little or too much medication. Plasma levels obtained at steady state help to assess dosage of some neuroleptics (see below; haloperidol and fluphenazine are most studied).

Compliance is a common problem with antipsychotic medications. All too often patients stop medications because of legitimately troublesome side effects and thus experience psychotic decompensation. To ensure acute compliance, administer intramuscular injections or observe the patient for 30 minutes after oral ingestion of liquid medications. For long-term maintenance, fluphenazine and haloperidol are available in slow-release depot forms that may be given intramuscularly every 2–4 weeks.

Ensure that troublesome **side effects** do not hinder the effectiveness of treatment, especially in akathisia, which can mimic or exacerbate psychotic agitation. Pseudoparkinsonism and oversedation may make patients look artificially depressed, and neuroleptic malignant syndrome may make patients suddenly look worse (e.g., catatonic or delirious). If a schizophrenic patient does not improve, it is also important not to miss a treatable depression. Finally, for patients who cannot tolerate or do not respond to typical neuroleptics, a trial of an atypical antipsychotic is indicated (see below).

10. How can blood levels of antipsychotic medications be helpful in the clinical management of patients?

There is evidence that at least some antipsychotic medications have a therapeutic window of ideal dosage or blood levels. Currently, haloperidol is the most thoroughly studied agent, with best therapeutic effects achieved at trough plasma levels of 5–12 ng/ml in most patients. Fluphenazine also is well studied, with recommended plasma levels of 1–2.8 ng/ml. For other agents, plasma levels are useful in ruling out subtherapeutic levels of medication in patients who "hypermetabolize," have poor absorption, or are noncompliant. If a laboratory reports a therapeutic range for a neuroleptic, it is reasonable to inquire how the laboratory arrived at its recommendations. For the atypical antipsychotic clozapine, patients should have improved clinical response at trough plasma levels of greater than 350–410 ng/ml.

11. Name possible problematic interactions between antipsychotic medications and other drugs.

- Anticholinergic agents may place patients at increased risk of anticholinergic delirium.
- Numerous agents may induce or worsen hypotension or orthostatic changes in combination with neuroleptics, including barbiturates and nonbarbiturate hypnotics, narcotics, benzodiazepines, angiotensin-converting enzyme inhibitors, antihypertensives, antidepressants, methyldopa, anesthetics, and epinephrine.
- Sedation may be worsened when antipsychotics are used with benzodiazepines, sedatives, narcotics, cimetidine, antidepressants, and antihistamines. In particular, chlorpromazine and meperidine used in combination may lead to hypotension and lethargy.
- Lithium and antidepressants may worsen extrapyramidal side effects (pseudoparkinsonism and acute dystonias). For a more complete listing of drug interactions with antipsychotic medications, including changes in plasma levels, see Maxmen and Ward.[5]

12. What is tardive dyskinesia? Why is it of concern with chronic use of antipsychotic medications?

Tardive dyskinesia is a syndrome of abnormal involuntary movements such as buccolingual masticatory movements, choreoathetoid movements of the limbs or even trunk and neck, and facial grimacing or tics. Long before the advent of antipsychotic medications, such movements were noted in schizophrenic patients, who probably are at increased risk of developing the syndrome. Tardive dyskinesia tends to develop after months to years of neuroleptic treatment and has been described in patients treated with all available typical agents. It occurs in about 15–20% of patients receiving chronic neuroleptic treatment; the incidence rises significantly in elderly populations. Curiously, it is temporarily masked by increased antipsychotic doses and tends to worsen acutely with decreased dosage.

13. How is tardive dyskinesia avoided or managed?

Patients treated with neuroleptics should be examined for abnormal involuntary movements before initiating therapy and every 6 months or with dosage changes or appearance of suspected movements. Patients should be maintained on the lowest effective dosage of medication. On examination, the abnormal movements are more apparent when patients do not know that they are being observed or when they are concentrating on tasks such as rapid alternating movements. In addition, a syndrome of withdrawal dyskinesias may occur briefly on withdrawal of neuroleptics. In a small but significant percentage of cases, tardive dyskinesia becomes permanent and disfiguring.

Unfortunately, there are no effective treatments for tardive dyskinesia, although vitamin E (400 IU 3–4 times/day) has been shown to decrease symptoms in some patients, especially those who are young and have had the syndrome briefly. The atypical antipsychotic clozapine appears not to cause this problem and may improve symptoms in patients who develop tardive dyskinesia (see below) and need continued antipsychotic treatment. Risperidone, olanzapine, and quetiapine appear to be much less likely to cause tardive dyskinesia than typical antipsychotics, though long-term use with these agents is limited at this time.

14. Define neuroleptic malignant syndrome.

Neuroleptic malignant syndrome (NMS) is a potentially fatal side effect that involves:
- Fever (up to 42°C) in the absence of infection
- Rigidity, which may be "lead pipe" and generalized, and other neurologic signs (e.g., akinesia and dyskinesia)
- Autonomic dysfunction leading to tachycardia, labile hypertension, diaphoresis, and pallor (mix of symptoms varies widely)
- Changes in mental status ranging from mild obtundation through stupor and coma (in approximately 70% of patients)
- Other possible symptoms: rhabdomyolysis (with elevated creatine phosphokinase in 40–90%), dysarthria, dysphagia, mutism, Babinski reflex, sialorrhea, opisthotonus

NMS usually occurs within 2 weeks of initiating typical antipsychotics or increasing dosage, but may occur after months of stable-dose treatment. It evolves over 24–72 hours and lasts 5–10 days with oral medications or considerably longer with depot intramuscular medications. NMS has an estimated mortality rate of 15–20%. Prompt diagnosis and discontinuation of neuroleptics are essential. Treatment is primarily supportive, although dantrolene and bromocriptine have been helpful. There have been isolated case reports of NMS associated with clozapine, risperidone, and olanzapine.

15. What is clozapine?

Clozapine (Clozaril) is a tricyclic dibenzodiazepine antipsychotic medication. It was synthesized in the 1960s but withdrawn from the market in the U.S. after 8 of 16 patients who developed agranulocytosis in Finland died in the 1970s. It has been used continuously in other countries since then. In 1990 it was reintroduced in the U.S. after it was shown that, in comparison to typical neuroleptics:

- Clozapine is more effective in treatment-resistant schizophrenic patients for both positive psychotic symptoms, such as delusions and hallucinations, and chronic negative symptoms, such as social withdrawal, anhedonia, blunted affect, and poor initiative.
- Clozapine is unlikely to cause dopaminergic side effects such as pseudoparkinsonism, tardive dyskinesia, and elevated prolactin levels.

16. What are the side effects of clozapine?

The FDA mandates weekly dispensing and CBC monitoring with initial treatment due to the risk of **agranulocytosis**. Most cases of agranulocytosis occur in the first 6 months of treatment. With weekly monitoring, the incidence of agranulocytosis has decreased from 1–2% in the initial studies to 0.38% in the first 5 years of use since U.S. reintroduction (versus 0.1% with typical antipsychotics). The FDA now allows every other week dispensing and CBC checks in stable patients after the first 6 months of treatment. There is still some risk of death from agranulocytosis despite this careful monitoring (19 deaths out of over 180,000 patients exposed to clozapine in the U.S. as of this writing; an approximate 1/10,000 risk of death).

Other side effects can include dose-related seizures (5% at doses above 600 mg/day), sedation, orthostatic hypotension, sialorrhea, and weight gain. The risk of seizures dictates low starting doses and slow dose increases, and if a patient has been off of clozapine for more than a few days, retitration back to previous dosage.

17. Why is clozapine considered the prototypic atypical antipsychotic medication?

Clozapine has been designated as an atypical antipsychotic because of its clinical profile and pharmacologic actions. Clozapine affects a large number of neurotransmitter systems. Its atypical properties currently are thought to be due to its relatively high 5HT2 blockade and weak D1/D2 blockade, with more dopamine effects in limbic systems (related to antipsychotic effects) than in striatal systems (leading to motor side effects). Average doses are 250–450 mg/day with a range of 100–900 mg/day.

Clozapine has been found useful in a number of psychotic conditions in addition to schizophrenia including treatment refractory bipolar affective disorders. It remains the gold standard for efficacy in antipsychotic medications, but its use is limited by side effects, cost, and monitoring requirements.

18. What other atypical antipsychotic medications currently are available?

As of this writing, the atypical antipsychotic medications available in the U.S. in addition to clozapine are (in order of introduction) risperidone (Risperdal), olanzapine (Zyprexa), and quetiapine (Seroquel). All three medications appear to be effective with both positive and negative symptoms of schizophrenia.

19. How do they compare to clozapine in atypical characteristics?

Risperidone has dose-dependent dopaminergic effects that are low at optimal doses of 4 mg/day (range 2–16/day). There is increasing pseudoparkinsonism, akathisia, and elevated prolactin with increased doses of risperidone, though usually less than that seen with typical antipsychotics.

Olanzapine (current range 7.5–20 mg/day) also has some risks for akathisia and elevated prolactin at higher doses, again less than that seen with typical antipsychotics. While tardive dyskinesia can occur with risperidone and olanzapine, the incidence with each appears to be considerably less than that seen with typical neuroleptics. Both of these medications also are showing promise in the treatment of other psychotic disorders, such as treatment refractory mania. While there are isolated case reports of mania induction attributed to risperidone, other data suggest that this is not likely to be a problem, especially if a mood stabilizer is also used.

Quetiapine (dose range 150–750 mg/day) is the closest to clozapine in being very unlikely to induce dopaminergic effects such as pseudoparkinsonism and elevated prolactin levels, but there are limited data on its efficacy.

20. Name the other common side effects of risperidone, olanzapine, and quetiapine.

Risperidone can cause insomnia, agitation, dizziness, orthostatic hypotension, and tachycardia in addition to its dose-related dopaminergic side effects. Olanzapine can cause somnolence, dry mouth, insomnia, weight gain, dizziness, orthostatic hypotension, and nausea in addition to less common dopaminergic side effects. Quetiapine can cause dizziness, orthostatic hypotension, dry mouth, constipation, dyspepsia, and somnolence, which can require a slower titration than risperidone or olanzapine, though not as slow as clozapine. Again, quetiapine appears to not have significant dopaminergic side effects.

21. Should the atypical antipsychotic medications be used first line in psychosis?

Clozapine, with its potential for agranulocytosis and seizures and monitoring requirements, is not a first-line agent. However, other, newer atypical antipsychotics increasingly are being used as first-line agents in the treatment of psychosis, with data supporting their greater efficacy, lower side effects, increased compliance, and fewer relapses when compared to typical antipsychotics. There also are preliminary data that these agents may be more effective for first-break patients, an important consideration given that schizophrenic patients tend to experience the greatest decline in the first 5 years of their illness. Because of their more favorable side-effect profiles, these agents also are recommended for elderly patients (who can be susceptible to hypotension and tachycardia) and patients with Parkinson's disease. There is little debate that these agents are indicated for patients who either can't tolerate or don't respond to typical antipsychotics.

Cost is an important consideration, as oral typical neuroleptics cost approximately $200 per year, as compared to $2000–3000 per year for atypicals, and more for clozapine with monitoring. There are a number of open trials that show overall cost savings when atypical antipsychotics are used in schizophrenic patients, due to decreased need for hospitalization and outpatient visits.

However, only a small number of randomized control studies are completed at this time; these show modest to significant cost savings.

BIBLIOGRAPHY

1. Arnt J, Skarsfeld T: Do novel antipsychotics have similar pharmacological characteristics? A review of the evidence. Neuropsychopharm 18:63–101, 1998.
2. Baldessarini RJ, Frankenburg FR: Clozapine: A novel antipsychotic agent. N Engl J Med 324:746–754, 1991.
3. Janicak PG, Davis JM, Preskhorn SH, Ayd FJ: Principles and Practice of Psychopharmacotherapy, 2nd ed. Baltimore, Williams & Wilkins, 1997.
4. Jenkins SC, Hansen MR (eds): A Pocket Reference for Psychiatrists, 2nd ed. Washington, DC, American Psychiatric Press, 1995.
5. Maxmen JS, Ward NG: Psychotropic Drugs Fast Facts, 3rd. New York, WW Norton and Co, 2000.
6. Schatzberg AF, Nemeroff CB: The American Psychiatric Press Textbook of Psychopharmacology, 2nd ed. Washington, DC, American Psychiatric Press, 1998.
7. Stahl SM: Essential Psychopharmacology. New York, Cambridge University Press, 1998.
8. Van Putten T, Marder SR,Wirshing WC, et al: Neuroleptic plasma levels. Schizophr Bull 17:197–216, 1991.

49. MOOD-STABILIZING AGENTS

James L. Jacobson, M.D.

1. What are mood-stabilizing agents?

Mood-stabilizing agents are medications with both antimanic and antidepressant effects. The ideal mood stabilizer would treat acute mania *and* depression, as well as prevent recurrence of both states. Currently available medications in this class tend to be better antimanic agents than antidepressant agents.

Mood stabilizers are sometimes called **thymoleptics**. This term implies the capacity to alter emotional or mental states, once (wrongly) thought to be influenced by the thymus gland. Hence the persistence of terms such as euthymic (normal mood range) and hyperthymic (excessively elevated mood).

2. Name some mood-stabilizing agents.

Lithium (as a carbonate or citrate salt) and valproate (valproic acid, divalproex sodium) are the only FDA-approved medications in this class. Both have proven antimanic benefits, and certainly may be useful in treating bipolar depression. Lithium has been shown to decrease recurrent mood episodes. It is widely believed that valproate also may prevent recurrent episodes in bipolar illness, but this has yet to be proven in controlled research studies. Carbamazepine has clearly demonstrated antimanic properties, but it has not yet gained FDA approval for this indication.

Dose Ranges and Therapeutic Levels of Mood-Stabilizing Agents

MEDICATION	DOSE RANGE (APPROXIMATE)	THERAPEUTIC BLOOD LEVELS*
Lithium	600–1800 mg/day	0.5–1.5 mEq/L
Carbamazepine	600–1600 mg/day	6–12 ng/ml
Valproate acid	750–3000 mg/day	50–100 µg/ml

* Based on trough values obtained 8–12 hours after the preceding dose of medication.

Other medications currently being investigated and used as mood-stabilizing agents include lamotrigine, gabapentin, calcium channel blockers (e.g., verapamil), and neuroleptic medications.

3. In what conditions are mood stabilizers used?
Bipolar I disorder
Bipolar II disorder
Cyclothymia
Schizoaffective disorder
Intermittent explosive disorder
Mania due to medical conditions (e.g., stroke, temporal lobe syndrome, cancer)
Major depressive disorder (adjunctive treatment or prophylaxis in recurrent disorder)

4. What assessment is necessary before initiation of treatment with mood-stabilizing agents?
A general medical assessment, including history, physical examination, and laboratory evaluation focusing on organ systems potentially affected by each agent, is important prior to starting these medications.

Mood-Stabilizing Agents: Side Effects and Laboratory Tests

MEDICATION	ORGAN SYSTEM AFFECTED	POTENTIAL SIDE EFFECTS	LABORATORY TESTS
Lithium	Cardiac	Conduction disturbance Sinus node dysfunction	EKG
	Hematologic	Elevated white blood cell count	Complete blood count with differential
	Renal	Diabetes insipidus/development of renal failure	Electrolytes, blood urea nitrogen (BUN), creatinine, urinalysis (specific gravity)
	Reproductive (women)	Fetal abnormalities	Pregnancy test
	Thyroid	Hypothyroidism/goiter	Thyroid-stimulating hormone (TSH)
Valproate	Hematologic	Anemia	Complete blood count with differential
		Leukopenia	Blood count
		Thrombocytopenia	Platelet count/bleeding time
	Hepatic	Hepatic dysfunction or failure	Hepatic enzymes
	Reproductive (women)	Fetal abnormality	Pregnancy test
Carbamazepine	Cardiac	Arrhythmia	EKG
	Hematologic	Agranulocytosis Aplastic anemia	Complete blood count with differential
		Thrombocytopenia	Platelet count
	Hepatic	Hepatitis	Hepatic enzymes
		Jaundice	Bilirubin
	Renal	Syndrome of inappropriate secretion of antidiuretic hormone	BUN/creatinine
		Hyponatremia	Electrolytes
	Reproductive (women)	Fetal abnormality	Pregnancy tests

Once treatment is initiated and efficacy is established, periodic blood level monitoring of the mood stabilizer, review of potential side effects, physical examination, and laboratory monitoring for side effects are recommended. The patient's general health and reliability should be taken into account in deciding the frequency of monitoring (generally no less than every 3 months). For example, in a healthy, reliable 35-year-old patient whose bipolar illness is well controlled, monitoring of medication, blood levels, and laboratory tests screening for side effects every 3 months is probably adequate in the absence of newly developed symptoms attributable to the medication. In a 50-year-old patient with bipolar disorder, a history of alcohol abuse, liver damage, and treatment noncompliance, blood level monitoring and screening laboratory tests may be needed every 2–4 weeks to ensure compliance and to decrease the risk of serious side effects.

5. Describe an acute manic episode.

The acute manic phase of bipolar illness is heralded by the rapid onset of a persistently elevated, expansive, or irritable mood accompanied by a cluster of symptoms such as inflated self-esteem, grandiosity, decreased need for sleep, increased talking, racing thoughts, easy distractibility, increased motor behavior, increased goal-directed activity, and increased involvement in high-risk, pleasure-seeking activities. The symptoms cause marked impairment in functioning and may have profound effects on others (e.g., intrusive, aggressive behavior, high risk-taking activities, impulsive spending). Additionally, frank psychotic symptoms may be present (e.g., delusions, hallucinations). Hospitalization often is necessary.

6. Discuss the pharmacologic management of an acute manic episode.

Medication is the primary mode of treatment. Lithium and valproate are the principal agents for mania, with response rates reported as high as 80% in bipolar I disorder. After appropriate medical and laboratory evaluation, **lithium** can be initiated at 300 mg orally 3 times/day (no parenteral form is available), then titrated according to side effects, clinical response, and blood level. A blood level of 0.8–1.2 mEq/L generally is required to treat acute mania. A steady-state, stable blood level generally is achieved in about 5 days and is measured 10–12 hours after the lithium dose (e.g., in the morning before the first dose of the day). Changes in dosage require monitoring of lithium levels at least every 5–7 days after the change. Some patients require (and tolerate) levels up to 1.5 mEq/L, although higher levels are not advisable because of the risk of toxicity. Treatment with lithium alone may have a relatively slow response rate (up to 2 weeks after a therapeutic blood level is established); hence adjunctive medication treatment usually is required. **Valproate**, used alternately or adjunctively, often provides more rapid antimanic response (e.g., 3–5 days). Valproate is the preferred treatment in rapid cycling and mixed bipolar states, as well as in mania caused by many medical conditions and in patients intolerant of lithium (e.g., due to allergy). Valproate may be initiated at 250 mg orally 3 times/day, or an oral-loading regimen may be used (e.g., 20 mg/kg/day in divided doses).

Carbamazepine also is effective in acute mania, although it may be slightly less effective than lithium. Treatment is started at 200–600 mg/day in divided doses and titrated as tolerated, usually to 800–1000 mg/day, striving for blood levels of 6–12 ng/ml. Blood levels should be monitored at least weekly initially, with the specimen drawn about 10 hours after the previous dose. Sedation and ataxia early in treatment may slow the upward titration and attainment of therapeutic blood levels. Dermatologic reactions also may occur early in treatment.

If psychotic symptoms are present, the addition of a **neuroleptic (antipsychotic) medication** may be essential. Neuroleptics generally result in rapid improvement (days as opposed to weeks) in agitation, thought disorder, and sleep. For example, haloperidol, 5–20 mg/day in divided doses, is a typical regimen. However, bipolar patients are at an increased risk of neuroleptic malignant syndrome and tardive dyskinesia. In addition, a syndrome of combined lithium-neuroleptic neurotoxicity (e.g., confusion, encephalopathy, delirium, ataxia, nystagmus, extrapyramidal side effects) can occur. Hence, these medications have to be monitored closely.

Atypical antipsychotic medications (e.g., olanzepine, risperidine, quetinpine, clozapine) are becoming the preferred choice due to lower risks of side effects. However, mood cycling and/or switching have been reported.

Benzodiazepines also are widely used in treating acute mania. Both clonazepam and lorazepam are effective in decreasing hyperactivity, controlling agitation, decreasing anxiety, and improving sleep during a manic episode. Both are effective orally (clonazepam, 4–20 mg/day; lorazepam, 4–30 mg/day in divided doses). Lorazepam may be given intramuscularly in severely agitated, noncompliant patients who require acute sedation (up to 4 mg IM). Benzodiazepines may decrease the total required dose of neuroleptic medications, resulting in a lowered risk of neuroleptic-related side effects. In addition, sedative-hypnotic agents often are needed to promote adequate sleep.

Hypomania may be managed with lithium or valproate and benzodiazepines. Doses can be lower than for mania, and treatment may forestall an incipient manic episode.

7. Describe bipolar depression.

Major depressive episodes in patients with bipolar type I and type II disorders are likely to occur more frequently than manic episodes (see Chapter 12). Such episodes are characterized by at least 2 weeks of depressed mood, loss of interest or pleasure in activities, weight loss or gain, insomnia or hypersomnia, psychomotor agitation or slowing, fatigue, loss of energy, feelings of worthlessness, difficulty in thinking, indecisiveness, and recurrent thoughts of death (often with suicidal ideas or attempts). Such patients are significantly distressed, and their functioning is impaired. Bipolar depressions often are characterized by hypersomnia, profound anergy, early age of onset, and/or postpartum onset. A family history of bipolar illness may be present.

8. Discuss the pharmacologic management of bipolar depression.

While one may be inclined to treat manifest depression with antidepressant medications, careful attention is necessary to discern a history of bipolarity, because antidepressants may adversely affect the course of illness in bipolar individuals. All antidepressants can induce switching from depression to mania, with rates of switching as high as 50%. In addition, in bipolar illness, antidepressants may induce rapid mood cycling and mixed mood states (mania and depression co-existing), as well as precipitate difficult-to-treat, severe depressive states.

Hence, treatment of bipolar depression should first make use of mood-stabilizing agents. **Lithium** alone may be used to treat bipolar depression; the response rate is 60–70%. However, response may be slow (6–8 weeks). Blood levels may need to be higher (> 1.2 mEq/L) than in mania. Thyroid augmentation (e.g., thyroxine) may be helpful, even if the patient has normal thyroid levels.

Valproate and **carbamazepine** also can be effective in treating bipolar depression. These medications should be initiated slowly to achieve antidepressant effectiveness, as rapid titration (as used in treating mania) may result in "mood stabilization" in a depressed state.

If depression persists despite a mood-stabilizer regimen, antidepressants may be added. When indicated (e.g., severe, life-threatening depression or depression unresponsive to mood stabilizers and psychotherapy), **buproprion** (75 mg 2 times/day–150 mg 2–3 times/day) or **tranyl-cypromine**, a monoamine oxidase (MAO) inhibitor (10 mg 2 times/day–20 mg 3 times/day) may be good choices; some studies have shown decreased rates of switching relative to other antidepressants. Buproprion may induce seizures; therefore, dosing schedules and total dose must be closely monitored. Tranylcypromine and all MAO inhibitors may interact with other antidepressants, carbamazepine, pressor agents, and food high in the amino acid tyramine to produce a potentially lethal hypertensive crisis. Monitor MAO inhibitors closely, and pay particular attention to patient education about diet restrictions.

Short-half-life **serotonin reuptake inhibitors** such as sertraline and paroxetine also may be reasonable choices; rates of switching may be relatively lower than with tricyclic antidepressants (TCAs). Other antidepressants (e.g., TCAs) clearly are effective in treating bipolar depression, but should be avoided because they have relatively increased rates of switching. Antidepressants should be used for the briefest period necessary to treat the depression, then gradually withdrawn.

Recent trials of **lamotrigine** and **gabapentin** (both anticonvulsants) have shown promise in treating bipolar depression and, perhaps, in stabilizing mood. While data is not yet conclusive, many anecdotal reports and a few controlled studies are supportive. Lamotrigine must be titrated very gradually due to the risk of Stevens-Johnson syndrome and of toxic dermal necrolysis. This risk is increased in the presence of concurrent valproate treatment.

Electroconvulsive therapy clearly is effective in bipolar depression and at times is the preferred treatment (see Question 16).

9. Why are long-term maintenance strategies important in bipolar disorders?

Bipolar disorder is a chronic, relapsing, and remitting illness. At this time there is no cure. In addition, recurrent episodes predispose toward more frequent and severe episodes (a phenomenon known as kindling). Therefore, long-term management is critical, and life-long treatment is extremely likely.

10. What are the goals of maintenance treatment?

The goals of maintenance treatment are to decrease the psychosocial impact of the illness (such as job loss, economic ruin, and loss of relationships), suicide risk, and frequency and severity of recurrence; to improve compliance to treatment regimens, and to achieve the most effective treatment regimen with the fewest possible side effects. Many people with bipolar illness also have significant impairment from mood fluctuation and other symptoms between identifiable episodes of illness (subsyndromal symptoms), which also can be improved with continuous pharmacologic intervention and psychotherapeutic efforts.

11. How is long-term maintenance executed?

Lithium maintenance decreases the frequency and severity of both manic and major depressive episodes. When lithium is stopped abruptly, more than 50% of patients relapse within 6 months. Maintenance therapy with lithium should focus on maintaining the blood level range that was effective in treating acute illness. Lower-dose maintenance has been associated with an increased relapse rate. Long-term lithium maintenance requires monitoring of lithium blood levels (which may change with age, diet, use of other medications, concurrent illness, and state of hydration) and periodic (e.g., every 6 months) assessment of thyroid (TSH) and renal function (BUN and creatinine; 24-hour creatinine clearance in patients with evidence of altered functioning).

Neither valproate nor carbamazepine has been carefully studied in the long-term management of bipolar illness. Some studies (none carefully controlled) suggest that these agents may be useful in decreasing the intensity of recurrent manic episodes. However, when lithium alone is ineffective for maintenance or acute treatment, the *addition* of either valproate or carbamazepine often is beneficial.

Interepisode management may require intermittent use of benzodiazepines during periods of sleep deprivation (e.g., at times of increased acute stress) to decrease the risk of precipitating a manic episode.

Antidepressants should be avoided in long-term management, when possible, because of the risk of inducing rapid-cycling disorders.

Neuroleptics also should be avoided because of the increased risk of tardive dyskinesia and neuroleptic malignant syndrome in patients with bipolar disorder. However, some bipolar patients and all patients with schizoaffective disorder require neuroleptic medications in maintenance regimens. The lowest effective dose should be established to minimize the risk of side effects. Clozapine may be a good choice, because of lower risk of tardive dyskinesia and emerging reports of mood stabilization. However, clozapine should not be the neuroleptic of first choice because of the risk of potentially fatal agranulocytosis. Atypical antipsychotic agents (e.g., olanzapine, risperidone) are becoming the preferred agents.

12. Describe the clinically pertinent pharmacodynamics of the mood-stabilizing agents.

Pharmacodynamic properties are helpful in understanding various clinically pertinent phenomena. For example, with a patient taking lithium, peak blood levels are more likely to be associated with transient side effects (e.g., tremor), and a decrease in total body water (i.e., dehydration) increases blood level and blood level-sensitive side effects (e.g., diarrhea).

When valproate or carbamazepine is used, competition for protein-binding sites and hepatic metabolic pathways affects the doses of concurrently used medications (see Question 13).

Pharmacodynamics of Mood-Stabilizing Agents

MEDICATION	PEAK BLOOD LEVEL (HR)	METABOLISM	HALF-LIFE (HR)	PROTEIN BINDING
Lithium	1–2	Renal excretion	14–30	No (distributed in total body water)
Valproate (Divalproex sodium)	2 3–8	Hepatic	6–16	Yes
Carbamazepine	4–8	Hepatic	18–55	Yes

13. Discuss some significant drug interactions of the mood-stabilizing agents.

Lithium. Blood levels of lithium are increased by thiazide diuretics and nonsteroidal antiinflammatory agents through renal mechanisms. Intracellular concentrations of lithium may be increased by neuroleptic agents. Dehydration also increases lithium levels. Calcium channel blockers may cause increased neurotoxicity.

Valproate. Valproate levels are decreased by inducers of microsomal enzymes, such as carbamazepine, and increased by inhibitors of microsomal enzymes, such as fluoxetine and paroxetine. Valproate increases the blood levels of protein-bound drugs, including phenobarbital, phenytoin, tricyclic antidepressants, digoxin, and warfarin and increases blood levels of lamotrigine.

Carbamazepine. Carbamazepine, an inducer of microsomal enzymes, decreases its own levels (autoinduction) as well as the levels of other drugs, including neuroleptics, benzodiazepines, other anticonvulsants, TCAs, and hormonal contraceptives. However, competition for protein-binding sites may increase blood levels initially when carbamazepine is added to ongoing treatment regimens.

14. Discuss the clinical presentation and management of lithium toxicity.

Lithium toxicity typically occurs at blood levels ≥ 2.0 mEq/L. Some individuals may experience toxicity at lower doses. Neuroleptics may synergistically cause increased neurotoxicity even at therapeutic blood levels. Patients with lithium toxicity may experience lethargy, clumsiness, nausea, vomiting, diarrhea, marked tremulousness, blurred vision, and confusion. Findings on physical exam may include nystagmus, increased deep tendon reflexes, and altered mental status. Such manifestations may progress to include seizures, coma, and cardiac arrhythmias. This progression is more likely to occur in patients with lithium levels > 2.5 mEq/L. Permanent CNS damage may ensue.

Lithium toxicity is a medical emergency and should be managed in an intensive care setting. Fluid and electrolyte monitoring, treatment of arrhythmias and respiratory compromise, and prevention of further gastrointestinal absorption may be required. Hemodialysis is the most effective way of acutely reducing the blood lithium level.

The best treatment of lithium toxicity is prevention, which often is achieved through patient education. Patients need to know the symptoms of lithium toxicity, drugs that may interact with lithium, and the necessity of careful monitoring of blood lithium levels. In addition they need to be aware that avoidable circumstances (such as dehydration and use of nonsteroidal anti-inflammatory agents) may increase lithium levels.

Lithium Toxicity

SYMPTOMS	SIGNS
Lethargy, fatigue	Nystagmus
Clumsiness	Ataxia
Weakness	Increased deep tendon reflexes
Muscle cramping	Altered mental status
Nausea	Cardiac arrhythmia
Vomiting	
Marked tremor	
Blurred vision	
Confusion	

15. Discuss the management of side effects of mood-stabilizing agents.

Side Effect	*Management Strategy*
Lithium	
Gastrointestinal distress (nausea, vomiting, diarrhea	Check blood level; decrease dose if clinically possible
	Take medication with meals
	Change to slow-release preparation
Poor concentration, confusion, sedation	Give majority of dose at bedtime; decrease if clinically possible
Tremor	As above, and add a beta blocker (e.g., propranolol, 10–20 mg up to 3 times/day)
Increased white blood count	Monitor, usually resolves with time
Polydipsia, polyuria (nephrogenic diabetes insipidus)	Decrease dose if severe
	Monitor electrolytes
	Consider adding nonthiazide diuretic
Renal insufficiency	Nephrology consultation
	Lower lithium dose; monitor blood level more frequently
	Consider change to alternate mood stabilizer
Hypothyroidism	Monitor thyroid functions
	Add T_4
Psoriasis	If moderate-to-severe, consider change to alternate mood-stabilizing agents
Acne	Topical antibiotics and retenoic acid
Weight gain	Advise about diet/exercise; lower dose, if possible
Valproate	
Gastrointestinal distress (change in appetite, nausea, vomiting, diarrhea)	May resolve with time
	Give drug with meals
	Change preparations
	Decrease dose
Sedation	As above
	Give bulk of dose at bedtime
Tremor	As above
	Add a beta blocker
Hair loss (usually transient)	B complex vitamins
	Folic acid
	Zinc (50 mg/day) and selenium (50 μg/day)
Minor hepatic transaminase elevation	Decrease dose
	Monitor hepatic enzymes
Asymptomatic thrombocytopenia or leukopenia	Decrease dose
	Monitor platelet and granulocyte counts; if significantly diminished, taper valproate and switch to alternate agent
Pancreatitis, agranulocytosis, severe transaminase elevation or hepatic failure	Potentially fatal
	Discontinue valproate
	Urgent medical consultation
Carbamazepine	
Gastrointestinal distress	Usually transient
	Decrease dose
	Give medication with meals
	Bulk of dose at bedtime
	Consider extended-release preparations

Table continued on following page

Side Effect	*Management Strategy*
Carbamazepine *(cont.)*	
Blurred vision, fatigue, ataxia, sedation, skin rash	As above, may require reduced dose
	Observe
	Antihistamines to control itching with mild rash
	Medical or dermatologic consultation to determine if drug should be discontinued (discontinue if associated with fever, wheezing respiration, or blisterlike skin lesions)
Mild leukopenia	Increase frequency of monitoring white blood cells
	Discontinue if leukopenia persists or worsens
Mild thrombocytopenia	Increase frequency of monitoring platelet counts
	Discontinue if thrombocytopenia persists
Hyponatremia	Monitor electrolytes
	Change mood stabilizers, if hyponatremia persists
Agranulocytosis, aplastic anemia, exfoliative dermatitis, or severe elevation of hepatic enzymes	May be fatal; discontinue drug
	Urgent medical consultation
	Discontinue medication

16. When is electroconvulsive therapy (ECT) used in bipolar disorders?

ECT is effective in treating both acute manic and depressive phases of bipolar illness. Efficacy rates equal or exceed those of lithium, and often with a more rapid onset of action. Although ECT generally is reserved for cases in which standard agents are not effective, it should be considered as a primary treatment when rapid response is necessary or when standard treatments are contraindicated.

ECT may be the primary treatment in manic delirium (a severe mania with identifiable delirium that may include hyperthermia), mania with neuroleptic malignant syndrome, and mania during pregnancy or other medical contraindications to mood-stabilizing medications (e.g., renal impairment, history of allergy to mood-stabilizing agents). ECT also may be used earlier in the course of treatment in patients with psychotic depression and when the risk of slower response may severely compromise the patient's health (e.g., ongoing serious suicide attempts, deteriorating nutritional status).

Lithium generally is discontinued before starting ECT because of an increased risk of delirium and intractable seizures when ECT and lithium are combined.

Indications for ECT as Primary Treatment in Bipolar Illness

Manic delirium
Mania or bipolar depression with neuroleptic malignant syndrome
Medical contraindications to using mood stabilizers
Psychotic bipolar manic or depressive episodes
Severely compromised health (e.g., serious, ongoing suicide attempts)

17. How does age affect the use of mood-stabilizing medications?

Metabolic differences in children, adolescents, and geriatric populations require altered dosing strategies. Hepatic metabolism generally is less efficient in these groups, and lower doses of carbamazepine and valproate are used to establish therapeutic blood levels. In elderly patients, renal function often is diminished; hence a lower dose of lithium is typical. In addition, elderly patients often take other medications (carefully review drug interactions) and are more sensitive to potential neurotoxic effects (blood levels should be maintained at the lower end of the therapeutic range).

18. What other medications are used for mood stabilization?

Although they are not widely used, evidence suggests that calcium channel blockers may be effective as mood stabilizers. For example, verapamil (120–360 mg/day) has been beneficial in bipolar illness. It probably works well in the same group of patients who respond best to lithium (bipolar type I). Newer anticonvulsant medications (e.g., lamotrigine, topiramate, gabapentin) also are being investigated for mood-stabilizing properties.

Some studies demonstrate that atypical antipsychotic agents, especially clozapine and olanzapine, are mood stabilizing.

Long-acting depointramuscular injections of neuroleptic medications (e.g., fluphenazine decanoate, haloperidol decanoate) sometimes are the only effective treatment for patients who are not compliant with oral medication and whose illnesses are severe enough to warrant this approach.

In patients whose mood or behavioral instability is caused by an underlying medical condition (e.g., thyroid disease, brain tumor), identification and aggressive treatment of underlying illnesses may cure the secondary mood disorder.

Intermittent explosive disorder and impulsive aggressive behavior in brain-injured patients also may respond to beta blockers (e.g., propranolol in widely variable doses has been used effectively).

19. How do mood-stabilizing medications work?

The mode of action is not yet known for any of the mood-stabilizing medications. Current research efforts are trying to determine the basic cellular mechanisms that correlate with clinical processes. For example, lithium attenuates neuronal signal transduction mediated by G-proteins, which may be associated with increasing mood stability. Current research also focuses on lithium inhibition of neurotransmitter-receptor–coupled adenylate or cyclase activity, cyclic adenosine monophosphate formation, and metabolism of phosphoinositide in relation to its effect on other significant second-messenger systems. Also under investigation are attenuation of dopamine receptor turnover and function, effects on serotonin synthesis and function and binding of certain serotonin receptors, interactions with protein kinase C, ion-channel function, intracellular calcium mobilization, and impact on gene expression.

With regard to anticonvulsant-type mood stabilizers (e.g., valproate, carbamazepine, lamotrigine, gabapentin), effects on voltage-gated sodium and calcium ion channels, ligand gated ion channels (e.g., GABA receptor/channel), NMDA/glutamate receptor are being investigated.

BIBLIOGRAPHY

1. American Psychiatric Association: Practice guidelines for the treatment of patients with bipolar disorder. Am J Psychiatry 15(Suppl), December, 1994.
2. Bowden CL, et al: Efficiency of divalproex vs. lithium and placebo in the treatment of mania. The Depakote Mania Study Group. JAMA 271:918–924, 1994.
3. Bowden CL, et al (eds): Practical Guidelines for the Management of Bipolar Disorder. Monograph on Treatment. Deerfield, IL, Discovery International, 1992.
4. Calabrese J, et al: A double-blind placebo-controlled study of lamotrigine monotherapy in outpatients with bipolar I depression. J Clin Psychiatry 60(2):79–80, 1999.
5. Freeman M, Stoll A: Mood-stabilizer combinations: A review of safety and efficacy. Am J Psychiatry 155(1):12–21, 1998.
6. Gerner RH, et al: Algorithm for patient management of acute manic states: Lithium, valproate, or carbamazepine? J Clin Psychopharmacol 12:576–635, 1992.
7. Goodwin FK, Jamison KR: Manic-Depressive Illness. New York, Oxford University Press, 1990.
8. Janicak P, Levy N: Rational copharmacy for acute mania. Psychiatric Ann 28(4):204–212, 1998.
9. Jefferson J (Chairperson): Lithium: The present and the future (report on symposium). J Clin Psychiatry 156:41–48, 1995.
10. McElroy SL, et al: Valproate in the treatment of bipolar disorder. Literature review and clinical guidelines. J Clin Psychopharmacol 12(Suppl):42S–52S, 1992.
11. Nemeroff C (ed): Lithium in the treatment of manic-depressive illness: An update. J Clin Psychiatry 59(suppl), 1998.
12. Solomon D, et al: The course of illness and maintenance treatments for patients with bipolar disorder. J Clin Psychiatry 56:5–13, 1995.
13. Suppes T, et al: Risk of recurrence following discontinuation of lithium treatment in bipolar disorder. Arch Gen Psychiatry 48:1082–1088, 1991.
14. Sussman N (ed): Anticonvulsants in Psychiatry. Roundtable Series, 64. London, Royal Society of Medicine Press, 1999.

50. ANTIANXIETY AGENTS

Robert D. Davies, M.D., and Leslie Winter, M.D.

1. What are antianxiety agents?

Antianxiety agents are medications that decrease the symptoms of anxiety and induce calm. The physical symptoms typically seen in anxiety include flushing, palpitations, hyperventilation or shortness of breath, tremulousness, sweating, nausea, diarrhea, urinary urgency, dizziness, and lightheadedness. This is not to say that antianxiety agents are medications whose *only* actions are to decrease anxiety. In fact, many drugs commonly used to treat anxiety also have other beneficial effects (such as inducing sleep, muscle relaxation, anticonvulsant effects, and antidepressant effects). The most widely used antianxiety agents are benzodiazepines. However, as new drugs are developed and the full ranges of their beneficial effects are understood, many unique compounds, as well as established classes of drugs, are being found to have significant anxiolytic effects.

2. How do benzodiazepines work?

Benzodiazepines are believed to exert their anxiolytic effect by binding to the GABA-benzodiazepine receptors in the brain. GABA (gamma-aminobutyric acid) is the primary inhibitory neurotransmitter. Benzodiazepines and GABA enhance the binding of each other to this receptor complex. Benzodiazepines are presumed to have no direct effect on this complex other than to increase GABA's effect on chloride channels. The binding of GABA to the receptor complex opens these channels, causing a decrease in neuronal excitability and thereby decreasing anxiety.

3. How do I choose which benzodiazepine to use in a given situation?

The two most important factors in choosing a particular benzodiazepine for a given clinical situation are the **onset of action** and the **half-life**. Benzodiazepines with rapid onsets of action and short half-lives typically are useful for inducing sedation and/or sleep (and are therefore referred to as sedative/hypnotics). Using benzodiazepines with long half-lives for sleep induction will likely result in early morning grogginess or a "hang-over" effect. When treating occasional panic attacks (regardless of the disorder in which they occur), benzodiazepines with rapid onsets of action afford the quickest relief of symptoms. For more persistent forms of anxiety (such as is seen in generalized anxiety disorder or panic disorder with frequent panic attacks and/or significant anticipatory anxiety), benzodiazepines with longer half-lives tend to be more beneficial. Benzodiazepines with longer half-lives also may allow an easier taper and discontinuation when they have been used in a more chronic fashion.

Pharmacokinetic Properties of Commonly Used Benzodiazepines

DRUG	ONSET OF ACTION (HRS)	HALF-LIFE (HRS)
Alprazolam	1–2	10–15
Chlordiazepoxide	2	> 50
Clonazepam	1–2	18–20
Clorazepate	1–2	> 50
Diazepam	1–2	> 50
Flurazepam	0.5–2	> 50
Lorazepam	1–2	10–15
Oxazepam	3	10–15
Temazepam	1–2	7–12
Triazolam	0.5–2	2–4

4. List the effects that benzodiazepines have on the stages of sleep.
- Increase total sleep time
- Increase amount of time spent in Stage 2
- Decrease amount of time spent in Stages 3 and 4
- Increase REM latency
- Decrease amount of time spent in REM sleep

5. What side effects are commonly seen with benzodiazepines?
As a rule, benzodiazepines have a more favorable side-effect profile than other medications used in the treatment of anxiety. The most obvious side-effect is sedation. Other side effects include weakness or fatigue, ataxia, dry mouth, clumsiness, slurred speech, confusion (particularly in the elderly), and depression.

6. What are the potential risks of chronic treatment with benzodiazepines?
The greatest concern about the chronic use of benzodiazepines is the development of **dependence**. Approximately 50% of people who have been on a regular benzodiazepine dose for 4–6 months develop dependence. Dependence becomes apparent when the drug is discontinued and withdrawal symptoms emerge. **Symptoms of withdrawal** include agitation, insomnia, moodiness, irritability, headaches, anorexia, sweating, tremulousness, nausea, and perceptual disturbances. Sudden discontinuation of a benzodiazepine is likely to precipitate a severe withdrawal reaction that may include seizures. A more gradual taper, however, might only elicit mild withdrawal symptoms. Withdrawal symptoms usually are time-limited—peaking shortly after they appear and then diminishing over the next several days. The onset of withdrawal symptoms varies depending on the length of action of the benzodiazepine being used. Withdrawal symptoms from short-acting drugs may begin within 24 hours. For intermediate-acting drugs, the onset is within 1–2 days, and for long-acting drugs the onset may not be until 3–7 days after discontinuation.

Concerns about patients abusing benzodiazepines are probably exaggerated. For those patients with alcohol or drug abuse histories, this is a reasonable concern. But the majority of people who are prescribed benzodiazepines do not have drug abuse histories and do not tend to abuse their medication. The most common cause of a "drug-seeking" patient, who uses up the prescription earlier than planned, is inadequate treatment of anxiety.

Other concerns about chronic treatment with benzodiazepines include the possibility of developing **memory impairment** and **depression**. In addition, as people age they become more sensitive to the effects of benzodiazepines (particularly to effects on cognition and balance), and the clearance of these agents is decreased. Dosage adjustments should be considered for aging patients on chronic benzodiazepine regimens.

7. How fast can I withdraw someone from a benzodiazepine?
It depends on which benzodiazepine is being tapered, the dose that the person has been taking, and how long he or she has been taking it. In those cases where the person has been taking a benzodiazepine for 2 weeks or less, it is safe to just stop the medication. When treatment has lasted 2–4 weeks, a fairly quick taper schedule can be employed, with doses reduced by 50% every 3–4 days.

When tapering a benzodiazepine that has been used for more than 12 weeks, decreases in dose should not exceed 25% of the total daily dose. For intermediate-acting agents, this can occur in weekly increments. For long-acting benzodiazepines, however, changes should not occur sooner than every 2 weeks. In cases where someone has been taking a benzodiazepine for more than 6 months, extending the time between dosage reductions even more may improve the success of the taper.

It is important to plan out the taper with the patient and educate them about the possibility of some mild, transient withdrawal symptoms occurring after each decrease in dose. Keep in mind the psychological aspects of dependence—many patients experience increased anxiety as they proceed with a taper because of their fear of not having the medication.

8. What is the difference between withdrawal, rebound, and recurrence?

Withdrawal is the time-limited development of unique symptoms (as described in Question 6) as the result of decreasing or discontinuing the use of a psychoactive drug. *Rebound* occurs when a drug is withdrawn and the individual experiences anxiety symptoms that are more severe than those experienced prior to treatment. *Recurrence* is when the person experiences the same symptoms and severity of symptoms that existed prior to treatment.

All of these phenomena can occur with the discontinuation of benzodiazepines, but they also have been described with nonbenzodiazepine treatments for anxiety (particularly SSRIs).

9. What other medications can be used to treat anxiety?

- **Beta-blockers**, such as propranolol, can be used to treat the physiologic symptoms of anxiety experienced in specific phobic situations. Their direct effect is to decrease autonomic arousal, although this may have an indirect effect on the cognitive components of the phobic response by interrupting the physiological feed-back loop that fuels catastrophic, distorted thought processes. Most commonly, these agents are used on an as-needed basis 30 minutes prior to the anxiety-producing situation. The typical dose range for propranolol is 10–40 mg.
- **Buspirone**, a selective agonist of the $5HT_{1A}$ receptor, is a safe and effective treatment for generalized anxiety disorder. It has not been shown, however, to be effective in treating panic disorder, specific phobias, or social phobia. Dependence does not occur with chronic buspirone treatment. The clinical response is often delayed for up to 2 weeks of regular, daily use, and it is not effective when used on an as-needed basis.
- **Tricyclic antidepressants** (TCAs) are effective treatments for panic disorder and generalized anxiety disorder—although they have not demonstrated efficacy in social phobia. Care must be taken when initiating treatment with a TCA, as many people experience palpitations which may trigger a worsening of anxiety symptoms. The side-effect profile of TCAs tends to limit their current use, as newer agents with more agreeable side-effect profiles (such as SSRIs) have become available.
- **Monoamine oxidase inhibitors** are useful in the treatment of panic disorder and social phobia. Despite their clear efficacy, their use is limited now because of the risk of hypertensive crisis induced by tyramine-containing foods and interactions with other medications.
- **Serotonin-specific reuptake inhibitors** (SSRIs) are quickly becoming the mainstay treatment of most anxiety disorders. They are effective in treating panic disorder, social phobia, generalized anxiety disorder, and obsessive-compulsive disorder. Anecdotal reports also suggest their efficacy in post-traumatic stress disorder. For the most part, they have a favorable side-effect profile (although certain side effects, such as sexual dysfunction, become prohibitive to their use in some cases). SSRIs may cause an initial worsening of anxiety and therefore treatment often is started at very low doses.
- **Venlafaxine**, which inhibits the reuptake of serotonin and norepinephrine, has been shown to be effective in treating panic disorder, social phobia, and generalized anxiety disorder.
- **Newer agents** that act on the GABA receptor complex, such as gabapentin, are showing promise as being effective antianxiety agents as well.

10. What benefits over benzodiazepines do these other agents offer?

Use of these agents does not lead to dependence, as is seen with chronic benzodiazepine use. Therefore, they tend to be considered safer for chronic treatment. They also are the better option for use in individuals with histories of drug abuse or dependence. The antidepressants have the added benefit of treating comorbid depression—a common occurrence in individuals with anxiety disorders.

11. What drawbacks do the use of these drugs have?

Neither the antidepressants nor buspirone offer immediate relief from symptoms. Often there is at least a 2-week lag in response. Delay in symptom relief may play some role in the development of phobic avoidance behaviors. As mentioned previously, the TCAs and the SSRIs both may cause some initial worsening of anxiety symptoms. For these two reasons, it often is necessary to initially start a person on an antidepressant along with a benzodiazepine, and then later discontinue the benzodiazepine.

BIBLIOGRAPHY

1. Keck PE, McElroy SL: New uses for antidepressants: Social phobia. J Clin Psychiatry 58(Suppl 14):32–36, 1997.
2. Pies RW: Handbook of Essential Psychopharmacology. Washington DC, American Psychiatric Press, Inc., 1998.
3. Schatzberg AF, Nemeroff CB: Textbook of Psychopharmacology, 2nd ed. Washington, DC, American Psychiatric Press, Inc., 1998.
4. Schnabel T: Evaluation of the safety and side effects of antianxiety agents. Am J Med 82:7–13, 1987.
5. Schweizer E: Generalized anxiety disorder: Longitudinal course and pharmacologic treatment. Psychiatr Clin North Am 18(4):843–857, 1995.
6. Uhlenhuth EH, Balter MB, Ban TA, Yang K: International study of expert judgment on therapeutic use of benzodiazepines and other psychotherapeutic medications: V. Treatment strategies in panic disorder, 1992–1997. J Clin Psychopharm 18(6 Suppl 2):27S–31S, 1998.

51. SEDATIVE-HYPNOTIC DRUGS

Kim Nagel, M.D.

1. What clinical situations provide clearcut indications for sedative-hypnotic drugs?
Transient insomnia and recurrent transient insomnia are the only clearcut indications for sedative-hypnotic drugs. Additional indications and longer-term use require careful clinical assessment and weighing other treatment options.

2. How is transient insomnia defined?
Transient insomnia is a period of insomnia usually 1–14 days in length and often in response to a specific stressor (e.g., loss, illness, hospitalization, long-distance travel). After a duration of 3 months, insomnia is considered to be subacute or chronic and requires further work-up to define underlying etiology.

Case study: A 34-year-old woman presents 7 days after the unexpected death of her father. She reports trouble getting to sleep before 2–2:30 AM, difficulty arising for work in the morning, and daytime fatigue. Although sad, she reports few vegetative signs of depression. She is given 20 tablets of zolpidem, 10 mg, to use as needed over the next 3–4 weeks. At follow-up she says that she took the medication nightly with good response and ran out 3 days before her appointment. She has slept only approximately 5 hours for the last 3 nights off medication and feels that continuing it would be helpful. A few times in the last week she woke up early and was unable to return to sleep, but overall she feels that her mood is good. Two additional refills of zolpidem, 10 mg, are given with follow-up as needed.

Her next visit occurs in 8 weeks, and she reports that early morning awakening has become more frequent. Occasionally she takes an additional one-half pill to get back to sleep at 3:00 AM. When she ran out of pills, sleep became much more difficult and impairment of concentration at work became more noticeable. She says that she has lost weight and feels less enthusiasm. Major depression is diagnosed, and sertraline is started at 50 mg and increased to 100 mg the next week. Four weeks after starting sertraline, her sleep returns to normal, and she stops zolpidem on her own. At this point she agrees that weekly psychotherapy would be beneficial to deal with issues arising from her father's death and that continuing sertraline is appropriate at this time.

3. What is the recommended treatment for transient insomnia?
A consensus paper published by the National Institute of Mental Health (NIMH) in 1984 stated that benzodiazepines (and closely related compounds) are the first choice of medication for transient insomnia because of safety, efficacy, and side-effect profiles. The consensus recommended use of the lowest possible dose for the shortest period of time until insomnia improves, with a maximum of 20 doses/month for 3 months.

4. Why is it important to avoid long-term use of sedative-hypnotic medication?

Long-term use of hypnotics should be avoided for several reasons. First, many cases of insomnia are truly transient, and patients need to be informed clearly that brief treatment may be adequate. Some patients develop a habit of regular sedative usage; when they stop, the may be disturbed by brief rebound insomnia and believe that they must stay on medication. Tolerance, which tends to develop to most sedatives over time, decreases their efficacy and may promote escalation of dosage. All sedative/hypnotics have side effects, including decreased dreaming and deep sleep and increased brief arousals at night, which make sleep less restful (see Question 8). Even more important is that long-term symptomatic treatment of insomnia may prevent the detection of an underlying medical or psychiatric condition that can be treated with better response.

Although a number of conditions may benefit from long-term sedatives, it is important to diagnose and treat them adequately. In general, nonaddictive agents are preferred to treat chronic insomnia. Some studies have supported long-term use of *nonbenzodiazepine* hypnotics as a safe and effective treatment. An open trial in France of 180 consecutive days of 10–20 mg of zolpidem for insomnia showed little tolerance and virtually no withdrawal or rebound insomnia after discontinuation.

5. What factors should be considered in deciding which hypnotic is most appropriate for a specific patient?

Assess the form of the patient's insomnia. The four most common types of insomnia are:
• Sleep onset or initial insomnia
• Frequent short awakenings
• One or two long awakenings
• Early morning awakening (early awakening is a common symptom in major depressive disorder)
Assess pertinent characteristics of the sedative-hypnotic:
• Rate of absorption
• Extent of distribution in body and CNS
• Affinity of CNS receptors
• Elimination half-life
• Route of metabolic biotransformation
For the sake of simplification, rate of absorption and elimination half-life can be used to guide drug choice.

GABA$_A$ Benzodiazepine Receptor Agonist Hypnotics

	HALF-LIFE (HRS)	ABSORPTION	TYPICAL DOSAGE
Zaleplon (Sonata)	1–1.2	Fast	5–10 mg
Zolpidem (Ambien)	1.5–4	Fast	2.5–10 mg
Triazolam (Halcion)	2–5	Fast	0.125–0.25 mg
Zopiclone	5–6	Fast	3.75–7.5 mg
Temazepam (Restoril)	8–12	Moderate	7.5–30 mg
Estazolam (Prosom)	12–20	Moderate	1–2 mg
Oxazepam (Serax)	5–15	Moderate	10–25 mg
Alprazolam (Xanax)	12–20	Fast	0.25–1.0 mg
Lorazepam (Ativan)	10–22	Moderate	0.5–2 mg
Clonazepam (Klonipin)	22–38	Slow	0.5–2 mg
Quazepam (Doral)	50–200	Fast	7.5–15 mg
Flurazepam (Dalmane)	50–200	Fast	15–30 mg

6. What drugs are most helpful for sleep onset or initial insomnia?

If the patient has trouble falling asleep initially, zolpidem, triazolam, zaleplon, and temazepam are the best choices. **Zolpidem** is effective, rapidly absorbed, cleared quickly from the system, and there is minimal evidence of memory loss, motor incoordination, tolerance, or withdrawal symptoms.

Zaleplon 10 mg has the same rapid onset of action and rapid clearing. Its short duration of action may convey even less risk of impairing coordination or cognition.

A number of studies have suggested that **triazolam** is equivalent in efficacy and side effects (except perhaps rebound insomnia) if not used above 0.25 mg. It is a reasonable next choice at one-third the price.

The fourth choice is **temazepam**, 15–30 mg, which is the least expensive of the four. Occasionally the three shorter-acting agents shift the patient's sleep pattern from sleep-onset insomnia to early morning awakening after the drug is mostly cleared from the system. Temazepam's longer duration of action may be helpful to combat this tendency. As temazepam is slowly absorbed, it may need to be taken 1–1½ hours before bedtime to aid getting to sleep. Elderly patients are generally given one-half the average adult dosage.

7. What drugs are most helpful for nocturnal and early morning awakening?

Temazepam is the first choice for nocturnal and early morning awakenings. It is slowly absorbed, but its peak effect begins about 1–1½ hours after administration and persists for 6–10 hours. This duration of action may be ideal to maintain sleep until morning without leaving the patient groggy the next day. Depending on the patient, shorter-acting (triazolam, zolpidem) or longer-acting (estazolam, oxazepam, lorazepam, clonazepam) may be more suitable.

The long-acting drugs, such as flurazepam, quazepam, and chlorazepate, are quite effective for nocturnal and early morning awakenings, but the patient may have daytime hangover, memory loss, or incoordination. These drugs are best for very anxious patients or for infrequent or intermittent usage.

Zaleplon offers unique benefits. Three to four hours after ingestion, patients are nearly free of impaired cognition or coordination; thus, depending on arising time, the patient may take zaleplon as late as 2–3 AM to return to sleep without fear of hangover. This allows the patient to take medication only if he or she needs it, rather than prophylactically at bedtime in case nocturnal or early morning awakening occurs.

8. What are the likely side effects of benzodiazepine receptor agonists?

The most common side effects of benzodiazepine receptor agonists are daytime sedation, motor incoordination, slow reaction times, anterograde and retrograde amnesia, confusional states, withdrawal states, rebound insomnia, respiratory depression, tolerance to drug effect, and potential for abuse.

9. With such side effects, why are benzodiazepine receptor agonists the drugs of choice?

They are easily tolerated by most patients and highly effective in 75–90% of cases. Side effects can be minimized by drug choice, regulation of dosage, and dosing schedules. One of the major advantages is their safety in overdose. The lethal dose is so large for all benzodiazepine receptor agonists death is unlikely even from a whole month's supply. A patient merely becomes highly sedated until the drug is cleared from the bloodstream.

10. What is anterograde amnesia? Discuss its cause and prevention.

Anterograde amnesia is impaired consolidation of new memories of experiences or learning after administration of a drug. In contrast, retrograde amnesia is impaired recall of previously consolidated memory. Anterograde amnesia may occur when high doses of long-acting or short-acting drugs are used. It generally is prevented by using as low a dose of a hypnotic as possible and avoiding concurrent usage of other drugs or alcohol. High-potency hypnotics are more likely to cause anterograde amnesia.

11. What are the guidelines for prescribing to elderly patients or other groups that may suffer from impaired liver metabolism?

For elderly patients or patients with liver impairment, very short-acting drugs such as triazolam, zaleplon, or zolpidem, or drugs that do not require hydroxylation by the liver, are preferred. Temazepam, lorazepam, and oxazepam are excreted by the kidneys without necessity of liver hydroxylation; therefore, their metabolism and excretion are not prolonged by age or liver dysfunction.

Unexpected falls may be an unfortunate consequence of motor incoordination induced by hypnotics used in the elderly. The weakened and brittle nature of their bones makes them highly prone to hip fractures if they fall. The likelihood of hip fracture in the elderly may be correlated with the half-life of a regularly used hypnotic. One study showed that flurazepam is twice as likely as triazolam to cause a hip fracture with regular use in elderly patients.

12. What are the effects of sedative/hypnotic drugs on sleep quality?

Benzodiazepine hypnotics generally increase total sleep time, tend to suppress and delay REM or dreaming sleep, increase the duration of stage 2 sleep, and decrease the amount of stage 3 and 4 or deep sleep. Most users feel more refreshed and alert in the daytime compared with periods of insomnia but less rested than in periods of normal, unmedicated sleep. Stopping such drugs after short or intermediate term usage may result in REM rebound (increase in REM sleep) and rebound insomnia for 0–3 days. Studies of zolpidem indicate that it increases total sleep time, increases deep sleep but does not suppress REM sleep or create REM rebound with discontinuation. Zaleplon decreases sleep latency, increases deep sleep, but may decrease REM sleep. Correct doses of most benzodiazepine receptor agonists enhance next day functioning.

13. What is the mechanism of action of benzodiazepine and nonbenzodiazepine hypnotics?

Both benzodiazepine and the newer nonbenzodiazepine hypnotics have an inhibitory effect on the central nervous system that is mediated through the stimulation of benzodiazepine receptors creating an agonist effect on the neurotransmitter, gamma-aminobutyric acid (GABA). The $GABA_A$ receptor complex in the brain contains two benzodiazepine receptor subtypes: omega-1 (ω_1) and omega-2 (ω_2). Agonistic stimulation of these receptors causes hyperpolarization of associated neural membranes which decreases the cell's excitability or response to stimulus. Omega-1 receptors seem to mediate sedation, whereas omega-2 receptors mediate anxiety reduction, anticonvulsant activity and, unfortunately, memory loss and motor incoordination. Most benzodiazepines stimulate both omega-1 and omega-2 receptors; therefore, their sedative effect correlates with an adverse effect on coordination and memory. Benzodiazepines typically stimulate a third receptor, omega-3 (ω_3), but these receptors are mostly located in the spinal cord and have no relevance to sleep, memory, or coordination. It should be that patients will feel an improvement in well-being from use of a hypnotic without an objective response in total sleep time. Changes in perception of sleep duration may be part of the drug's mode of action.

14. Is it possible to create a drug with fewer side effects by stimulating only the benzodiazepine omega-1 receptors?

Theoretically, yes. At least three drugs have shown a pharmacological profile of selective binding to omega-1 receptors. These include quazepam, zolpidem, and zaleplon. Quazepam itself is ω_1-selective, but its two long-acting metabolites are approximately 150 times more potent and not ω_1-selective. Zolpidem is ω_1-selective and has no significant active metabolites. It has the theoretical advantage of ω_1 selectivity but has not been shown to have a statistically significant advantage in reduction of motor incoordination or memory impairment over non–ω_1-selective, short-acting benzodiazepines (e.g., triazolam) at typical therapeutic dosages. Evidence does suggest that zolpidem may offer a more physiologically normal sleep, produce fewer withdrawal symptoms, and be less prone to induce tolerance.

Zaleplon is another nonbenzodiazepine sedative hypnotic with ω_1 receptor selectivity. It differs from other short-acting sedatives in that its elimination half-life is only one hour. Studies have shown very little effect on cognition or coordination at 3–4 hours post ingestion. This implies the possibility of using zaleplon not only to treat sleep onset insomnia but also to treat nocturnal or early morning awakenings as long as there is still 4 hours till arising time.

15. In addition to transient insomnia, what other common diagnoses or conditions may benefit from the use of sedative-hypnotic agents?

- Chronic insomnia due to:

  Age. One's ability to remain asleep decreases with age. In severe cases, after encouraging physical activity and sleep hygiene, the clinician may give a 2-week trial of zolpidem, 5 mg; triazolam, 0.125 mg; or temazepam, 7.5–15 mg. If the drug is clearly helpful and side effects are not severe, it may be continued with attempts to shift to intermittent dosing if tolerance begins to develop.

Chronic pain. Many nocturnal arousals from sleep are caused by pain. Tricyclic antidepressants (e.g., amitriptyline, 10–50 mg, doxepin, 10–50 mg) are first choices in patients with chronic pain, because they reduce pain sensations as well as frequency or duration of awakenings.

Chronic medical condition. Congestive heart failure is an example of a chronic medical condition that induces severely fragmented sleep. Temazepam, 15 mg, has been shown to decrease nighttime awakening and arousals and to improve daytime alertness with no compromise of the medical condition.

Medication side effects. For example, in a 38-year-old asthmatic woman taking long-acting theophylline (300 mg/day) and using a metaproterenol sulfate inhaler (2 puffs 4 times/day), the stimulating effects of medication may induce severe insomnia and occasional symptoms of anxiety. Flurazepam, 15 mg, can be used at bedtime 3–6 times/'week to inhibit insomnia and daytime anxiety.

Fibromyalgia, chronic fatigue syndrome. First choices are doxepin, 10–50 mg at bedtime; amitriptyline, 10–50 mg at bedtime; or nortriptyline, 10–50 mg at bedtime (if anticholinergic effect of doxepin or amitriptyline is too strong). Studies show that sleep improvement is correlated with improvement in pain or fatigue in some patients. Patients who are intolerant of tricyclic antidepressants may consider trazodone, 25–100 mg, short-acting benzodiazepines, or mirtazapine, 15–60 mg qhs.

- Major depression
- Bipolar affective disorder
- Dysthymic disorder
- Panic disorder
- Generalized anxiety disorder
- Posttraumatic stress disorder

• Psychophysiologic insomnia. This is a conditioned negative response to one's sleep environment. Sleep hygiene, sleep restriction, stimulus control, and relaxation training often are effective. Short-acting benzodiazepine receptor agonists may aid psychological intervention as well as low-dose sedating tricyclics or trazodone.

• Restless leg syndrome. This crawling discomfort in the legs makes one feel a need to stretch or move the legs and causes sleep onset insomnia. It may be associated with iron or B12 deficiency anemia, renal disease, or pregnancy after week 20.

• Periodic leg movements of sleep. Leg-jerking movements accompany restless leg syndrome but also may occur up to 2–3 times/minute during sleep in patients without restless leg symptoms. The arousals that they cause may make sleep nonrestorative.

Recommended order of treatment for restless leg syndrome and periodic leg movements is Sinemet (the combination of carbidopa [15 mg] and levodopa [100 mg]), 1–2 tablets at bedtime. (This works about 50%of the time but may induce nightmares.) If it fails, try an alternative dopamine agonist like bromocriptine or pergolide. Other alternatives include:

Temazepam, 15–30 mg at bedtime

Clonazepam, 0.5–2 mg at bedtime

Percocet (the combination of oxycodone HCL and acetaminophen), 1–2 tablets at bedtime. This may be the most effective treatment, but the addictive nature of the drug requires that the leg movements must be severe and documented by nocturnal polysomnogram. Studies have shown that Percocet and other opiates actually eliminate the leg-jerking movements rather than just allow the patient to sleep through the disturbance of the movement. Dosage can be held steady for many years without significant tolerance to benefits.

• Circadian/rhythm disturbances

Melatonin is a hormone created by the pineal gland at night in concert with the calm phase of the body's daily rhythm. Evidence suggests that 1–2 tablets of 2.5-mg Melatonin given in early afternoon help to maintain or reregulate an out-of-sync circadian rhythm.

Triazolam, 0.125–0.25 mg, or zolpidem, 5–10 mg, also may be used to help reestablish a normal circadian sleep pattern.

Bright light therapy can be used to reset circadian rhythm.

16. What changes in strategy can be used in prescribing hypnotics for chronic conditions?

• Use benzodiazepines on an intermittent basis 1–4 times/week to decrease tolerance and maintain potency.

• Strictly reinforce daily routine and relaxation techniques to enhance efficacy of medication.

• In appropriate populations for either primary or adjunctive treatment, consider alternatives, such as:

Antidepressants (see Question 18)
Mood stabilizers (see Question 19)
Antihistamines (see Question 20)
Antipsychotics (see Question 20)

17. How does one approach the evaluation of the patient who has chronically used benzodiazepines and/or alcohol for treatment of a chronic insomnia?

Sedative-hypnotics and alcohol are estimated to be the *cause* of 10–15% of cases of insomnia due to withdrawal symptoms and tendency to cause arousal and nonrestorative sleep. Alcohol has no place in chronic treatment of insomnia, and abstinence should be recommended. If this is difficult, formal detoxification and enrollment in substance abuse treatment may be needed. More compliant patients can stop alcohol and reduce their sedative/hypnotic by one therapeutic equivalent/week (e.g., 0.125 mg triazolam, 15 mg temazepam, or 5 mg zolpidem). During this period one should closely evaluate the patient for symptoms beyond the expected mild withdrawal symptoms (e.g., panic attacks, mood instability). The purpose of the taper and discontinuation is to allow better diagnosis of any underlying etiology of the insomnia and potentially to provide more effective treatment.

18. List antidepressant medications that may be used for their sedative properties.

Antidepressant Medications with Sedative Properties*

DRUG	DOSAGE	USES
Mirtazapine (Remeron)	18–60 mg	Fibromyalgia, adjunctive use with SSRI, can inhibit nausea, but often increases appetite
Amitriptyline (Elavil)	10–100 mg	Chronic pain, peripheral neuropathy, fibromyalgia
Doxepin (Sinequam)	10–200 mg	Chronic fatigue syndrome, fibromyalgia, post alcohol withdrawal insomnia, as adjunct with nonsedating selective serotonin reuptake inhibitors (SSRIs)
Trazodone (Desyrel)	25–200 mg	Adjunct to nonsedating SSRI; make sure to warn men about risk of priapism and potential need for immediate withdrawal from drug; also warn of orthostatic hypotension
Nortriptyline (Pamelor)	25–200 mg	Often helpful for mild-to-moderate anxiety disorder and insomnia
Nefadazone (Serzone)	100–500 mg	Less sedation than trazodone without risk of orthostatic changes or priapism; no REM sleep suppression
Fluvoxamine	25–300 mg	Most sedating of serotonin reuptake inhibitors

* From most sedative to least sedative.

19. How are mood stabilizers used as hypnotics?

Adequate sleep is essential to stabilize a bipolar affective disorder. Carbamazepine is moderately to highly sedating and a typical sedating dose is 100–400 mg at bedtime. Bedtime doses of 100–400 mg may be used adjunctively with other primary mood stabilizers like lithium or valproate. Valproate is mildly to moderately sedating and may be used at doses of 125–1500 mg at bedtime. Both often may be used as adjunctive medicine for sedation or mood stabilization in patients still suffering from insomnia while treated with lithium carbonate or another mood stabilizer. In addition, they may be desired as primary agents in mixed or rapid cycling bipolar disorders with severe insomnia. These show some utility in patients with posttraumatic stress disorder, insomnia, nightmares, night terrors, and agitated drug withdrawal states. Although responses can be varied, Neurontest (gabapentin 100–200 mg) or Lomictal (lamotrigine 235–400 mg) can show distinctly sedative properties which may improve sleep and stabilization of bipolar disorder.

20. What other drugs are of occasional usefulness as sedative-hypnotic agents?

Other Drugs With Sedative-Hypnotic Properties

DRUG	DOSAGE	USES
Antihistamines		
Diphenhydramine	25–100 mg	Allergies, mild insomnia, patients at risk to abuse medications, patients on antipsychotic medication with extrapyramidal symptoms such as muscle dystonia or parkinson-like tremor
Cyproheptadine	4–40 mg	Posttraumatic stress disorder, cluster headaches with insomnia, nightmares
Atypical Neuroleptics		
Quetapine (Seroquel)	25–600 mg	First-line treatments for psychotic disorders; often useful in
Olanzapine (Zyprexa)	2.5–20 mg	bipolar disorder or in borderline personality disorder; atyp
Risperidine (Risperdal)	0.9–10 mg	ical neuroleptics commonly used for insomnia, agitation, or paranoia in elderly demented patients
Traditional Neuroleptics		
Thioridazine (Mellenil)	10–800 mg	
Penphenazine (Tailafon)	2–66 mg	
Haloperidol (Haldol)	0.5–40 mg	
Others		
Buspirone	5–40 mg	Shown to be effective occasionally for nocturnal agitation in elderly patients
Clonidine	0.1–1.2 mg	Opiate withdrawal insomnia, refractory posttraumatic stress disorder, and treatment-resistant bipolar disorder
Valerian	400–900 mg	Limited evidence of mild hypnotic effect; little safety data and no comparisons to other drugs

21. Which agents should *not* be prescribed for sleep?
    Ethchlorvynol, methaqualone, and barbiturates no longer have a place as sedative/hypnotic agents alone. They have greater risk of abuse, dependence, and lethal overdose and tend to lose effectiveness much more rapidly than benzodiazepines. Alcohol is sedating but promotes nocturnal awakenings, and severely impairs sleep quality; tolerance develops rapidly. Chloral hydrate is now felt to be of only brief, limited usefulness because of overdose potential, rapid tolerance, GI disturbance, and interactions with other drugs. A review of all evidence about melatonin's efficacy found no evidence that it improves sleep. There are also concerns that melatonin may inhibit ovarian function, alter immune system, or cause vasoconstriction of cerebral and coronary arteries. Patients taking steroids, those with an immune disease, cancers of the immune system, and women of childbearing age should be counseled not to use it.

22. Are sedative-hypnotics associated with homicidal behavior, psychotic reactions, or agitation?
    Short-acting hypnotics have been associated with agitated states, sleepwalking, psychotic reactions, and at least two cases of homicide. Triazolam has been associated with at least two cases of homicide. It is suspected that the underlying pathology that caused the insomnia may have been a major factor. A committee of the U.S. Institute of Medicine thoroughly reviewed all studies and literature related to triazolam and concluded they ". . . do not support clearly the existence of a unique profile or syndrome of adverse events." Zolpidem has been associated with sleepwalking and pyschotic reactions that are unrecallable the next day. With the million of users of these drugs, it is unlikely that they represent a significant hazard. It is prudent to avoid short-acting sedatives in patients

with history of severe agitation, highly anxious states, and impulsiveness and to keep sedative hypnotic dosages within accepted parameters.

BIBLIOGRAPHY

1. Bunney WE Jr, Azarnoff DL, et al: Report of the Institute of Medicine Committee on the Efficacy and Safety of Halcion. Arch Gen Psychiatry 56:349–352, 1999.
2. Greenblatt DI, Harmatz JS, von Moltke LL, et al: Comparative kinetics and dynamics of zaleplon, zolpidem, and placebo. Clin Pharmacol Ther 64(5):553–561, 1998.
3. Kryger M, Roth T, Dement WD (eds): Principles and Practice of Sleep Medicine, 3rd ed. Philadelphia, W.B. Saunders, 1999.
4. Lobo BL, Greene WL: Zolpidem: Distinct from triazolam? Ann Pharmacother 31(5):625–632, 1997.
5. Mendelson WB: Efficacy of melatonin as a hypnotic agent. J Biol Rhythms 12(6):651–656, 1997.
6. National Institute of Mental Health, National Institutes of Health: Drugs and Insomnia. Consensus Development Conference Summary, vol 4, no 10. Bethesda, MD, U.S. Department of Health and Human Services, 1984.
7. Nolen TM: Sedative effects of antihistamines: Safety, performance, learning, and quality of life. Clin Ther 19(1):39–55, 1997.
8. Poceta JS, Mitler MM: Sleep Disorders: Diagnosis and Treatment. Totowa, NJ, Humana Press, 1998.
9. Reite ML, Nagel KE, Ruddy JR: Concise Guide to the Evaluation and Management of Sleep Disorders. Washington, DC, American Psychiatric Press, 1997.
10. Wagner J, Wagner ML, Hening WA: Beyond benzodiazepines: Alternative pharmacologic agents for the treatment of insomnia. Ann Pharmacother 32(6):680–691, 1998.

52. THE USE OF STIMULANTS IN PSYCHIATRIC PRACTICE

Hubert H. Thomason, Jr., M.D.

1. List the common stimulants prescribed in psychiatric practice.

Generic Name	Trade Name	Dose Range
Dextroamphetamine	Dexedrine; Dextrostat	5–60 mg/day
Dextroamphetamine/amphetamine (mixture)	Adderall	5–60 mg/day
Methylphenidate	Ritalin; Ritalin SR; Metadate; Metadate ER	5–60 mg/day
Modafinil	Provigil	100–400 mg/day

2. Describe the physiologic effects of stimulants.

Stimulants increase catecholaminergic activity in the brain through inhibition of monoamine oxidase (MAO), blockade of neuronal catecholamine reuptake, and direct release of catecholamine from nerve terminals. Serotonin (5HT) activity at the neuronal level also is altered. The resultant physiologic state is characterized on electroencephalography (EEG) by increased power, especially in the alpha range. This finding is related to the clinical state of arousal associated with the use of stimulants. Patients taking stimulants typically report activation, increased motivation, improved mood, and even euphoria (which may be followed by a dysphoric crash when catecholamine stores are depleted in the brain), suppression of drowsiness, and decreased need for sleep. Blood pressure and heart rate may be increased, and appetite suppression is common.

Among the unpleasant physiologic effects of stimulants are increased sweating, restlessness and agitation, and stereotypic movements such as teeth grinding, jaw-clenching, and skin picking. Sexual functioning may be impaired, with decreased libido in both men and women, inability to maintain an erection in men, and anorgasmia in women.

3. What are the common uses of stimulants in psychiatric practice?

The most common use of stimulants in psychiatric practice is in the treatment of **attention deficit/hyperactivity disorder** (ADHD) in children and occasionally adults. (ADHD is common in children, but rare in adults). The Food and Drug Administration (FDA) sanctions the use of stimulants in this disorder.

Also approved by the FDA is the use of stimulants to treat **narcolepsy**, a rare disorder in which the sufferer is plagued by sleep "attacks." Modafinil is specifically approved for narcolepsy.

Important uses of stimulants beyond those approved by the FDA center on the treatment of **mood disorders** and **amotivational states**.

Stimulants may be added to a partially effective **antidepressant regimen** to augment the antidepressant action (see Chapters 47 and 49) when it is impractical to increase the antidepressant dose, either because of adverse effects or because the maximal dose already has been reached without sufficient improvement.

Amotivational states (which may or may not be tied to depression) may respond acutely to the use of stimulants. Such states include **medically compromised patients** who are not participating actively in treatment and therefore are at risk of further deterioration of functioning. The typical scenario involves elderly persons, persons who are having difficulty with weaning from a ventilator, patients infected with the human immunodeficiency virus (HIV), poststroke victims or postoperative neurosurgical patients, and terminally ill patients. Behavioral control and cognition have improved with stimulant treatment in chronic closed-head-injury patients.

Clinical Pearl: Using a stimulant (5 mg of dextroamphetamine) helps to differentiate between depressed and demented patients. Depressed patients are likely to respond with improved mood, cognition, and alertness, whereas demented patients may show increased alertness but worsened cognition.

4. What are inappropriate uses of stimulants?

Stimulants are not effective as the primary treatment for depression. Additionally, stimulants should not be used to relieve normal fatigue states. In general, weight control and appetite suppression are not clinically appropriate uses for stimulants because of lack of efficacy over time and risk of adverse effects. Behaviorally based treatments are better than stimulants for weight control.

5. List and discuss some of the common problems associated with prescription of stimulants.

Tolerance. The sympathomimetic effects of stimulants diminish quickly at a steady dose. Thus persons using stimulants to produce euphoria, appetite suppression, energy, and wakefulness become quickly disappointed and seek to increase the dose to achieve the former level of stimulation. Of interest, tolerance does not develop to the therapeutic benefit of stimulants in ADHD, or to their antidepressant effects when used to augment treatment of depression, or in medically ill patients maintained on stimulants for amotivational states.

Abuse. Stimulants have been extensively abused in the past because they are known to produce euphoria, energy, and wakefulness. An historically important form of stimulant abuse occurred during World War II. Allied and Axis forces used amphetamine extensively. Japanese fighter pilots, on suicide missions in the Pacific, used amphetamine. Postwar Japan experienced an epidemic of amphetamine abuse when large stockpiles of amphetamine from the military were placed on the open market. The potential for abuse has caused stimulants to become heavily regulated in the United States.

Adverse effects. Common or important stimulant-induced side effects include:

Anxiety	Increased heart rate and blood pressure
Irritability	Palpitations
Insomnia	Tics and other involuntary movements
Dysphoria	(teeth grinding/jaw clenching)
Emotional lability	Transient growth suppression in children
Decreased appetite	Paranoia

Psychological dependence   Hallucinations
Physical dependence   Psychosis
Exacerbation of other illnesses such as glaucoma, hypertension, anxiety disorders,
     psychotic disorders, and seizure disorders

Drug–drug interactions. Stimulants may decrease metabolism (and thus increase plasma level) of certain drugs:

Tricyclic/tetracyclic antidepressants   Phenobarbital
Warfarin (Coumadin)   Phenytoin (Dilantin)
Primidone (Mysoline)   Phenylbutazone (Butazolidin)

Use stimulants with extreme caution in the presence of MAO inhibitors because of the possibility of a hypertensive crisis. In addition, exercise extreme caution when prescribing stimulants to patients with bipolar affective disorder, as these compounds may induce mania or rapid-cycling.

6. Summarize governmental regulation of stimulants.

All stimulants (except modafinil, which has a schedule IV designation) are classified by the U.S. Drug Enforcement Agency (DEA) as schedule II, along with certain narcotics. Additional regulations may vary from state to state, including the use of triplicate prescriptions for stimulants (one copy is filed with a state governmental agency). A proper state medical license and DEA certification are required for physicians to prescribe stimulants. Internationally there is much variability in the regulation of stimulants. Sweden has banned stimulants, whereas they are available without prescription in other countries.

7. Summarize practical information about prescribing stimulants.

Prescription of Stimulants*

	DEXEDRINE	RITALIN/METADATE	PROVIGIL	ADDERALL

How supplied (Tablets)	5, 10 mg
	Oral suspension:
	  5 mg/ml
	Sustained release: 5,
	  10, and 15 mg
		10 and 20 mg	100, 200 mg	5, 10, 20, and
				  30 mg

Pretreatment evaluation	Cardiac, liver, and
	  renal function
		Cardiac, liver, and
		  renal function
			Cardiac, liver, and
			  renal function
				Cardiac, liver, and
				  renal function

Concurrent monitoring	None	None	None	None

Starting dose (mg)
  Adults
  Children
	
	2–5–10
	2–5 (3–5 yrs)
	5 (6 yrs and older)
		
		5–10
		5
			
			100–200 mg
			No data in chil-
			  dren under 16
				
				5–10
				5

Increase dose weekly by	5 mg	5–10 mg	100 mg	5–10

Daily schedule	Twice daily divided
	  dose except in
	  sustained release
	  form (once daily)
		Two to three times
		  daily except
		  longer acting
		  form (once or
		  twice daily)
			Once daily in AM	Twice or three
				  times daily

Maximal recommended dose	60 mg	60 mg	400 mg	60 mg

* There is no indication for the use of stimulants during pregnancy. Dextroamphetamine (Dexedrine) and methylphenidate (Ritalin) pass into breast milk.

8. What are useful strategies for managing common stimulant-induced adverse effects?

*Management of Common Stimulant-Induced Adverse Effects
in Attention Deficit/Hyperactivity Disorder*

ADVERSE EFFECTS	MANAGEMENT
Anorexia, nausea, weight loss	Administer stimulant with meals. Use caloric-enhanced supplements. Discourage forcing meals.
Insomnia, nightmares	Administer stimulants earlier in day. Change to short-acting preparations. Discontinue afternoon or evening dosing. Consider adjunctive treatment (e.g., antihistamines, clonidine, antidepressants).
Dizziness	Monitor blood pressure. Encourage fluid intake. Change to long-acting form.
Rebound phenomenon	Overlap stimulant dosing. Change to long-acting preparation or combine long- and short-acting preparations. Consider adjunctive or alternative treatment (e.g., clonidine, antidepressants).
Irritability	Assess timing of phenomena (during peak or withdrawal phase). Evaluate comorbid symptoms. Reduce dose. Consider adjunctive or alternative treatment (e.g., lithium, antidepressants, anticonvulsants).
Growth impairment	Attempt weekend and vacation holidays. If severe, consider nonstimulant treatment.
Dysphoria, moodiness, and agitation	Consider comorbid diagnosis (e.g., mood disorder) Reduce dose or change to long-acting preparation. Consider adjunctive or alternative treatment (e.g., lithium, anticonvulsants, antidepressants).
Poor or variable absorption	Avoid citric and ascorbic acid for 1 hour prior to the stimulant dose.

From Wilens TE, Biederman J: The stimulants. In Shaffer D (ed): Pediatric Psychopharmacology: The Psychiatric Clinics of North America. Philadelphia, W. B. Saunders, 1992, with permission.

BIBLIOGRAPHY

1. Arieti S (ed): American Handbook of Psychiatry, 2nd ed. New York, Basic Books, 1986.
2. Evans RW, Gualtieri CT, Patterson D: Treatment of chronic closed head injury with psychostimulant drugs: A controlled case study and an appropriate evaluation procedure. J Nerv Mental Dis 175:106–110, 1987.
3. Fernandez F, Levy JK: Psychopharmacology in HIV spectrum disorders. Psychiatr Clin North Am 17:135–148, 1994.
4. Gilberg C, et al: Long-term stimulant treatment of children with attention-deficit hyperactivity disorder symptoms: A randomized, double-blind, placebo-controlled trial. Arch Gen Psychiatry 54:857–864, 1997.
5. Goodwin K, Jamison KR: Manic Depressive Illness. New York, Oxford Press, 1990.
6. Greenhill LL, et al: Medication treatment strategies in the MTA: Relevance to clinicians and researchers. J Am Acad Child Adolesc Psychiatry 35:1304–1313, 1996.
7. Hales RE, Yudofsky SC: Textbook of Neuropsychiatry. Washington, DC, American Psychiatric Press, 1987.
8. Kaplan HI, Sadock BJ: Pocket Handbook of Psychiatric Drug Treatment. Baltimore, Williams & Wilkins, 1993.
9. Kaplan HI, Sadock BJ: Comprehensive Textbook of Psychiatry, 6th ed. Baltimore, Williams & Wilkins, 1995.
10. Massie MJ, Shakin EJ: Management of depression and anxiety in cancer patients. In Breithart W, Holland JC (eds): Psychiatric Aspects of Symptom Management in Cancer Patients. Washington, DC, American Psychiatric Association, 1994, pp 1–21.

11. Pickett P, Masand P, Murray GB: Psychostimulant treatment of geriatric depression disorders secondary to medical illness. J Geriatr Psychiatry Neurol 3(3):146–151, 1990.
12. Spencer T, et al: Pharmacotherapy of attention-deficit hyperactivity disorder across the life cycle. J Am Acad Child Adolesc Psychiatry 35:409–432, 1996.
13. Woods SW, Tesar GE, Murray GB, Cassem NH: Psychostimulant treatment of depressive disorders secondary to medical illness. J Clin Psychiatry 47:12–15, 1986.

53. UNDERSTANDING MEDICATION INTERACTIONS

Dee Opp, R.Ph., BCPP, and Lyle Laird, PharmD, BCPP

1. Why are drug interactions important to consider?

To maximize therapeutic outcome and minimize adverse side effects, a prescriber needs to understand how a drug works, how it is metabolized, and what side effects are common with the use of the medication. When you consider a new medication for use, you must know how it will interact both **dynamically** and **kinetically** with other medications. For example, if a patient is currently on clonidine for hypertension, and a tricyclic antidepressant (TCA) is being considered for therapy, the prescriber should know that the TCA could antagonize the alpha-2 agonist property of the clonidine and negate its antihypertensive effects. This is an example of a pharmacodynamic interaction. Thus, it is important to have an understanding of the mechanisms of action of medications to determine if one is likely to antagonize or block the therapeutic effect of another.

In many therapeutic regimens, physicians are faced with using more than one agent to treat or ameliorate symptoms. All combinations need to be assessed for the presence of both **kinetic** and **dynamic** interactions.

2. What are the mechanisms of psychotropic medication metabolism?

Most of the psychotropic medications are metabolized by a process known as **phase I metabolism**. This type of metabolism is carried out hepatically by a group of enzymes known as the cytochrome P450 (CYP450) mixed oxidase system. CYP450 enzymes break down the medications into more water-soluble metabolites, which then are more easily excreted into the urine and eliminated from the body. In addition, **phase II metabolism** involves another group of enzymes in the liver. This system primarily results in glucuronidation of drugs, which also allows them to be excreted in the urine.

A clinically important example is the interaction between the anticonvulsants, lamotrigine and valproic acid. When these two medications are used together, valproic acid inhibits the phase II process of glucuronidation, causing up to a 50% decrease in lamotrigine's clearance and a significant increase in its half-life. This effect on the pharmacokinetic parameters of lamotrigine can increase blood levels and, hence, side effects (most significantly, increasing the risk of Steven-Johnson's syndrome).

3. Are there other ways medications interact beside via metabolism in the liver?

Medications can interact through multiple mechanisms, and all concurrently. The difficult task is to evaluate which one will influence the success of drug treatment the most. There are two main types of drug interactions: **pharmacokinetic** and **pharmacodynamic**. Pharmacokinetic interactions involve how one drug influences the normal movement of another drug in the body.

For example, one medication may inhibit the **absorption** of another. Ascorbic acid inhibits the absorption of amphetamines and therefore decreases their effectiveness in the treatment of attention deficit hyperactivity disorder. Another type of interaction is how one medication may influence the volume of **distribution** of another. If one medication like warfarin is highly protein bound and another highly protein-bound medication is added (e.g., valproic acid or carbamazepine), they could interact via a competition for albumin-binding sites, resulting in a rise in unbound, active components of one of the medications in the blood. If the medication freed from its protein binding sites from this interaction is warfarin, the patient could be at risk for bleeding episodes.

With carbamazepine, after the initial increase in blood levels and INR values secondary to protein binding displacement, **metabolic** effects will occur due to the enzyme **induction** properties of this anticonvulsant. Warfarin will then be metabolized more readily, and INR values will drop. Valproic acid on the other hand can initially bump INR values and may continue to increase warfarin's effect through **inhibition** of warfarin's main route of metabolism (the CYP450 isoenzyme, 2C9).

Excretion is another mode of interaction and occurs when one medication interferes with the excretion of another. For example, nonsteroidal antiinflammatory drugs (NSAIDs) inhibit prostaglandin synthesis, which is responsible for normal renal function. If NSAIDs (except sulindac) are used with lithium, one could observe a 30% or higher increase in lithium levels. Given lithium's narrow therapeutic index, such a consequence could result in lithium toxicity. Other medications that also affect lithium disposition in this way are the so-called ACE inhibitors and thiazide diuretics.

Mechanisms of Drug Interactions

PHARMACOKINETIC	PHARMACODYNAMIC
Absorption	
Distribution	Duplication in effect or antagonistic interactions between medications
Metabolism (includes the ability of medications to induce or inhibit P-450 isoenzymes)	Side effects common with medications (can exacerbate or complicate other medical symptoms or disease states)
Excretion	

4. How do patient-specific factors play a role in predicting clinical significance of drug-drug interactions?

Age, gender, race, and co-morbid medical conditions can complicate medication outcomes. **Age** plays an important role in how we choose medications and dose them. The elderly tend to become more easily toxic on water-soluble medications or medications with a low volume of distribution. Hence, lithium should be prescribed in lower doses in a geriatric patient than in a younger patient. These lower than expected doses can readily result in therapeutic blood levels. Blood levels will require closer monitoring. Liver function can be decreased in the elderly, especially phase I type reactions. If benzodiazepines are used that undergo phase I metabolism (e.g., temazepam), this may cause toxicity and increased risk of falls. Phase II reactions such as glucuronidation are usually intact. Lorazepam and oxazepam are better benzodiazepine choices in the elderly because they undergo phase II metabolism and have shorter half-lives.

Race is also important to consider when prescribing psychotropics. Phase I hepatic metabolism can be influenced by genetic polymorphism of an isozyme. For example, some racial groups are more likely to be poor metabolizers of drugs that require the isozyme, CYP450 2D6. It has been found that 5–10% of Causcasians and 1–3% of Asians and African-Americans possess genetic polymorphism for this isozyme. Clinically this could mean that if individuals who are poor metabolizers at CYP450 2D6 are given medications (substrates) that rely on this isozyme for metabolism, they could be at risk for elevated levels of these drugs with the resultant clinical consequences (be that enhanced therapeutic effects or adverse effects and toxicity). Certain antipsychotics (e.g., phenothiazines, clozapine, and risperidone) rely on CYP 2D6 to varying degrees for their metabolism. Another type of a clinically significant CYP450-related interaction is the case of codeine, a "prodrug" that requires CYP450 2D6 to be metabolized to the active analgesic component. If the 2D6 enzyme is inhibited, for example by a drug such as paroxetine, codeine will not be an effective analgesic medication.

Finally, **comorbid medical diseases** can greatly influence how a patient responds to medication. A patient with impaired renal function clears lithium less effectively than the patient without kidney impairment. In this example, the renally compromised individual has a greatly increased chance of becoming lithium toxic. Similarly, patients with severe liver dysfunction (e.g., cirrhosis) are more likely to become toxic on many medications, since the majority of them rely on intact hepatic function for effective elimination from the body.

5. When assessing patient medication regimens, what are two important mechanisms of metabolic interaction?

There are two drug interaction mechanisms that are crucial to determining whether medications will interact. **Induction** is the propensity of certain substances to increase the production of isozymes in the liver. For example, phenytoin (relying on CYP450 1A2, 2C9, 3A4 for metabolism), carbamazepine (relying on 2C9, 3A4), and phenobarbital (relying on 1A2, 2B6, 2C9, 2C19, and 3A4) are enzyme-inducing antiepileptics. When these medications are used, they increase production of certain subfamilies of isozymes in the liver. This enzyme induction effect reaches its full potential when the inducer medication itself reaches steady-state conditions (based on the half-life of each inducer) and adequate time has elapsed for the new production of enzymes. Carbamazepine, for instance, takes at least 2 weeks to see an induction effect. Other inducers include caffeine (1A2), omeprazole (1A2), nicotine (1A2), rifampin (2C9, 2C19, 3A4), ritonavir (1A2, 3A4), and phenobarbital (1A2, 2C9, 3A4).

Once more enzymes are produced, they metabolize substrates more efficiently, resulting in decreased levels of the substrate compared to the pre-induction period. Thus, to maintain therapeutic effects of the substrate drugs, their doses need to be increased. The opposite holds true if an inducer is discontinued from a patient's regimen, necessitating a reduction in the dose of the substrate medication to avoid potential toxicity. This type of interaction may take awhile to diminish until the inducer is completely eliminated from the body. An example is the discontinuation of carbamazepine from a regimen that includes haloperidol. Once induction has subsided, increased haloperidol blood levels could place the client at greater risk of adverse drug effects.

In contrast to induction, **inhibition** can occur and is usually competitive in nature. It results from one substrate having greater affinity for an isozyme in the liver than another medication. For example, erythromycin is an effective inhibitor of the 3A4 isozyme. If cisapride is given along with erythromycin, the metabolism of cisapride is effectively impaired, resulting in an increased probability of cardiac toxicity, such as Torsades de pointes, from the cisapride. Thus, toxicity of certain medications can be greatly increased by the concomitant administration with medications that inhibit CYP450 isozymes. Inhibition can be immediate, but is dose dependent. The higher the dose of inhibitor, the more likely the interaction with other substrates (medications). The full effect can be seen after one dose, but does not reach full effect until the inhibitor has reached steady-state levels.

6. Discuss the implications of therapeutic index.

Therapeutic index refers to the range of blood level concentrations of a medication in which the probability of desired clinical benefits is relatively high and risk of unacceptable side effects (toxicity) is relatively low. A wide therapeutic index is preferable.

Not all psychotropic medications have well-established therapeutic indices. Selective serotonin reuptake inhibitors (SSRIs; fluoxetine, sertraline) have broad therapeutic indices; hence, severe toxicity is unlikely. Tricyclic antidepressants (e.g., nortriptyline, imipramine) and lithium carbonate have narrow therapeutic indices; hence, greater caution is needed (e.g., blood level monitoring) to avoid toxicity. It is well established that therapeutic blood levels of lithium of 0.5–1.2 mEq/L are needed for clinical response. This narrow range can easily be exceeded by dehydration, age, or adjunctive medications, resulting in potentially dangerous toxicity.

7. What are common psychotropic drug interactions?

Interactions involving the CYP450 system are currently receiving a great deal of attention because of burgeoning discoveries regarding how these metabolic systems function and the potential for drug-drug interactions within these systems. For example, we now know that some of the SSRIs (e.g., fluoxetine, paroxetine) are potent inhibitors of the CYP450, 2D6, and/or CYP450, 3A4 systems.

Hence when used concomitantly with medications metabolized by the enzyme systems (e.g., cisapride, nortriptyline, some antipsychotic medications) significant toxicity can occur.

With complex, multi-medication regimens it may be prudent to consult with a clinical pharmacist or pharmacologist to understand the relative risks with different drug choices, or if problems arise with side effects. Keeping track of trends in side effects (e.g., time course) after adding a new medication may provide clues to these drug interactions. Educating patients and family members about these risks (including risks with over-the-counter and nontraditional medications) and conferring with other prescribers are essential in providing safe, effective pharmacologic treatment.

The following table is not complete, but provides a guideline to assessing potential drug interactions (see next page).

8. How do psychiatrists minimize adverse effects secondary to drug interactions?

As a rule of thumb, it is prudent to add only one medication at a time. While in practice this is often difficult to do given the enormous number of variables with any given patient, it does allow the practitioner to observe which medication is working while minimizing chances of drug-drug interactions.

Likewise, it is advisable to titrate dosages of only one medication at a time. If one medication's dosage has been maximized for an adequate period of time but the patient is not clinically benefitting, consider the possibility of a drug-drug interaction complicating the situation. When you find yourself adding medications to treat side effects, always ask yourself if lowering or discontinuing another medication is warranted before the addition.

Consider antidepressant-induced sleep disturbance. If a patient being treated for depression is complaining of sleeplessness, evaluate drug-induced reasons for this occurrence as well as sleep hygiene issues *before* the addition of a sleep medication. The reason may be as simple as changing the time of administration of a medication. For example, fluoxetine, bupropion, and venlafaxine should not be given at bedtime secondary to the risk of activation and insomnia. The addition of another medication is prevented which in turn decreases the likelihood of drug-drug interactions.

BIBLIOGRAPHY

1. Anderson G: A mechanistic approach to antiepileptic drug interactions. Ann Pharmacother 32:554–563, 1998.
2. Evans WE, Schentag JJ, Jusko WJ: Applied Pharmacokinetics, 3rd ed. Vancouver, Washington Applied Therapeutics, Inc., 1992.
3. Jefferson J: Drug interactions—Friend or foe? J Clin Psychiatry 59(suppl 4):37–47, 1998.
4. Michalets EL: Update: Clinically significant cytochrome P-450 drug interactions. Pharmacotherapy 18(1):83–112, 1998.
5. Shen W: The metabolism of psychoactive drugs: A review of enzymatic biotransformations and inhibition. Biol Psychiatry 41:814–826, 1997.
6. Winans E, Cohen L: Assessing the clinical significance of drug interactions in psychiatry. Psychiatric Ann 28(7):399–405, 1998.

Potential Drug Interactions

ISOENZYME	SUBSTRATES	INHIBITORS	INDUCERS
CYP1A2 *Genetic Polymorphism: 1–3% Caucasians & 18% AA*	*Caffeine* * Clomipramine Clozapine Cyclobenzaprine Fluvoxamine * Imipramine Methadone (racemic mix) Mirtazapine *Olanzapine* Ondansetron Propranolol Sibutramine Tacrine * Tamoxifen Theophylline R-Warfarin Valproic acid Zileuton	Cimetidine Ciprofloxacin Disulfiram Ethinyl Estradiol **Fluvoxamine** Grapefruit Juice Isoniazid (INH) Mexilitine Norethindrone Tacrine Verapamil Zileuton	Caffeine & Smoking Charcoal-broiled meat Cruciferous Veggies Omeprazole Phenytoin & Barbiturates **Ritonavir**
CYP2C9 *Genetic Polymorphism: 1–3% Caucasians & 18% AA*	Clozapine Diclofenac Dronabinol Fluvastin Glipizide Ibuprofen Indomethacin Losartan Naproxen Nelfinavir Phenytoin Piroxicam Sibutramine Tolbutamide Torsemide S-Warfarin * potent anticoagulant form * Valproic acid	Cimetidine Cotrimoxazole Disulfiram Fluconazole Fluoxetine Fluvoxamine Isoniazid (INH) Itraconazole Ketoconazole Metronidazole Ritonavir Sulfinpyrazone Ticlopidine Zafirlukast	Barbiturates Carbamzepines Phenytoin Primidone Rifampin
CYP2C19 *Genetic Polymorphism: 18–20% Asians & 3–5% Caucasians*	* Amitriptyline Carispodol Chlordiazepoxide Citalopram * Clomipramine Clorazepate *Diazepam* * Imipramine Lansoprazole Mephenytoin/phenytoin Omeprazole * Pentamidine Propranolol R-Warfarin Valproic acid	Citalopram Felbamate Fluconazole Fluoxetine Fluvoxamine Omeprazole Paroxetine Sertraline Ticlopidine Tranylcypromine	Rifampin
CYP2D6 *Not liver specific, extrahepatic locations include the brain* *Genetic Polymorphism: 5–10% Caucasians & 1–3% Asians/AA*	* Amitriptyline Buspirone (&3A4) Carvedilol Citalopram (minor) * Clomipramine Clozapine Codeine-Morphine (prodrug) * **Despiramine** Dextromethorphan Donepazil (& 3A4) Fluoxetine Fluvoxamine * Haloperidol Hydrocodone * Imipramine * **Maprotiline** Methamphetamine Metoprolol Mexilitine Mirtazapine m-CCP (metabolite of nefazadone & trazodone) * Nortriptyline Oxycodone Olanzapine Paroxetine * Perphenazine Propafenone *Propranolol* * Risperidone Sertraline * Thioridazine Tramadol Trazodone Venlafexine	Amiodarone Cimetidine Citalopram (weak) **Fluoxetine** Fluphenazine * Haloperidol Methadone **Paroxetine** * Perphenazine Propafenone Propoxyphene * **Quinidine** Ramitidine **Ritonavir** Sertraline (weak) Yohimbine * Thioridazine	**Note:** CYP2D6 appears to be relatively resistant to enzyme induction

Table continued on following page

Potential Drug Interactions (Continued)

ISOENZYME	SUBSTRATES		INHIBITORS		INDUCERS
CYP3A4	Alfentanil	* Erythromycin	Cimetidine	Nifedipine	Aminoglutethimide
Most abundant in liver and intestinal mucosa	*Alprazolam*	Ethinyl Estradiol	Clarithromycin	Norethindrone	Barbiturates
	Amlodipine	Etoposide	Cyclosporin	Norfloxacin	Carbamazepine
	Amiodarone	Felodipine	Danazol	Norfluoxetine	Dexamethasone
	Atorvastatin	Fexofenadine	Delaviridine	(Prozac metb)	Efavirenz
No genetic poly- morphism known	* Bedepril	Fentanyl	**Erythromycin**	Omeprazole	Ethanol (with chronic use)
	Bromocryptine	Finasteride	Ethinyl Estradiol	Oxicanozxole	Glutethimide
	Carbamazepine	Flutamide	Fluconazole (weak)	Prednisone	Griseofulvin
	Chlordiazepoxide	Ifosfamide (podrug)	Fluoxetine	Quinine	Nafcillin
	* *Cisapride*	Indinavir	Fluvoxamine	**Ritonavir**	Nalfinavir
	Citalopram	Isradipine	Grapefruit juice	Saquinavir	Nevirapine
	Clarithromycin	Itraconazole	Indinavir	Troleandomycin	Phenytoin
	Clorazepate	Ketoconazole	Isoniazid	(TAO)	Primidone
	Clozapine	Lidocaine	Itraconazole	Valproic acid	Rifabutin
	Cocaine & metabolite	Loratidine	**Ketoconazole**	Inhibits 2C9	Rifampin
	Cyclophosphamide	Losartan	Methadone	and 2C129 &	Ritonavir
	Cyclosporine	Lovastatin	Metronidazole	epoxide hydro-	
	Dapsone	Methadone	Methylprednisolone	lase	
	Delaviridine	Methylprednisolone	Mibefradil	Verapamil	
	Dexamethasone	Miconazole	Miconazole	Zafirlukast	
	Diazepam	*Midazolam*	Miconazole		
	Diltiazem	*Nefazodone*	**Nefazodone**		
	Disopyramide	Nicardipine	Nelfinavir		
	Doxorubicin	*Nifedipine*	Nicardipine		
	Ergotamine	Nimodipine			
	Nisoldipine				
	Nitrendipine				
	Paclitaxel				
	* Pimozide				
	Prednisolone				
	Quetiapine				
	* Quinidine				
	Quinine				
	Rifabutin				
	Ritonavir				
	Saquinavir				
	Sertraline				
	Sibutramine				
	Sildenafil				
	Simvastatin				
	Tacrolinus				
	* *Tamoxifen*				
	Testosterone				
	Trazadone				
	Triazolam				
	Verapamil				
	Vinblastine				
	Vincristine				
	R-Warfarin				
	Ziprasidone				
	Zolpidem				

Italic substrate = main route of metabolism
Boldface = drug is a potent inhibitor
* = risk of QTc prolongation

54. ELECTROCONVULSIVE THERAPY

Kerry L. Bloomingdale, M.D.

1. Has electroconvulsive therapy (ECT) become a less clinically advantageous psychiatric treatment now that such a wide spectrum of psychoactive medications is available?

No, but its role has changed over the years. In fact, ECT dominated somatic treatment of major mental illness until the introduction of the phenothiazines in the 1950s. As neuroleptics, antidepressants, and mood stabilizers were made increasingly available, the "market share" of ECT naturally diminished. However, since the mid 1970s refinement in awareness of when and how to use ECT safely has given it an established and respected place alongside medications in the armamentarium of somatic treatments for mental illness.

2. True or false: ECT is useful primarily in treating the most severe forms of major depressive disorder.

False. It is a misconception that ECT is useful only or primarily in severe and psychotic forms of major depressive disorder. It is highly effective not only in these disease entities, but also in moderate and even mild forms of bona fide major depressive disorder. Confusion sometimes arises because, compared with antidepressants alone (without antipsychotic drugs), ECT is much more effective in treating psychotic depression. Furthermore, many clinicians find ECT easier to use than combinations of antipsychotics and antidepressants. Moreover, whenever significant suicidal ideation, intent, or planning occurs, regardless of the presence or absence of psychotic features, clinicians generally choose the most expeditious treatment. Although ECT does not work immediately, it typically works faster than antidepressants.

3. For what psychiatric conditions other than major depressive disorder is ECT useful?

Mania: ECT probably is not used more often for this condition because of the potentially rapid effectiveness of mood stabilizers and antipsychotics. However, ECT has a particularly appropriate role in the treatment of mania when (1) the patient is in the first trimester of pregnancy (because of concerns about the teratogenicity of mood stabilizers) or (2) the patient has a history of neuroleptic malignant syndrome.

Schizophrenic decompensation: Transient benefit can be obtained in treating acute forms with many positive symptoms, such as hallucinations, delusions, or floridly bizarre behavior. It may be particularly appropriate in the context of a time-limited stressor, such as loss of a loved one or disruption of a living situation, because of the possible brevity of the schizophrenic patient's response to ECT.

Lethal catatonia: This is a "final common-pathway" disorder probably caused by various affective and psychotic conditions and marked by extreme rigidity. Such rigidity may lead to muscle breakdown, acute renal failure, and death.

A variety of other conditions, including **Parkinson's disease** with significant rigidity and **neuroleptic malignant syndrome**, also can benefit from ECT.

Possible Indications for ECT

- Major depression (unipolar or bipolar)
- Mania, especially in the context of first-trimester pregnancy or history of neuroleptic malignant syndrome
- Schizophrenia, especially in the setting of floridly positive symptoms and/or a time-limited stressor
- Miscellaneous conditions
    - Lethal catatonia
    - Parkinson's disease
    - Neuroleptic malignant syndrome

4. Is ECT useful in depressive conditions marked by features of both axis I major depressive disorder and axis II personality disorders?

To the extent that the clinician can separate the symptoms of major depressive disorder from those of a personality disorder, ECT should be useful in treating the depressive symptoms. However, such discriminations typically are difficult to make. In practice, the decision of whether to proceed with ECT in the face of this combination often is better made by using your clinical sense of whether an autonomous, somatically treatable depressive syndrome exists than by counting cookbook criteria. Moreover, when considering ECT in patients with symptoms of both major depressive disorder and personality disorder, consider the patient's post-treatment subjective sense of well-being as well as the treatment team's objective criteria for response. For instance, even if the major depressive symptoms respond to ECT, the patient may experience almost as much dysphoria after ECT as before because of the relatively refractory problems of personality disorder.

5. Should psychoactive medications be stopped when ECT is started?

The combination of psychoactive drugs with ECT has been the subject of much interest in the recent literature. Whereas there has been no conclusive demonstration that any medication or class of medication consistently adds to the therapeutic effects of ECT, reports have documented patients who seemed to do better clinically with the combination of ECT and a psychoactive medication than with either alone.

However, there are reasons to be cautious about the concurrent use of ECT and each class of psychoactive medications. Lithium carbonate, for example, may cause increased neurotoxicity when combined with ECT. Benzodiazepines and anticonvulsant mood-stabilizers, such as carbamazepine and valproic acid, make the elicitation of seizures more difficult. Thus, these medications may be tapered or discontinued (see Question 9). Antidepressants generally lower the seizure threshold, which may increase the duration of seizures or the probability of status epilepticus and spontaneous seizures. Certain antidepressants, such as tricyclics, may increase cardiac irritability when combined with ECT. Antipsychotic medications lower the seizure threshold and, when combined with ECT, may cause greater neurotoxicity.

6. Does ECT cause an excessive cardiovascular response (e.g., hypertension, tachycardia) or a diminished cardiovascular response (e.g., bradycardia)?

At different stages in the physiologic response to ECT, the procedure may cause either a heightened or an attenuated cardiovascular reaction. Initially, the ECT stimulus may produce a vagally mediated bradycardia, sometimes associated with a sinus pause. This response is replaced, upon elicitation of the seizure, by a catecholaminergically mediated hypertensive and/or tachycardic reaction. Finally, a compensatory bradycardia may then ensue.

Obviously, each of these stages has different treatment implications (see table). If the patient is refractory to the electrical stimulus and does not experience a seizure, he or she will be particularly susceptible to the original sinus pause and/or bradycardia, because the sinus pause or bradycardia will not be counterbalanced by the seizure-induced, catecholaminergically mediated tachycardia.

Cardiovascular Reactions to ECT

STAGE OF ECT	CARDIOVASCULAR RESPONSE	PRETREATMENT OR ACUTE THERAPY
Electrical stimulus	Sinus pause and/or bradycardia	Atropine or similar anticholingeric drug
Seizure	Tachycardia and/or hypertension	Short-acting beta blocker (e.g., esmolol) or alpha and beta blocker (e.g., labetalol)
Postictal	Compensatory bradycardia	Atropine or similar anticholinergic drug

7. What are the contraindications to ECT?

There are no absolute contraindications to ECT.

Relative Contraindications to ECT

SYSTEM	SIGN, FINDING, OR SYMPTOM	POSSIBLE INTERVENTIONS FOR SAFE AND EFFECTIVE ECT
Cardiovascular	Ischemic heart disease	Reduction in anticipated oxygen consumption by heart (e.g., with preadministration of beta blocker)
	Tachycardia	Reduction of heart rate (e.g., with preadministration of beta blocker)
	Hypertension	Reduction of blood pressure before and/or during ECT
	Ventricular ectopy	Administration before and/or just after induced seizure of antiarrhythmic agents. Avoid IV lidocaine if possible before seizure because it may raise seizure threshold
Pulmonary	Gastroesophageal reflux, surgical history, gastro-paresis—all of which may predispose to aspiration	In addition to standard NPO precaution, preadministration of metoclopramide; intraprocedural pressure on cricoid cartilage; intubation
Orthopedic	Recent fracture, particularly vertebral compression	Use of increased dose of muscle relaxant (e.g., succinyl-choline) and/or curare
Neurologic	Space-occupying intracranial lesion (see Question 8)	Neurologic and/or neurosurgical consultation indicating that intracranial pressure not likely to rise to dangerous level during ECT
	Seizure disorders (see Question 9)	Consider lowering dose of anticonvulsant drug in consultation with neurologist

8. Is a space-occupying intracranial lesion a contraindication to ECT?

Yes, but only relatively, not absolutely. At one time they were considered absolute contraindications, and clinicians avoided ECT because of concern over the sometimes already elevated intracranial pressure. They anticipated that the pressure would go even higher with ECT-induced seizures, putting the patient at risk of complications such as herniation. However, experience has dictated that such lesions can be compatible with safe and effective ECT; clinicians have administered ECT without complications to patients in whom imaging studies subsequently revealed pre-existing space-occupying intracranial lesions.

If these lesions are discovered before ECT in patients who are candidates for the procedure (e.g., after work-up for a localizing finding on neurologic examination for ECT), appropriate consultation should be sought. If there is no evidence of a mass effect, such as papilledema on funduscopic examination, or edema and midline shift on imaging studies, and if the lesion appears relatively small, it may be possible to administer ECT safely. In this instance the potential dangers must be balanced carefully against the potential benefits of ECT.

9. Is a patient taking anticonvulsants for seizure disorder a viable candidate for ECT?

Yes, in many cases. Consult with a neurologist. The seizure disorder itself is not an absolute contraindication to ECT, although careful consideration should be given to the possibilities that ECT may destabilize an epileptic condition or precipitate status epilepticus. Conversely, of course, ECT may make a patient with epilepsy temporarily more refractory to spontaneous seizures. Anticonvulsants typically do not interfere with ECT, although they may require higher electrical dosing. If it is impossible to elicit adequate seizures in patients taking anticonvulsants for seizure disorder, consult with the patient's treating neurologist about cautious titration downward of the anticonvulsant dose. If the patient is taking anticonvulsants purely for their mood-stabilizing effects, the decision to taper them before ECT is less weighty.

In addition, before proceeding with ECT, consider tapering and discontinuing drugs such as benzodiazepines that are not used for anticonvulsant purposes, but raise the seizure threshold.

10. Does ECT cause permanent structural or functional brain damage?

No compelling evidence indicates that ECT causes *structural* brain damage. When animals are given electroconvulsive shock using parameters analogous to those used in ECT, histopathologic studies reveal no structural neuronal damage. Imaging studies before and after patients have received ECT also reveal no structural brain damage. Moreover, autopsies of patients who received ECT do not suggest a pattern of CNS damage caused by ECT.

It is more difficult to rule out permanent *functional* CNS damage resulting from ECT. In fact, limited numbers of patients note cognitive changes persisting for extended periods. Studies based on neuropsychological testing of ECT patients show that interference with the ability to form new **memories** (anterograde amnesia) can persist for at least 3 months after a course of ECT. Patients have difficulty laying down permanent memories of some events that take place just before, during, and immediately after a course of ECT. Neuropsychologically documented retrograde amnesia for events that took place more than several weeks before the start of ECT is rare. In general, then, it is difficult to document ECT interference with memory for events that take place more than a few months before or more than a few months after a course of ECT.

11. Is the suprathreshold approach to dosing in ECT the best way to administer the treatment?

Suprathreshold ECT is defined as the use of electrical charge or energy in excess of the amount minimally needed to elicit a seizure. The parameters for suprathreshold ECT are established by first titrating upward to the minimal electrical charge or energy necessary to elicit a seizure; for subsequent seizures that amount is multiplied by a factor greater than 1, such as 1.5. The universal appropriateness of suprathreshold ECT is not fully clear. Clinical research seems to indicate that higher-than-necessary quantities of charge or energy are often more effective than threshold amounts, particularly in unilateral ECT. It has not yet been firmly established whether the cognitive side effects of suprathreshold ECT are greater than those of threshold ECT.

12. Should electrode placement in ECT be unilateral or bilateral?

The choice of which electrode placement to use for ECT is controversial. In *unilateral ECT*, one electrode is placed midline and the other is placed temporally over the nondominant hemisphere (generally presumed to be the right). In *bilateral ECT*, both electrodes are placed temporally, one over each hemisphere. Bilateral ECT often seems to work more effectively and rapidly than unilateral ECT, but it also may produce more cognitive side effects. Some practitioners believe that bilateral ECT is universally advantageous, if cognitive impairment does not preclude its use. Other clinicians believe that it is appropriate in many cases to initiate ECT treatment with a unilateral approach and then switch to bilateral ECT in patients with poor or sluggish clinical response.

13. What is the optimal number of treatments in a course of ECT?

There is no magic number of ECT administrations per course of treatment. In treating patients who manifest a prompt and full response to ECT for major depressive disorder, experienced practitioners may administer 5–10 treatments, generally at the rate of 3 per week.

If patients with major depressive disorder do not respond promptly or adequately to ECT, clinicians may give 10–20 treatments, assuming that each treatment results in an adequate seizure. However, in giving such an extended course of treatment, the ECT practitioner also is likely to manipulate key variables such as electrode placement or amount of electrical charge or energy. If the seizure durations are inadequate, the clinician administering the ECT should: (1) if possible, make sure that the patient is off all drugs that could raise the seizure threshold; (2) adjust the dose or type of anesthetic agent; (3) hyperventilate the patient; and/or (4) use agents such as intravenous caffeine to lower the seizure threshold.

14. How does the clinician know that a patient is responding to ECT?

Generally, objective signs of improvement precede subjective signs. For example, if the patient is treated for major depressive order, other inpatients on the psychiatric unit or, if on an outpatient basis, the family may report that the patient acts more spontaneously, eats more, or sleeps better before doctors or nursing staff observe changes. Clinical staff then may notice similar neurovegetative changes. Finally, the patient may note improved self-esteem, hopefulness, or physical well-being.

Occasionally, the clinician encounters a difficult and awkward period in his or her alliance with the patient, perhaps between approximately the third and seventh treatments, in which objective signs of improvement are relatively clearcut, but the patient is discouraged about the lack of perceived improvement and wants to stop ECT. At such a time, the ECT practitioner's alliance with the patient's family or friends may prove critical in ensuring the continuation of treatment.

15. Is the electroencephalograph (EEG) the best way to assess the duration of a seizure in ECT?

If accessible, an EEG printout readily provides a way to quantify the duration of the seizure. However, a two-lead EEG produced by an ECT apparatus may be difficult to interpret, especially in documenting an exact seizure duration. Accordingly, the EEG printout should be used in conjunction with **visual monitoring** of seizure duration, especially if the cuff method is used. This technique consists of inflating a blood pressure cuff to a greater than systolic pressure around an extremity before infusion of the muscle relaxant, to prevent the extremity from being paralyzed during the seizure. The visually monitored duration of the convulsion in the extremity generally provides an accurate measure of seizure length.

Another way to corroborate seizure duration is to record the rate of change in heart rate. If IV beta blockers are not used, the heart rate will peak in approximate conjunction with the visually and EEG-monitored durations of the seizure.

16. What are continuation ECT and maintenance ECT?

Continuation ECT is administered after a successful, acute course of ECT, but during the interval when the patient would still be suffering from the index episode of illness if the treatment had been unsuccessful. Such a period may be presumed to last for at least several months. *Maintenance ECT* is administered after the patient is no longer suffering from the underlying episode of illness originally treated acutely with ECT. Continuation and maintenance ECT treatments usually are given less frequently than ECT to treat an acute episode of illness. Preferred schedules of maintenance ECT vary considerably: some experienced clinicians use a fixed schedule, such as weekly, then biweekly, then monthly, assuming that the patient remains symptom-free; others plan follow-up ECT on a less frequent basis, but increase the frequency if symptoms recur.

17. Are continuation and maintenance ECT always indicated when a patient responds acutely to ECT?

They are only one follow-up treatment option for the patient who responds acutely to ECT. If the patient was treated for major depressive disorder, antidepressant or mood-stabilizing medications typically are used for follow-up. Some form of supportive or insight-oriented psychotherapy usually should accompany follow-up ECT or medications.

The decision about the form of follow-up treatment after a successful acute course of ECT is complicated. It should be made on the basis of anticipated **safety** and **efficacy** as well as **patient preference**. One strategy for patients treated effectively with ECT for an episode of major depressive disorder is to consider medication follow-up after the first episode of illness; if the patient breaks through such follow-up, ECT may be offered again. Follow-up ECT is instituted if the breakthrough, relapse, or recurrence is treated successfully with further acute ECT.

18. Is ECT too complicated from a medical standpoint to be done on an outpatient basis?

Except in limited cases, ECT can be done safely and effectively on an outpatient basis. In fact, outpatient ECT may be preferable to inpatient ECT, because the patient is able to remain in his or her home environment and the costs are lower. Obviously, the severity of a patient's psychiatric condition may preclude outpatient ECT.

Note that the periods of greatest physical risk from ECT are usually the treatment and post-treatment recovery phases. Assuming that the patient is carefully monitored during these phases, outpatient ECT may be considered even for mild-to-moderate medical risk factors. The clinician should give specified pre- and post-treatment suggestions to the patient and responsible family members, such as avoiding oral ingestion before ECT and refraining from activities such as driving, operating machinery, and making major decisions.

19. True or false: The patient's informed consent is unnecessary because most candidates for ECT suffer from diminished cognitive acuity.

False! Although the illnesses that respond to ECT commonly affect mental status, it is essential, for legal and ethical reasons, that the patient understand the risks and benefits of ECT before agreeing to the procedure. If the patient is unable to give such informed consent, the clinician should be sure to satisfy the state's legal conditions for alternative means of obtaining permission (see Question 20).

20. If a patient is truly unable to give informed consent for ECT, should you obtain the written informed consent of the patient's nearest relative?

Not necessarily. Inexperienced ECT practitioners may believe that the consent of the nearest relative is automatically an acceptable alternative to informed consent of an incompetent patient. However, the state in which ECT is to be administered may require court appointment of a guardian (who in fact may be the nearest relative) to make treatment decisions for the patient who is unable to do so.

21. Should transcranial magnetic stimulation (TMS), which has few side effects, be used instead of ECT?

No. TMS, an electromagnetic technique that stimulates certain areas of the brain in a more specifically targeted fashion than ECT, may be effective for certain psychiatric disorders, including depression. However, its definitive efficacy for psychiatric disorders is still unproven. It remains a significant investigational technique which may help to shed light on important questions about the etiology of depression and the mechanism of action of such treatments as ECT.

TMS ultimately may prove to be a useful treatment for psychiatric disorders such as major depression, because TMS does not require general anesthesia and is not intended to induce seizures (although seizures can be a side effect).

BIBLIOGRAPHY

1. American Psychiatric Association: The Practice of Electroconvulsive Therapy: Recommendations for Treatment, Training, and Privileging. Task Force Report. Washington DC, American Psychiatric Association, 1990.
2. Beyer J, Weiner R, Glenn M: Electroconvulsive Therapy: A Programmed Text. 2nd ed. Washington DC, American Psychiatric Association, 1998.
3. Coffey C (ed): The Clinical Science of Electroconvulsive Therapy. Washington DC, American Psychiatric Association, 1993.
4. Devanand D, Lisanby S, Nobler M, et al: The relative efficiency of altering pulse frequency or train duration when determining seizure threshold. J ECT 14:227–235, 1998.
5. Kellner C, Bourgon L: Combining ECT and antidepressants: Time to reassess. J ECT 14:65–67, 1998.
6. Kellner C, Pritchett J, Beale M, et al: Handbook of ECT. Washington DC, American Psychiatric Association, 1998.
7. Post R, Kimbrell T, McCann U, et al: Repetitive transcranial magnetic stimulation as a neuropsychiatric tool: Present status and future potential. J ECT 15:39–59, 1999.
8. Royal College of Psychiatrists: The ECT Handbook. London, Royal College of Psychiatrists, 1995.
9. Sackeim H: The anticonvulsant hypothesis of the mechanisms of action of ECT: Current status. J ECT 15:5–26, 1999.
10. Sackeim H, Prudic J, Devanand D, et al: Effects of stimulus intensity and electrode placement on the efficacy and cognitive effects of electroconvulsive therapy. New Engl J Med 328:839–846, 1993.

VII. Diagnosis and Treatment of Psychiatric Disorders in Childhood and Adolescence

55. AUTISM SPECTRUM DISORDERS

Loisa Bennetto, Ph.D., and Sally J. Rogers, Ph.D.

1. What is autism?

Autism is a developmental disability marked by significant impairments in social relatedness, communication, and the quality, variety, and frequency of various activities and behaviors. The onset of autism is generally before age 3, and impairments persist throughout the lifespan. Autism may occur across a range of functioning, and often is associated with mental retardation.

2. What are the main symptoms of autism in childhood and adulthood?

Autism involves a constellation of primary symptoms that are present in all individuals, plus a variety of other symptoms that often are associated with the disorder. The presentation of symptoms varies greatly among individuals and across age and developmental levels, and no single symptom is pathognomonic.

Symptoms of Autism

PRIMARY SYMPTOMS (present in all individuals)	ADDITIONAL SYMPTOMS (may not be present in some individuals)
Abnormal social relatedness	Abnormal movement patterns
Abnormal communicative development	Cognitive impairment
Abnormal capacity for symbolic play	Abnormal sensory responses
Restricted and odd behavioral repertoire	Stereotypic behaviors
Onset before age 3	Neurological abnormalities
	Extreme behavioral problems

3. How is social relatedness affected?

Social relatedness is always impaired in autism. The degree of impairment, however, may range from an oddness in social interaction, as in Asperger's syndrome, to an almost complete detachment and lack of responsiveness to others' social initiations. Social deficits are most obvious with strangers and with peers; many children with autism show differential preferences for familiar people and demonstrate attachment to their primary caregiver. Social abnormalities may include poor use of eye contact, lack of social initiation (as opposed to response), and little apparent interest in sharing exciting or pleasurable experiences with others.

Individuals with autism often have difficulty in both reading others' and signaling their own emotional states through body movements and facial expressions. They also have difficulty understanding others' mental states and perspectives. Finally, children with autism demonstrate a marked deficit in imitating others' actions, which may impede the development of interpersonal synchrony, communication, symbolic play, and the learning of new behaviors.

4. In what way is communicative development abnormal?

Much of the literature on autism has focused on deviance in the development of spoken language. However, the communication deficit is much more profound than deviant speech patterns. Some children with autism seem to lack the understanding that behavior can be communicative. For example, the most severely affected children do not seem to comprehend the meaning of a parent's smile, frown, or gesture. Furthermore, they rarely use behavior communicatively (e.g., no pointing, showing, seeking to hold the parent's attention with eye contact). At the milder end of the spectrum are people who are highly verbal, but impaired in pragmatic aspects of language. They may be quite "chatty" and very socially motivated; yet they rarely engage in the typical back-and-forth pattern of normal conversation and lack a grasp of humor and irony.

5. How is the symbolic play of childhood affected?

Children with autism rarely engage in the pretend play typical of preschool-aged children, including doll play, role play, and dramatic play. Those who have some ability to carry out this kind of play do so in a repetitive and simplistic manner, and they rarely seek out play partners or engage in interactive symbolic play.

6. What kinds of odd behaviors are characteristic of the autistic individual?

Typical toy play, marked by curiosity, creativity, and interest in novelty, usually is lacking in children with autism. Much time is spent in a very limited range of activities, which may consist of a few highly ritualized or repetitive ways of handling a few objects (e.g., sucking, shaking, arranging, carrying around). When age-appropriate play skills are present, they often are inappropriately repetitive. Water play, watching things move or spin, and repeatedly watching television commercials or videos are typical interests of young children with autism.

For those with well-developed language skills, preferred topics of conversation may be highly ritualized and repetitive, focusing on very specific themes. The interests, activities and conversational topics of adolescents and adults may seem quite restricted and idiosyncratic either in content or in intensity of involvement. Finally, changes in familiar routines or aspects of the environment may be very upsetting.

7. Describe the typical age and symptoms of onset.

Children with autism usually have symptom onset within the first 3 years of life. In the first year of life, commonly reported symptoms include either passivity or unusually difficult behavior (e.g., irritability, poor feeding and sleeping patterns) and a lack of interest in imitative mother-baby games. However, a number of children do not show specific symptoms in the first year of life. For those with apparent onset after 12 months, deviance in language development often is the first symptom reported. These children may not develop any speech, or they may display a pattern of normal first words at 12–14 months, but do not develop further language and may lose already acquired words. This usually is accompanied by decreased social interest and engagement. Additional symptoms, often including repetitive behavior, rituals, and intense emotional reactions, may develop in the third and fourth years.

8. What is the evidence for cognitive impairment?

Mental retardation, ranging from mild to severe, is present as an additional primary handicap in approximately 75% of children with autism. Overall cognitive ability, or IQ, tends to be stable across the lifespan and is predictive of long-term outcome. However, individuals with autism often show a distinct and uneven pattern in the development of specific cognitive abilities. Language and social development are the slowest areas to develop and demonstrate the most deviance. Other facets of development, such as visuospatial skills and memory for facts, tend to be the least delayed. Research on the neuropsychology of autism points to additional impairments in organizational skills, in shifting from one idea or behavior to another, and in the planning and execution of complex motor movements.

9. Elaborate on additional symptoms that may be present.

Abnormal sensory responses: Persons with autism often display either hyper- or hyporeactivity to sensory stimulation of all types (e.g., visual, auditory, tactile, pain).

Stereotypic behaviors: Persons with autism often display repetitive actions that appear to provide sensory stimulation (e.g., finger and hand movements, teeth grinding, jumping and flapping, rocking, and peculiar movement patterns when excited or anxious).

Neurological abnormalities: Abnormal muscle tone and movement patterns are common in children with autism. In addition, 20–35% of persons with autism develop seizures during adolescence or early adulthood, which are associated with greater impairments in intellectual functioning.

Extreme behavioral problems: A minority of persons with autism exhibit extreme behavioral difficulties such as self-abuse, and high levels of aggression and destruction.

10. What is the range of severity in autism?

Each of the primary and related symptoms of autism varies in severity, making this disorder quite different from one individual to the next. Similarly, the level of intellectual impairment may vary from severe mental retardation to normal or even superior intelligence. Individuals at both ends of the spectrum often are the most difficult to diagnose accurately. Those with severe autistic symptoms and severe mental retardation may be hard to differentiate from individuals with severe to profound mental retardation alone. Similarly, those with the mildest symptoms may appear similar to individuals with social problems due to personality disorders, nonverbal learning disabilities, pragmatic language disorders, and social anxiety.

11. What is pervasive developmental disorder, not otherwise specified (PDD-NOS)? How is it related to autism?

PDD-NOS is a term that engenders some confusion among parents and others trying to understand diagnoses. It sometimes is used interchangeably with autism, particularly with higher functioning or milder cases. It also is sometimes incorrectly interpreted as a qualitatively different diagnosis than autism. PDD-NOS is used if a child's behavior does not meet the full range of diagnostic criteria for autistic disorder. While these children may be functioning at a higher level than most children with autism, the nature of their symptoms still constitutes a significant impairment and often necessitates intervention.

PDD refers to a broad category of disorders that begin in infancy or early childhood and are characterized by qualitative impairment in social interaction, impairment in communication skills, and the presence of stereotyped behavior, activities, or interests. Autism is the most familiar of the PDDs. The other disorders in this category all have different features and courses, and include Asperger's syndrome, Rett's syndrome, and childhood disintegrative disorder. The term **autism spectrum disorder** is also used to connote autism and its milder variants, including PDD-NOS and Asperger's syndrome.

12. Describe Asperger's syndrome.

The diagnostic criteria generally are similar to those for autism. Individuals with Asperger's syndrome have severe and **sustained impairments in social interaction**, which are particularly marked in interactions with peers, and a **restricted and repetitive range of activities, behaviors, and interests**. In contrast to autism, there are no clinically significant delays in language or adaptive behavior early in development, and IQs are in the normal or borderline range. However, individuals with Asperger's syndrome do tend to show **pragmatic abnormalities in language** (e.g., poor conversational skills) and **impairments in nonverbal expressiveness** (e.g., gestures, facial expression). The symptoms of Asperger's syndrome often lead to significant difficulties in personal and occupational functioning.

Prevalence estimates indicate that Asperger's syndrome occurs in as many as 3–4 per 1000 school-aged children, with a higher rate in boys than girls. Young children may be identified for significant motor delays or motor clumsiness, but their perseverative tendencies and odd way of relating to others may be less noticeable. By school age, however, impaired social interaction skills become more obvious, and children often have few or no peer friendships. These children typically develop idiosyncratic or circumscribed interests, which are pursued quite perseveratively through reading, collecting, or memorizing facts.

Many researchers and practitioners consider Asperger's syndrome to be a milder form of autism. In fact, the differential diagnosis may be difficult to make for very young children. By later childhood and adolescence, however, these children may be distinguished from those with autism by their history of relatively intact language skills, their cognitive profiles, and the presence of well-developed perseverative interests.

13. Describe Rett's syndrome.

Rett's syndrome is a progressive neurological disorder that occurs only in females. It is quite rare, occurring in 1 per 12,000–15,000 live female births. Early in development, these girls may show many autistic characteristics, including withdrawal, social isolation, and cognitive delays, which often lead to an early diagnosis of autism. However, Rett's syndrome can be distinguished from autism by its **degenerative course** and certain striking characteristics.

Girls with Rett's syndrome show normal development until between 6 and 18 months, at which point their development appears to stop or regress. Most notably, they show a **loss of purposeful hand movement, severely impaired expressive and receptive communication skills, decelerated head growth, and severe cognitive deficits**. Loss of hand use is replaced by characteristic **stereotyped midline movements**, including hand wringing, hand washing, and hand biting. As girls with Rett's syndrome grow older, their overall motor skills deteriorate, with about half losing independent walking abilities altogether. In contrast, the autistic features of social isolation and withdrawal often improve with age. Other symptoms associated with Rett's syndrome include seizures in early childhood, feeding difficulties, and abnormal breathing patterns including hyperventilation, breath holding, and air swallowing.

14. Describe childhood disintegrative disorder.

Childhood disintegrative disorder is characterized by a significant regression in two or more areas of functioning, after a period of at least **2 years of normal development**. The regressions can be gradual or abrupt, and may affect social skills, expressive or receptive language, motor skills, play, toileting, or other adaptive behaviors. Like children with autism, those with childhood disintegrative disorder exhibit qualitative impairments in social interaction and communication, have a restricted range of behaviors, and tend to exhibit motor stereotypes. This disorder can be differentiated from autism by its course; the delays in autism are usually evident within the first year or two of life. However, after symptoms have developed, these children have the same symptom pattern as those with severe autism and significant mental retardation.

15. Are there tests to assist in the diagnosis of autism?

There is no specific medical test for autism. Diagnosis is based on parental report of developmental history and current functioning and observations of the child's behavior. However, the reliability and validity of diagnosis have improved greatly with the recent development of standardized methods of assessment. One of the most widely used diagnostic tools is the **Childhood Autism Rating Scale** (CARS).[13] The CARS is based on clinician's observations of a child's behavior. It requires only minimal training, and is particularly appropriate for an initial screening of autistic symptoms.

A formal diagnostic evaluation should include a more comprehensive evaluation of symptoms from multiple sources. One of the best-validated methods, the **Autism Diagnostic Interview-Revised** (ADI-R),[11] is a semi-structured interview with the child's primary caretaker that provides a lifetime assessment of the behaviors central to autism. The ADI-R is excellent in identifying autism in individuals from mental ages of 18 months through adulthood, and yields a diagnosis based on DSM-IV and ICD-10 criteria.

The **Autism Diagnostic Observation Schedule-Generic** (ADOS-G)[12] was developed to complement the ADI-R by providing a semi-structured and standardized interview with the patient in which to observe social, communicative, and play behaviors. The ADOS-G comprises several different modules designed for nonverbal, preschool children through high-functioning adults. Like the ADI-R, observations are scored in the context of DSM-IV and ICD-10 criteria. Both the ADI-R and ADOS-G provide rich information for diagnosis and treatment planning, but require a substantial amount of experience and training.

16. What factors should be considered in formulating a differential diagnosis?

For children who may have autism, the differential diagnosis must rule out the presence of severe language disorder, nonverbal learning disability, mental retardation (without autism), deafness, and reactive attachment disorder as alternative explanations for the difficulties with social, communicative, and play behavior. *For adults*, the differential diagnosis must rule out schizoid or schizotypal personality disorder, mental retardation (without autism), nonverbal learning disabilities, and neurological disorder.

17. Elaborate on the assessment process.

Whereas the purpose of diagnosis is to determine the existence of autism, assessment is the process of identifying the individual's strengths, weaknesses, and needs. A full interdisciplinary assessment is helpful in making the initial diagnosis and in therapeutic and educational planning. The **assessment team** ideally involves psychology, pediatrics, psychiatry, occupational therapy, social work, and speech and language pathology (neurology and physical therapy also are often included, depending on the presenting medical symptoms). A full assessment during the elementary school years is recommended to aid in optimal educational planning and curriculum development. Adolescents with autism may benefit from a comprehensive assessment as issues of vocational training, further education, and planning for independence from the parental home arise. A tertiary facility such as a university hospital or children's hospital, or a university-affiliated program for developmental disabilities, can provide comprehensive interdisciplinary assessments and recommendations.

18. How common is autism?

The prevalence of autism in the general population is approximately 10–12 per 10,000 live births. If one considers the broader PDD spectrum (including milder variants such as Asperger's syndrome and PDD-NOS), the prevalence estimate rises to over 20 per 10,000. Autism occurs more often in boys than girls, with a gender ratio of approximately 4:1 males to females.

19. What causes autism?

The precise pathogenesis of autism is unknown. We do know, however, that autism has a biological basis, related to neurological or neurophysiological factors. Historical theories about psychosocial etiologies (such as inadequate or poor parenting) have been rejected empirically.

Research clearly indicates that in many cases, autism has a **genetic basis**. The symptoms of autism appear to be associated with several genetic conditions, including **fragile X syndrome**, **tuberous sclerosis**, and **Moebius syndrome**. Family studies have demonstrated that autism is both familial and heritable. Subsequent siblings born to a family with an autistic child have a recurrence risk of 3–7%, compared to the population risk of 0.1%. The concordance rate is 9% for dizygotic twins, and roughly 60% for monozygotic twins. Recent research also suggests that the features of autism may be present in a milder form in nonaffected relatives of individuals with autism. This "broader autism phenotype" may include social reticence or shyness, pragmatic language difficulties, mood disturbances, and subtle neuropsychological deficits.

The pattern of transmission and specific genes responsible for autism are still unknown. Statistical models suggest that at least two to five genes are acting together to produce the autism phenotype. Based on the heterogeneity of symptoms and unpredictable inheritance patterns, it also is likely that these genetic factors are not inherited in a simple fashion and may be influenced by genetic or environmental modification.

Neuroanatomical and neuropathological studies of autism have identified several abnormalities, but findings in this area are still inconclusive. The most commonly reported findings include hypoplasia of specific brainstem nuclei, reduction in Purkinje cells, hypoplasia of the cerebellar vermis, neuronal immaturity, and increased cell packing density in the amygdala and hippocampus. Taken together, these findings suggest that autism may involve developmental abnormalities very early in the gestational period. Functional imaging studies using PET and SPECT have been inconsistent, but point to some reduction in metabolic rates in frontal and temporal regions. Finally, several neurochemical studies have reported possible abnormalities in dopamine and serotonin metabolism. Immunological abnormalities also have been documented.

20. Is there treatment for autism?

Autism generally is considered a lifelong, chronic disability. Nevertheless, **appropriate, intensive, and early intervention** is critical for stimulating development in all areas and improving functioning across settings.

For children with autism, intervention should begin as early as the diagnosis is made, in the toddler and preschool period. Specific interventions should focus on developing language, cognitive and imitation skills, social responsiveness, and appropriate behavior. A recent review of early intervention in autism describes several common elements of effective programs, which include **many hours per week of intervention, appropriate curriculum content, highly structured and predictable teaching environments, strategies to help generalize skills** across environments and people, and **a functional, positive approach to behavioral problems.**[8]

The school-aged child with autism needs a curriculum that is tailored to individual strengths and needs. With appropriate educational approaches, virtually all children with autism can be expected to make clear, measurable progress in learning. The educational programs that are helpful vary from individualized instruction in regular school classrooms to specialized programs for students with autism. There is an array of educational choices for families, but all effective education programs are highly individualized, using well-structured, systematic teaching routines, consistency and repetition, and concrete, functional learning objectives.

Adolescents and adults with autism frequently need specific help in negotiating the complexities of life demands. Social skills groups, recreational activities, individual psychotherapy, and vocational coaching and assistance can help them acquire skills necessary for a satisfying adult life. Participating in recreational activities with typical peers is an important part of community life for adults with autism. People with autism often have areas of strength that should be supported through further teaching and extracurricular activities, since they may represent abilities that will be respected and valued by peers or be important in establishing vocations or avocations in adult life.

21. Specifically which techniques are beneficial in the treatment of autism?

Intervention techniques that are effective in treating core symptoms of autism include cognitive/behavioral approaches, systematic instruction, and concrete, pragmatic approaches to life's challenges. Educational professionals and psychologists often play key roles in developing comprehensive intervention plans for individuals with autism. Speech and language therapy also is important in helping individuals with autism develop their communicative capacities to their fullest. Occupational therapy and physical therapy are important in treating motor abnormalities involving both motor development and sensory processing dysfunction. Attention to the mental health of the entire family is an important aspect of intervention programs as well, often involving social workers or psychologists on a treatment team.

A variety of alternative and sometimes controversial treatment approaches frequently are promoted in the popular press. The symptoms of autism are very complex, and it can be difficult for parents (and professionals) to judge the relative importance of enthusiastic endorsements versus empirical validation. *It is therefore critical to evaluate the scientifically reported effectiveness and safety of new treatments before recommending them to families.*

22. What medications are helpful in autism?

At present, there is no pharmacological treatment to "cure" autism. However, several classes of medications have been used to treat specific associated behavioral problems.

Antidepressants, particularly the selective serotonin reuptake inhibitors, have been used with some success in treating preoccupations and ritualized behaviors, as well as the mood disorders and anxiety that are sometimes evident in autism. Although they do not directly address social and communicative deficits, these symptoms may improve as rituals and anxiety decrease.

Stimulant medications have been used to decrease the activity levels and improve the attention span of some children, which may then lead to a better response to behavioral and educational treatments. While anecdotal reports have suggested some effectiveness in certain children with autism, a review of the research on stimulant medications suggests little or no clinical improvement.

Antipsychotic medications also have been considered in treating some symptoms of autism. The preponderance of the research has been done with haloperidol, which has been reported to improve hyperactivity, aggression, agitation, stereotypic behaviors, and mood lability in some studies. Newer atypical antipsychotic medications may be useful in treating aggressive and hyperactive behavior with fewer side effects.

Finally, **anticonvulsant medications** are used to treat individuals with autism who suffer from seizures. These medications also may be effective in decreasing aggressive behavior and episodic behavioral outbursts, particularly in children with seizure disorder.

23. What is the prognosis for children with autism?

With appropriate and intensive educational and treatment services, children with autism show improvements. The **preschool years** are typically the most difficult, because children with autism tend to be the least social, least communicative, and have the most behavioral difficulties. The severity of the social and communicative deficits tends to diminish as children grow older. Learning continues throughout childhood and adolescence, as long as children are receiving appropriate services and environmental supports. **Adolescence** can be a difficult time for some individuals with autism, because of increased social and organizational demands. In addition, some high-functioning adolescents and adults with autism may experience depressed mood.

A number of followup studies have been conducted with autistic individuals. These studies typically are based on samples of individuals who did not receive the intensive treatment services that are available today, and may therefore underestimate positive outcomes. These studies suggest that 5–17% of individuals with autism can work and live independently as adults. The most important positive prognostic indicators are functional (i.e., useful) language before age 5 and cognitive abilities above the mentally retarded range (i.e., IQ > 70). In addition, individuals with autism appear to do best in environments that are well suited to their specific needs.

The good news is that in today's culture of early intensive interventions, it appears that a number of children with autism grow up to have **unexpectedly positive outcomes**.

24. How is autism related to other mental disorders?

Individuals with autism may demonstrate symptoms of other psychiatric disorders. Treatment of comorbid conditions is likely to improve the response to interventions aimed at symptoms of autism. Some of the more common comorbid conditions include:

Affective disorders: Mood and anxiety disorders occur in autism with some frequency. There appears to be a higher rate of depression in individuals with autism, as well as their first-degree relatives. Higher levels of anxiety also have been observed in autism, and may be responsible for some of the behavioral outbursts, resistance to change, and need for repetitive routines. Because many individuals with autism do not have the verbal skills to describe their symptoms, clinicians must be sensitive to vegetative signs and other nonverbal markers of these conditions.

Attention-deficit/hyperactivity disorder (ADHD): ADHD is present in some, but certainly not all, children with autism. Many children with autism display some of the characteristic symptoms of ADHD, such as hyperactivity and distractibility.

Mental retardation: Mental retardation frequently co-occurs with autism. However, children with autism often demonstrate intact skills in certain areas, so *it is quite important that psychological testing be conducted by clinicians who are familiar with the diagnosis*, and that the intelligence tests used are appropriate to the individual's abilities and understanding. For example, nonverbal intelligence tests or nonverbal adaptations of tests are appropriate for younger children with autism and those who have limited verbal skills. For individuals with autism who do not have mental retardation, there is a common pattern of cognitive strengths and weaknesses, in which visual perceptual skills often are significantly better than verbal abilities, and concrete problem solving is better than abstract knowledge. Thus, in high-functioning individuals with autism, there often is a learning disability profile, which necessitates individual approaches to education.

BIBLIOGRAPHY

1. Attwood T: Asperger's Syndrome: A Guide for Parents and Professionals. London, Jessica Kingsley Publishers, 1998.
2. Bailey A, Phillips W, Rutter M: Autism: Toward an integration of clinical, genetic, neuropsychological, and neurobiological perspectives. J Child Psychol Psychiatry 37:89–126, 1996.
3. Bryson S, Smith I: Epidemiology of autism: Prevalence, associated characteristics, and implications for research and service delivery. Ment Retard Dev Disabil Res Rev 4:97–103, 1998.
4. Cohen DJ, Volkmar FR (eds): Handbook of Autism and Pervasive Developmental Disorders, 2nd ed. New York, John Wiley & Sons, 1997.
5. Cook EH: Genetics of autism. Ment Retard Dev Disabil Res Rev 4:113–120, 1998.
6. Courchesne E: Brainstem, cerebellar, and limbic neuroanatomical abnormalities in autism. Curr Opin Neurobiol 7:269–278, 1997.
7. Dawson G (ed): Autism: Nature, Diagnosis, and Treatment. New York, Guilford Press, 1989.
8. Dawson G, Osterling J: Early intervention in autism. In Guralnick MJ (ed): The Effectiveness of Early Intervention. Baltimore, Paul H. Brookes, 1997, pp 307–326.
9. Hagerman RJ, Cronister A (eds): Fragile X Syndrome: Diagnosis, Treatment, and Research. 2nd ed. Baltimore, Johns Hopkins University Press, 1996.
10. Lindberg B: Understanding Rett's Syndrome. Toronto, Hogrefe and Huber, 1991.
11. Lord C, Rutter M, LeCouteur A: Autism Diagnostic Interview—Revised: A revised version of a diagnostic interview for caregivers of individuals with possible pervasive developmental disorders. J Autism Dev Disord 24:659–685, 1994.
12. Lord C, Rutter M, Di Lavore PC: Autism Diagnostic Observation Schedule—Generic. Chicago, University of Chicago Department of Psychiatry, 1998.
13. Schopler E, Reichler RJ, Renner BR: The Childhood Autism Rating Scale (CARS). Los Angeles, Western Psychological Services, 1988.

56. ATTENTION DEFICIT–HYPERACTIVITY DISORDER

William W. Dodson, M.D.

1. What is attention deficit–hyperactivity disorder (ADHD)?

The first descriptions of ADHD appeared at the turn of the century, and the current medication treatment was first described in 1937. Our understanding of the disorder has developed over time, and the name and diagnostic criteria for ADHD have changed with that understanding. The current diagnosis as it is described in the DSM-IV is: (1) a persistent pattern of inattention/easy distractibility, (2) behavioral and emotional impulsivity, and *sometimes* (3) hyperactivity or severe restlessness. These symptoms are significantly more severe than is typical in persons of a similar developmental level. Inattention, impulsivity, and restlessness must cause significant impairment in at least two areas of function (school, peer relationships, family relationships, and work, mood regulation, and self-esteem) and must have been continuously present for at least 6 months. For example, a child who misbehaves in the classroom and is disruptive, but does not exhibit similar problems on the playground or at home, does not meet diagnostic criteria.

DSM-IV Criteria for Attention Deficit–Hyperactivity Disorder

Inattention

Six or more of the following, manifested *often*:

Inattention to details/makes careless mistakes	Difficulty organizing
Difficulty sustaining attention	Avoids tasks requiring sustained attention
Seems not to listen	Easily distracted
Loses things	Forgetful
Fails to finish tasks	

Impulsivity/Hyperactivity

Six or more of the following, manifested *often*:

Impulsivity	Hyperactivity
Blurts out answer before question is finished	Fidgets
Difficulty awaiting turn	Unable to stay seated
	Inappropriate running/climbing
	"Always on the go"
	Restlessness
	Difficulty in engaging in leisure activities quietly
	Talks excessively
	Interrupts or intrudes on others

The symptoms of inattention *or* impulsivity/hyperactivity:
- have persisted for 6 months or longer
- are more frequent and severe than is typical of the individual's level of development
- have onset prior to age 7
- cause some impairment in two or more settings (i.e., cause significant impairment in social, academic, or occupational functioning)
- are not better accounted for by another mental disorder

---

2. What are the behavioral signs of ADHD?

The presentation of ADHD varies depending on the age and developmental level of the patient.

Preschool (Ages 3–5)	Elementary School-Age (Ages 6–12)
"Always on the go"	Easily distracted, hard to stay on task
Aggressive (hits or pushes others)	Homework poorly organized, incomplete, and contains careless errors
Dangerously daring	
Noisy, interrupts	Impatient, blurts out answers, fails to wait turn in games
Excessive temper tantrums	
Insatiable curiosity	Often out of seat
Low levels of compliance	Perceived as immature
Adolescent (Ages 13–18)	**Adulthood**
Restless, rather than hyperactive	Disorganized, fails to plan ahead
School work disorganized and incomplete	Forgetful, loses things
Procrastination on most tasks	Multiple jobs, relationships
Engages in risky behavior (speeding, drug experimentation)	Misjudges time available, frequently late
	Mood lability and flash anger outbursts
Poor peer relationships	Many projects started but few completed
Poor self-esteem	
Difficulty with authority figures	

3. Is hyperactivity required for the diagnosis?

No. While the hyperactive features are unmistakable when present (and, therefore, were the main focus of earlier diagnostic frameworks), we now know that fewer than half of persons with

ADHD are hyperactive. True hyperactivity is much more common in boys, leading them to be identified and treated much more frequently than girls. When hyperactivity is absent, the individuals still are restless, talk incessantly, commonly lose the point of what they are saying, fidget, may be out of their seats walking around, pat their feet or fingers tirelessly, and/or cannot "turn off their minds to fall asleep" at night.

4. What causes ADHD?

The exact cause remains unknown, but there usually is a clear genetic clustering of cases in families. Adoption studies identify that genetics are far more important than environment in the manifestation of the disorder. Twin studies do not show complete concordance, indicating that other factors contribute to the etiology of ADHD. However, to date the only factor clearly demonstrated to be linked to the disorder is maternal smoking during pregnancy. Six studies of twins with ADHD show concordance rates of 60–80%.

5. Does ADHD persist into adulthood?

In the time when diagnostic schemes heavily focused on hyperactivity, it was believed that ADHD was a lag in developmental maturation that would go away with age. In the years that followed, however, as the genetic basis was identified and as children with ADHD grew up to be adults with continuing symptoms and impairment, it was recognized that adults can have ADHD. There still are no formal DSM criteria for adults, who must be given the diagnosis of ADHD–In Partial Remission or Not Otherwise Specified.

The rate of persistence depends on how "persistence" is defined. If using the strictest definition of being diagnosed as a child and continuing to meet full criteria as an adult, the persistence rate is about 33%. If persistence is defined as "probably" having met criteria in childhood and currently meeting 5 out of 9 criteria (instead of 6 out of 9), the persistence rate jumps above 80%. Luckily, adults continue to respond to the same medications and interventions as children do.

Often, people diagnosed as adults have additional therapy to do as they mourn all of the time and opportunities lost due to not being treated for their condition. They must also rework a sense of who they are as people with ADHD: they are not "lazy, stupid, or crazy."[5a]

6. How common is ADHD?

ADHD is the most common behavioral condition diagnosed in children. The DSM-IV reports a prevalence in children of 3–5%. When studies were done, however, to determine the impact on prevalence rates of the DSM-IV's emphasis on inattention, researchers were surprised to discover much higher rates both in Tennessee, where every child of school age in an entire county was screened, and in Germany, where the identical study had been performed a year earlier. Both studies demonstrated rates in excess of 10%.

Based on new criteria, studies have shown prevalence rates for purely inattentive individuals (4.9–9%) in addition to the impulsive/hyperkinetic (3.4–3.9%) and combined subtypes (4.4–4.8%). More girls are identified using the DSM-IV criteria than ever before.

7. Is ADHD over-diagnosed and over-treated?

This perception has arisen from a number of factors:
- Increased awareness of the condition by the public
- Acceptance of a broader set of diagnostic criteria
- Greater appreciation of the course of the illness and its ultimate impact on adult life, which justifies lengthier and uninterrupted treatments
- Diminished concern about growth retardation, predisposition to drug use, and long-term effects of stimulant class medications
- Increased treatment of adults.

In fact, the condition still goes unrecognized and untreated most of the time. Even assuming the lower end of the traditional prevalence estimates (3%), fewer than one in three affected children ever get diagnosed and treated.

8. How is ADHD diagnosed?

The diagnosis of ADHD is a clinical diagnosis derived from a careful history taken from many individuals and sources. The more data available to the clinician, the better. The process begins by taking a history—either from the child's parents or from the adult patient directly—of persistent, lifelong behavioral patterns that cause significant impairment in every area of the patient's life. Various researchers have assembled the common symptoms of ADHD into scales and checklists. Among the best available are:

ADHD Rating Scales

For Clinicians:	For Teachers:	For Parents:
Brown scales	Connors Teacher's List	Conners Parent's Checklist
Auchenbach scale	Vanderbilt Teacher's Rating Scale	
	ADHD Comprehensive Teacher	
	Rating Scales (ACTeRS)	

School records and report cards are helpful to establish longitudinal patterns of distractibility, behavior problems, and failure to perform up to potential.

9. What is the differential diagnosis of ADHD?

A careful history must be taken to rule out conditions that may be mistaken for ADHD. This is complicated by the fact that ADHD may coexist with any of these conditions.

Differential Diagnosis of ADHD

Coexisting Conditions	**Differential Conditions**
Conduct disorder	Age-appropriate high activity
Oppositional defiant disorder	Mental retardation
Learning disabilities	Thyroid disorders
Anxiety disorder	Absence seizures
Mood disorder	Sensory deficits
Speech/language disorder	Tourette's syndrome
	Tic disorder
	Sleep disorders
	Asperger's or autism
	Psychosis
	Substance abuse
Possible Etiologic Conditions	**Environmental Conditions**
Chronic lead poisoning	Abuse or neglect
Post-traumatic or infectious	Family adversity
Encephalopathy	Situational stress
Fetal alcohol syndrome	High intelligence with inappropriate
Fragile X syndrome	school placement
Phenylketonuria	

10. Which laboratory tests are helpful?

None. Sometimes standard IQ test subtests that involve attention (e.g., Digit span) draw scores that are significantly lower than other subtest scores, or there may be "subtest scatter" in which the subtest scores vary by more than 4 points. IQ testing scores may be available due to previous academic failure, but should not be obtained as part of an ADHD assessment unless comorbid specific learning disorders also are suspected. Computer-based continuous performance tests (e.g., the TOVA [Test of the Variables of Attention] or Conners test), which measure attention span and impulse control directly, are available. These tests cannot be used to make or deny the diagnosis since they have many false-negative tests and measure inattention/impulsivity from any etiology, not just ADHD. Their utility lies in research and in objective determination of the optimal dose of medication. EEG rhythm analysis and various scans (e.g., SPECT, PET) currently are being studied, but have not yet demonstrated sufficient validity to justify their high cost. They are not considered a part of the evaluation of ADHD except in the most complicated cases.

Once medication therapy has begun, blood levels of stimulant class medications are not useful, since there is no correlation between blood level and effect upon the symptoms of ADHD.

11. Discuss the controversies surrounding the diagnosis of ADHD.

The diagnosis often is difficult to make for a number of reasons:
• No specific diagnostic test is available.
• The symptoms are nonspecific and can be found in a number of medical and psychiatric conditions.
• The core symptom of inattention is invisible. (Only the patient is aware that his or her attention has wandered. Learned social behaviors mask the fact that the person is no longer paying attention.)
• There often is a low rate of agreement between different informants (patient, teachers, parents, and spouses).
• Many people do not make a clear distinction between having an *explanation* and having an *excuse* for misbehavior and failure. It is a cornerstone of American values that any problem can be overcome if you buckle down, work hard enough, and have sufficient self discipline. The reality that some people are born hardwired to be inattentive, impulsive, and fidgety goes against this tenet of faith.
• The best treatment for ADHD is the stimulant-class medications. These schedule C-II drugs make many physicians and parents uncomfortable and are inconvenient to prescribe; hence there is reluctance to diagnose.
• The diagnosis, treatment planning, and patient/parent education are time consuming and do not fit well into the busy schedules of physicians, parents, and teachers.

12. What is the impact of ADHD on patient's lives and the consequences of not treating the condition?

Almost without exception, every study of the impact of ADHD on people with the condition has shown compelling evidence that ADHD has a detrimental effect upon the individual's life. Twenty-five percent of affected individuals must repeat at least one grade in spite of adequate academic ability. Despite similar IQ scores and educational attainment, individuals with untreated ADHD have lower occupational attainment and job satisfaction. Adolescents with ADHD who do not take medication have been shown in three studies to be four times more likely to have injury-producing accidents than adolescents with ADHD who do take medication. An old joke that ADD actually stands for "Accidental Death and Dismemberment" illustrates the strong connection between ADHD and traumatic injury.

Adolescents with ADHD have much higher risk for self-inflicted injuries than do adolescents without ADHD (1.3% vs. 0.1%).

By the age of 27 the rate of substance use disorders in persons with ADHD who do not take medication is 300% higher than the general population (47% vs. 15%). Patients who continue to take stimulant-class medication for their ADHD have the same risk of developing substance use disorders as does the general population. Stimulant-class medication is protective against the development of these disorders in adolescents and young adults with ADHD.

It is becoming more clear as time goes on that *the risk lies in not treating ADHD*, rather than in using stimulant-class medications.

13. What constitutes optimal treatment for ADHD?

The current gold-standard treatment for ADHD is stimulant-class medications. There are now over 170 controlled studies demonstrating that these medications are most effective, as well as safe. Additionally, they continue to be effective without the development of tolerance. It is this latter factor that leads many researchers to look for a mechanism of action other than their stimulant properties. For now, we must say that their mode of action for persons with ADHD is unknown.

14. Elaborate on the stimulant-class medications.

Stimulants have been used to treat ADHD for a long time. Since Bradley's original article in 1937, we have had more than 60 years of experience with amphetamine and 30 years of experience with methylphenidate, with no negative effects identified from chronic administration.

There are three commonly prescribed stimulant-class medications. They come in various immediate and long acting forms:

Generic Name	Trade Name	Dosage
Methylphenidate	Ritalin, Methylin	5, 10, 20 mg
	Ritalin SR	20 mg
	Metadateer	10, 20 mg
Dextroamphetamine	Dexedrine, Dextrostat	5, 10 mg
	Dexedrine Spansule	5, 10, 15 mg
d, l Amphetamine salts	Adderall	5, 10, 20, 30 mg

15. Which stimulant is best for ADHD?

Methylphenidate (Ritalin) is by far the most commonly prescribed medication for ADHD, but this pattern is changing as clinicians become familiar with the long-acting preparations of amphetamine (Dexedrine Spansule, Adderall). Five recent double-blind studies comparing methylphenidate directly to Adderall seem to show that the amphetamine product is superior to methylphenidate in treating the core symptoms of ADHD—but more research is needed.

The sustained release (SR) formulations of methylphenidate are unreliable and come in only one dosage strength (20 mg), which cannot be cut without losing the sustained release effects. Consequently, the Ritalin SR formulation is not recommended or used by most practitioners.

Note that medication alone is rarely enough to treat the many impairments of ADHD adequately. *Pills don't give skills.* Medication levels the neurologic playing field so that individuals with ADHD can have an equal chance at life and begin to do the remedial work necessary to rebuild their lives, work, and relationships.

16. How is the optimal dose of medication determined?

For many years practitioners used weight-based nomograms to determine the dose of stimulant. This was largely a misunderstanding. The nomograms had been taken from the original blinded studies that demonstrated the effectiveness of this class of medications. The nomograms were intended to protect the double-blind conditions and were not recommended as the best way to determine the right dose of medication. We now know that the dose at which a unique individual gets optimal benefit varies widely from as low as 1 mg per dose to as high as 40 mg per dose. There is no known way to predict the optimal dose. It usually is found through a trial-and-error titration.

Take home message: Optimal doses vary widely and must be fine-tuned to each patient. Most patients detect a difference in their function even at a dosage change of 2 mg. More is not better. The dose that achieves optimal focus of attention, impulse control, mood stability, and no side effects is different for each patient!

17. Describe a trial-and-error titration.

A typical titration protocol starts with just 2.5 mg of medication every 4 hours for methylphenidate or immediate release dextroamphetamine, and every 5 to 7 hours for long-acting amphetamine products. The dose is then increased by 2.5 mg of medication every 1–3 days. With each increase in dose the patient should notice a clear improvement in performance, impulse control, and mood stability, without side effects other than mild appetite suppression. At some point, the dose is increased by 2.5 mg but the patient doesn't notice any improvement over the previous dose. At that point, the optimal dose for that individual is the lower of the two doses. This dose does not change for many years; tolerance does not develop.

Clinical Pearl: All of the stimulant-class medications are moderately strong bases (pH 12–13). If these medications are present in the lumen of the gut with organic acids such as citric acid or ascorbic acid (vitamin C), the stimulant medication is ionized and cannot be absorbed from the gut into the blood stream. The following foods should be avoided for 1 hour before and after taking a dose of stimulant class medication:

Citrus fruit	Kool Aid, lemonade, Gatorade
Citrus juices	Poptarts, granola bars, breakfast bars
Fruit juices with citric acid as a preservative	Oral suspension medications
Sodas/carbonated beverages	Vitamins and food supplements containing vitamin C

18. What are the adverse effects of stimulant-class medications?

At the dose that is optimal for a given individual, there should be no side effects other than a transient loss of appetite. The adverse effects that do occur generally are mild, short lived, and responsive to small decreases in dose or adjustments in the timing of doses.

The more common adverse effects reflect overdosage and include insomnia, jitteriness, irritability, headache (especially as a dose wears off), mild hand tremor, and palpitations. Stimulants may unmask a tic disorder, but do not cause tics. In very rare instances, stimulants can precipitate a psychosis. When psychosis occurs, a coexisting diagnosis of either bipolar mood disorder or schizophrenia must be considered.

There was once a concern that stimulants caused growth retardation in children. When this has been found, compensatory growth always has occurred, and each subject has ultimately reached their full predicted stature.

19. Does treatment of ADHD with stimulant-class medication lead to future drug abuse?

Several prospective studies demonstrate that treatment of ADHD with first-line stimulant class medications seems to **protect against** the development of substance use disorders. The risk comes from *not* treating ADHD.

20. Are there other stimulant medications used to treat ADHD?

Pemoline (Cylert) is a derivative of methylphenidate that is effective for about 70% of persons with ADHD. In multiple clinical trials, pemoline has been shown to be effective in doses of 75–100 mg given once a day in the morning. Unlike the other stimulants which are completely effective as soon as they are absorbed, pemoline often requires 3 weeks to accumulate effectiveness.

The major side effect is difficulty falling asleep. Rarely, children develop **hepatotoxicity**, which has been fatal in more than 20 cases worldwide. Although liver function studies are recommended every 2–4 weeks for at least the first year of treatment, several cases of hepatotoxicity have been so quickly progressive that LFTs would not have caught the hepatitis in time. Due to the potential for fatal hepatotoxicity, the FDA no longer recommends pemoline as a first-line medication. Nonetheless, it is a good alternative for the patient at risk of substance abuse or who is so disorganized and forgetful that once-a-day dosing is all they can manage.

21. Discuss the use of second-line medications.

The second-line medications are second for two reasons: (1) they are only about half as effective as the first-line stimulants, and (2) their effectiveness commonly decreases over time and may suddenly stop altogether. Since their mechanism of action is unknown, it is not known why this "tachyphylaxis" occurs.

The tricyclic antidepressant (TCA) medications **imipramine** and **desipramine** have been used longest. Some research recommends doses of 2–4 mg/kg, while other literature recommends low doses of no more than 60 mg/day even for adults. Either way, TCAs slow cardiac conduction, and an EKG is recommended before initiation of therapy. TCAs may be the best choice for the patient with mild to moderate ADHD and comorbid depression or panic.

Buproprion (Wellbutrin) is an antidepressant that has metabolites similar in clinical structure to amphetamine. Three studies report that buproprion improved the core symptoms at doses up to

400 mg/day in adults and 150–250 mg/day in children. Buproprion usually is well tolerated, with mild headache, nausea, and insomnia the most commonly reported side effects.

One study reports a significant benefit for adults with ADHD from **venlafaxine (Effexor)** at 75 mg bid.

22. What is the role of alpha-2 agonists?

The two alpha-2 adrenergic agonists currently on the market—**clonidine (Catapres)** and **guanfacine (Tenex)**—have been extensively studied. The hyperactive symptoms respond best to the alpha agonists, but they have no effect on other core symptoms of inattention and impulsivity. Consequently, the alpha agonists almost always are used *in conjunction with stimulant-class medications*, especially in the treatment of children with significant hyperactivity.

The alpha agonists have extra utility for patients with coexisting tics and/or Tourette's syndrome. Their side effects of sedation also may be useful to help patients with ADHD shut off their brains and bodies to fall asleep at night.

Treatment is started at low doses (one-half of a 0.1 mg-tablet of clonidine twice a day) and increased gradually to allow development of tolerance to the sedative side effects and because the decrease in hyperactivity may take 2 weeks or more to develop. Once the optimal dose is determined (0.2–0.4 mg/day of clonidine), it can be administered by a transdermal patch. Alpha agonist treatment should not be discontinued abruptly due to the potential for hypertensive rebound.

The combination of stimulants and clonidine was studied extensively following reports of five deaths of children prescribed this combination. The medications seemed to have no causal linkage to the deaths, and the combination is now considered to be both safe and effective.

23. What modalities are not effective for the treatment of ADHD?

More than 20 studies have refuted the claims of dietary manipulations, such as the Feingold diet or elimination diets. Other interventions that have been shown to be largely ineffective in treating core symptoms are:

Individual psychotherapy	Chiropractic manipulation
Cognitive therapy	Megavitamins
Play therapy	Eye movement therapy
EEG biofeedback	Trying harder
Allergy treatments	

BIBLIOGRAPHY

1. American Academy of Child and Adolescent Psychiatry: Practice parameters for the assessment and treatment of attention-deficit hyperactivity disorder. J Am Acad Child Adolesc Psychiatry 36(Suppl 10):85S–121S, 1991.
2. Biederman J, Wilens TE, Mick E, et al: Pharmacotherapy of attention deficit/hyperactivity disorder reduces risk of substance use disorder. Pediatrics 104(2), Internet edition, p e20, 1999.
3. Diagnostic and Statistical Manual of Mental Disorders, 4th ed. Washington, DC, American Psychiatric Association, 1994.
4. Elia J, Ambrosini PJ, Rapoport JL: Treatment of attention-deficit-hyperactivity disorder. N Engl J Med 340:780–788, 1999.
5. Goldman LS, Genel M, Bezman RJ, et al: Diagnosis and treatment of attention-deficit/hyperactivity disorder in children and adolescents. JAMA 279:1100–1107, 1998.
5a. Kelly K, Ramundo P: You Mean I'm Not Lazy, Stupid, or Crazy? New York, Scribner, 1995.
6. Pliszka SR: Comorbidity of attention-deficit/hyperactivity disorder: An overview. J Clin Psychiatry 59(Suppl 7):50–58, 1998.
7. Wolraich ML, Hannah JN, Pinnock TY, et al: Comparison of diagnostic criteria for attention-deficit hyperactivity disorder in a county-wide sample. J Am Acad Child Adolesc Psychiatry 35:319–324, 1996.
8. Zametkin AJ, Ernst M: Problems in the management of attention-deficit-hyperactivity disorder. N Engl J Med 340:40–46, 1999.
9. Zametkin AJ, Liotta W: The neurobiology of attention-deficit/hyperactivity disorder. J Clin Psychiatry 59(suppl 7):17–23, 1998.

57. CONDUCT DISORDER

Paula DeGraffenreid Riggs, M.D., and Elizabeth A. Whitmore, Ph.D.

1. Define conduct disorder.

Conduct disorder is a psychiatric disorder of children and adolescents characterized by a persistent and repetitive pattern of behavior that violates the basic rights of others or major age-appropriate societal norms or rules. According to the specific diagnostic criteria in DSM IV, three (or more) characteristic behaviors must have been present during the past 12 months, with at least one behavior present in the past 6 months (criterion A). Such behaviors generally are present in various settings and cause clinically significant impairment in social, academic, or occupational functioning (criterion B).

The diagnostic criterion behaviors of conduct disorder fall into four main groupings:

Aggressive conduct that causes or threatens harm to other people or animals (bullying, fighting, use of weapons, physical cruelty to people or animals, stealing with confrontation of victim, forced sex)

Nonaggressive conduct that causes property loss or damage (deliberate destruction of property or fire-setting)

Deceitfulness or theft (breaking and entering, "conning" others, theft of nontrivial items without confrontation of victim)

Serious violations of rules (staying out late at night despite parental prohibitions before age 13, running away from home overnight at least twice, truancy from school before age 13).

2. Are there subtypes?

Yes. Conduct disorder is subdivided into two main subtypes:

Childhood-onset type—defined by onset of at least one conduct disorder behavior before age 10. Youths with this type of conduct disorder are usually male and aggressive, with disturbed peer relationships, and meet full criteria for conduct disorder before puberty. The prognosis for these individuals is worse, because these behaviors are more likely to persist into adulthood, and many of these individuals will develop antisocial personality disorder.

Adolescent-onset type—defined by the absence of any criterion of conduct disorder before age 10. Patients are generally less aggressive than those with childhood-onset conduct disorder and have more normative peer relationships. Youths with adolescent onset are less likely to have persistent conduct disorder evolving into antisocial personality disorder. Thus, they more often have adolescent-limited conduct disorder, and their prognosis is better. Girls with conduct disorder are more likely to have this type.

3. How common is conduct disorder?

Conduct disorder is the most common reason for referral of children for psychiatric evaluation and treatment. It is about 2–3 times more common in boys (6–16% prevalence) than in girls (2–9% prevalence).

4. What causes conduct disorder?

There is no single cause of conduct disorder. Generally, factors associated with and contributing to conduct disorder can be categorized as intrinsic and extrinsic. Intrinsic factors are more likely to influence the childhood-onset type than the adolescent-onset type.

Intrinsic factors include:

- **Genetics**. Although definitive studies on the genetics of conduct-disorder have been lacking, at least one behavioral genetics study (that accounts for both environmental and genetic effects) indicates that there is a substantial genetic influence on conduct disorder (accounting for as much as 70% of the variance).

- **Temperamental features**. Hyperactivity, early aggression, impulsivity, sensation seeking, lack of empathy, and guilt have all been associated with the development of conduct disorder.
- **Cognitive impairment and distorted information processing**. Conduct-disordered children have been noted to have verbal and planning skills deficits. They also have a marked tendency to misperceive the intentions of others as hostile and aggressive, especially in ambiguous situations.
- **Dysregulation of serotonin levels** (see Question 9).
- **Autonomic hyporeactivity**. Low reactivity may make it more difficult to influence conduct-disordered children with positive and negative reinforcement.

Extrinsic factors include:

- **Family factors** such as (1) low maternal affection; (2) father's deviance (alcoholism or criminality); (3) substance use disorders in parents or parental surrogates; (4) parental aggression, violence, harsh discipline and/or physical or sexual abuse of children; (5) inability of the parents to provide adequate supervision, consistent structure, and limits; and (6) lack of consistent parental emotional investment, support, and affection.
- **Sociocultural factors**, such as low socioeconomic status, unemployment, and association with delinquent peers.

5. What is the differential diagnosis of conduct disorder?

Oppositional defiant disorder includes some features of conduct disorder but does not include the persistent pattern of more serious deviant behavior in which the basic rights of others or age-appropriate societal norms or rules are violated. According to DSM IV, when an individual meets criteria for both conduct disorder and oppositional defiant disorder, the diagnosis of conduct disorder supersedes the diagnosis of oppositional defiant disorder.

Children with **attention deficit-hyperactivity disorder** (ADHD) often exhibit hyperactive and impulsive behavior and low frustration tolerance, which may be disruptive. Yet this behavior does not violate age-appropriate societal norms and does not usually meet criteria for conduct disorder. The key features of ADHD are inattentiveness, motoric hyperactivity, and poor concentration. Such features distinguish ADHD from conduct disorder.

The irritability and impulsivity of a manic or hypomanic episode, characteristic of **bipolar disorder**, may contribute to behavioral problems. These features usually are distinguished from the disruptive behavioral pattern of conduct disorder based on episodic course and other symptoms, such as pressured speech, reduced need to sleep, and racing thoughts.

The diagnosis of **adjustment disorder** (with disturbance of conduct and emotions) should be considered if clinically significant conduct problems, not meeting criteria for another specific disorder, develop in clear association with the onset of a psychosocial stressor.

For individuals over the age of 18 years, conduct disorder may be diagnosed only if the criteria for **antisocial personality disorder** are not met. The diagnosis of antisocial personality disorder cannot be given to individuals under the age 18 years. On the other hand, the diagnosis of antisocial personality disorder requires evidence of conduct disorder before age 15 (DSM IV).

Aggression, impulsivity, and behavioral problems may be manifestations of various **neurologic problems**, including seizures. Usually such disorders are easily distinguished from conduct disorder by considering longitudinal course and associated features. The same is true for **chronic psychotic disorders**. However, both psychosis and neurologic disorders may be separately comorbid with conduct disorder.

Moreover, many different kinds of psychiatric disorders may present with behavior problems, and the diagnostic criteria for conduct disorder are broad. Therefore, it is essential for the clinician to perform a detailed comprehensive psychiatric evaluation before making the diagnosis of conduct disorder. It is equally essential to assess thoroughly for comorbid disorders.

6. What other disorders are associated with conduct disorder?

Substance use disorders and conduct disorder are highly associated both in adolescence and later adulthood. Although the exact prevalence of substance abuse or dependence with conduct disorder in adolescence is not clear, the Epidemiologic Catchment Area study demonstrated that 84% of individuals with antisocial personality disorder (vs. 17% of the general population) had diagnoses of a substance use disorder in adulthood, and all had conduct disorder as youths.[9] Most antisocial adults with substance use disorders begin substance abuse in adolescence. As the number of conduct symptoms increases, so does the incidence of associated substance use disorder.

ADHD occurs in 30–50% of cases of conduct disorder in both epidemiologic and clinically referred samples. Although both conduct disorder and ADHD are classified as disruptive behavior disorders and may have some symptoms in common, recent studies support that they are separate disorders and that ADHD does not "cause" conduct disorder. If the diagnostic criteria for both disorders are met, both should be diagnosed and treated.

Depressive disorders occur with conduct disorder in 15–24% of cases in both epidemiologic and clinically referred samples.

Anxiety disorders are also more prevalent among youths with conduct disorder (15–24%) than among those without conduct disorder (5–11%).

There are few data regarding the co-occurence of **bipolar disorder** with conduct disorder, partly because of the low prevalence of bipolar disorder in adult populations (approximately 1%). A manic or hypomanic episode with prior depression presenting before age 15 is even more rare. Some studies indicate that adolescents with bipolar disorder may have higher rates of conduct disorder than found in the general population. However, large community-based or multicenter studies will be necessary to address this comorbidity more adequately.

Learning disabilities (especially reading disabilities) are comorbid with conduct disorder in 10–90% of cases. The broad range is most likely due to differences in assessment and diagnosis of learning disorders. Nevertheless, the literature supports high rates of comorbid learning disabilities with conduct disorder overall. Most conduct-disordered children are not severely retarded, but many score in the low normal or borderline ranges of intelligence. Conduct-disordered individuals show a pattern of having lower verbal IQ scores compared to their performance IQ scores, suggesting that they may have specific verbal deficits. Language deficits may contribute to a tendency to express feelings and attitudes physically instead of verbally.

7. Are there gender differences in conduct disorder?

As mentioned, conduct disorder is about 3 times more common in boys than in girls. Boys are also more likely to have the childhood-onset type of conduct disorder and associated ADHD than are girls. Boys are more likely to have persistence of conduct disorder, evolving into antisocial personality disorder in adulthood. Girls may be more likely to have associated depressive disorders than boys.

Gender differences are also found in specific types of conduct problems. Boys with a diagnosis of conduct disorder frequently exhibit fighting and other aggressive acts, stealing, vandalism, and school discipline problems. Girls with a diagnosis of conduct disorder are more likely to exhibit lying, truancy, running away, and prostitution. Conduct disorder in girls also places them at much higher risk for adolescent pregnancy, promiscuity, and contracting sexually transmitted diseases. Both boys and girls with conduct disorder have a high prevalence of comorbid substance use disorders.

8. Are there effective treatments for conduct disorder?

Several recent reviews have highlighted the four major intervention strategies used to treat conduct disorder: (1) parent- and family-targeted programs, especially parent management training; (2) social-cognitive programs; (3) peer- and school-based programs; and (4) community-based programs.

Parent management training (PMT) is aimed at redirecting interactional processes between the parent and child or within the family that may inadvertently develop and sustain aggressive and antisocial behavior. PMT has been demonstrated to be effective in clinically referred populations. A potential problem with PMT, however, is that parents of conduct-disordered children are often not able to participate because of their own psychopathology, substance abuse, marital discord, or family dysfunction.

Social-cognitive and problem-solving skills training assume that changing cognitions and affects will lead to changed or enhanced behavioral adjustments. Children and adolescents with conduct disorder have been shown to have deficits in problem-solving skills, perceptions, self-statements, and self-attributions. For instance, aggressive children are more likely to interpret the intentions and actions of others as hostile and to have poor social relations with peers, teachers, and parents. They often have a limited verbal and behavioral repertoire from which to draw their reactions to strong affects or situations. Thus, a cognitive-behavioral therapeutic approach is aimed at enhancing and broadening this repertoire to help conduct-disordered youths better deal with anger-provoking situations as well as their own impulsive behaviors. Although cognitive and social skills training therapies appear to have some usefulness, their long-term efficacy has not been established. Practical behavioral approaches targeting problem-solving skills appear to be more successful.

Peer- and school-based interventions are focused on the role of peer relations and schools in the development of conduct disorder and antisocial behavior. The theoretical basis is that parental factors are more important in the development of conduct disorder in the preschool years, but that school and peer factors may become ascendent in the early to middle school years. Forty percent of peer-rejected children are aggressive and at high risk to develop antisocial behavior in adolescence. Thus, this treatment focuses on prosocial skills training aimed at reducing aggressive behavior, improving peer and teacher relations, and preventing the development of antisocial behavior. Some evidence supports the short-term effectiveness of this intervention, but no long-term benefit has been demonstrated.

Community intervention strategies are aimed at strengthening the ability of the community to promote prosocial behavior and to deter antisocial and delinquent behavior through changing or enhancing existing systems. Some of the most promising, empirically-supported approaches (e.g., multisystemic therapy and functional family therapy) combine aggressive community case management, intensive family therapy, and specific behavioral approaches to reduce criminality, deviant peer associations, substance use, and out-of-home placements. These types of therapy appear to have the greatest long-term impact on the youth's behaviors.

Treatment of comorbid disorders such as substance use disorders, depression, ADHD, and learning disorders is essential. Specific treatment modalities for comorbidities must be used in conjunction with the behavioral management of the conduct problems; concurrent treatment of the comorbid disorder(s) may enhance the effectiveness of management and treatment of conduct disorder.

Overall, the available literature indicates that early intervention and treatment may be more effective than later intervention. Individual, psychodynamic therapy does not appear to be effective in this population. Because no single intervention works to treat severe conduct disorder, multimodal interventions that target problem behaviors/areas (i.e., criminality, family dysfunction, poor parenting, interactions with deviant peers, school performance) appear to be the most effective.

9. Is there evidence of a specific neurochemical abnormality in conduct disorder and its associated features?

Yes. A growing database supports abnormalities of serotonin in the modulation of brain functions in the disruptive behavior disorders of childhood. A low serotonin syndrome has been associated with early onset of impulsive violent behavior, chronic impulsivity, aggression, and substance abuse—all clearly associated with conduct disorder. Depression and suicidality occur at high rates among conduct-disordered youth and are associated with low central serotonin. Current data are insufficient to determine whether serotonergic agents are helpful in the treatment of conduct disorder. Data indicate that lithium, a nonselective serotonergic agent enhancing 5HT function, is better than placebo in improving the behavior of children with aggressive conduct disorder as well as aggression in adult felons. Additional neuroimaging and neurochemical studies are needed to explore other potential structural or neurotransmitter (e.g., dopamine) abnormalities.

BIBLIOGRAPHY

1. Bukstein OG, Brent DA, Kaminer Y: Comorbidity of substance abuse and other psychiatric disorders in adolescents. Am J Psychiatry 146:1131–1141, 1989.
2. Crick NR, Dodge KA: A review and reformulation of social information processing mechanisms in children's social adjustment. Psychol Bull 115:74–101, 1994.

3. Crowley TJ, Riggs PD: Adolescent substance use disorder with conduct disorder, and comorbid conditions. In Adolescent Drug Abuse: Clinical Assessment and Therapeutic Interventions. NIDA, Research Monograph Series, 1995.
4. Kazdin AE: Psychosocial treatments for conduct disorder in children. J Child Psychol Psychiatry 38:161–178, 1997.
5. Lewis DO: Conduct disorder. In Lewis M (ed): Child and Adolescent Psychiatry: A Comprehensive Textbook. Baltimore, Williams & Wilkins, 1991.
6. Moffitt TE: The neuropsychology of conduct disorder. Dev Psychopathol 5:135–151, 1993.
7. Moffitt TE: Adolescence—limited and life-course-persistent antisocial behavior: A developmental taxonomy. Psychol Rev 100:674–701, 1993.
8. Offord DR, Bennett KJ: Conduct disorder: Long-term outcomes and intervention effectiveness. J Am Acad Child Adolesc Psychiatry 33:1994.
9. Raine A, Lenez T, Bihrle S, LaCass L, Colletti P: Reduced prefrontal gray matter volume and reduced autonomic activity in antisocial personality disorder. Arch Gen Psychiatry 57:119–127, 2000.
10. Riggs PD, Whitmore EA: Substance use disorders and disruptive behavior disorders. In Henderson R (ed): Disruptive Behavior Disorders in Children and Adolescents. Washington, DC, American Psychiatric Association Press, 1999.
11. Robins LN, Regier DA (eds): Psychiatric Disorders in America. The Epidemiologic Catchment Area Study. New York, Macmillan, 1991.
12. Rutter M, Giller H, Hagell A: Antisocial Behavior in Young People. Cambridge, UK, Cambridge University Press, 1998.
13. Steiner H: Practice parameters for the assessment of children and adolescents with conduct disorder. J Am Acad Child Adolesc Psychiatry 36(10 Suppl):122S–139S, 1997.
14. Zubieta JK, Alessi NE: Is there a role of serotonin in the disruptive behavior disorders? A literature review. J Child Adolesc Psychopharm 3:1993.

58. OBSESSIVE-COMPULSIVE DISORDER IN CHILDREN AND ADOLESCENTS

Frederick B. Hebert, M.D.

1. Define obsessive-compulsive disorder.

Obsessive-compulsive disorder (OCD) was formerly thought to be rare and to have a poor prognosis. It is now known to be one of the most treatable of psychiatric disorders. OCD is a lifelong condition that waxes and wanes and often is complicated by depression and anxiety. Defined as a type of anxiety disorder, the symptoms of OCD consist of obsessions or compulsions, and sometimes both.

2. What are obsessions?

Obsessions are demonstrated by recurrent and persistent **ideas, thoughts, impulses**, or **images** that are felt as intrusive and recognized as senseless. The person attempts to ignore, suppress, or neutralize the obsessions with some other thought or action. The obsessions are recognized as the product of the person's own mind rather than imposed from without (except perhaps in children). If another disorder is present, the content is not related (i.e., the obsession is not about guilt or depression). Typical themes are aggression, fear of contamination, doubting, or ordering of objects.

3. What kinds of behavior demonstrate compulsions?

Compulsions consist of **repetitive behaviors** that appear purposeful and intentional, performed in response to an obsession or according to certain rules in a stereotyped fashion. The behavior is designed to neutralize or prevent discomfort or some dreaded event; however, the activity is not connected in a realistic way or is clearly excessive. The person recognizes that the behavior is excessive or unreasonable (children may not). Common compulsions are hand-washing, checking, counting, hoarding, or touching performed in a rigid manner.

4. Since almost everyone has a few obsessions or compulsions, does everyone have OCD?

No. The obsessions or compulsions must cause marked distress and take more than 1 hour/day or significantly interfere with occupational or social functioning to meet DSM IV criteria for diagnosis.

5. How often does OCD occur? What is the prognosis?

OCD occurs frequently in most ethnic groups, with a 2.5% prevalence rate. The onset is in childhood in 33–50% of the cases, with an average onset at age 15. Onset over age 40 is rare. Typically, onset is gradual and follows some trivial precipitant. The family may have a scrupulous religious background; the disorder is recognized among all major religions and is known as *scrupulosity*. Girls are afflicted more frequently, but boys have an earlier onset. In families with one affected member, 20% of relatives meet OCD criteria, and another 20% meet criteria for compulsive personality disorder. A patient's prognosis worsens with concurrent cluster A personality traits (schizoid, schizotypal, paranoid), but a patient's prognosis is not worsened with compulsive personality or passive traits.

As an example, an 11-year-old boy became depressed. When he gradually became obsessed with the idea that his mother would be harmed and simultaneously had suicidal thoughts, he was hospitalized. On the ward, he would pace around the perimeter of the day room. At each corner, he would stop for a ritual of hand wringing. This ritual decreased when it was interrupted by staff, and an antidepressant was started. While one of his siblings also suffered from obsessive thoughts, the mother was quite organized in her work and suffered no disabling rituals.

6. What's the cause of OCD?

The underlying mechanism causing OCD is unknown. Recent biologic, clinical, radiologic, and physiologic evidence of problems in the caudate nucleus or connections from the caudate to prefrontal area of the brain point to an ultimate organic or biologic cause. Self-grooming problems in dogs, particularly canine acral lick disorder (ALD), suggest overstimulation of parallel CNS pathways from a disturbed serotonin balance. Canine ALD is helped by use of selective serotonin reuptake inhibitors (e.g., fluoxetine).

7. What other disorders frequently are associated with OCD?

Depression frequently is associated with OCD; a significant number of children with OCD have major depression. As many as one-half suffered from some other anxiety disorder; 20% have tics, and 5% have Tourette's disorder, which is otherwise rare among the general population.

8. How does OCD present to other health care practitioners?

OCD often is initially seen by family practitioners, pediatricians, and dermatologists. Pediatricians see parents exhausted by the stress of the cleaning or checking rituals of their children. Sometimes a child will use an entire roll of toilet paper for a single bowel movement. If the child cannot attend school or is repeatedly late to school, truancy officials may make the first intervention. Family practitioners or dermatologists may see OCD presenting as nonspecific dermatitis. In children and adolescents, OCD often takes the form of multiple daily showers, an otherwise uncommon behavior in this age group. Children are sometimes noticed when they erase and reerase until they have worn holes in their school papers. Pediatric neurologists may see OCD when consulting for children with repetitive movements after a streptococcal infection. Sydenham's chorea may thus present as a compulsion in the form of repetitive leg movements. Such patients often have radiologic abnormalities. Surgeons frequently are asked by patients with OCD to perform cosmetic surgery for minimal disfigurement (more specifically defined as body dysmorphic disorder). This obsessive demand for bodily perfection is especially seen in adolescent performing artists. Dentists may be the first to see children with OCD, when they present with bleeding gums secondary to repetitive brushing.

9. What is the differential diagnosis of OCD?

In generalized anxiety disorder, the patient has anxiety most of the time, but it is not focused on one idea or behavior. In specific phobias, the patient is symptom-free except from a particular stimulus that causes anxiety. In OCD, the patient is focused on the symptom, yet the patient is also upset by it. Adolescents with OCD know their symptoms come from their own mind. Children with OCD may not know that their symptoms are the product of their own thinking, making the diagnosis more difficult. It is necessary to rely instead on a history of time-consuming rituals from the parents. Patients with OCD generally are not considered psychotic. Major depressive episodes may present with concurrent obsessional thinking; however, the mood disturbance dominates the clinical picture, with obsessing occurring later and remitting with successful treatment of depression.

10. What are the so-called OCD spectrum disorders?

Several disorders that may be related to OCD are called spectrum disorders. Compulsive hair pulling or trichotillomania, urinary and bowel obsessions, and body dysmorphias (obsessive concern that one part of the body is misshapen) are most likely variants of OCD, and are referred to as spectrum disorders. Ritualistic vomiting associated with bulimia is under active debate as a variant, because the vomiting often continues without significant weight loss or obvious personal gain. All of these disorders may have their onset in childhood or adolescence.

11. Are there different types of OCD?

Yes. Most patients (up to 85%) are "cleaners" at some time in their illness. Some are "checkers," endlessly testing whether they have shut doors or turned off a switch. Other children "classify" baseball cards in endless ways or count ceiling tiles over and over. Some patients must have a special symmetry, such as lining up pencils, colored crayons, or shoes; others balance everything that they do or say, such as reading until the number of pages is divisible by two. Far less commonly, the child cannot enter a doorway without a ritual behavior or taps out a rhythm on a fence while repeatedly walking a certain route. A common presentation in many children is to ask questions over and over. Adolescents who need to have the last word may have an obsessive fear that things will not be evened out if they do not.

12. What are the nonmedication treatments?

OCD is particularly interesting among psychiatric disorders, because research indicates an overall low response to both placebo and psychotherapy. In **behavior therapy**, successes and failures have been noted. Systematic desensitization techniques (gradual increase in the presentation of a feared stimulus) were tried first, but failed. Other behavioral techniques also have been demonstrated to reduce anxiety, but not obsessions. **Exposure in vivo (stimulus exposure)** has been known to be effective for some time. This technique requires the patient to come in contact with the obsessive stimulus, such as door handles or toilet seats. **Response prevention** (interrupting or interfering with the patient's response after the obsessive stimulus) keeps the patient from performing the usual cleaning ritual. Several studies, both controlled and uncontrolled, have demonstrated 70–80% rates of effectiveness. Individuals who receive both imagined and actual exposure tend to maintain their gains more successfully over time. Patients with prolonged stimulus exposure do better than those with less exposure.

In response prevention, there were no differences between patients who received 24-hour supervision and patients with minimal supervision. A cotherapist, including a family member, who works with the practitioner has improved results.

One author found that about 60% of patients could be treated overall as outpatients with assigned homework, which stressed an opportunity to learn new strategies. He also found that most of the treatment needed to be carried out in the patient's immediate environment where the rituals take place. However, up to 25% of patients drop out of behavior therapy, and many refuse to follow through with the treatment. The 75% success rate is obtained in the 75% of patients who complete treatment (for an overall response rate of 50%).

Persistent reductions in compulsive rituals over time have been seen most often with behavior therapy, but it is less effective with obsessions, because it is impossible to deal with them in vivo. For such patients, particularly those with severe obsessions, medications are indicated.

13. What medications should be used?

Most antidepressant medications with serotonergic mechanisms of action have been shown to be beneficial in treating OCD. **Clomipramine**, a tricyclic antidepressant with prominent serotonergic effects, was first noted to reduce obsessions in 1968 in a European study. Several double-blind comparisons with other medications have substantiated these results. In one early study combining clomipramine and behavior therapy, medication improved depression, anxiety, social adjustment, and rituals as well as compliance with behavior therapy. In other studies, clomipramine in lower doses reduced obsessive thoughts, but lower doses had no effect on rituals. Clomipramine has a typical tricyclic antidepressant side-effect profile: dry mouth, constipation, and tremor are frequent. Less often, dizziness, sedation headache, and fatigue occur. Sometimes sweating, weight increase, and ejaculation failure are seen. All side effects are reported less frequently by children and adolescents.

Clomipramine remains the drug most often used in studies. Onset of action is in 2–4 weeks, with final improvement over 8–10 weeks. The dose of clomipramine is up to 200 mg/day or 3 mg/kg for children or adolescents.

Selective serotonin reuptake inhibitors (SSRIs) are effective in the treatment of OCD. Of the SSRIs, only **sertraline** and **fluvoxamine** have been approved for the treatment of childhood OCD. Doses often are double that used for the treatment of depression. A dose of 100 mg of sertraline per day or 100–300 mg/day of fluvoxamine often is necessary. Fluvoxamine usually is given in divided doses because of its shorter half-life, and because it is more sedating. Whatever drug is used, starting at a low dose and moving slowly upward works best.

Monoamine oxidase inhibitors have been noted to reduce OCD behavior in patients who also had panic attacks.

Overall, symptoms are reduced by 70%. Less than 10% of children can be expected to drop out of treatment, but children and adolescents include a greater number of placebo responders; thus, children actually may not respond as well as adults. Patients with OCD and an avoidant style or sexual themes in their obsessions have poorer response.

14. All of the medications are antidepressants. Does the patient have to be depressed?

No. The antiobsessive effect is independent of antidepressant effect and is usually maintained with treatment.

15. What if the patient does not respond in 8–10 weeks?

If behavior therapy and clomipramine are not effective, augmentation of the medication with lithium or buspirone may be effective. If side effects limit use of clomipramine, fluoxetine may be administered after tapering clomipramine over 1 week. Fluoxetine is long-acting and frequently competes with other plasma-bound medications for receptor sites; thus care must be taken if other drugs are given. Fluoxetine alone often works well; only 16% of patients report insomnia or anxiety. Stomachaches are frequent if the drug is taken without food. It is best not to start with fluoxetine, because treatment failure may require a drug-free period of up to 5 weeks. Sertraline has a shorter duration of action and may interact less with other drugs than fluoxetine because of less interference with cytochrome P-450 metabolic pathways. Patients with tics and OCD often need an additional neuroleptic or clonidine for sustained response. Neuroleptics may increase the blood levels of clomipramine significantly.

16. Do patients with OCD need hospitalization?

Very few. Treatment of OCD usually can be accomplished on an outpatient basis, with a combination of behavior therapy and medication.

17. What is a PANDA?

PANDA is a pediatric autoimmune neuropsychiatric disorder associated with streptococcal (group A beta-hemolytic streptococcal) infections. Swedo and her group first reported on these children in 1998. All the children had the five working diagnostic criteria: presence of OCD or a tic disorder, prepubertal onset, episodic course of symptom severity, association with group A beta hemolytic infections, and association with neurological abnormalities. The presence of abnormal movements in children following streptococcal infection has been known for years as Saint Vitus dance. It was thought to be a rare complication. Swedo's group was the first to make the connection that this is a form of OCD caused by an autoimmune response.

BIBLIOGRAPHY

1. Flament MF, et al: Obsessive compulsive in adolescents: An epidemiological study. J Am Acad Child Adolescent Psychiatry 27:764–771, 1988.
2. Geller DA, et al: Similarities in response to fluoxetine in the treatment of children and adolescents with obsessive-compulsive disorder. J Am Acad Adolescent Psychiatry 34:36–44, 1995.
3. Insel TR, Akiskal HS: Obsessive-compulsive disorder with psychotic features: A phenomenologic analysis. Am J Psychiatry 143:1527–1533, 1986.
4. Jenike MA, et al: Obsessive-compulsive disorder: A double-blind, placebo-controlled trial of clomipramine in 27 patients. Am J Psychiatry 146:1328–1330, 1989.
5. Kirk JW: Behavioral treatment of obsessive-compulsive patients in routine clinical practice. Behav Res Ther 21:57–62, 1983.
6. Marks I, O'Sullivan J: Drugs and psychological treatment for agoraphobia/panic and obsessive-compulsive disorders: A review. Br J Psychiatry 153:650–658, 1988.
7. March JF, et al: Sertraline in children and adolescents with obsessive-compulsive disorder. JAMA 280:1752–1756, 1998.
8. Perse T: OCD: A treatment review. J Clin Psychiatry 49:48–55, 1988.
9. Reynynghe deVoxrie G: Anafranil in obsession. Acta Neurol Belg 68:787–792, 1968.
10. Rapoport JL: The Boy Who Couldn't Stop Washing. New York, Plume, 1989.
11. Rasmussen SA: Obsessive-compulsive disorder in dermatologic practice. J Am Acad Dermatol 13:965–967, 1985.
12. Swedo SE, et al: Pediatric autoimmune neuropsychiatric disorders associated with streptococcal infection: Clinical descriptions of the first 50 cases. Am J Psychiatry 155:264–271, 1998.
13. Zak JP, et al: The potential role of serotonin reuptake inhibitors in the treatment of obsessive-compulsive disorder. J Clin Psychiatry 49(Suppl):23–29, 1988.

59. ENCOPRESIS AND ENURESIS

Benjamin P. Green, M.D.

ENCOPRESIS

1. Define encopresis. How common is it?

As defined by the Diagnostic and Statistic Manual–IV (DSM–IV), encopresis is the repeated involuntary or intentional passage of feces into inappropriate places, such as into clothing or onto the floor, at a frequency of at least monthly for a duration of 3 or more months. To qualify for this diagnosis the patient must be at least 4 years old (corrected for mental and developmental age), and the condition must not be due to a medication (e.g., laxative) or caused by a general medical (somatic) condition other than constipation.

Although encopresis may occur at any age—especially among individuals with severe organic brain disease—it is primarily an affliction of childhood. Approximately 15% of 8 year olds and 0.8% of 11 year olds suffer from this disorder; the male:female ratio is 3:1.

2. Are there clinically significant subtypes?

Although historically much has made of the distinction between primary encopresis (in which bowel continence has never been achieved) and secondary encopresis (in which incontinence has been established but then lost), the most useful clinical subtyping is organized around the presence or absence of constipation with overflow incontinence. Constipated or retentive encopresis is usually associated with small, soft, poorly formed stools that leak out both day and night. When constipation is absent, the stools tend to be large, well formed and intermittently deposited, often in particularly offensive places. The nonretentive type is more likely associated with oppositional and defiant behavior.

3. How important is encopresis in the context of psychotherapy?

Careful study of clinical case material derived from psychoanalysis and psychotherapy has convincingly demonstrated the centrality of anal phenomena and their far-reaching influences on human psychic development. The physical functions of the rectum and the anal sphincter—i.e., storing, withholding, hiding, expelling, soiling, controlling/losing control—are infantile bodily experiences that remain important in a literal sense throughout the lifespan. They also serve as metaphors, paradigms, and experiential templates that tend to impose powerful a priori patterns of meaning and relationship configurations on a wide variety of subsequent life events. Anal preoccupations are normative for 18–36-month-old children. Undue focus on these matters by older individuals suggests temporary or persistent ego regressions, developmental arrests, psychosexual fixations, or post-traumatic reenactments.

As a caveat that anticipates the discussion of treatment that follows, it is imperative that these anxiety-provoking psychodynamic realms only be probed and explored with the patient by a qualified clinician and even then only within the context of an empathetic, child-oriented therapeutic relationship. This symptom tends to elicit intense feelings and a heightened sense of urgency, and you may feel strongly tempted to let fly with premature interpretations and piercing insights; to yield to this temptation would quite likely be both unproductive and even quite hurtful to the patient.

4. Which causes encopresis—psyche or soma?

Over the past several decades, writings from the fields of behavioral pediatrics have increasingly defined thinking about the resource-efficient, symptom-focused treatment of encopresis. This is not to say that psychosocial variables are not significant risk factors; children ranked by parents' questionnaires in the top decile for behavioral problems are five times more likely to soil. The direction of causality—if any—between encopresis and emotional/behavioral problems is less certain, however (e.g., one may soil because of angry obstinacy, or one may become angry and defiant because of bowel failure and the consequent interpersonal conflicts and societal rejection).

By contrast, the temporal primacy of physiologic variables is all but undeniable in many cases. Infantile "early colonic inertia" and an imperforate or stenotic anus and/or rectum strongly predispose a child toward later fecal difficulties. Rather than to assert causality per se, however, it is more rigorously correct to assess the relative etiologic weighting of the various predisposing, potentiating, and perpetuating factors.

The muscular ability to defecate a rectal balloon (an approach commonly used in experiments to quantify rectal mobility) evaluates one of the primary somatic, constitutional aspects of encopresis. It has been used to predict both the presence of encopresis and the likely response to treatment. In one study, 43% of encopretic boys, compared with 10% of controls, could not extrude a distal rectal balloon because of tightening of the muscles near the anal canal. Furthermore, failing at balloon defecation lowered the probability of treatment success from 63% to 15%.

Ultimately, most authorities conclude that causality is best explained in terms of both psyche and soma. The most elegant pathogenic models are interactive, contemplating the ways in which constitutional and acquired physiologic factors influence outcome in conjunction with individual and familial psychosocial variables. One conceptualization describes the interaction in terms of developmental stages:

	Physiologic Factors	Psychosocial Factors
1. Infancy and toddler (0–2 years)	Simple constipation	Parental overreaction
	Early colonic inertia	Overzealous anal manipulations
	Congenital anorectal problems	
	Other anorectal condition	
2. Early childhood (3–5 years)	Painful or difficult defecation	Idiosyncratic toilet fears
		Psychosocial stresses during training period
		Coercive or extremely permissive toilet training

3. Early school years (6–11 years)	Prolonged or acute gastro-enteritis Food intolerance, lactose deficiency	Attention deficit/task impersistence Frenetic life style Psychosocial stresses Avoidance of school bathrooms

For the sake of completeness, several rare pediatric conditions that can—in and of themselves—cause colonic encopresis should be mentioned: Hirschsprung's disease (and the still controversial variant known as ultrashort segment Hirschsprung's), hypopthyroidism, spinal cord lesions, Crohn's disease, malnutrition, and disorders of voluntary muscle function, such as amyotonia congenita, infectious polyneuritis, and cerebral palsy.

5. What data should a competent evaluation include?

Resources permitting, a full pediatric and psychiatric evaluation should be undertaken.

The **history of present illness** should begin with the child's and then the parents' description of the problem and their explanations of causality. Often, surprising issues are raised that may help to focus and prioritize the treatment plan.

A **developmental history** should be taken of the child's bowel habits and the environment's response to same over time. Particular attention should be paid to the timing, characteristics, and outcome of initial toilet training efforts and to subsequent epochal events, such as relapses, exacerbations, or progressions. For each significant period, data should include biomedical, social/contextual, and individual psychological factors.

Biomedical questions should cover the frequency, chronology, volume, viscosity, and caliber of stooling as well as the presence or absence of defecatory pain.

Social/contextual data should include the health and stresses of the caretakers, marriage and family, parental history for elimination disorders, expectations of the child, attempts at teaching continence, response to successes and failures, utilization of help (from both professional and lay sources), and the variability of caretakers' behaviors across different settings (e.g., grandparents, day care providers, school staff).

Individual psychological evaluation should emphasize the assessment of global developmental projectory, acquisition of adaptive intelligence, quality of relatedness generally and with primary caretakers specifically, negativism, oppositionality, dependence and counterdependence, inattention, forgetfulness, self-monitoring, depression, guilt, peer relationships, and self-esteem.

While taking the history of present illness and developmental history, the clinician should observe carefully the interaction between the child and caretakers with regard to empathy, ability to discuss difficult subjects openly, degree of agreement regarding the encopresis, conflict resolution skills, interdependence, intimacy, demoralization, anger, shame, guilt, and frank potential for violence and abuse.

The **physical exam** should evaluate the child's general health, thyroid, lower limb neurologic status, abdomen, and the perianal area to evaluate, respectively, for (the wasting of) Hirschsprung's disease, hypothyroidism, neuromuscular disorders, retained stool, and perianal fissures, sores, or group A streptococcal cellulitis. Impactions may not be detected by a rectal exam; experienced practitioners know that the midline suprapubic area is the most frequent location of retained stools.

Barium enemas and manometric evaluation of sphincter function are seldom contributory, but a **plain film** of the abdomen should be ordered routinely to assess for fecal retention. Rectal or colonic biopsies should be considered only for extreme cases. Radiographic studies should be repeated after the initial bowel clean-out, because 30% of the disimpacted patients once again will be found to have retained stools.

6. When should toilet training begin?

Crosscultural studies demonstrate that the ability for self-initiated toileting can be consolidated by 10½ months of age! The timing of training is primarily influenced by social values and assumptions. Surveys in the United States, for instance, document that in 1947, 95% of children had completed toilet training by 33 months of age, whereas by 1975 this figure had fallen to 58%. A child who can crawl or walk is probably neurologically ready for training.

7. What is the significance of toilet training?

Many health care professionals have a minimal understanding of optimal toilet training. This knowledge is critical for both prevention and treatment of disorders of elimination. Developmentally, toilet training is anything but trivial. Successful training is a source of pride and of a growing sense of developmental mastery for both child and family. Conversely, problems in this area may result in intense conflicts, low self-esteem, and even violence; in one study, toilet training failure was the second most common precipitant of fatal child abuse. Given humankind's recent, belated focus on child maltreatment, it is not surprising that assertions have been made regarding the association between encopresis and child abuse.[9] A careful statistical comparison with baseline rates have, however, detected no significant differences.[4]

8. How should toilet training be carried out?

The usual recommendations for parents include the following:

1. Children are usually ready for toilet training between 18 and 24 months (corrected for mental age). Signs of readiness include verbal awareness of "poop" and "pee," understanding the "potty chair" and how its use can prevent being wet or soiled, expressed preference for being dry (which should be encouraged by the parents), and a demonstrated ability to postpone elimination.

2. The parental approach should be characterized by praise, patience, and encouragement. Punishment and pressure should be avoided. Parents are teaching a skill, not attempting to subjugate an adversary.

3. Helpful equipment includes a floor-level potty chair offering good foot support, training pants, food rewards, stickers or stars, and an educational picture book to make the process more friendly and familiar.

4. The potty chair should be selected by the child and parent together and then decorated and individualized. It can be used outside the bathroom as a chair (with clothes on) during enjoyable activities (e.g., watching television) for a week or so before being used for its designated function.

5. "Practice runs" should be used to rehearse the interrupting of play activities, going to the bathroom, undressing, sitting, waiting, wiping, and redressing. Reading stories or watching television on the potty can make the process more pleasant. Such sessions should not exceed five minutes, but they should happen several times a day, especially right after meals (thus taking advantage of the gastrocolonic reflex).

6. Rewards of praise, food, stickers, stars, or even money should be given for compliance with practice runs, for successful toileting, and especially for self-initiated toileting.

It is important to assess whether the parent understands this basic approach to toilet training. If not, parental education and support should be the first order of business. Sometimes, of course, the problem may be more serious than lack of knowledge. Any child over 2½ years of age who is not continent after several months of training can be assumed to be resistant rather than undertrained. Intermittent minor underwear wetting or small fecal smears should be considered part of the learning process and as pathological resistance, unless the frequency or degree is extreme.

9. Describe difficulties that may be encountered during toilet training.

Entrenched power struggles over toileting may occur. Parental behaviors that exacerbate such a conflict include repeated nagging, long periods of enforced toilet sitting, use of shame-inducing techniques, excessive physical punishment, and inappropriate use of enemas and/or digital disimpaction. Suggestive behaviors on the part of the child may involve daytime incontinence, refusal to sit on the toilet, wetting and soiling immediately after enforced toilet sitting, and apparent indifference to the problem. When such an impasse is detected, referral should be made to a mental health professional or to a pediatrician specializing in behavior disorders.

10. When and how should pharmacologic treatments be used?

Despite a few anecdotal reports of successful treatment with imipramine, pharmacotherapeutic agents of established efficacy include only enemas, laxatives, and stool softeners. Before any of these are used, however, it is imperative that nonretentive soiling be distinguished from retentive, constipated soiling; the treatment of the former should *not* involve medicines but, instead, the same psychotherapeutic and behavioral strategies used with oppositional-defiant disorders and protracted parent-child conflicts.

The use of **enemas** to treat retentive encopresis carries a certain degree of psychological stress, but it is absolutely necessary to ensure initial bowel emptying. Fleet's hyperphosphate enemas should be used, 1 ounce for every 20 pounds of body weight, up to a maximal dose of 4 ounces. A second dose should be given 1 hour later. An optional third enema may be administered after another 12–24 hours if continued soiling or persistent abdominal mass suggests incomplete evacuation. Ultimate treatment failure is inevitable unless the fecal impaction is cleared from the onset. Once this is accomplished, however, subsequent enemas should be unnecessary (unless severe reimpaction occurs) and may even be countertherapeutic. It is wise to have the child drink 1–2 glasses of water before an enema to minimize dehydration.

Once the impaction has been treated, relapse can usually be prevented with **stool softeners**. Mineral oil is most commonly used; it tastes best when refrigerated and chased by the fruit juice of choice. A vitamin pill should be given each day that mineral oil is used to prevent nutritional leeching. The alternatives to plain mineral oil are the better tasting emulsified oils such as Retrogalas, plain Agoral, Metamucil, and Kondremul. Because of the risk of aspiration and pulmonary complications, none of these oils should be given to children who have gastrointestinal reflux vomiting or who are not yet walking.

If stool softeners prove inadequate in promoting daily evacuations, **laxatives** may be used to stimulate colonic motility. Laxatives can be prescribed with relative impunity; "laxative dependency" is an unfounded concern. Recommended products include Senokot, Fletcher's Castoria, Milk of Magnesia, Haley's M-O, and Ducolax.

Definitive treatment in all but the mildest cases requires a minimum of 6 months. The relapsing of symptoms and the lapsing of therapeutic compliance are more the rule than the exception; persistent, gentle support and redirection from the physician are usually necessary.

11. Should the child be reminded to toilet?

Normal children and adults perceive when their rectum is full, but chronic constipation causes stretching and desensitization of the lower gastrointestinal tract. Psychological reluctance and constitutional inattention also may contribute to the child's failure to initiate trips to the bathroom. It is therefore recommended that the child be gently reminded to adhere to scheduled sittings on the toilet after breakfast and dinner either until a bowel movement has occurred or until 10 minutes have expired. To take full advantage of the gastrocolic reflex, 5–30 minutes after eating is optimal. Bending forward while sitting, relaxing the anus and buttocks, and pushing gently with the abdomen may help. For shorter children, a foot stool is recommended to enhance pushing leverage and to provide a greater sense of security. If recurrent soiling occurs (indicating a full rectum) or if the child complains of stomachache, cramping, or feeling blocked up, a more intensive program of sitting on the toilet is indicated. On weekends and after school, 10 minutes of every hour should be dedicated to sitting on the toilet until a large bowel movement has been produced.

Individuals in the child's other significant environments (e.g., school, day care, family relatives) should be advised to allow the child unfettered access to bathrooms and to offer gentle reminders when there are indications of flatulence, abdominal cramping, or frank soiling. Lectures, harsh criticism, and shame induction should be avoided.

12. How should a caregiver respond to soiling?

Evidence (either olfactory or visual) of soiling should be met with an immediate, firm but restrained request that the child clean him- or herself and put on fresh clothing. Spare undergarments should be available at school or at day care. The child should be involved in scraping off (e.g., with a spatula or spoon) solid waste and then washing the soiled underwear in the toilet. A bucket of water with bleach and a lid can be left for this purpose in the bathroom. This procedure reinforces the message that soiling is not catastrophic but neither is it to be tolerated.

13. Is diet important?

Absolutely. Milk products and cooked carrots tends to be constipating, whereas fruits and vegetables —especially raw ones—promote healthy defecation. Particularly recommended are figs, dates, raisins, peaches, pears, apricots, celery, cabbage, broccoli, cauliflower, peas, and beans. The cereal food groups also provide much fiber, including popcorn, nuts, bran flakes, bran muffins, shredded wheat, oatmeal, brown rice, and whole wheat bread. Copious consumption of water and fruit juices also should be encouraged, although—as with all of these items—in a manner gentle enough to avoid conflict.

ENURESIS

14. Define enuresis.

DSM-IV defines enuresis as the intentional or involuntary voiding of urine into clothes or any other inappropriate place by a child at least 5 years old (corrected for mental and developmental age). The condition cannot be caused by a substance (e.g., a diuretic) or by a medical condition (epilepsy), and the frequency must equal or exceed 2 times/week for a duration of at least 3 consecutive months. Finally—as with any disorder of clinical significance—the symptoms must result in significant subjective distress and/or dysfunction (e.g., social failures).

15. Are there clinically important subtypes?

Subtypes include nocturnal, diurnal, and combined. Another distinction is primary vs. secondary enuresis. Primary enuresis denotes life-long incontinence, whereas in secondary enuresis continence was achieved for at least 1 year but then lost. Among school-age children primary and secondary enuresis are roughly equal, but three times as many children have nocturnal rather than diurnal enuresis. Daytime and secondary enuresis are more likely to be related to emotional and behavioral problems and times of psychosocial stress: ages 5–7 and the onset of adolescence are developmental periods at highest risk for these subtypes.

16. What is the incidence rate?

The total incidence of enuresis by age is roughly as follows:

Age	Percentage of the Population
3	40
4	30
5	20
8	7
12	3
18	1

17. What is known about the cause of enuresis?

As with encopresis, causality is best explained by simultaneous consideration of both psychosocial and physiologic factors and their interactions. Enuretic children appear to suffer from developmental delays across multiple domains; they tend to have smaller bladders, immature bone-age scores, learning disabilities, and disturbances of behavior. The presence of enuresis doubles the risk for an additional **psychiatric diagnosis**, although the association is not specific to any particular concurrent disorder.

The numerous **sleep stage and sleep arousal theories** are at present more suggestive than definitive. **Genetic predisposition** is significant; having one enuretic parent increases the life-time risk to 45%, whereas having two afflicted parents increases the likelihood to 75%. Twin studies estimate that 70% of the symptom variance is attributable to genetic factors. Note that the male:female ratio is 2:1.

Among the numerous **organic causes** that should be ruled out, the most important is urinary tract infections. Also to be considered are diabetes mellitus and insipidus, constipation, ectopic ureter, lower urinary tract obstruction, neurogenic bladder, bladder calculi (or other foreign bodies), epilepsy, and sleep apnea due to enlarged adenoids. However, in the absence of such phenomena as a weak or dribbly urinary stream, excessive urine production, or manifestations of convulsive diathesis, a simple urinalysis is the only laboratory evaluation recommended to augment the routine history and physical exam. More intrusive studies (e.g., intravenous pyelography) tend to be expensive, traumatizing, and noncontributory.

18. How similar to encopresis is enuresis?

Very similar. To avoid redundancy, the reader is referred to the section about encopresis for discussion of the psychosocial factors to be assessed in an evaluation, the psyche-soma controversy, toilet training procedures, and behavioral management. Apart from the obvious differences in physiologic factors, the major phenomenologic difference between the two disorders of elimination is the propensity of enuresis to be nocturnal. The behavioral management of diurnal enuresis is virtually identical with that described for encopresis. The pharmacologic treatments of enuresis—as one would expect—are also quite different.

19. What are the behavioral treatments for nocturnal enuresis?

The fundamental problem causing nocturnal enuresis is the combination of a small bladder and an inadequate capacity for self-arousal during sleep. Either or both traits can be heritable.

Bladder capacity is measured by asking the child to try on three separate occasions to hold his or her urine for as long as possible and then to void into a container. The maximal quantity should equal in ounces a child's age + 2; a smaller quantity suggests small bladder size. In such cases, it may well help to prescribe bladder-stretching exercises, which encourage the child to hold his or her urine for as long as possible during the day. Whenever the urge to void is felt, self-distracting techniques should be used in an effort to override the bladder spasms for a minimum of 10 seconds. Physiologically, this exercise may increase the functional bladder capacity while psychologically the child is learning to resist and postpone the first urge to urinate. Parents are encouraged to challenge the child playfully to try to break the record for maximal single-void volumes.

Several strategies also may be used to address the child's **inability to self-awaken** in response to bladder fullness. First, fluid intake should be gently discouraged for the 2 hours prior to bedtime; however, heated arguments over a few swallows are unwarranted. Secondly, the bladder must be emptied just before the child goes to sleep. The majority of nocturnal urine is produced in the first third of the night. One implication of this fact is that parents who stay up several hours later than their child may routinely wake the child for a second voiding just before their own bedtime. Even small bladders may then be adequate to contain the urine produced during the remainder of the night. If this technique is used, it should be carefully discussed with the child in advance and the child's co-operation should be rewarded with praise, stickers, stars (put on a chart or calendar), or even small food treats or toys (to avoid over-stimulating the child, these rewards should be given the next morning). Optimally, the child should learn to self-awaken. An alarm clock can be set for 3 hours after bedtime; in many ways, this approach is preferable because it encourages more autonomous functioning. (Another more technically demanding procedure—"bladder biofeedback"—involves multiple training sessions using a transurethral catheter. This treatment has proven itself successful with 70% of patients, but it is made available by only a small number of interested urologists.)

Another helpful approach focuses on **teaching the child to attend and respond** to nocturnal bladder sensations. The child and parent(s) practice three times each night before bedtime the sequence of lying down, closing eyes, pretending to perceive bladder fullness in the middle of the night, feeling the ache, getting up, running to the bathroom, urinating, and then returning to bed. This sequence should be rehearsed physically as if one were practicing for the theater. It is more realistic if the child voids a small amount during each repetition before finally emptying his or her bladder completely before being tucked in. Appealing to the child's developmentally appropriate magical thinking, one can personify the bladder and describe it as trying to wake up the child "before it's too late." Another helpful metaphor is to suggest that the child is a fireman or firewoman who needs to respond to the alarm and get up in time to put out the fire with their urinary stream. Both compliance with practicing and nocturnal successes should be rewarded. Also, putting a nightlight or flashlight in the child's room and/or in the bathroom may add a measure of safety and control.

20. When should a nocturnal alarm be used?

Enuresis alarms should used when the simpler behavioral techniques have been unsuccessful and when the child is sufficiently motivated and mature to cooperate. This approach tends to work best when the child is at least 8 years of age and when the prescribing physician is comfortable with and knowledgeable about the treatment. Caveats notwithstanding, it is the opinion of many experts that nocturnal alarms are the most definitive therapy for nocturnal enuresis. Compared with imipramine treatment, the use of enuresis alarms is associated both with a higher cure rate (70% vs. 60%) and a dramatically lower relapse rate (10–15% vs. 50–100%); it is therefore curious that less than 5% of physicians recommend nocturnal alarms.

The newer alarms are lightweight, comfortable to wear, inexpensive, and widely available. (If local pharmacies do not stock them, the Nyton Alarm can be ordered from Nyton Medical Products, 2424 South 900 West, Salt Lake City, UT 84119, or the Nite Train'r Alarm can be ordered from Koregon Enterprises, 9735 SW Sunshine Court, Beaverton, OR 97005.)

21. How are nocturnal alarms used?

These alarms fit into or clip onto underwear and generally do not impede sleep. Parents and children should be encouraged to experiment with the alarm before putting it into use; it is important to demonstrate that a few drops of fluid result in an auditory signal but not—as some may imagine— any form of shock or pain. The child should be encouraged to feel ownership for both the alarm and the treatment program. Again, practicing before sleep helps to make the requisite response to the alarm more automatic. The child can rehearse by setting off the alarm with a few drops of water, getting up, voiding, putting on dry underwear, resetting the alarm, and returning to bed. The goal of awakening before wetting should be underscored; it can become a game to "beat the buzzer."

Parents should be told to wait several seconds after the alarm has begun before trying to wake their child (e.g., by stroking the face with a cold washcloth) and to let child turn off the alarm. The child's participation should be maximized. The alarm should be used until a month has elapsed without incontinence—usually after 2–3 months of treatment. Relapses, if they occur, usually respond to a few additional months of the program.

22. What are the pharmacologic treatments for enuresis?

If the more benign nonpharmacologic methods have failed, **imipramine** and **desmopressin** (DDAVP) should be considered.

23. Describe the treatment of enuresis with imipramine.

Several dozen studies since 1960 have demonstrated the efficacy of imipramine as a treatment for enuresis. The initial starting dose is 25 mg/day; low-dose responders should not be overmedicated. If necessary, the dosage should be increased at a rate of 25 mg/week until therapeutic success is realized, adverse side effects (e.g., anticholinergic symptoms) become intolerable, or the maximal daily recommended dose of 5 mg/kg of body weight is reached. The usual therapeutic daily dose is 75–125 mg. For children who wet early in the night, the total dose may be divided into a midafternoon dose and another dose 1 hour before bedtime; for children with other enuretic patterns, the entire dose should be given 1 hour before sleep.

An electrocardiogram (EKG) should be obtained during the baseline period and for every dosage increase over 3.5 mg/kg of body weight. Although various EKG parameters may be monitored, the primary concern is that the quinidine-like effect of imipramine will result in cardiac dysrhythmia if the corrected (for heart rate) QT duration (i.e., the QTc) exceeds 450 ms. Several studies suggest that successful treatment is most likely when the combined imipramine plus desipramine serum level is at least 80 ng/ml.

Some children seem to respond transiently to imipramine (e.g., for 2–3 weeks) but then demonstrate tolerance to each successive dosage increase up to and including the maximal recommended daily dose. As many as 60% of enuretic children are successfully treated with imipramine; however, the relapse rate is 50–100% once the medicine is discontinued. Imipramine has a rather narrow therapeutic index; numerous pediatric tragedies have resulted from accidental tricyclic overdoses, many related to lack of precaution regarding medication storage.

24. Describe the treatment of enuresis with desmopressin.

Desmopressin is a more recent addition to the therapeutic armamentarium. Supplied as a nasal spray, DDAVP has efficacy and relapse rates similar to imipramine without the concomitant unpleasant side effects and the risk of cardiac conduction delays. Treatment with DDAVP, however, is quite expensive (i.e., 3–6 dollars per night). Note also that there have been case reports of desmopressin-induced hyponatremia, some involving iatrogenic seizures. To prevent this, children should be restricted to 8 oz of fluid intake during evenings when desmopressin is to be administered. Parents should be instructed that nausea, vomiting, or headaches in a child taking desmopressin should be evaluated with a serum electrolyte determination—with a temporary cessation of treatment pending diagnostic clarification.

25. Do the benefits of these agents outweigh the risks?

Both medicines have their pros and cons. Some clinicians believe that successful treatment (e.g., for 3 months) results in permanent cures at rates greater than one would expect from spontaneous remission alone. Others point to the lack of empiric support for this claim. Temporary use of either medicine—e.g., for summer camp or overnight stays with a friend—are much less controversial and may well be a real boon to a child's social life. For a number of patients, the risks and costs of these medicines given continuously may be more than offset by the psychosocial benefits; in such cases, drug tapering every 3 months should be scheduled to detect as soon as possible maturationally driven remissions.

26. Are other medications helpful?

There are several published anecdotal reports about successful treatments involving other pharmaceuticals. The SSRIs (specifically fluoxetine and sertraline, given in doses comparable to anti-depressant therapy) seem promising although it's not clear whether they act by increasing ADH release, inducing bladder smooth muscle relaxation, or other, as yet unidentified mechanisms. In a recent Finnish study, indomethacin in doses of 100 mg/day also resulted in "improvement" in 76% (but only absolute continence in 14%) of their sample of 29 children—this comparing with 93% improvement in the desmopressin group. The benefit noted appeared related to the decrease in the serum and urine concentrations of the (bladder-contracting) prostaglandin PGE.

27. How should a parent respond to bed wetting?

• The child should be encouraged to try to stop the urinary flow as soon as he or she realizes that wetting has begun. At this juncture, the child should hasten to the toilet to eliminate whatever urine remains.

• The child should change into dry nightclothes and place a dry towel over the wet part of the bed; to encourage the child's independence, clean pajamas and a towel should be laid out the night before on a chair near the bed.

• In the morning the child should wash him- or herself and the pajamas.

• As with soiling, pains should be taken to avoid criticism, humiliation, or punishment by parents or siblings. Support and encouragement for attaining developmental mastery minimize psychological trauma and accelerate the learning process.

A few more practical recommendations may help to reduce the family's aggravation and frustration: Extra thick underwear may be provided for nighttime use. Sheets and bedding may be protected with a towel placed under the child's buttocks and a plastic mattress cover. Sheets may be allowed to air dry and then laundered twice weekly. Remind the parents that the problem is esthetic, not sanitary (i.e., urine is sterile). To discourage infantilization, diapers and plastic pants should be discontinued by age 4 years (corrected for mental age).

ACKNOWLEDGMENTS

The author gratefully acknowledges the contributions of Carol Green, Janet Nakata, Bart Schmitt, and Lin Borden.

BIBLIOGRAPHY

1. Aladjem M, Wohl R, Boichis H, et al: Desmopressin in nocturnal emesis. Arch Dis Child 57:137–140, 1982.
2. Feeney D, Klykylo W: SSRI treatment of enuresis (letter). J Am Acad Child Adol Psychol 36:1326–1327, 1997.
3. Fergusson DM, Horwood LJ, Shannon FT: Factors related to the age of attainment of nocturnal bladder control: An 8-year longitudinal study. Pediatrics 78:884–890, 1986.
4. Foreman D, Thambirajah M: Letter to the Editor. Child Abuse Negl 22:337, 1998.
5. Hoekx L, Wyndaele J, Vermandel A: The role of bladder feedback in the treatment of children with refractory nocturnal enuresis associated with idiopathic detrusor instability and small bladder capacity. J Urol 160:858–860, 1998.
6. Kaplan SL, Breit M, Gauthier B, et al: A comparison of three nocturnal enuresis treatment methods. J Am Acad Child Adolesc Psychiatry 28:282–286, 1989.
7. Levine MD, Bakow H: Children with encopresis: A study of treatment outcome. Pediatrics 58:845–852, 1976.
8. Levine MD: Encopresis: Its potentiation, evaluation and alleviation. Pediatr Clin North Am 29:315–330, 1982.
9. Morrow J, Yeager C, Lewis D: Encopresis and sexual abuse in a sample of boys in residential treatment. Child Abuse Negl 21:11–18, 1997.
10. Schmitt BD: Toilet training refusal: Avoid the battle and win the war. Contemp Pediatr 4(12):32–50, 1987.
11. Schmitt BD: Your Child's Health, 2nd ed. New York, Bantam Books, 1991.
12. Rapoport JL, Mikkelsen EJ, Zavadil A, et al: Childhood enuresis. II: Psychopathology, tricyclic concentration in plasma, and antienuretic effect. Arch Gen Psychiatry 37:1146–1152, 1980.

60. ADOLESCENT DRUG ABUSE

Frederick B. Hebert, M.D., and Gordon K. Farley, M.D.

1. How common is adolescent substance abuse?

The use and abuse of alcohol and other drugs by adolescents in the United States is a common, serious, and sometimes life-threatening problem. In a study of consecutive appearances at a large city psychiatric emergency room, 35% of the adolescent admissions were for suspected or confirmed drug abuse. About one-third of eighth graders and about two-thirds of twelfth graders use alcohol. Over one-half of twelfth graders report that they drive after drinking. More than 50% of fatal car crashes involving drivers under 20 are alcohol-related. Well over one-half of twelfth graders report marijuana use. Cocaine and crack use are reported to be high among teenagers. It is estimated that 10–15% of all teenagers will develop serious problems with drug and alcohol abuse.

With the frequent use of psychoactive substances by adults to change their moods and emotions, it is not surprising that substance abuse is among the most common problems of adolescents. Adults use substances to wake up in the morning, to sleep at night, to enjoy sex more, to improve their alertness, and to self-medicate their psyches. By the time an adolescent is 15, he or she will have had thousands of experiences of seeing respected and admired adults smoking, ingesting, and perhaps even injecting psychoactive substances, both in person and the media.

2. List the most commonly abused drugs.

Commonly abused drugs in rough order of frequency include:

Substance	Street Names
Alcohol (most commonly used drug by adolescents)	—
Tobacco/Nicotine (second most commonly used drug by adolescents; accounts for more adult deaths than any other drug)	—

Table continued on next page

Substance	Street Names
Marijuana	Dope, grass, stash, hash, Mary Jane, M.J., pot, reefer
Stimulants	
Amphetamines	Speed, ice, meth, crystal, crank, glass
Dexedrine	Bennies, white crosses
Methylphenidate (Ritalin)	—
Cocaine	Coke, cocoa, paste, snow, powder, crocks, quarter rock, crack
Anorectic drugs either by prescription (Preludin, Tenuate) or over the counter, such as phenyl-propanolamine and pseudoephedrine	
Hallucinogens	
Lysergic and diethylamide	LSD, acid
Psilocybin	Magic mushroom, boomers, shrooms
Mescaline	Peyote, cactus, button
Phencyclidine	Angel dust, PCP
Ketamine	Special K, Vitamin K
Narcotics and Analgesics	
Morphine	Morf, Miss Emma
Codeine	—
Heroin	Smack, stuff, horse, junk, China white
Volatile Substances (inhaled)	
Solvents (gasoline, paint thinner, benzene, acetone)	—
Toluene (Rustoleum clear paint, plastic and rubber cement)	—
Aerosol sprays (paint, hair spray, cooking oil)	—
Cryogenic chilling fluids (Freon)	—
Sedative Hypnotics	
Barbiturates	Reds, yellows, rainbows
Barbiturate-like drugs	—
Methaqualone	Soapers (even though now only illegally manufactured)
Benzodiazepines (e.g., Librium, Valium, Xanax, Halcion)	—
Anticholinergic Drugs	
Atropine, some antihistamines, antiparkinsonian medications (Artane, Kemadrin)	—
Scopolamine	Scope
Club Drugs	
Methylenedioxymethamphetamine (MMDA)	Ecstasy, XTC, clarity, lover's speed
Gammahydroxybutyrate (GHB)	G, liquid ecstasy

3. What are the general concerns in treating acute intoxication with any drug?

The major concern in the acutely intoxicated is to maintain life-support systems until it is known what specific drug has been ingested. The acute treatment of intoxication or acute drug abuse is a highly specialized activity and best done in inpatient medical or psychiatric settings where medical support is readily and immediately available.

4. What makes alcohol intoxication dangerous?

Alcohol intoxication is extremely common and often occurs in combination with other substances, most frequently sedative hypnotics. The symptoms vary with route of administration, amount used, specific substance, previous history of use and addiction, and period of time over which the substance has been consumed. Alcohol intoxication should be suspected with a history of rapid change in mental status, because alcohol is rapidly absorbed through the gastric mucosa. Laboratory confirmation of alcohol use is easily obtained; however, behavioral symptoms correspond only roughly to blood alcohol levels. Nystagmus on extreme lateral gaze, mild dysarthria, and mild ataxia are relatively early signs.

The most important part of treatment is to follow the patient carefully to avoid coma. Some adolescents have died from high alcohol blood levels when their breathing stopped, apparently because levels were high enough to block the medullary breathing centers. Social risks include impulsive and unprotected sex, fighting, and automobile accidents.

5. What about hallucinogens?

Psychomimetics include marijuana, LSD, psilocybin, and phencyclidine (PCP). These agents cause a cognitive disorder with illusions ("trails" with marijuana), frank visual hallucinations (color and shape changes with LSD), and disordered thinking (body image changes progressing to thought blocking and delirium with PCP). What is not generally known is that all hallucinogens produce anxiety, ranging from mild transient dysphoria with marijuana to anxious irritability with PCP and genuine panic with LSD ("bad trips").

Physical changes include injected conjunctivae with marijuana, and dilated but reactive pupils with LSD and psilocybin. PCP, however, produces more prominent physical signs. Paresthesias in the limbs, initially or at low doses, progress to analgesias (cigarette burns are common), then muscular rigidity, myoclonus, or even convulsions or coma. When seen in the emergency department, the patient taking PCP may be mute and amnestic with catatonic posturing. Ptosis and nystagmus may be the only clues to diagnosis.

Lab tests may be helpful, but most hallucinogens are cleared quickly; hence negative drug screens are common. However, urine screens for marijuana may be positive for several days after a single dose.

6. Is sniffing glue dangerous?

Solvents produce a giddy delirium that may progress to coma with prolonged inhalation. Despite newspaper reports, few youths have died from acute inhalation, but many have suffered long-term brain damage by repeated use. Usually this damage takes the form of dementia, but sometimes presents as pure cerebellar degeneration. The diagnosis is suspected when a patient has a ketone breath and body odor, and swollen mucous membranes but no other cold symptoms. Poverty and depression frequently are associated with solvent abuse. Initial medical treatment is supportive.

7. Why is abuse of stimulant drugs harder to treat?

Stimulants are known as "body" drugs for their ability to produce physiologic changes. Cocaine in its many forms is now the best known illicit stimulant, but even caffeine produces many symptoms if sufficient amounts are taken. Symptoms include dilated but reactive pupils with a host of Ts: tremor, tachycardia, tachypnea, talkativeness, temperature (elevated), and tension (muscular and nervous). Grand mal convulsions and a high temperature may lead to shock. Deaths have been related to strokes, cardiac irregularities, and delirium. Initial euphoria is followed by anxiety and irritability, then anger and rage with higher doses. Speeded-up thinking may become maniacal acutely or paranoid over prolonged periods. In this case a urine toxicology screen or hospitalization for longer term observation is the only method for distinguishing chronic stimulant abuse from schizophrenia.

Acute treatment for mild reactions requires only general support, or, at most, single-dose neuroleptics (e.g., haloperidol [Haldol], 5 mg intramuscularly) to calm the patient. Serious toxicity requires major supportive measures in a structured medical setting, with ice packs and diazepam (Valium) to control temperature and seizures. Physical and mental depression frequently follow withdrawal; thus the tendency to increase the dose of the drug is high. With the advent of lower melting point cocaines through freebasing and high-tech marketing (pagers, cell phones, and crack houses), the drug has come into widespread use. Cocaine, particularly in its newer form as cocoa paste, is a highly concentrated and dangerous drug.

8. Do adolescents who take drugs have other problems?

Most of these youngsters were breaking rules before they began using substances. There are only three methods of supporting an expensive drug habit—theft, prostitution, or distribution—and none is legal. Current methods of distribution emphasize use of youngsters on the front lines, because they face less severe penalties when caught. Although most adolescents do not become addicts, the U.S. leads all industrialized nations in percentage of young people involved with illicit drugs.

9. Can drugs be detected without blood or urine tests?

Cocaine recently has been shown to be excreted in saliva at levels parallel to plasma levels. It may be possible to develop a saliva screening test using a dipstick method.

10. What are the basics of long-term treatment for drug abuse?

No one method is more effective than others; thus, treatment reflects a plethora of methods. Basic approaches emphasize the goals of acceptance, education, and usually abstinence. More recent approaches have emphasized addiction as a family disease and focused on sexual abuse as a common theme. Inpatient programs emphasize a stepwise approach, last 4–6 weeks, and make frequent use of videos and films. Patients are taught to increase self-esteem and to recognize their individuality; return to the community is gradual.

When in denial and/or uninformed, the family's attitude toward substance abuse ("Don't talk, don't trust, don't feel") can lead to specialized roles in the family as well as emotional abuse and passage of substance abuse to the next generation. Multisystemic and multimodal treatment programs that attend to individual, family, peer, school, and community factors associated with drug abuse have achieved recent prominence. These programs are especially effective for the treatment of juvenile offenders who also have a drug abuse problem. All comprehensive treatment programs should attend to comorbid psychiatric conditions. Note that Alcoholics Anonymous and Narcotics Anonymous are helpful, long-term support systems.

11. What can the physician do to help the cessation and prevention of tobacco use?

From the standpoint of lifetime mortality and morbidity, tobacco use is undoubtedly the most serious addiction. More than 450,000 Americans die each year because of tobacco use, and a much larger number suffer chronic illness. There is evidence that maternal smoking during pregnancy may put the offspring at additional risk for specific psychopathology (e.g., attention deficit-hyperactivity disorder [ADHD]). For most smokers, tobacco use begins during the juvenile years. The National Cancer Institute recommends that physicians use a five-step program when treating adolescents. All steps begin with the letter A. The steps are: 1. Anticipatory guidance. 2. Ask. 3. Advise. 4. Assist. 5. Arrange follow-up. These steps have been described in great detail by the American Academy of Pediatrics. Nicotine addiction treatment using nicotine-containing gum and transdermal patches as a substitute for cigarettes has had some success. The use of medications such as bupropion (Wellbutrin, Zyban) to decrease nicotine craving also has been useful.

12. What factors predict adolescent drug abuse?

A number of contributors to adolescent drug abuse have been identified by workers in the field:

Social sanction	Cultural and ethnic factors
Previous risk-taking behavior	Family patterns
Abuser personality characteristics	Family dysfunction
Economic feasibility	Modeling
Family history, genetic loading	Peer influences
Poverty	Alienation
Psychiatric co-morbidity, e.g., ADHD, bipolar mood disorder, depression, anxiety, conduct disorder)	Reinforcing chemical properties of the substance
Environmental reinforcement (family, societal, and media influences)	

13. What stages of drug abuse have been identified?

The National Commission on Marijuana and Drug Abuse describes these patterns or stages:

1. Experimental drug use
2. Social or recreational use
3. Circumstantial or situational drug use
4. Intensified drug use
5. Compulsive drug use

The American Medical Association describes the following patterns of drug use:

1. Drug experimentation
2. Drug use, first recreational, then regular
3. Drug abuse
4. Drug dependency

A common pattern of cocaine use and abuse by groups includes the following steps:

1. Curiosity
2. Initiation
3. Pleasure
4. Group identification
5. Group prestige
6. Family isolation
7. Psychopathic behavior
8. Ritualistic behavior
9. Dependency tolerance
10. General physical deterioration
11. Severe sociopathic personality destruction

Despite the different labels, each of these progressions notes a movement from curiosity and controlled casual use to uncontrolled obligatory use (addiction).

14. How can the stages help to identify at-risk adolescents?

To treat adolescent drug abuse effectively, many experts believe that the stage of the abuser or potential abuser must be recognized. Many questionnaires purportedly reveal adolescents who are at risk for or already in the early stages of abuse. The questions revolve around parent and peer relations, school adjustment, and observed drug use.

Drug abuse by teenagers is believed by many to be seriously underestimated because of numerous factors, including **denial by physicians, mental health professionals, and family members**, as well as the often episodic nature of drug abuse. The use of routine questions about family and individual patterns of drug abuse and use can aid in detection.

15. Can treatment during early stages be helpful?

During the early stages of drug curiosity and experimentation, parental and peer attitudes are crucial. Parents must present appropriate questions and expectations to the adolescent and let the adolescent know what their actions will be if drug use is observed. Group sessions to explore attitudes toward drug use and anticipated consequences and alternatives may be helpful, because adolescents are susceptible to peer influences.

16. How successful is treatment during the middle stages?

During middle stages of adolescent drug use and abuse, traditional mental health approaches have been relatively unsuccessful. By contrast, many different kinds of self-help and peer-support groups claim remarkable success. Some of these groups include: Parents, Peers, and Pot; Palmer Drug Abuse Program (PDAP); Channel One; Alcoholics Anonymous (AA); Al-Anon Family Groups; Families Anonymous; Narcanon Family Groups; and Narcotics Anonymous. Often, a traditional psychotherapeutic approach combined with chemically enforced abstinence and a self-help peer-support group leads to the best results. Note that treatment of co-morbid psychiatric illness is important at any stage of abuse.

BIBLIOGRAPHY

1. American Academy of Child and Adolescent Psychiatry: Practice parameters for the assessment and treatment of children and adolescents with substance use disorders. J Am Acad Child Adolesc Psychiatry 36(suppl):140S–156S.
2. Brook JS, Cohen P, Brook DW: Longitudinal study of co-occurring psychiatric disorders and substance use. J Am Acad Child Adolesc Psychiatry 37:322–330, 1998.
3. Epps RP, Manley MW, Glynn TJ: Tobacco use among adolescents: Strategies for prevention. Pediatr Clin North Am 42:389–402, 1995.

4. Galanter M, Gleaton T, Marcus CE, McMillen J: Self-help groups for parents of young drug and alcohol abusers. Am J Psychiatry 141:889–891, 1984.
5. Henggler SW, Borduin CM: Family Therapy and Beyond: A Multisystemic Approach to Treating the Behavior Problems of Children and Adolescents. Pacific Grove, CA, Brooks/Cole, 1990.
6. Kaminer Y: Adolescent Substance Abuse: A Comprehensive Guide to Theory and Practice. New York, Plenum, 1994.
7. Kandel DB, Chen K, Warner LA, Kessler RC, Grant B: Prevalence and demographic correlates of symptoms of last year dependence on alcohol, nicotine, marijuana and cocaine in the US population. Drug Alcohol Depend 44:11–29, 1997.
8. Kandel DB, Johnson JG, Bird HR, et al: Psychiatric disorders associated with substance use among children and adolescents: findings from the Methods for the Epidemiology of Child and Adolescent Mental Disorders (MECA) Study. J Abnorm Child Psychol 25:121–132, 1997.
9. Riggs DD: Depression in substance-dependent delinquents. J Am Acad Child Adolesc Psychiatry 34:764–771, 1995.
10. Weissman MM, Warner V, Wickramaratne PJ, Kandel DB: Mental smoking during pregnancy and psychopathology in offspring followed to adulthood. J Am Acad Child Adolesc Psychiatry 38:892–899, 1999.
11. Zoccolillo M, Vitaro F, Tremblay RE: Problem drug and alcohol use in a community sample of adolescents. J Am Acad Child Adolesc Psychiatry 38:900–907, 1999.

61. PRINCIPLES OF CHILD AND ADOLESCENT PSYCHOPHARMACOLOGY

Frederick B. Hebert, M.D.

1. Why are physicians concerned about child and adolescent medications?

Practitioners sometimes avoid giving medications to children and adolescents because they are concerned about unusual responses or dosage requirements. However, except for the lack of a euphoric response to stimulants in children, there are few qualitative differences between children and adults in their response to medication. Children's younger organs frequently clear medications more quickly, whereas adolescents generally need adult doses.

2. What are major issues for the family practitioner?

Families sometimes focus all difficulties on unlikely medical causes or past injuries and expect that medications either will not work at all or will work miracles. Medications may allow a seriously ill child to be treated as an outpatient; this is an important point, but hardly a miracle. Medications are part of a total treatment plan. Parents and practitioners need to be supportive, never using medications as a punishment. Children and adolescents need to remember that medications do not excuse them from the need to work on their problems. Below are specific principles for treatment of attention deficit-hyperactivity disorder, depression, psychosis, conduct disorders, and anxiety disorders.

ATTENTION DEFICIT-HYPERACTIVITY DISORDER

3. Why is so much attention paid to attention deficit-hyperactivity disorder (ADHD)?

ADHD is a common and well-researched childhood disorder. The central notion of a short attention span and hyperactivity has been around since a German poet wrote about "Fidgety Phil" a hundred years ago. In the ensuing years, over 10,000 articles have been published in the scientific literature. Although stimulant medications have been used for over 50 years, from time to time splinter groups have raised questions about their use. From the standpoint of the scientific community, stimulants remain one of the safest and most effective of all psychotropic medications. The increase in use of stimulants is probably the result of an increased recognition that 15% of patients with

ADHD continue to show signs and symptoms in adolescence. Girls suffer from ADHD only one-fourth as often as boys. In the differential diagnosis, mood disorders are most difficult to rule out. A positive family history of mood disorder and lack of learning disability are more likely in bipolar patients. Thirty to 50% of the mental health referrals for children are for ADHD.

4. Are stimulant medications still the mainstay of the medication treatment for ADHD?

Absolutely. Stimulants remain the best medications for ADHD. Recent concern over the short duration of action of methylphenidate (Ritalin) and the small dose size of dexedrine tablets has led to the development of mixed salts of a single-entity amphetamine product, marketed as Adderal. Adderal showed greater efficacy than methylphenidate at mid-day and day's end across several behavioral measures. Side effects were similar to other stimulants: anorexia, insomnia, stomach pain, headache, irritability, and weight loss. Adderal often is titrated up to 0.75 mg/kg, or 75% of the dose of methylphenidate.

In addition, bupropion, marketed as an antidepressant, has been shown to be equal to methylphenidate in at least one study of ADHD when it was given at doses of about 3 mg/kg body weight. The larger tablet sizes available in Adderal (10, 20, 30 mg, scored) and Wellbutrin (75, 100, 100 SR, 150 mg SR, unscored) permit dosing in heavier adolescents and young adults but may pose a problem in children. Risk of seizure with bupropion also is a consideration (especially with a history of head injury or seizure disorder).

5. What can we tell parents about ADHD?

The physician must take a careful history and have parents and teachers fill out checklists, because only 20% of children show signs of ADHD in the office. Historical factors in ADHD known to be associated with the mother's pregnancy include heavy metal exposure, chronic drug abuse, moderate alcohol use, or smoking more than 4 cigarettes/day. Once the diagnosis is made and before medication is started, an explanation to the parents is helpful. Compare the brain to a machine, and tell parents that the medication lubricates the system and makes it run more smoothly; it does not offer a cure. Physician and parents can tell the child that the medication is like a baseball glove; if the child takes the medication, it will help him or her, but the child must still try to play the game.

6. What is the role of clonidine in the treatment of child and adolescent behavior disorders?

Clonidine is useful in treating patients with ADHD and oppositional defiant disorders who have not responded to more conservative treatment with stimulants and behavioral therapy. It is a centrally acting drug that inhibits release of norepinephrine and acts centrally to reduce brain arousal; its effects on attention are indirect. Its antihypertensive effects are not clinically evident in children and adolescents, despite a 10% decrease in measured blood pressure. Clonidine reduces arousal and irritability, improving frustration tolerance. Parents have noted improvement in doing chores, and teachers have seen a reduction in classroom aggression.

Clonidine is rapidly absorbed, peaking in 60–90 minutes. If inactive, such as sitting on a school bus, patients may fall asleep for up to 30 minutes afterwards. When active, patients are alert and not sedated. The clinical effects last only 3–4 hours because of rapid metabolism by both liver and kidneys. The dose ranges from 4–6 μg/kg/day. A typical starting dose is one-half of a 0.1-mg tablet at bedtime for 3 days. Another half tablet is added in the afternoon or morning, increasing gradually to a dose of 2–4 tablets given 2–3 times/day.

Clonidine has been used as a test for growth hormone release, but it is not clear whether it actually increases growth. It increases appetite, however, and this effect is helpful in reducing weight loss when clonidine is combined with methylphenidate hydrochloride (Ritalin). Clonidine also reduces energy and stamina, and these effects, along with lowered blood pressure, should be monitored.

Clonidine is available in the form of a skin patch (Catapres TTS) in doses of 1, 2, and 3 mg; the patch lasts for about 5 days. Young patients adapt easily and wear the patch on their back. The patch tolerates brief exposure to water (as in the shower), but if submerged or pulled at, it loosens. An overlay patch, which comes with each medication patch, may be used. A new area of the back should be chosen each week. About 25–50% of patients react with local irritation, itching, and erythema. The reaction is more commonly to the gum in the patch than to the medication itself. Older children and adolescents frequently want to demonstrate their own control by "improving" or removing the patch. Some adolescents explain its presence as a way of staying off nicotine, although clonidine was not effective for this indication in adult trials.

7. Can clonidine be combined with methylphenidate hydrochloride?

For patients with both oppositional or conduct disorders and ADHD, clonidine may be combined with methylphenidate hydrochloride. Such children often are highly distractible and explosively aggressive; combined medication helps to avoid institutional placement. Often patients take high (> 1 mg/kg) doses of methylphenidate hydrochloride in the morning and at noon and are difficult to control in the afternoon and evening. The addition of clonidine allows an afternoon nap for younger children and more controlled bedtime behavior. In the evening, clonidine should be given at bedtime; otherwise, some patients awaken later in the evening and cannot return to sleep. Frequently, the dose of methylphenidate hydrochloride can be reduced by one-third or more. Side effects such as anorexia and insomnia are relieved whether clonidine is given concurrently or separately later in the day.

Clonidine also has been combined clinically with tricyclic antidepressants (TCAs) and neuroleptics. In one case report a patient with only a 1-day wash-out from propranolol had a serious drop in heart rate when clonidine was started. Heart rate rebounded when clonidine was discontinued. Propranolol and clonidine should not be given simultaneously.

8. Can Tourette's disorder (TD) in children be treated with clonidine?

It is important to establish the correct diagnosis. Many children have motor tics, but the diagnosis of TD requires additional vocalizations (grunts, yelps, explosive sounds, or words). TD in adults most often is treated with haloperidol, but child psychiatrists often start with clonidine. Clonidine has a slower onset of action and lower response rate than haloperidol or pimozide, but a lower incidence of side effects and no risk for tardive dyskinesia.

DEPRESSION

9. Do children become depressed like adults?

Depression is now recognized in children, although it may not be the same disorder as in adults. Because larger numbers of children respond to placebo, it is difficult to tell whether medications are effective. Symptoms of depression in children include self-deprecation, inhibition, sleep disturbance, morning tiredness, decreased activity, difficulty in concentrating, and poor school performance. But they also may exhibit aggression, enuresis, and hypochondriasis—symptoms not predicted from the adult model. TCA doses have ranged from 1–5 mg/kg, usually of imipramine, after an initial EKG. Blood levels and serial EKGs are performed weekly when patients take doses > 4 mg/kg to monitor the quinidine-like effect of imipramine. Responders had higher plasma levels (about 150 ng/ml) than nonresponders, with optimal response at blood levels of about 200 ng/ml of imipramine and its metabolites. Higher levels were associated with decreased efficacy and delirium on some occasions.

10. Is monitoring of blood levels necessary in every child?

It is important to measure TCA blood levels routinely in children, because clinical response is related to blood level, not dosage, and a 40-fold difference may exist in the plasma concentration of different patients receiving the same dose. Because children differ from adults in body fat, percent of total body water, and protein-binding characteristics, and have more active enzyme systems, they may create and accumulate more metabolites than adults. Available studies indicate that both beneficial and serious side effects of TCAs are related to plasma concentration and that the therapeutic range is relatively narrow; thus monitoring of plasma levels is necessary in the treatment of childhood depression. A 1-week baseline period should be obtained in all children before treatment, as about 20% will no longer be depressed after this interval. There is no benefit in monitoring blood levels of other antidepressants, as blood levels are not well correlated with clinical response.

11. What about adolescent depression?

Although scientific evidence is lacking, most clinicians agree that adolescents whose depression resembles adult endogenous depressions respond to TCAs. Adolescent major depressions are characterized by gradual onset, anorexia, weight loss, middle- and late-night insomnia, psychomotor disturbance, and family history of serious depression. Early morning wakening is so strikingly different from the usual "stay-up late and sleep-in" style of adolescents that it should raise the clinician's suspicion. Many adolescents also no longer appear depressed after a short hospital stay without medication. There are no reliable laboratory studies for diagnosing depression (e.g., dexamethasone suppression test). As in adults, diagnosis is based upon history and presentation. Be alert to family histories of mood disorder.

12. What controversies exist in the treatment of adolescent mood disorders?

The problems stem from diagnostic issues. Most adolescents don't present with depressions that look like adult depressions. When they do have symptoms of adult depression (e.g., weight loss, decreased sleep and energy) they also may have auditory hallucinations. Some evidence suggests that these adolescents may be at risk for bipolar disorder. Therefore, adolescent patients with hallucinations may be helped by putting them on mood stabilizers before, or in addition to, antidepressants or antipsychotics.

Another diagnostic issue occurs when adolescents present with aggression and irritability, but no grandiosity or hallucinations. The diagnostic manual, DSM IV, allows the diagnosis of manic disorder without euphoria or hallucinations. However, the combination of irritability and aggression most often presents in adolescents who suffer from conduct disorder, and this is the diagnosis typically given by child psychiatrists. Adult or general psychiatrists are likely to make the diagnosis of bipolar disorder and commence treatment with a mood stabilizer (e.g., valproic acid). This places the patient at some risk because valproate has known side effects for adolescents; while hair loss is only a temporary problem, polycystic ovaries, a life-long concern, have been reported in adolescent girls. It is the opinion of many child psychiatrists that bipolar disorder should not be diagnosed in the absence of psychosis or euphoria, even if irritability is present. Epidemiological studies show that conduct disorder is many times more frequent than bipolar. Giving a sedating medication like valproate to every irritable adolescent does not prove the diagnosis of bipolar disorder, but may create a patient who appears "improved" largely because he or she is sedated.

13. Are adolescents at risk for overdosing on medications?

The adolescent's ability for rapid behavior change necessitates caution. Adolescents attempt suicide more than other age groups, many by drug overdose. This fact emphasizes the need for careful assessment of suicide risk and follow-up of adolescents taking medications with a high potential for lethal overdose (e.g., TCAs, lithium).

14. What about outpatient follow-up for adolescent depression?

When the adolescent is followed as an outpatient, only small amounts of antidepressants are prescribed at one time; thus the patient must be seen frequently or a responsible adult must be in control of dispensing. In follow-up visits, the patient is asked routinely about sleep disturbance. If middle or late insomnia recurs, the patient should resume therapeutic doses and may be on maintenance treatment for 1 year. Such long-term therapeutic regimens are extrapolations of prescribing patterns for adults; there are no comparable adolescent studies. To date, drug studies in adolescents do not demonstrate the superiority of antidepressant over placebo in the treatment of depression, but practitioners continue to see clinical improvement after careful diagnostic screening for major depression.

15. Are newer medications safer?

Yes. Many of the newer antidepressants (e.g., fluoxetine and sertraline) have been used with adolescents and are less toxic in overdosage than TCAs; hence they are safer to use. Fluoxetine is the selective serotonin reuptake inhibitor (SSRI) that has been used most often with adolescents who are depressed, as an extrapolation of its wide use in adults. Trazodone also has been successfully used in doses up to 400 mg/day. Because trazodone is initially quite sedating and may cause light-headedness, it was originally given in divided doses after meals. Now it is most often used as an adjunct to fluoxetine to help the patient sleep. It is given at bedtime after a snack. Anticholinergic and cardiac effects are unlikely, but priapism shortly after initiating treatment has been reported; this side effect is a relative contraindication for adolescent boys. Like all currently known antidepressants, trazodone is excreted in breast milk and should not be given to nursing mothers; it is considered a category C drug because of increased fetal absorption in rats. Overall, these medications are much safer than older tricyclics, are at least as effective, and often are better tolerated.

16. Do all classes of depression in adolescents look like depression in adults?

Although major depressions respond to regular antidepressants, many depressed adolescents do not meet criteria for major depression. Atypical depressions present with dysphoric mood, but patients maintain mood reactivity while depressed; that is, they respond to comments by the interviewer with a change of mood. In addition, patients may have a history of sensitivity to rejection. Instead of weight loss and inability to sleep, they may show increased appetite or weight gain and sleep over 10 hours/day. Any sleep disturbance in adolescents needs to be distinguished from the common habit of staying up late and sleeping in with overall adequate sleep time. Patients also may complain of severe fatigue, sometimes manifested by complaints of leaden weights in arms or legs.

17. What medications are useful in atypical depression?

Earlier studies demonstrated that for atypical depression in young adults, monoamine oxidase inhibitors (MAOIs) were better than TCAs. Of adolescents unresponsive to TCAs, 75% responded to phenelzine in one study. Side effects were numerous, but dietary compliance was a problem for less than one-third. Most patients had no significant side effects, even with dietary indiscretion. Later studies concluded that atypical depression may reflect primarily the age of the patient. A more recent study found that adolescents who fail to respond to treatment with TCAs often improve when lithium carbonate is added. At therapeutic doses of lithium, adolescents took up to 2 weeks to respond, but improvement persisted. Atypical depressions may also represent depression in individuals with bipolar disorder; hence treatment may need to be modified. Atypical depressions may also respond to SSRIs and venlafaxine.

18. Can newer medication be used for atypical depression?

Concern over lethal overdose led to a search for treatments of adolescent depression of all types with agents that are less likely to be harmful. Fluoxetine has gained wide use in adults, but few studies are available in adolescents. Bupropion, which is unrelated to both TCAs and SSRIs, has been effective in atypical depression in adults. It has shown stimulant effects and was withheld from introduction because of seizures in bulimic patients who took the drug. Overall risk is low if the dose is below 400 mg per day and any single dose is less than 150 mg. The usual adult dose is 150 mg SR, two times/day; a typical dose in adolescents is 250 mg/day or less. Menstrual irregularities were seen infrequently with bupropion. Both medications are safer in overdose than TCAs, MAOIs, or lithium carbonate.

PSYCHOSIS

19. What kinds of psychoses are seen in children and adolescents?

Psychosis in children and adolescents may be reflective of primary psychiatric illness or secondary to medical problems (e.g., toxicity). Delirium is usually the result of drug ingestion, either accidental in children or recreational in adolescents. In either case, treatment is directed to the underlying cause, but delirium-induced agitation may need separate treatment.

20. How is delirium treated in children and adolescents?

Treatment usually takes the form of a structured and locked setting, including the use of a seclusion room or restraints if necessary. Delirium-induced agitation also may require judicious medication. A child who is thrashing about may need to be sedated for brain scan, EEG, or radiograph.

Adolescents who have taken hallucinogens usually can be talked down. Patients who have taken phencyclidine (PCP) may become agitated if a therapeutic encounter is attempted. Such patients may seriously harm themselves and others because the anesthetic properties of PCP keep them from knowing that they have painful injuries.

Agitated and delirious patients can be sedated with haloperidol, 0.1–0.3 mg/kg, over 1 hour; dystonia is the only likely acute side effect. This side effect frequently is more frightening to the patient and family than the original delirium. Any child or adolescent given haloperidol should be observed closely for 24 hours so that dystonic reactions can be treated. Benadryl (diphenhydramine), 25–50 mg orally or intramuscularly, and reassurance once the dystonia subsides usually are the only treatments needed for dystonias.

21. What about chronic psychotic disorders that accompany autism and head injuries?

More recently, medications have been used to treat the obsessive-repetitive behaviors in autistic children. Clomipramine and fluoxetine have reduced stereotypic behaviors. Patients with chronic psychoses due to head injury, autism, or pervasive developmental disorders may respond to low doses of haloperidol, which reduce stereotyped and aggressive behavior.

22. Can short-term use of antipsychotic medications cause serious side effects?

A major concern is the potential for movement disorders, especially tardive dyskinesia (TD). Acute use of antipsychotic medications is unlikely to cause TD. However, children and adolescents may develop a time-limited form of TD after taking antipsychotics only 6 months. Symptoms appear in the extremities as choreiform movements or as ataxia and usually disappear 2 weeks after the medication is discontinued, but movements may persist from 3–12 months. Many chronically ill children and adolescents may need to be on neuroleptics for years and, like adults, are at risk for long-term oral-buccal tardive dyskinesia. One of the newer atypical neuroleptics, resperidone, has also caused dyskinesias. Olanzapine has led to large weight gain and akathisia. Quetiapine has been associated with cataracts in dogs.

23. What primary psychiatric illnesses can present as psychosis?

Mania, schizophrenia, and depression can all present as psychosis. Psychotically depressed children and adolescents have more auditory hallucinations than adults; these can be treated by adding neuroleptics to the antidepressants. Hallucinations usually remit in less than 1 month, and the neuroleptics can be discontinued. Adolescents and children with psychotic depressions are at risk for bipolar disorder. Although mania is quite uncommon in children, 20% of all bipolar disorders have their onset before the age of 20, most often presenting initially as major depression.

24. How is mania treated?

Mania in children and adolescents presents more commonly with irritability than euphoria and also has a high incidence of hallucinations, making differentiation from schizophrenia difficult. Clinicians should err in favor of the least disabling diagnosis; thus the diagnosis frequently is mania, even if not all hallucinations are related to mood. Agitation and hallucinations respond to neuroleptics, but the grandiosity usually requires lithium carbonate. Baseline kidney and thyroid function studies are done to confirm the patient's ability to clear lithium and euthyroid status. Lithium carbonate is begun at up to 30 mg/kg in divided doses. Lithium carbonate, 300 mg in sustained-release form, avoids the gastric upset and dizziness associated with regular lithium. Within 5 days the patient should be in range of 0.8–1.2 mEq/L. Children and many adolescents need to reach levels of 1.5 mEq/L for a good serum level. Doses which maintain a serum range of 0.8–1.2 mEq/L are also appropriate for maintenance. The serum level is followed at gradually greater intervals. Thyroid studies should be repeated at 6-month intervals, because a few patients become hypothyroid. If a good response ensues, with tolerable side effects, chronic maintenance is recommended as bipolar illness tends to get worse over repeated episodes. Preventing recurrence is extremely important to the long-term prognosis.

25. What are the alternative medications for mania?

Carbamazepine and valproic acid have been used as alternatives because 30–40% of adult manic patients do not respond to or cannot tolerate lithium carbonate. The use of carbamazepine is less common in children than in adults. Sodium divalproex is used for dysphoric mania, rapid cycling, and patients whose presentation includes psychotic symptoms or substance abuse in addition to mania. Many adolescents present with psychotic symptoms, and sodium divalproex often is added to lithium carbonate, but also may be used alone.

After baseline liver and platelet studies, sodium divalproex is given in divided doses of 20 mg/kg. It is rapidly absorbed with a peak action at 4–6 hours. The dose is gradually increased until levels of 50–120 mg/ml are reached. Patients frequently respond in 5–10 days. The most common side effects are GI upset, mild tremor, and initial lethargy. A decrease in platelets and an increase in liver enzymes may occur. An increase of liver function values to 300% of baseline is acceptable, and thrombocytopenia usually is not seen until blood levels exceed 100 mg/ml of valproate. Hair thinning is transient and dose-related but may be particularly disturbing to adolescents. Sodium divalproex also is available in pull-apart capsules as a sprinkle that can be used in soft foods with younger children or patients who cannot take capsules by mouth. Unlike lithium, sodium divalproex is 80–95% protein-bound and thus competes with other protein-bound medications, such as carbamazepine or fluoxetine. As a result of the interaction, the less tightly bound drug is displaced and its side effects are increased. Although sodium divalproex and carbamazepine have been used in combination in adults, their interaction is complex. Little experience is available in adolescents; it is safer to use one or the other by itself. Sodium divalproex is a recent addition to the child psychiatry armamentarium and, if polypharmacy is avoided in younger children, a safe alternative to lithium. However, use of valproate in girls poses a risk of polycystic ovary; hence it should be used only when other options have failed or are contraindicated.

26. How is schizophrenia treated?

Schizophrenia frequently begins in adolescence. A gradual decline in functioning with the onset of suspiciousness and auditory hallucinations that comment on one's behavior are ominous signs. A baseline CT scan is done to check ventricular size. Atrophy is associated with poor prognosis. This also screens for lesions that could cause psychosis. Treatment with neuroleptics requires a minimal dose of 300 mg of chlorpromazine or 5 mg of haloperidol. Chlorpromazine and thioridazine cause problems with sexual side effects (retrograde ejaculation or galactorrhea) and general inhibition of movement (akinesia). The potent neuroleptics tend to induce dystonia, particularly if large doses are given early in treatment. The newer, atypical antipsychotic medications are rapidly becoming the first-line treatments because of more tolerable side effects and greater efficacy.

Akathesia, which may appear later with any neuroleptic, requires a reduction in dose or the addition of propranolol, 40–120 mg/day. If the patient's agitation or perplexity persists, the dose of neuroleptic is gradually increased, and the patient is observed for approximately a week before increasing the dose again. Over a period of approximately 6 weeks the patient's hallucinations and psychosis gradually come under control. A significant portion of psychoses in adolescents seems to result from severe external stresses and remit without further recurrence. Mania and schizophrenia, on the other hand, are considered life-time illnesses.

BEHAVIOR OR CONDUCT DISORDERS

27. Is there a practical way of classifying behavior disorders?

Behavior disorders can be divided into "good kid" and "bad kid" styles. The **"good kid"** has discrete episodes of anger, usually with little or no precipitant. "Good kid" adolescents trash their rooms, throw things, or hit whoever happens to be close. Once over this episode, they are contrite and apologetic. An EEG may be helpful, because some patients have an epileptic focus, usually in the temporal lobe. However, up to 40% of EEGs are false negatives, and nasal pharyngeal leads are not well tolerated.

Sometimes diagnosed as having explosive disorders, such patients do better on carbamazepine. A baseline CBC with reticulocyte count is necessary, because carbamazepine usually reduces the WBC initially. If carbamazepine is started at a low dose of 200 mg/day and increased by 200 mg each week with weekly blood counts for the first month, there are few problems. If the dose is increased too quickly, the patient often complains of upset stomach. In almost all cases, the reticulocyte count decreases, with a later decrease in overall white cell count. A petechial rash rarely appears. Therapeutic carbamazepine levels of 0.8–1.2 µg/ml are associated with a reduction in outbursts after 1 month with adequate drug serum levels. If the white cell count drops below 4000, the clinician may consider the trial a failure. Patients who respond need regular white counts with gradually decreasing frequency. As in adults, blood levels may drop over time because of enzyme induction. Clinically, some adolescents show increased irritability on carbamazepine, particularly those with an associated affect disorder.

28. Are the "bad kids" more commonly diagnosed?

The "bad kids" are classified as conduct disorders. DSM-IV lists 15 symptoms of conduct disorder, requiring at least three for the diagnosis:
- Often bullies, threatens, or intimidates others
- Often initiates physical fights
- Used a weapon that can cause serious physical harm to others
- Has been physically cruel to people
- Has been physically cruel to animals
- Has stolen, with confrontation of the victim
- Forced sexual activity on someone
- Deliberately engaged in fire setting with intention of serious damage
- Deliberately destroyed others' property
- Has broken into someone else's property
- Often lies, to obtain favors or avoid obligations (cons)
- Has stolen without confrontation of victim more than once
- Stays out at night, with onset before age 13
- Has run away from home overnight at least twice
- Often truant from school, with onset before age 13

The diagnosis of conduct disorder is much more common than explosive disorder ("good kid"), because only three symptoms from the list above are required.

29. What other diagnoses should be considered?

Even when the patient meets the criteria for diagnosis of conduct disorder, a careful review of the possibility of **ADHD** and affective disorders should be performed. ADHD is commonly associated with conduct disorder and worsens the overall prognosis. It is worthwhile to consider a trial of clonidine if the aggression is mostly verbal and ADHD is prominent; clonidine seems to reduce irritability in patients with ADHD. Of delinquent populations, 23–30% meet the criteria for **major depression** and deserve treatment. In one study of depressed conduct-disordered male adolescents, behavior improved as the depression lifted after treatment with imipramine.

Bipolar disorder also should be ruled out, with particular attention to family history. Clinicians have increasing awareness of bipolar disorder in adolescents with the understanding that the offspring of bipolar parents also are at risk for mania. Mania in adolescents frequently presents as irritability, and underlying irritability frequently accompanies conduct disorder behavior; thus, lithium was tried in the treatment of conduct disorder. One study comparing lithium with haloperidol found both to be equally effective, but lithium caused fewer side effects, including no detrimental effect on learning. Although responsiveness to lithium does not prove a bipolar diagnosis, it is reasonable to give a conduct-disordered adolescent a trial of lithium if other treatable disorders are unlikely. Only one controlled study has shown that youth with affective symptoms are more responsive to lithium.

30. What are the general principles of treating conduct disorder with medication?

Treatment for conduct disorder with lithium follows the regimen for bipolar disorder with kidney and thyroid studies and with gradual increase in the lithium level to the range of 1.0–1.5

mEq/L. An EEG should be obtained before lithium is started, because lithium in the system creates EEG artifacts. Hand tremor and gastric distress are common but mild. Sustained-release lithium may be used to reduce gastric distress, and beta blockers may reduce tremors. *Medications frequently are necessary for conduct disorder, but never sufficient.* Structure and control during inpatient care and follow-up are always necessary. Many, if not all, patients with conduct disorders need remedial education for reading and learning disabilities.

GENERAL ANXIETY AND OBSESSIVE-COMPULSIVE DISORDER

31. Why were childhood anxiety disorders not treated in the past?
Child psychiatrists traditionally have not treated anxiety disorders with medications because of a belief that anxiety was part of the developmental process and a concern that medication may interfere with the process. Until recently, medications used to treat anxiety also carried some potential for addiction or at least psychological dependence among adults. The introduction of buspirone allows the treatment of anxiety disorders with a medication that has no addiction liability and does not produce sedation. There are few reports of its use in children or adolescents. Case reports have found it useful in treating anxiety in adolescents. Additional reports have shown it to be a useful adjunct in reducing aggression in autistic adolescents. Currently the indications are clinical; its efficacy has not been established for general use.

32. Does increasing evidence suggest that obsessive-compulsive disorder (OCD) is an organic medical problem?
One specific type of anxiety associated with obsessions and compulsions has responded to agents that increase serotonin in the CNS. Such agents markedly reduce behaviors associated with this particular anxiety. Although the cause is unknown, recent biologic, clinical, radiologic, and physiologic evidence strongly implicates problems in the caudate or connections from caudate to the prefrontal area of the brain. Patients with Sydenham's chorea and postencephalitic patients have OCD more often than the general population, and both disorders have obvious organic causes. OCD is much more common than previously thought. As much as 2–3% of the U.S. population is estimated to be affected—more than 4 million people. Clues in children include erased school papers (sometimes so repeatedly that holes are worn through the paper) and/or retraced letters. Clues in adolescents include bleeding gums from overbrushing and extreme religiosity.

33. What treatments have been used for OCD?
Many treatments have been tried. Psychotherapy is ineffective. Behavior therapies have been variably effective. Stimulus exposure with response prevention is effective, but 25% of patients drop out, and many do not follow through on exposure-response prevention. Antianxiety agents, neuroleptics, and antidepressants have been tried without much success. Infrequently, children respond to imipramine and, rarely, clonidine. Clomipramine is a strong serotonin reuptake blocker often used for OCD in children. Clomipramine has a typical tricyclic side-effect profile of dry mouth, constipation, tremor, dizziness, somnolence, headache, and fatigue, but such effects are seen less often in children. As much as 200 mg/day or as little as 3 mg/kg may be used for children or adolescents. Fluvoxamine is now also indicated in the pediatric age group (8–17) for the treatment of OCD. Doses start with 25 mg at bedtime, titrated up to 200 mg per day in divided doses, with the largest dose given at bedtime. Behavior therapy with parental assistance helps.

BIBLIOGRAPHY

1. Campbell M, et al: Lithium in hospitalized children with conduct disorder: A double-blind and placebo-controlled study. J Am Acad Child Adolesc Psychiatry 34:445–453, 1995.
2. Conners CK: Rating scales in attention-deficit disorder: Use in assessment and treatment monitoring. J Clin Psychiatry 59:24–30, 1998.
3. Cowart VS: The Ritalin controversy: What's made this drug's opponents hyperactive? JAMA 259:2521–2523, 1988.

4. Cyranowski JA, et al: Adolescent onset of the gender difference in lifetime rates of major depression: A theoretical model. Arch General Psychiatry 57:21–27, 2000.
5. DeVane CL, Sallee FR: Serotonin selective reuptake inhibitors in child and adolescent psychopharmacology: A review of published experience. J Clin Psychiatry 57(2):55–56, 1996.
6. Farley GK, Hebert FB, Eckhardt LO: Handbook of Child and Adolescent Psychiatric Emergencies and Crises, 2nd ed. New York, Elsevier, 1986.
7. Finding RL, Dogin JW: Psychopharmacology of ADHD: Children and adolescents. J Clin Psychiatry 59(Suppl 7):42–49, 1998.
8. Gualtieri CT, et al: Tardive dyskinesia and other clinical consequences of neuroleptic treatment in children and adolescents. Am J Psychiatry 41:20–23, 1984.
9. Hunt RD, Minderaa RB, Cohen DJ: Clonidine benefits children with attention deficit disorder and hyperactivity: Report of a double-blind placebo-crossover therapeutic trial. J Am Acad Child Adolesc Psychiatry 24:617–629.
10. Jensen PS: Ethical and pragmatic issues in the use of psychotropic agents in young children. Can J Psychiatry 43(6):585–588, 1998.
11. Ryan ND, et al: Mood stabilizers in children and adolescents. J Am Acad Child Adolesc Psychiatry 38(5):529–536, 1999.
12. Satterfield JH, et al: Therapeutic interventions to prevent delinquency in hyperactive boys. J Am Acad Child Adolesc Psychiatry 26:56–64, 1984.

VIII. Disorders Associated with Pregnancy and Menstruation

62. PREMENSTRUAL SYNDROME AND PREMENSTRUAL DYSPHORIC DISORDER

Doris C. Gundersen, M.D.

1. What is premenstrual syndrome (PMS)?

Premenstrual syndrome describes a cluster of nonspecific psychological, behavioral and somatic symptoms, which occur in the luteal phase of the menstrual cycle. The *timing* of the symptoms, between ovulation and the onset of menses, distinguishes PMS from other psychiatric conditions experienced by women of reproductive age. PMS symptoms include depression, irritability, and rejection-sensitivity. Bloating (related to fluid retention), increased appetite, weight gain, breast tenderness or swelling, and headache also are commonly reported. The symptoms are generally severe enough to interfere with performance and interpersonal relationships.

2. What is premenstrual dysphoric disorder (PMDD)?

In 1994, the diagnosis of PMDD was classified in the DSM IV under Mood Disorders Not Otherwise Specified. PMDD replaced late luteal phase dysphoric disorder, a diagnosis included in the DSM III-R (1987). Whereas many women experience premenstrual psychological and physical discomfort, a much smaller percentage develop symptoms severe enough to meet diagnostic criteria for PMDD. Due to poor reliability of retrospective symptom reports, DSM IV clinical criteria stipulate that the diagnosis of PMDD be made prospectively, over at least two consecutive menstrual cycles. The luteal phase symptomatology must be of sufficient severity to interfere with functioning and must be distinguished from the exacerbation of co-occurring medical or psychiatric disorders.

DSM IV Criteria for Premenstrual Dysphoric Disorder

A. In most menstrual cycles during the past year, five (or more) of the following symptoms were present for most of the time during the last week of the luteal phase, began to remit with a few days after the onset of the follicular phase, and were absent in the week postmenses, with at least one of the symptoms being either (1), (2), (3), or (4):

   (1) markedly depressed mood, feelings of hopelessness, or self-deprecating thoughts
   (2) marked anxiety, tension, feelings of being "keyed up," or "on edge"
   (3) marked affective lability (e.g., feeling suddenly sad or tearful or increased sensitivity to rejection)
   (4) persistent and marked anger or irritability or increased interpersonal conflicts
   (5) decreased interest in usual activities (e.g., work, school, friends, hobbies)
   (6) subjective sense of difficulty concentrating
   (7) lethargy, easy fatigability, or marked lack of energy
   (8) marked change in appetite, overeating, or specific food cravings
   (9) hypersomnia or insomnia
  (10) a subjective sense of being overwhelmed or out of control
  (11) other physical symptoms, such as breast tenderness or swelling, headaches, joint or muscle pain, a sensation of "bloating," weight gain

Table continued on following page

_____
DSM IV Criteria for Premenstrual Dysphoric Disorder (Continued)
_____

B. The disturbance markedly interferes with work or school or with usual social activities and relationships with others (e.g., avoidance of social activities, decreased productivity and efficiency at
   work or school).

C. The disturbance is not merely an exacerbation of the symptoms of another disorder, such as major
   depression, panic disorder, dysthymic disorder, or a personality disorder (although it may be superimposed on any of these disorders).

D. Criteria A, B, and C must be confirmed by prospective daily ratings during at least two consecutive
   symptomatic cycles. (The diagnosis may be made provisionally prior to this confirmation.)

Note: In menstruating females, the luteal phase corresponds to the period between ovulation and the
onset of menses, and the follicular phase begins with menses. In nonmenstruating females (e.g., those
who have had a hysterectomy), the timing of the luteal and follicular phases may require measurement
of circulating reproductive hormones.
_____
From The American Psychiatric Association: Diagnostic and Statistical Manual of Mental Disorders, 4th ed.
Washington DC, APA, 1994, pp 717–718; with permission.

3. How common are these conditions among menstruating women?

Epidemiological surveys estimate that approximately 75% of women with regular menstrual
cycles report minor or isolated premenstrual symptoms, and 20–50% of women experience PMS.
According to DSM IV, PMDD afflicts approximately 3–5% of all menstruating women.

It is important to consider the high incidence of **comorbid psychiatric conditions** in this age
group. Premenstrual aggravation of a primary mood disorder may be mistakenly diagnosed as PMS
or PMDD unless careful prospective rating scales are employed to distinguish these conditions. Of
significance, about 70% of women with bipolar disorder have dysphoric PMS, and 30–60% of
women with premenstrual dysphoria have a history of major depression. This tremendous symptom
overlap contributes to the ongoing difficulty in establishing whether PMS or PMDD are truly independent disorders versus premenstrual magnification of preexisting affective disorders.

4. Are there specific risk factors for developing PMS?

Yes. A prior history of clinical depression confers some heightened risk for developing PMS. A
history of postpartum depression and/or mood changes related to oral contraceptive use also increases
the risk for developing the condition. Finally, a family history of PMS is an independent risk factor.

5. Describe the proposed etiology for PMS.

Despite extensive research in this area, no precise etiology for PMS has been identified. A
number of theories continue to be entertained and vigorously explored. Because of the heterogeneity
associated with PMS, the majority of investigators agree that the etiology is likely **mulifactorial**.

Prospective evaluations of stressful life events in women with PMS have failed to demonstrate a
link between environmental stress and symptom severity. Biological factors appear to play a more
substantial role in the development of this condition. There exists a high familial incidence of PMS,
supporting some genetic contribution. Women with afflicted mothers and/or sisters are at greater risk
for developing PMS. Finally, monozygotic twin concordance rates for PMS exceed those observed
in dizygotic twins.

6. What is the postulated role of endogenous sex hormones in the pathogenesis of PMS?

Earlier theories were based on the premise that abnormal levels of gonadal steroids contributed
to the development of premenstrual symptoms. The diminished secretion of progesterone in the
luteal phase of the menstrual cycle was previously implicated as a potential etiologic factor in the
development of PMS. However, many well-designed studies do not support this theory. Luteal phase
progesterone supplementation is no more effective than placebo in the treatment of PMS.

Hypoestrogenism also has been proposed as a factor in the pathogenesis of PMS. In the peri-
ovulatory phase of the menstrual cycle, a subtle, transient decline in circulating estradiol is observed
and is temporally related to mood changes and hot flushes in some women.

The importance of **gonadal steroids** is most clearly illustrated by studies in which women with PMS are given gonadotropin releasing hormone (GnRH) agonists. The resulting ovarian "shutdown" is accompanied by a dramatic reduction in PMS symptoms. Interestingly, these women showed no differences in levels of ovarian steroids, estrogen to progesterone ratios, gonadotropins, or ovarian steroid binding globulins when compared to control subjects. This suggests that **hormone cyclicity**, not absolute levels of circulating sex hormones, is a more important factor in the development of PMS. Genetically predisposed women may possess supersensitivity to the normal, monthly fluctuations in these hormones. The absence of symptomatology before puberty, during pregnancy, and post menopause (i.e., periods of anovulation) lends support to this premise.

Results of a more recent study conducted by Schmidt et al. challenge the notion that premenstrual symptoms are related to luteal phase fluctuations of estrogen and progesterone. Women meeting (prospectively confirmed) criteria for PMS were given the antiprogesterone agent, RU 486 (mifepristone). Despite premature termination of the luteal phase, the research subjects experienced their usual premenstrual syndrome well into the synthetically-induced follicular phase of their menstrual cycles. This suggests that hormonal events *preceding* the luteal phase may trigger PMS. Alternatively, PMS may represent a cyclic disorder, independent of the menstrual cycle and associated hormonal changes.

7. What other endogenous substances have been implicated?

Both progesterone and estrogen affect **endorphin** levels. Disturbances in endogenous opioid systems are associated with PMS-like symptoms including, but not limited to, irritability, sleep disruption, and headache. Furthermore, opiate antagonists tend to magnify PMS symptoms in susceptible women, suggesting a possible link between endorphin abnormalities and the expression of PMS.

Variability in **thyroid hormone** measures has been noted in women with PMS. However, no specific thyroid disorders have been diagnosed in this population.

Mastalgia is a symptom commonly reported by women with PMS. For this reason, **prolactin** is suspected to be a factor in the development of the syndrome. The involvement of prolactin is also supported by two research findings. Women with PMS demonstrate a blunted prolactin response to tryptophan challenge in both the follicular and luteal phases of the menstrual cycle. Additionally, a blunted prolactin response to the administration of buspirone during the follicular phase has been observed in these women.

Central nervous system deficiencies of the **prostaglandin** PGE-1 are associated with headache, fatigue, and a craving for sweets. The accumulation of prostaglandin PGE-2a in the uterine myometrium plays a role in the development of dysmenorrhea. These findings lead some investigators to conclude that disturbances in prostaglandin synthesis and/or functioning likely contribute to PMS.

Follicular stimulating hormone (FSH), lutenizing hormone (LH), melatonin, cortisol, and testosterone also have been identified as potential etiological agents. Again, no definitive link between PMS and any of these substances have been established.

8. Are the neurotransmitters associated with mood regulation thought to play a role in the etiology of PMS?

Contemporary hypotheses point to a link between fluctuations in ovarian steroids and dysregulation of central neurotransmission in women predisposed to PMS. Investigators have established that estrogen, progesterone, and metabolites of these parent compounds alter **noradrenergic, serotonergic**, and **GABA** (gamma-aminobutyric acidergic) neurotransmission.

In animal studies, hypothalamic estrogen induces a diurnal pattern of serotonin (5HT) rhythm. Administration of serotonin agonists, such as m-chlorophenylpyperazine (m-CPP) may induce mood elevation, whereas serotonin antagonism is associated with some behavioral changes (also observed in women with PMS), including irritability and social withdrawal.

Human clinical data also supports that PMS may be related to the apparent effects of ovarian hormones on central serotonin neurotransmission. Studies have determined that, premenstrually, women with PMS possess heightened sensitivity of 5HT-1a receptors. Reduced whole blood concentrations of serotonin have been observed in the luteal phase of women meeting criteria for PMS.

Decreased platelet serotonin uptake also has been noted in this same population, but not in healthy controls. Some investigators suspect that women with PMS who report food cravings in the late luteal phase of their cycles and engage in carbohydrate binging may be attempting to self-medicate a mood disturbance by boosting tryptophan levels and, ultimately, central serotonin supplies.

9. What is the differential diagnosis for PMS?

PMS and/or PMDD should be considered diagnoses of exclusion. Of all the women presenting with complaints of premenstrual symptoms, 25–75% will actually meet criteria for another underlying medical or psychiatric condition.

Differential Diagnosis of Premenstrual Symptoms

MEDICAL	PSYCHIATRIC
Migraines	Affective disorders
Seizures	Anxiety disorders
Endocrinopathies	Eating disorders
Irritable bowel syndrome	Substance abuse
Chronic fatigue syndrome	
Anemia	
Pelvic inflammatory disease	
Endometriosis	
Perimenopause	
Idiopathic edema	
Fibrocystic breast disease	

10. What steps should be taken to confirm the diagnosis of PMS or PMDD?

Begin with thorough psychiatric, medical, and family histories. A physical examination, including pelvic examination, should be pursued routinely in women presenting with both physical and psychological complaints. As emphasized previously, premenstrual magnification of both medical and psychiatric disorders are common and should be ruled out before a diagnosis of PMS or PMDD is assigned. No specific laboratory testing is recommended to make the diagnosis. However, in women complaining of fatigue or depression, a complete blood count to rule out anemia in addition to thyroid screening is recommended. If breast tenderness is severe and/or the menstrual cycle irregular, a prolactin level can be obtained. For women in their 40s, consider the possibility of perimenopause. Estradiol levels and FSH screening are recommended.

In one study, it was found that fewer than 50% of women seeking treatment for presumed PMS actually had a cycle-dependent constellation of symptoms. This illustrates the importance of **prospective daily rating** to confirm that the symptoms are isolated to the luteal phase and recur with most cycles. Once other medical and psychiatric illnesses are ruled out, at least two months of prospective daily rating should be pursued.

Prospective Daily Rating Scales

Daily Record of Severity of Problems
Patient Self-Report Scale (PSRS)
Moos Menstrual Distress Questionnaire (MMDQ)
Patient Record of Increased Symptoms with Menses (PRISM)
Premenstrual Experience Assessment (PEA)
Premenstrual Assessment Form (PAF)
Calendar of Premenstrual Experiences (COPE)

If the prospective charting reveals luteal-phase symptoms in the absence of follicular phase complaints, the diagnosis of PMS (or PMDD, depending on the severity of reported symptoms) can be made. However, persistent follicular phase symptomatology without dramatic magnification in the luteal phase should prompt the clinician to continue a search for occult medical and/or psychiatric conditions. Finally, persistent follicular phase complaints accompanied by significant luteal phase worsening points to the presence of an underlying disorder and comorbid PMS, or simply premenstrual magnification of an untreated medical or psychiatric condition. *Identify all confounding conditions, and treat them aggressively.*

11. Once the diagnosis is confirmed, what treatment strategies can be employed?

Given the lack of a precise etiology, the treatment of PMS and PMDD generally focuses on attempts to ameliorate isolated symptoms. Treatment should begin with conservative interventions, including psychoeducation, support, and healthy lifestyle changes. The process of prospective rating allows a woman to participate in her own treatment, thereby reducing apprehension by providing greater predictability. When a woman is able to establish a pattern of recurring symptoms, it allows her to anticipate the more difficult days of her cycle and make plans to minimize stress during that time period. **Cognitive, behavioral, and relaxation therapies** have been found to decrease the severity of PMS. Additionally, physical (aerobic) exercise promotes endorphin release, which is believed to have a positive effect on mood and promote relaxation. **Increased exercise** should be encouraged in the late luteal phase of the menstrual cycle for women who complain of lethargy, tension, anxiety, and depression.

A nutritional assessment can be helpful. Excessive **alcohol** consumption can exacerbate mood and sleep disturbances in women with PMS. Eliminating **caffeine** is suggested for women complaining of irritability, anxiety, and breast pain. Finally, reducing **sodium** intake, at least in the luteal phase of the cycle, may minimize bloating due to fluid retention. Wurtman et al. found that low-protein, high-carbohydrate diets consumed during the luteal phase led to a greater reduction in postmeal depression, tension, anger, confusion, and fatigue in PMS patients compared to their controls.

Evening primrose oil (linoleic acid) has been reported to relieve premenstrual symptoms of depression, bloating, headache, breast pain, and irritability. A review of the literature reveals seven placebo-controlled trials, five of which were randomized. Inconsistent scoring and response criteria employed in these studies limit their usefulness. However, two of the better-designed studies failed to demonstrate the efficacy of this proposed remedy.

12. What is the role of vitamin and mineral supplementation in the treatment of PMS?

Vitamin and mineral supplementation is frequently recommended as part of the overall treatment strategy for women with PMS despite the fact that no actual vitamin or mineral deficiencies have been reported in this patient population. Many earlier studies were methodologically flawed due to poor subject selection and the failure to use valid prospective rating scales for establishing an accurate diagnosis. More recently, a handful of well-designed clinical trials have demonstrated efficacy for some nutritional supplements.

Results of a double-blind, placebo-controlled study[14] confirmed that **calcium** is effective in alleviating both the physical and psychological symptoms of PMS. By the third treatment cycle, subjects receiving 1200 mg of calcium daily experienced a significant reduction in muscle aches, depression, food cravings, and fluid retention. The researchers hypothesized that the same hormones involved in calcium regulation also interact with reproductive hormones. Premenstrual symptoms may reflect a calcium deficiency in some women.

Vitamin B6 (pyridoxine) is a cofactor in the synthesis of dopamine and serotonin. It has been reported to reduce depression, irritability, fatigue, edema, and headache in some premenstrual women. The scientific data concerning the value of B6 (pyridoxine) supplementation is mixed. Pooled data from ten randomized, double-blind trials revealed that approximately 30% of subjects experience a beneficial response. Two-thirds showed ambiguous results or no benefit compared to placebo. Effective doses range from 50 mg to 100 mg per day. Patients should be warned of the risk of developing an irreversible peripheral neuropathy if the recommended doses are exceeded.

Magnesium deficiencies are associated with depletion of central nervous system dopamine, and also increased peripheral aldosterone. Magnesium is involved in prostaglandin synthesis and affects glucose-induced insulin secretion. Well-designed trials support magnesium supplementation during the luteal phase, (360 mg to 1080 mg per day) to minimize fluid retention, depression, and fatigue. Vitamin E modulates prostaglandin synthesis, and 400 IU daily may be helpful for reducing premenstrual depression and pain, although scientific data on efficacy is mixed.

13. What pharmacological treatments are helpful in the treatment of PMS or PMDD?

Nonpsychotropic Agents For Severe, Disabling Symptoms of PMS and PMDD

MEDICATION	DOSE	CYCLE PHASE	TARGET SYMPTOM(S)
Ibuprofen	600 mg bid–tid	As needed	Dysmenorrhea, headache
Bromocriptine	2.5 mg bid–tid	Luteal	Breast pain, edema
Spironolactone	25 mg–100 mg qd	As needed	Edema, weight gain
Naltrexone	25 mg bid	Days 9–18	Irritability, anxiety, depression
Atenolol	50 mg qd	Entire cycle	Irritability
Clonidine	17 mcg/kg qd*	Entire cycle	Irritability, hostility, anxiety

* Divided doses are recommended.

Nonsteroidal anti-inflammatory drugs (NSAIDs), when given several days before the onset of menses, reduce pelvic pain, cramping, and headaches. For severe breast pain, the dopamine agonist (and prolactin inhibitor) bromocriptine can be prescribed. One double-blind, randomized, crossover trial supports the use of bromocriptine to alleviate premenstrual edema, weight gain, and bloating.[9] It is reported to be less effective in relieving mood symptoms. Nausea is a common side effect, especially at higher doses, and may preclude its use.

Several well-designed trials support the use of the potassium-sparing, aldosterone antagonist **spironolactone** to reduce severe edema and bloating. Some investigators believe the antiandrogenic properties of this diuretic are responsible for improving mood in addition to alleviating somatic symptoms. Diuretics should be used judiciously because of the risk of secondary aldosteronism and rebound edema.

The opiate antagonist **naltrexone** may reduce luteal phase irritability, anxiety, depression, lethargy, bloating, and headaches in women suffering from PMS or PMDD. Nausea, dizziness, and appetite suppression are potential side effects.[3]

The beta-blocker **atenolol** has been reported to alleviate premenstrual irritability. Similarly, the alpha-blocker **clonidine** has demonstrated efficacy in the treatment of premenstrual symptoms including irritability, hostility, and anxiety.

14. Which psychotropic agents are used to treat PMS and PMDD?

The use of psychotropic drugs in the treatment of PMS is based on the premise that a dysregulation in the hypothalamic-pituitary-gonadal axis affects central neurotransmitter physiology.

Some Psychiatric Medications Currently Used in the Treatment of PMS and PMDD

MEDICATION	DOSE	CYCLE PHASE
Dextroamphetamine	10 mg–20 mg qd	As needed in luteal phase
Alprazolam	.25 mg–2.0 mg qd	As needed in luteal phase
Buspirone	15 mg–60 mg qd	Continuous or luteal phase
Fluoxetine	20 mg qd	Continuous or luteal phase
Sertraline	50 mg–100 mg qd	Continuous or luteal phase
Citalopram	10 mg–30 mg qd	Continuous or luteal phase

Table continued on following page

Some Psychiatric Medications Currently Used in the Treatment of PMS and PMDD (Continued)

MEDICATION	DOSE	CYCLE PHASE
Paroxetine	10 mg–30 mg qd	Continuous
Clomipramine	25 mg–75 mg qd	Continuous
Nortriptyline	50 mg–100 mg qd	Continuous
Nefazadone	100 mg–600 mg qd	Continuous
Mirtazapine	7.5 mg–15 mg qd	Continuous

Note: For women with early age onset of PMS, documented mood or anxiety disorders, or severe symptoms of PMDD, intermittent SSRI dosing is *not* recommended.

For pronounced premenstrual lethargy and hyperphagia, time-limited treatment with low-dose dextroamphetamine can be helpful. Anxiolytics are effective in alleviating prominent luteal phase anxiety, nervous tension and irritability. Specifically, alprazolam has been studied and found effective when prescribed in the week preceding menses. Average doses range from .75 mg to 2.25 mg per day. The medication should be tapered with the onset of menses. Caution must be exercised when prescribing stimulants or benzodiazepines in women with histories of substance abuse. Buspirone, a nonhabituating alternative, is also used to treat the anxiety and irritability associated with PMS and PMDD. Continuous dosing (15 mg to 60 mg per day), is recommended.

15. What about antidepressants?

Currently, no antidepressant agents are FDA-approved for the treatment of PMS or PMDD. However, numerous controlled studies have established that a variety of antidepressant medications dramatically reduce or ameliorate premenstrual symptoms. These agents are particularly useful for women diagnosed with comorbid depressive and anxiety disorders, or who have failed to respond to more conservative treatment interventions, including other pharmacotherapies.

16. What is the evidence for successful treatment with SSRIs?

Selective serotonin reuptake inhibitors (SSRIs) have been researched extensively in the treatment of these conditions. Carefully controlled studies demonstrate that **fluoxetine** is superior to placebo in abolishing behavioral, psychological, and, interestingly, somatic symptoms. Fluoxetine administered at 20 mg per day appears to be as effective as 60 mg per day, and research subjects reported fewer side effects on the lower dose. One long-term study (i.e., 1 year of treatment with fluoxetine) showed continued benefit.

Similar controlled studies of sertraline have established its efficacy in the treatment of PMS and PMDD. Open trials of paroxetine,[15] mirtazapine, and nefazadone[7] support the efficacy of these antidepressants as well. However, controlled, double-blind studies are needed to verify these promising preliminary results. Additionally, serotonergic antidepressants including desipramine, clomipramine, and nortriptyline have been used successfully, however with less tolerability than the SSRIs.

Flexible dosing regimens (e.g., drug administration limited to the luteal phase) have been studied for fluoxetine,[13] sertraline,[8] and citalopram. In the absence of psychiatric comorbidity, half-cycle dosing is as effective as continuous dosing for the treatment of premenstrual symptoms. The psychopharmacologic reasons for the efficacy of intermittent dosing are not known. These intriguing findings suggest the mechanism underlying PMS or PMDD may differ from that of affective disorders. Alternatively, the efficacy observed with the use of SSRIs may be a function of some action independent of the antidepressant effect.

17. Describe hormonal therapies used to treat premenstrual symptoms.

Oral contraceptives have have been proposed as a therapy for PMS based on the theory that the monophasic preparations supply steady doses of estrogen and progesterone throughout the menstrual cycle, thereby eliminating the natural hormonal fluctuations thought to contribute to premenstrual symptoms. Available studies reveal that about 25% of women improve, 50% report no change, and 25% experience an exacerbation of symptoms. Women with significant dysmenorrhea or heavy bleeding may benefit most from this intervention. Triphasic preparations, which provide hormonal cyclicity, should be avoided in women with PMS and PMDD.

The decline in progesterone during the luteal phase has been suspected as a potential trigger for premenstrual symptoms. Unfortunately, numerous clinical trials, including large, randomized, placebo-controlled studies, have failed to demonstrate the efficacy of progesterone.[6]

Estrogen, administered continuously, may blunt the normal late luteal phase decline of this hormone and, at least theoretically, prevent associated premenstrual mood and somatic symptoms. Given subcutaneously or transdermally, estrogen is more effective than placebo. However, potential side effects include nausea, breast tenderness, and weight gain, precluding its use in some women. Furthermore, unless a woman has undergone hysterectomy, oral progestins also must be prescribed to prevent uterine hyperplasia. Progestins can induce PMS-like symptoms in some women.

For women with severe PMDD, refractory to other available treatments, suppression of the hypothalamic-pituitary-ovarian axis to halt ovulation provides dramatic relief. **Danazol, a synthetic androgen**, works by inhibiting progesterone binding and estrogen synthesis. It suppresses the midcycle surges of FSH and LH, creating an anovulatory state. It has been reported to reduce premenstrual depression, irritability, anxiety, edema, and breast tenderness. Potential androgenic side effects include hirsutism, acne, and weight gain. About 10% of women develop hepatic dysfunction on this synthetic steroid.[8]

Similar symptomatic relief has been observed with **gonadotropin-releasing hormone** (GnRH) **agonists** like **leuprolide**. This agent produces a chemical menopause through downregulation of GnRH receptors, followed by the cessation of the cyclic release of estrogen and progesterone.

Although highly effective, these latter two treatments are expensive. Additionally, danazol and leuprolide create hypoestrogenic environments with the associated risks of menopause, including symptoms of hot flashes and vaginal dryness, osteoporosis, and cardiac disease. For this reason, prolonged treatment (i.e., greater than 6 months) is not advised at this time.

Hormonal Therapies For Premenstrual Symptoms

MEDICATION	DOSE	CYCLE PHASE
Oral contraceptives*	Variable	Continuous
Estrogen patches	200 μg q 3 d	Continuous
Danazol	200–400 mg	Onset of symptoms to menses
Leuprolide	3.75 mg im	q 4 weeks (< 6 months)

* Monophasics = Brevicon, Loestrin, Demulen

Researchers are exploring the possibility of using GnRH agonists in conjunction with steady-dose estrogen and progestin hormone replacement therapy. Preliminary findings are encouraging.

18. Is surgery an option?

Surgical menopause (i.e., ovariectomy) is a very *last* resort, and should be explored only if all other interventions are ineffective, diagnostic accuracy has been established, and future pregnancies are not desired.

BIBLIOGRAPHY

1. American Psychiatric Association: Diagnostic and Statistical Manual of Mental Disorders, 4th ed. Washington DC, American Psychiatric Association, 1994.
2. Blackstrom T, Hansson-Malstrom Y, Lindhe B, et al: Oral contraceptives in premenstrual syndrome: A randomized comparison of triphasic and monophasic preparations. Contraception 46:253–268, 1992.
3. Chuong CJ, Coulam CB, Bergstralh EJ, et al: Clinical trial of naltrexone in premenstrual syndrome. Obstet Gynecol 72:332–336, 1988.
4. Dubovsky SL, Giese A: Selected issues in the psychopharmacologic treatment of women with psychiatric disorders. J Pract Psychol Behav Health 277–282, 1997.
5. Facchinetti F, Borella P, Sances G, et al: Oral magnesium successfully relieves premenstrual mood changes. Obstet Gynecol 78:177–181, 1991.

6. Freeman EW, Rickels K, Sondheimer SJ, Polansky M: Ineffectiveness of progesterone suppository treatment for premenstrual syndrome. JAMA 264:349–353, 1990.
7. Freeman EW, Rickels K, Sondheimer SJ, et al: Nefazadone in the treatment of premenstrual syndrome: A preliminary study. J Clin Psychopharmacol 14:180–186, 1994.
8. Halbreich U, Rojanksy N, Palter S: Elimination of ovulation and menstrual cyclicity (with danazol) improves dysphoric premenstrual syndromes. Fertil Steril 56:1066–1069, 1991.
9. Moden-Vrtovec H, Vujc D: Bromocriptine in the management of premenstrual syndrome. Clin Exp Obstet Gynecol 19:242–248, 1992.
10. Menkes DB, Taghavi E, Mason PA, Howard RC: Fluoxetine's spectrum of action in premenstrual syndrome. Int Clin Psychopharmacol 8:95–102, 1993.
11. Schmidt PJ, Nieman LK, Grover GN, et al: Lack of effect of induced menses on symptoms in women with premenstrual syndrome. New Engl J Med 324:1174, 1991.
12. Steiner M, Wilkins BA: Diagnosis and assessment of premenstrual dysphoria. Psychiatric Ann 25(9):571–575, 1996.
13. Steiner M, Korzekwa M, Lamont J, et al: Intermittent fluoxetine dosing in the treatment of women with premenstrual dysphoria. Psychopharmacol Bull 33(4):771–774, 1997.
14. Thys-Jacobs S, Starkey P, Bernstein D, Tian J: Calcium carbonate and the premenstrual syndrome: Effects of premenstrual and menstrual symptoms. Premenstrual Syndrome Study Group. Am J Obstet Gynecol 179:444–452, 1998.
15. Yonkers KA, Gullion C, Williams A, et al: Paroxetine as a treatment for premenstrual dysphoric disorder. J Clin Psychopharmacol 16:3–8, 1994.
16. Young SA, Hurt PH, Benedek DM, Howard RS: Treatment of premenstrual dysphoric disorder with sertraline during the luteal phase: A randomized, double-blind, placebo-controlled crossover trial. J Clin Psychiatry 59:76–80, 1998.

63. PSYCHIATRIC DISORDERS AND PREGNANCY

Doris C. Gundersen, M.D.

1. How common are eating disorders in pregnant women?

Few reports of anorexia nervosa associated with pregnancy are found in the literature. To some extent, the two conditions are mutually exclusive. The endocrine abnormalities associated with anorexia nervosa substantially diminish fertility. The paucity of published information on bulimia in pregnancy may reflect the failure of physicians to identify the problem, despite an incidence of up to 13% in women of childbearing age.

2. How are pregnant women with eating disorders diagnosed and managed?

The possibility of an eating disorder should be considered in any woman whose pregravid weight is subnormal or who fails to gain weight as pregnancy progresses. Any patient who casually mentions that she has an eating problem should be carefully questioned. An eating disorder should be suspected in patients who are excessively preoccupied with weight gain and body image during pregnancy. A history of persistent vomiting before or during pregnancy should be investigated. A psychosocial history may reveal comorbidity with other psychiatric conditions, such as depression or chemical dependency in bulimic women.

Hospitalization is recommended for the eating-disordered pregnant patient with excessive weight loss, severe metabolic disarray, or prominent symptoms of depression. Psychotherapy and nutritional counseling should complement prenatal care. Enlisting the support of families to monitor weight gain and nutrition is helpful. Ideally, eating disorders should be identified before conception. The afflicted woman should be advised to delay pregnancy until the eating disorder is truly in remission.

3. How might issues specific to pregnancy affect the eating-disordered patient and, thus, the fetus?

Psychological conflicts thought to be important in the development of eating disorders concern adult sexuality, body image, autonomy, dependency, and relationships with parents. Because such issues become highlighted during pregnancy, exacerbations of eating disorders are likely. Women with active eating disorders at the time of conception typically experience many difficulties during pregnancy. They gain less weight and have smaller babies with lower Apgar scores. Serious complications of bulimia include acid-base disturbances, electrolyte imbalances, and disruption of normal intestinal motility. Anorexic women with reduced weight gain during pregnancy have associated intrauterine growth retardation. In one Danish study of 50 pregnant women treated for anorexia nervosa, 7 perinatal deaths were reported, with 6 attributed to prematurity.

4. What risks do illicit substances, tobacco, and alcohol pose to the child exposed in utero?

The incidence of substance abuse in women of childbearing age is high. The risk for developmental abnormalities in the fetus of a drug abusing mother is significant.

Cocaine-abusing women have a significantly higher rate of spontaneous abortion, abruptio placentae, and stillbriths.

Infants of **opiate-dependent mothers** face greater perinatal morbidity and mortality. In the first trimester, a common complication is spontaneous abortion. A 30–50% increased risk for growth retardation is observed.

Heavy tobacco use doubles the rate of spontaneous abortion. Smoking is linked to intrauterine growth retardation, premature labor, and low birth weight.

Cannabis abuse also is associated with negative effects on fetal growth.

Alcohol and its metabolite acetaldehyde have direct toxic effects on cellular growth and metabolism.

Summary of Major Risks of Drug Use During Pregnancy

Cocaine	Maternal depression, cerebrovascular accident
	Fetal cerebral hemorrhage
	Spontaneous abortion
	Low birth weight
	Increased rate of sudden infant death syndrome
	Neurobehavioral problems in neonates
Opiates	Increased perinatal morbidity and mortality
	Spontaneous abortion
	Fetal growth retardation
	Premature labor
	Neonatal septicemia, liver damage, cerebrovascular accidents
	Neonatal addiction and withdrawal
Cannabis	Slowed fetal growth
	Fetal hypoxia
Tobacco	Spontaneous abortion
	Slowed fetal growth
	Low birth weight
	Premature labor
Alcohol	Fetal alcohol syndrome includes
	• Mental retardation
	• Cardiac defects
	• Growth retardation
	• Facial and limb deformities

5. What specific effects does cocaine use have on the fetus?

Peripherally, cocaine causes a marked rise in maternal catecholamines with concomitant increases in blood pressure and heart rate. Acute myocardial infarction or cardiac arrhythmias may result. Maternal brain hemorrhage has been reported. Prolonged administration of cocaine results in depletion of presynaptic intraneuronal neurotransmitters, which is associated with profound depression. Increased levels of circulating catecholamines also lead to increased uterine vascular resistance and decreased uterine blood flow. Fetal hypoxia is produced by the diminished placental perfusion. Cocaine freely crosses the placenta. Fetal hypertension and tachycardia are direct effects of the cocaine. The cocaine-exposed fetus risks hemorrhagic cerebral lesions. Intrauterine growth retardation is common.

Neonates of cocaine-abusing mothers demonstrate low birth weight and low Apgar scores. They have a higher than expected rate of genitourinary tract malformations and cardiac anomalies. An increased frequency of sudden infant death syndrome (SIDS) is reported. Neonates with in utero exposure to cocaine exhibit transient neurobehavioral symptoms, including tremulousness, hyperreflexia, and hypertonicity. They are irritable and less consolable and have abnormal sleep patterns. They are at high risk for abuse and neglect. Cocaine appears in significant quantities in breast milk. Long-term administration of cocaine may result in irreversible decreases in dopamine, persistent mood dysfunction, and an inability to experience pleasure.

6. How do opiates harm pregnancy?

The majority of drug-dependent pregnant women must rely on the street supply of narcotics. Because of the irregularity of with which they receive opiates, intermittent withdrawal may occur, leading to uterine irritability. The incidence of premature labor is increased. Meconium aspiration is a common complication. Infants born to drug-addicted mothers often suffer from septicemia, hyperbilirubinemia, intracranial hemorrhage, and hypoglycemia. They demonstrate a withdrawal syndrome, characterized by irritability, poor feeding, respiratory difficulties, and tremulousness. Such infants are difficult to console and, like cocaine-exposed babies, are at high risk for abuse and neglect.

7. Give an example of the evidence for negative effects of tobacco on unborn children.

One study assessed over 700 children of mothers who smoked during pregnancy. At the age of 3 years, the children demonstrated decreased height and weight compared with unexposed 3-year-old controls. Statistically significant cognitive impairment in the tobacco-exposed children persisted, even after controlling for environmental variables.

8. How does cannabis cause risks?

Delta-9-tetrahydrocannabinol elevates carbon monoxide levels in the mother, resulting in poorer oxygenation in the fetus. Elevations in maternal heart rate and blood pressure reduce placental blood flow to the fetus. Finally, delta-9-tetrahydrocannabinol freely crosses the placenta and is exceptionally fat-soluble, requiring up to 30 days for the fetus to excrete.

9. How much alcohol is safe for a pregnant woman to consume?

Five to six drinks of hard liquor per day are associated with the most serious teratogenicity, called "fetal alcohol syndrome." Abnormalities include mental retardation, cardiac defects, growth retardation, and facial and limb deformities. Irritability in infancy and attention deficit symptoms during childhood are characteristic findings. The severity of the syndrome depends on the amount of alcohol exposure, the gestational age of exposure, and the genetic constitution of the infant. No safe level of alcohol consumption has been determined.

10. How can substance abuse be detected and managed in the pregnant woman?

Clinical management of substance-abusing women during pregnancy can be challenging. Drug-abusing women commonly neglect health care in general. Up to 75% fail to seek prenatal care. Drug abuse should be suspected in women who present late for prenatal care or have poor weight gain or other signs of compromised health. The patient also should be screened for other psychiatric conditions that predispose to substance abuse, such as anxiety and depression. Most pregnant women will disclose a history of drug or alcohol abuse if questioned in a nonjudgmental, straightforward manner. Authoritarian moralizing leads to an avoidance of prenatal care altogether. Providing an opportunity for treatment is the most effective strategy.

The first intervention should be to **educate the patient** about the hazards of drug use during pregnancy. Some will discontinue use on their own in response to the counseling. They should be offered prenatal care in conjunction with treatment for substance abuse. Outpatient care is usually indicated, but hospitalization may be needed for more severe cases, such as mothers addicted to tranquilizers or barbiturates in addition to opiates. In some cases it is necessary to pursue involuntary commitment to protect the fetus.

11. What sort of issues should be addressed in treatment?
Treatment goals should include developing a strong support system to allow the woman to break ties with the drug culture. Social stressors such as poor housing and inadequate income must be remedied. Emotional problems, including depression, low self-esteem, and poor coping skills, should be addressed in individual as well as group therapy. Urine toxicology screening detects relapse.

12. Describe the pharmacotherapy for a pregnant substance abuser.
Pharmacotherapy during pregnancy may be used to prevent or lessen withdrawal symptoms, to diminish cocaine craving, and/or to treat comorbid psychiatric disorders. The benefits of using a particular drug must be carefully weighed against the risks posed to the fetus. If possible, avoid medication in the first trimester. Administer it in the lowest effective doses for the briefest periods possible.

Dopamine agonists decrease acute cocaine craving. **Bromocriptine** has been used in pregnancy to treat hyperprolactinemia and pituitary adenomas. Multiple studies show no increase in pregnancy complications or untoward effects in the fetus. For severe cocaine craving, bromocriptine, 2.5 to 10 mg/day, may be a reasonable short-term intervention to facilitate abstinence after acute withdrawal. The tricyclic antidepressant **desipramine** also reduces cocaine craving and appears to be effective in facilitating longer-term abstinence. It should be avoided in the first trimester and during the few weeks before delivery.

Detoxification from opiates during pregnancy is possible but extremely difficult and fraught with possible hazards of abortion in the first trimester and fetal distress in the third. If detoxification is requested, it should be attempted from the 14th to 28th weeks of gestation and should not exceed a taper of more than 5 mg/week.

The absolute safety of **methadone** during pregnancy is uncertain. Infants have a lower birth weight, shorter length, and smaller head circumference. They suffer from a greater incidence of SIDS. However, methadone likely poses less risk to the fetus than do severe withdrawal, infectious diseases contracted by the mother from contaminated needles, and absence of prenatal care. Research suggests that the results for patients receiving methadone maintenance along with good prenatal care and counseling are comparable to those for nonaddicted mothers.

A vulnerable period for relapse is the postpartum period. Treatment and supportive measures should continue. Note that the pediatrician must consider relapse in the mother of any infant exhibiting signs of neglect and/or abuse. Child protective services should be notified.

13. Which psychotropic agent should be considered most carefully before deciding on use in pregnancy?
In most industrialized nations, about 0.1% of the population receives maintenance **lithium** therapy for bipolar illness; 50% are women, many in the fertile age range. Of all the psychotropic agents, lithium warrants the most caution during pregnancy. It should be avoided altogether, if possible, because of the potential risks to the developing fetus and neonate. However, note that lithium is the safest mood-stabilizing agent currently available.

14. Describe the potential hazards of in-utero exposure to lithium.
Lithium is a known teratogen in the first trimester. An increased rate of cardiovascular abnormalities is observed. The most recent epidemiologic data suggest a relative risk of 1:1000 for

Ebstein's anomaly—ten times lower than previously estimated. The risk for any congenital abnormality in lithium-exposed infants is estimated to be between 4 and 12%, a rate 2–3 times greater than that in untreated comparison groups. Stillbirth and Down's syndrome are associated with lithium exposure during the first 12 weeks of pregnancy.

In the last trimester, lithium inhibits hormone release from the thyroid gland of the developing fetus, thereby stimulating increased TSH production and resulting in goiter. Lithium exerts an insulin-like effect on carbohydrate metabolism, leading to macrosomia. Premature delivery and increased perinatal mortality are potential complications.

Neonates exhibit decreased renal clearance. The half-life of lithium is generally prolonged, increasing the risk for toxicity. Lithium toxicity in the newborn is characterized by hypothermia, bradycardia, shallow respiration, and cyanosis. Hypotonia and feeding difficulties are not uncommon. Such effects are presumed to be reversible, but conclusive studies are lacking.

Animal studies suggest that behavioral teratogenicity may result from in-utero exposure to lithium. In one study, rats with in-utero exposure demonstrated significant impairment in performance on T-mazes.

A large Scandinavian study of lithium-exposed children who were born without physical malformations and reached the age of 5 years or older revealed no significant neurobehavioral differences compared with unexposed but genetically similar siblings. The study does not rule out the possibility of behavioral teratogenicity in humans but suggests that, if present, the changes are subtle. This data is encouraging for pregnant women who require maintenance lithium treatment. Finally, it is not clear whether in-utero exposure to lithium increases the risk for behavioral or affective abnormalities later in life.

15. What are the risks of other mood stabilizers?

Carbamazepine is associated with craniofacial abnormalities (11%), developmental delay (20%), and digital hypoplasia (26%). First-trimester exposure to carbamazepine has been associated with spina bifida, with a 0.5–1% risk. The risk of spina bifida with valproic acid is 1–4%. The use of these anticonvulsants during pregnancy is not justified except perhaps in the clinical setting of nonresponse to other treatment modalities and severe, life-threatening illness. If they are used during pregnancy, the mother should receive folate supplementation.

Clonazepam, a benzodiazepine with anticonvulsant and antimanic properties, has proved to be the least teratogenic of six anticonvulsant agents in mice. Whether this holds true for humans is yet to be determined. Lee Cohen, et al. (unpublished data, 1995) found no evidence of neonatal malformations in infants born to 25 mothers prescribed clonazepam during pregnancy.

Some of the data regarding neurobehavioral effects of in-utero exposure to these anticonvulsants are difficult to interpret due to a failure to control for variables such as parental IQ, seizures occurring during pregnancy and psychological and/or social factors. However, a recent study comparing children with and without prenatal exposure to carbamazepine failed to demonstrate any adverse neurobehavioral effects (i.e., lowered IQ) in the exposed children.

16. What is known about the safety of tricyclic antidepressants (TCAs) in pregnant women?

TCAs are the most studied class of antidepressants. During pregnancy, they are considered relatively safe. However, because they readily cross the placenta, the developing fetus is vulnerable to anticholinergic side effects, including tachyarrhythmias. Thus the less anticholinergic compounds nortriptyline and desipramine are recommended for pregnant women needing somatic treatment for depression.

After delivery, the neonate no longer has the support of maternal circulation to metabolize drugs. Toxicity may result, characterized by respiratory distress, cyanosis, hypertonia, irritability, and even seizures. In addition, a tricyclic withdrawal syndrome has been described, consisting of colic, irritability, difficulty with feeding, and tachypnea. The medication may be gradually withdrawn several weeks before the estimated date of delivery to provide a washout period for the fetus and to lessen the risk for anticholinergic complications. If necessary, the antidepressants may be reinstated immediately after delivery.

The effect of TCAs on the developing central nervous system of humans is not known. Neuro-behavioral sequelae have been demonstrated in animals. Studies have revealed decreased exploratory responses, delayed reflex development, and changes in hypothalamic dopamine levels in rats exposed to imipramine. The changes in behavioral response persist into adulthood. Although no human studies have conclusively clarified this issue, pooled analysis of 414 children with known first-trimester exposure to TCAs failed to reveal a significant association between fetal exposure and high rates of congenital malformations. Furthermore, normal motor and behavioral development was found in children (followed from birth to the age of 3 years) exposed to TCAs in utero.

17. What is known about the safety of selective serotonin reuptake inhibitors (SSRIs) in pregnant women?

Data on the safety of SSRIs during pregnancy is promising. In humans, the safety of **fluoxetine** in pregnancy has been evaluated in several prospective and retrospective studies and surveys consisting of over 2000 women. The incidence of major malformations in infants exposed in-utero does not appear to exceed the rate (2–7%) observed in the general population. The tendency for spontaneous abortion in fluoxetine-treated pregnant women was similar to that observed for TCAs (13.5%) and not greater than the rate of spontaneous abortion found in historical controls (15%). The outcomes of all prospectively identified, spontaneously reported pregnancies with confirmed fluoxetine exposure during the third semester suggest that fluoxetine use during pregnancy is unlikely to result in significant postnatal complications. Finally, one prospective study conducted by Nulman and colleagues demonstrated normal cognitive, language, and behavioral development in children exposed in-utero to fluoxetine.

Similar data exists for **sertraline**. In one study of 267 pregnant women, 147 were exposed to sertraline. No difference was found in the exposed women compared to controls with respect to rates of miscarriage, congenital malformations, stillbirth, prematurity, weight, or gestational age. Preliminary data for paroxetine points to a similar safety profile.

Less is known about the newer antidepressant agents, including citalopram, venlafaxine, and nefazodone. Data is also lacking for trazadone and buprorion. Until a more substantial database is established for these medications, supporting their safety in pregnancy, they should be avoided.

18. What is known about the safety of monoamine oxidase inhibitors (MAOIs) in pregnancy?

MAOIs are known teratogens in animals. Preclinical studies suggest that this teratogenicity may also apply to humans. Given the risk of an MAOI-precipitated hypertensive crisis and the availability of safer alternatives, MAOIs are *contraindicated* in pregnancy.

19. What is known about the safety of antipsychotic agents during pregnancy?

Reviews of the literature, including several prospective studies of tens of thousands of women exposed to high-potency neuroleptics in the first trimester, do not support an increased rate of malformations. Low-potency neuroleptics are associated with a 2.4% risk of congenital malformations.

Neuroleptics, like TCAs, readily cross the placenta. Toxicity is similar to that seen in adults. Extrapyramidal symptoms, including hypertonicity, restlessness, and tremor, are observed in neonates of mothers taking antipsychotic agents at the time of delivery. Tachycardia, urinary retention, and functional bowel obstruction are seen in infants of mothers taking low-potency (and therefore strongly anticholinergic) antipsychotic drugs. Maintaining pregnant on high-potency neuroleptics such as Haldol, with gradual discontinuation 5–10 days before delivery, minimizes complications in the newborn.

Postnatal behavioral changes, including poor performance in maze learning and shock avoidance, have been demonstrated in animals, whether or not exposure occurred before or after the completion of organogenesis. Rats exposed to Haldol have decreased dopamine receptor activity.

Data about long-term behavioral consequences in humans are lacking. One study of 14 children exposed to antipsychotics in utero failed to reveal memory or learning deficits by age 4 years. Another study of 52 children exposed prenatally to thorazine failed to identify behavioral abnormalities or changes in IQ scores compared with controls. A cohort of 3,056 infants exposed to phenothiazines at various times during gestation showed no statistically significant differences in IQ scores by age 4 years. More prolonged prospective follow-up studies are needed to establish the possible relationship between such drugs and subtle long-term behavioral or cognitive abnormalities.

Little is known about the safety of atypical antipsychotic drugs such as clozapine, risperidone, and other newer agents. They should be avoided during pregnancy until adequate data is available to support their safe use.

20. Is prophylaxis against extrapyramidal symptoms of antipsychotic therapy a good idea?

Prophylaxis against extrapyramidal symptoms (dystonias, tremor, akathisia) is not recommended. Anticholinergic agents used to treat the side effects of antipsychotic drugs are best prescribed on an as-needed basis and withdrawn at the earliest possible time to avoid complications in the neonate. In one study, a possible association between the use of these drugs and malformations was found. Risk for malformations has not been associated with diphenhydramine. Amantadine exposure in-utero has been linked to congenital malformations and should be avoided during pregnancy.

21. What is known about the effects of benzodiazepines on the developing fetus?

Pregnant women should be advised that pooled data analysis of several small studies points to a positive association between first-trimester exposure to benzodiazepines and oral cleft anomalies. Estimating the strength of that association is difficult secondary to the heterogeneity of the study subjects, different benzodiazepine drug use, and variations in reports of malformations. As with all drugs, benzodiazepines should be withheld in the first trimester of pregnancy or at least until the tenth week of gestation when palate closure is complete. In addition to cleft palate abnormalities, a syndrome reminiscent of fetal alcohol syndrome has been reported in infants with in-utero exposure to benzodiazepines. However, the most recent prospective data are contradictory.

The literature suggests that use of benzodiazepines in the second and third trimesters is probably safe. However, with prolonged administration, cord plasma concentrations in the fetus may become greater than in the maternal circulation. Transient neurologic deficits, hypotonia, and respiratory depression have been reported in neonates born to mothers medicated in the later stages of pregnancy. In addition, neonates are at risk for withdrawal symptoms within a few days to 3 weeks after birth. Gradual discontinuation several weeks before delivery is recommended.

Abnormalities of motor and arousal processes in rodents exposed to diazepam in utero have been demonstrated. The significance of these findings in humans is not known. Some studies suggest that in-utero exposure to benzodiazepines is associated with developmental delay.

22. What legal considerations must be kept in mind when prescribing medication for a pregnant woman with psychiatric illness?

Remember that you are treating two patients: the psychiatrically impaired pregnant woman and her unborn child. The literature about psychotropic drug use in pregnant women is primarily retrospective and to some extent anecdotal. Thus the decision to prescribe such medications during pregnancy must be made based on a thoughtful risk-benefit analysis. Be sure to document the specific benefits that justify the risk. In documenting consent, indicate the patient's competence to understand the specific risks, benefits, and alternative treatments, including no treatment. Ideally, a course of action should be agreed upon *before* conception and when the woman is psychiatrically stable. It should be documented clearly in treatment records. If the woman deteriorates during the course of pregnancy and becomes incompetent to participate in treatment decisions, temporary guardianship must be pursued so that appropriate psychiatric care can proceed.

23. Describe the management of the bipolar patient who desires pregnancy.

Bipolar disorder (manic-depressive illness) has a mean age of onset in the early twenties, coinciding with childbearing years. Bipolar women need prenatal counseling to be advised of the risk of fetal anomalies associated with psychotropic medication. The prospective mother also must be made aware of her risk for manic decompensation when somatic therapy is withdrawn.

Ideally, psychotropic medications should be discontinued several weeks before conception. For the woman who has had a single episode of mania with complete recovery and a long period of stability, slowly tapering medication before attempting to conceive is a reasonable course of action. When a woman taking lithium conceives unknowingly, the drug should be gradually discontinued because abrupt withdrawal is associated with manic relapse. Close observation should follow. With early and mild relapse, hospitalization with structure, reduced environmental stimulation, and elimination of exacerbating stressors may avert worsening of symptoms. If conservative measures fail, low-dose antipsychotics should be instituted to ameliorate the most severe symptoms, for example, insomnia. An adjuvant benzodiazepine such as clonazepam may reduce the total required dose of either medication used alone. If such measures fail to stabilize the patient, lithium may be reinstated—ideally in the second trimester after organ formation is complete.

Bipolar patients are 4–5 times more likely to develop mania in the postpartum period than at any other time. Clinicians should follow such women closely. Extending the postpartum hospital stay for longer observation is warranted. Provisions for continued monitoring and support by family or professional agencies should be arranged before discharge.

24. Is management different for bipolar patients with brittle illness?

A more difficult decision must be made for women with brittle illness, which is characterized by high relapse risk in the absence of mood-stabilizing medication. The potential morbidity associated with the drugs must be weighed against the likelihood of severe psychiatric symptoms and the associated danger to the mother and her developing child. The decision to continue psychotropic medication through pregnancy must be made jointly by the physician and the carefully informed couple wishing to conceive. The consent process, which outlines risks, benefits, and alternative treatments as well as the planned course of action, should be documented carefully in the patient's records.

25. Describe some specifics of lithium therapy for the pregnant, bipolar woman.

For women maintained on lithium in the first trimester, fetal ultrasound should be obtained at 18 weeks to rule out cardiac malformations. Women need to understand the prognosis of Ebstein's anomaly. The literature suggests that up to 50% of affected infants die in the first week of life.

If lithium is used during pregnancy, it must be administered in several small doses to decrease the risk of toxicity associated with peak serum levels. Lithium levels should be monitored frequently. In the second trimester, higher doses may be necessary because of the increased glomerular filtration rate in the mother. Minimal effective serum levels should be maintained. The dosage should be reduced by at least 50% at the onset of labor to avoid toxicity due to abrupt falls in renal filtration rates and pronounced fluid shifting.

26. Is depression a problem in pregnant women?

Several recent prospective studies have demonstrated an incidence of depression during pregnancy as high as 20%. Symptoms are generally of less severity than those observed with postpartum mood disorders. Risk factors for developing depression during pregnancy include prior history of depression, family history of mood disorders, negative feelings about the pregnancy, and unrelated bereavement. Impoverished social supports and negative life events are also risk factors.

27. Describe the management of women who experience depression during pregnancy.

Despite the the relatively high number of women who experience depression during pregnancy, not all require pharmacotherapy. Many women develop minor depressive symptoms in the first trimester of pregnancy that are more consistent with an adjustment disorder. They usually respond to support, reassurance, and efforts to minimize psychosocial sources of distress. Pharmacotherapy is generally reserved for the most severe depressions characterized by neurovegetative dysfunction, including poor appetite and sleep disturbance. As with all psychotropic medications, the risks associated with pharmacotherapy must be weighed against the risks of withholding treatment.

TCAs and SSRIs can be given to pregnant women requiring pharmacologic intervention. Nonbiological interventions including cognitive-behavioral therapy and interpersonal therapy have proven efficacy and may provide adequate support to delay initiation of medication. Serum TCA levels should be monitored frequently as the pregnancy progresses and maternal fluid shifts occur. The medication may need to be tapered before or at the onset of labor to avoid adverse effects in the newborn.

A severely depressed woman expressing suicidal intent and/or showing signs of nutritional or physical deterioration represents a *psychiatric emergency*. Electroconvulsive therapy is the treatment of choice in such patients, who require rapid response.

28. Describe the management of women with psychotic illnesses during pregnancy.

Women with schizophrenia are at high risk of exacerbation during pregnancy and poor fetal outcome. For each month medication is withheld, approximately 10% of schizophrenics will relapse. It is estimated that 65% of unmedicated schizophrenics and 26% of those maintained on psychotropics will relapse during pregnancy.

Schizophrenia is the most difficult psychiatric disorder to deal with both during pregnancy and in the postpartum period. Psychotic women often have exaggerated and distorted responses to the somatic changes associated with pregnancy. Not infrequently, psychotic denial of the pregnancy prevents participation in prenatal care. Health professionals caring for them may develop intense and conflicting feelings toward the patient, ranging from anger to sadness.

When pregnancy is confirmed, if the patient is stable, a trial of no medication in the first trimester, with a plan to reinstitute treatment at the first sign of psychosis is recommended. A woman who first becomes psychotic during pregnancy should be thoroughly evaluated to identify reversible organic causes. Hospitalization or intense care management is desirable to ensure compliance with prenatal care and perhaps to reduce the total amount of medication required for adequate stabilization.

High-potency neuroleptics, such as perphenazine or haloperidol, should be given at the minimal effective dose for controlling the most disabling symptoms. As with other psychiatric disorders, complete amelioration of symptoms is not the goal in managing a pregnant woman with schizophrenia. Maintenance of self-care and moderately good functioning are more realistic achievements. Antiparkinson agents, such as Cogentin or Artane, should be given in the smallest effective dose on an as-needed basis.

A close obstetric-psychiatric liaison must be established and maintained throughout the pregnancy and postpartum period. When the patient is transferred to the obstetrics department for labor and delivery, she should be accompanied by psychiatrically trained nursing staff.

29. What issues are concerning postpartum in the schizophrenic mother?

During the postpartum period, schizophrenic mothers often demonstrate limited ability to attend to the infant or to recognize its needs. This should be anticipated by making provisions for supervised feedings and visits with the infant. The decision must be made about the appropriateness of a referral to child protective services for ongoing evaluation and monitoring of the mother's ability to care for her infant. If the mother shows gross inability or severely impaired reality testing, it may be necessary for the infant to be temporarily placed in foster care.

Schizophrenic patients have an increased risk of postpartum psychotic decompensation. Extended hospitalization should be planned. Many schizophrenic mothers are unmarried and have impoverished support systems. Before discharge, arrangements for a visiting nurse and involvement of social agencies should be made.

Note that contraception should be strongly encouraged to prevent a close succession of pregnancies in vulnerable women. Noncompliance with oral contraceptives and barrier methods is common. The patient should be informed of the availability of long-acting injectable preparations such as Depo-Provera and Norplant. The option of tubal ligation should be discussed.

30. How is the patient with anxiety disorder managed during pregnancy?

Anxiety disorders are common in women and tend to aggregate in those of childbearing age. Historically, it was believed that pregnancy was a time of quiescence for women with pregravid histories of anxiety. More recent literature suggests that although pregnancy may ameliorate symptoms of panic disorder in some women, such conditions tend to worsen during pregnancy, especially in the last trimester and postpartum period. For example, several studies have associated the onset of obsessive-compulsive disorder (OCD) with pregnancy and childbirth. Pre-existing disease typically is exacerbated by pregnancy.

Women with moderate to severe symptoms of anxiety during pregnancy and delivery experience more complications. Preterm labor, preeclampsia, placental abruption, stillbirths, and fetal hypoxia have been reported. Such complications may be related to increases in catecholamine secretion, which result in transient elevations in blood pressure and vasoconstriction of the fetoplacental unit.

The goal of managing anxiety-disordered women during pregnancy is to minimize risk to the mother and infant, not to achieve complete control of symptoms. Before instituting pharmacologic treatment, behavioral techniques such as progressive relaxation or biofeedback should be attempted. Such measures, in addition to supportive psychotherapy, may prevent the need for medication or at least minimize the required amount.

If psychotropic medication is required, fluoxetine, sertraline, and paroxetine are options. The TCA nortriptyline is also an option. Benzodiazepines should be avoided, if possible. If employed, the smallest effective dose for the shortest period of time is the goal. A reduction of benzodiazepine and TCA doses may be required before the estimated date of confinement to avoid toxicity and/or withdrawal in the neonate.

31. Is electroconvulsive therapy safe for pregnant women?

Electroconvulsive therapy (ECT) is an underutilized treatment modality in pregnant as well as nonpregnant patients. It is an excellent therapeutic alternative when psychotropic medications have failed or are contraindicated. *ECT is considered the first-line treatment in pregnant women requiring a rapid therapeutic response.*

Studies suggest that ECT is safe for women in any stage of pregnancy. Mortality associated with ECT is less than that observed for inadequately treated depression during pregnancy. The ECT complication rate of 5–6% is less than that for untreated pregnant psychotic women and pregnant women without psychiatric illness. Finally, the rate of miscarriage in the general population is considerably higher than that observed in pregnant women undergoing ECT, suggesting that ECT does not increase the likelihood of miscarriage.

32. Describe the management of the pregnant patient undergoing ECT.

The following steps decrease potential risk to the mother and fetus:

• Pelvic examination to rule out vaginal bleeding or cervical dilation is performed before a course of ECT.

• The prolonged gastric emptying time in pregnant women increases the risk of aspiration. Nonessential anticholinergic medications are discontinued to avoid further slowing of gastric transit. A nonparticulate antacid, such as sodium citrate, is administered to raise gastric pH, and thus to minimize the risk of aspiration pneumonitis. After the first trimester, some anesthesiologists recommend intubation.

• Fetal circulation may be compromised if the gravid uterus is large and heavy enough to compress the inferior vena cava when the patient is in a supine position. Elevating the patient's right hip to displace the uterus to the left can prevent this complication. Pretreatment intravenous hydration is also recommended.

• Excessive hyperventilation, usually done to lower the seizure threshold, is not recommended. Respiratory alkalosis in the mother hinders oxygen unloading from maternal to fetal hemoglobin. Fetal hypoxia is a real risk.

• Transient hypertension during a seizure may increase the risk for placental abruption. Intravenous Labetalol is recommended to control blood pressure.

• Self-limited fetal cardiac arrhythmias may occur during the seizure. External fetal cardiac monitoring is performed through the procedure and recovery period.

• An anticholinergic agent is administered before ECT to prevent excessive vagal bradycardia and to decrease oropharyngeal and tracheal secretions. Atropine, which quickly crosses the placental barrier, may produce fetal tachycardia. Glycopyrrolate has a more limited rate of transfer across the placenta and thus reduces risk to the fetus; it is the preferred anticholinergic drug for pregnant patients undergoing ECT.

• Adequate relaxation in the mother is essential to prevent injury to the fetus. Fortunately, succinylcholine in ordinary doses does not cross the placenta.

33. How do psychotropic medications affect breastfeeding?

The benefits of breastfeeding are well documented. Human milk possesses antimicrobial and unique trophic properties that benefit the infant. Breastfeeding enhances the process of maternal bonding. Unfortunately, the literature contains little information about psychotropic drug excretion in breast milk. However, all major classes of psychotropic drugs have been isolated in breast milk. Concentrations vary depending on the properties of the individual compound. Drugs that have protein binding tend to remain in the mother's plasma. Low-molecular-weight compounds and compounds with high lipid solubility diffuse into breast milk. Weak bases undergo ion trapping in the relatively acidic milk.

34. Discuss the effects of specific psychotropic agents on breast milk.

Lithium concentration in breast milk is about 30–50% of that in the mother's serum. Because an infant's regulatory and excretory mechanisms are not fully developed, toxicity is a real risk. Breastfeeding is contraindicated for women requiring maintenance lithium treatment.

Carbamazepine and **valproic acid** are listed with the American Academy of Pediatrics as drugs considered compatible with breastfeeding. Valproic acid should be used with caution due to an associated risk of hepatotoxicity in infants.

In general, **benzodiazepines** should not be given to breastfeeding mothers because of the risk of prolonging physiologic jaundice in the infant and because withdrawal syndromes have been observed in nursing infants exposed to benzodiazepines. However, intermittent, judicious use of benzodiazepines by highly anxious women is less likely to lead to accumulation and adverse effects in the nursing infant. Short-acting compounds lacking active metabolites (i.e., lorazepam) are preferred.

Antidepressants should be used with caution in the nursing mother. Imipramine, nortriptyline, and desipramine are not excreted in breast milk in appreciable quantities. If a mother taking these medications insists on nursing her infant, care should be taken to minimize the infant's exposure. This can be accomplished by having the mother take the medication immediately after the breastfeeding that precedes the infant's longest period of sleep. The infant should be observed for signs of drug effect, such as sedation or inexplicable irritability.

Fluoxetine is likely compatible with breastfeeding. While one case study revealed a lactating mother's infant developed watery stools, crying, and sleep disturbance, there is evidence that the infant's hepatic metabolism was immature. The serum levels of fluoxetine and norfluoxetine in the infant were much higher than expected for the amount ingested by the mother. A case series of 11 nursing infants exposed to fluoxetine revealed no adverse effects. A similar case series for sertraline revealed no adverse effects in the infants exposed to the drug via breastmilk.

If a mother requires **antipsychotic medication**, she is best advised to bottle-feed her infant.

BIBLIOGRAPHY

1. Altushuler LL, Cohen L, Szuba MP, et al: Pharmacologic management of psychiatric illness during pregnancy: Dilemmas and guidelines. Am J Psychiatry 1996;153(5):592–606.
2. Appleby L, Warner R, Whitton A, Faragher B: A controlled study of fluoxetine and cognitive behavioral counseling in the treatment of postnatal depression. BMJ 1997;314(7085):932–936.
3. Brunel P, Vial T, Roche I, et al: Follow-up on 151 pregnancies exposed to an antidepressant treatment (excluding MAOIs) during organogenesis. Therapy 1994;49:117–122.
4. Burch KJ, Wells BG: Fluoxetine/norfluoxetine concentrations in human milk. Experienced Reason 1992; 676–677.
5. Chambers CD, Johnson KA, Dick LM, et al: Birth outcomes in pregnant women taking fluoxetine. N Engl J Med 1996;335:1010–1015.
6. Chasnoff IJ, Burns WJ, Schnoli SH, Kayreen AB: Cocaine use in pregnancy. N Engl J Med 313:666–669, 1985.

7. Chelmow D, Halfin VP: Pregnancy complicated by obsessive-compulsive disorder. J Maternal-Fetal Med 1997;6(1):31–34.
8. Cohen LS: The use of psychotropic drugs during pregnancy and the puerperium. Curr Affect Illness 11:9, 1992.
9. Cohen LS, Friedman JM, Jefferson JW, et al: A reevaluation of risk of in utero exposure to lithium. JAMA 1994;271(2):146–150.
10. Cohen LS, Rosenbaum JF: Birth outcomes in pregnant women taking fluoxetine (letter). N Engl J Med 1997;336(12):872.
11. Cooper PJ, Murray L, Stein A: Psychosocial factors associated with the early termination of breast-feeding. J Psychosom Res 1993;37(2):171–176.
12. Duffull SB, Begg EJ, Ilett KF: Fluoxetine distribution in human milk (letter). J Clin Pharmacol 1996;36(11): 1078–1079.
13. Feingold M, Lyons B, Kaminer Y, et al: Bulimia nervosa in pregnancy. Obstet Gynecol 71:1025–1027, 1988.
14. Flaherty B, Krenzelok EP: Neonatal lithium toxicity as a result of maternal toxicity. Vet Hum Toxicol 1997; 39(2):92–93.
15. Goldstein DJ: Effects of third-trimester fluoxetine exposure on the newborn. J Clin Psychopharmacol 1995; 15:417–420.
16. Goldstein DJ, Corbin LA, Sundell KL: Effects of first-trimester fluoxetine exposure on the newborn. Obstet Gynecol 1997;89(5 Pt 1):713–718.
17. Goldstein DJ, Marvel DE: Psychotropic medications during pregnancy: Risk to the fetus. JAMA 1993;270 (18):2177.
18. Haynes JS: An update on psychotropic drugs in breastfeeding. Psychiatr Times June 1994.
19. Isenberg KE: Excretion of fluoxetine in human breast milk. J Clin Psychiatry 1990:51(4):169.
20. James ME: Cocaine abuse during pregnancy: Psychiatric considerations. Oral presentation, 1990.
21. Kulin NA, Pastuszak A, Sage SR, et al: Pregnancy outcome following maternal use of the new selective serotonin reuptake inhibitors. JAMA 1998;279:609–610.
22. Lester BM, Cucca J, Andreozzi BA, et al: Possible association between fluoxetine hydrochloride and colic in an infant. J Am Acad Child Adolesc Psychiatry 1993;32(6):1253–1255.
23. McCance-Katz EF: The consequences of maternal substance abuse for the child exposed in utero. Psychosomatics 32:268–274, 1991.
24. McIntosh R, Merritt KK, Richards MR, et al: The incidence of congenital malformations: A study of 5964 pregnancies. Pediatrics 1954;14:505–521.
25. McDonald AD: Maternal health and congenital defect. N Engl J Med 1958;258:767–774.
26. MeElhatton PR, Garbis HM, Elefant E, et al: The outcome of pregnancy in 689 women exposed to therapeutic doses of antidepressants. The collaborative study of the European network of the teratology information services (ENTIS). Reprod Toxicol 1996;10:285–294.
27. Miller LJ: Clinical strategies for the use of psychotropics during pregnancy. Psychiatr Med 2:275–298, 1991.
28. Milner G, O'Leary MM: Anorexia nervosa occurring in pregnancy. Acta Psychiatr Scand 77:491–492, 1988.
29. Miller LJ: Use of electroconvulsive therapy during pregnancy. Hosp Community Psychiatry 45:444–450, 1994.
30. Misri S, Sivertz K: Tricyclic drugs in pregnancy and lactation: A preliminary report. Int J Psychiatry Med 1991;21(2):157–171.
31. Muqtadir S, Hamann MW: Management of psychotic pregnant patients in a medical-psychiatric unit. Psychosomatics 1986;27(1):31–33.
32. Murray L, Stein A: The effects of postnatal depression on the infant. Baillieres Clin Obstet Gynecol 1989; 3(4):921–933.
33. Nulman I, Rovet J, Stewart DE, et al: Neurodevelopment of children exposed in utero to antidepressant drugs. N Engl J Med 1997;336:258–262.
34. Nurnberg HG: An overview of somatic treatment of psychosis during pregnancy and postpartum. Gen Hosp Psychiatry 1989;11(5):328–338.
35. Nurnber HG, Prudic J: Guidelines for treatment of psychosis during pregnancy. Hosp Community Psychiatry 35:67–71, 1984.
36. Oates MR: The treatment of psychiatric disorders in pregnancy and the puerperium. Clin Obstet Gynecol 13: 385–395, 1984.
37. O'Hara MW: Social support, life events, and depression during pregnancy and the puerperium. Arch Gen Psychiatry 43:569–573, 1986.
38. O'Hara MW, Schlechte JA, Lewis DA, Varner MW: Controlled prospective study of postpartum mood disorders: Psychological, environmental, and hormonal variables. J Abnorm Psychol 1991;100(1):63–73.
39. Pastuszak A, et al: Pregnancy outcome following first trimester exposure to fluoxetine. JAMA 269:2246–2248, 1993.
40. Rattan DA, Friedman T: Antidepressants in pregnancy and breastfeeding. Br J Psychiatry 1995;167(6):824.
41. Repke JT, Berger NG: Electroconvulsive therapy in pregnancy. Obstet Gynceol 63:39–41, 1984.

42. Riccardi VM: The genetic approach to human disease. New York, NY, Oxford University Press, 1977, pp 3–4.
43. Robert E: Treating depression in pregnancy. N Engl J Med 1996;335;1056–1058.
44. Roberts RJ, Blumer J, Gorman R, et al: Transfer of drugs and other chemicals into human milk. Pediatrics 84:924–936, 1989.
45. Robinson GE: The rational use of psychotropic drugs in pregnancy and postpartum. Can J Psychiatry 31: 183–190, 1986.
46. Robinson L: Cognitive-behavioral treatment of panic disorder during pregnancy and lactation. Can J Psychiatry 37:523–626, 1992.
47. Schou M: Lithium treatment during pregnancy, delivery and lactation: An update. J Clin Psychiatry 51:410–412, 1990.
48. Sitland-Marken PA, Rickman L, Wells B, et al: Pharmacologic management of acute mania in pregnancy. J Clin Psychopharm 9:78–87, 1989.
49. Spencer MJ: Fluoxetine hydrochloride (Prozac) toxicity in a neonate. Pediatrics 1993;92:721–722.
50. Stewart DE, Raskin J, Garfinkel P, et al: Anorexia nervosa, bulimia and pregnancy. Am J Obstet Gynecol 157:1194–1198, 1987.
51. Susman VL, Katz JL: Weaning and depression: Another postpartum complication. Am J Psychiatry 145: 498–501, 1988.
52. Williams KE, Koran LM: Obsessive-compulsive disorder in pregnancy, the puerperium, and the premenstruum. J Clin Psychiatry 1997;58:330–334.
53. Willis DC, Rand CS: Pregnancy in bulimic women. Obstet Gynceol 71:708–710, 1988.
54. Wisner KL, Perel JM: Serum levels of valproate and carbamazepine in breastfeeding mother-infant pairs. J Clin Psychopharmacol 1998;18:167–169.
55. Wisner KL, Perel JM, Blumer J: Serum sertraline and N-desmethylsertraline levels in breast-feeding mother-infant pairs. Am J Psychiatry 1998;155(5):690–692.
56. Wisner KL, Perel JM, Wheeler SB: Tricyclic dose requirements across pregnancy. Am J Psychiatry 1993;150(10):1541–1542.

64. POSTPARTUM PSYCHIATRIC DISORDERS

Doris C. Gundersen, M.D.

1. What psychiatric disorders are seen in the postpartum period?

Maternity blues, postpartum psychosis, and postpartum depression are the psychiatric diagnoses most often made after delivery.

2. Define maternity blues.

Maternity blues, or baby blues, is a term used to describe a self-limiting, relatively mild mood syndrome experienced by 30–80% of all postpartum women. Symptoms include lability of mood, anxiety, sadness, crying spells, insomnia, and fatigue. The onset of maternity blues is usually 3–10 days after parturition. The symptoms typically remit within 2 weeks.

3. Which risk factors predispose women to maternity blues?

Many regard maternity blues as a normal postpartum phenomenon because of its frequency and spontaneous remission. However, some women appear to be at higher risk. Major predictive factors include primiparous pregnancy, history of late luteal phase dysphoria (PMS), personal history of depression, or first-degree relative with depression.

4. What causes maternity blues?

The precise cause of maternity blues is unknown. Because the condition is common in all cultures and races and appears to occur independently of psychosocial factors, a biologic cause is likely. Studies have demonstrated that estrogen and progesterone influence the sensitivity of neurotransmitter-binding sites much like chronic administration of antidepressant drugs. With the delivery of the placenta, the elevated estrogen and progesterone levels maintained throughout pregnancy fall precipitously, and pregravid serum concentrations are reached within 3 days, coinciding with peak symptoms of maternity blues. It is hypothesized that this rapid decline in reproductive hormones after delivery destabilizes neurotransmitter mechanisms involved in mood regulation.

5. Describe postpartum psychosis.

Postpartum psychosis is sometimes called peurperal psychosis or postpartum psychotic depression. It develops in 1–2 per 1000 postpartum women worldwide. In the majority of cases, the symptoms are manifest within the first 2 weeks after delivery. However, a second peak has been observed 1–3 months after delivery.

A common prodrome for postpartum psychosis is worsening insomnia in the absence of a crying infant or physical discomfort in the mother. Psychomotor agitation may precede the psychosis. Women experience confusion, memory impairment, irritability, and anxiety. Intrusive thoughts, usually about harming the infant, are not uncommon. Paranoid and religious delusions, auditory hallucinations, thought insertion, thought withdrawal, and thought broadcasting have been reported. Faulty interactions with the infant, either misreading cues or blatant disinterest, also may be manifestations.

A unique feature of postpartum psychosis is the **mercurial changeability of the symptoms**. A brief period of elation characterized by incessant talking, increased energy, and euphoric mood may shift rapidly to profound, inexplicable sadness or rage. Lucid intervals are common and may give a deceptive impression of recovery. Abrupt episodes of floridly psychotic behavior may resurface after weeks of calm. Postpartum psychosis may resolve abruptly, but more often it evolves into serious, protracted depression. Postpartum psychosis frequently resembles mania and may prove to be a variant of bipolar affective disorder.

6. How frequently do women with postpartum psychosis harm their infants?

The level of infant morbidity correlates well with the severity of psychiatric symptoms in the mother. Infants of mildly to moderately impaired mothers may demonstrate difficulty with feeding or bonding. Infants of more severely afflicted mothers present with failure to thrive or evidence of frank physical abuse. Infanticide occurs in an estimated 4% of cases. Approximately 80–120 infanticides are committed by psychotic new mothers in the United States each year. At least 50% of the infant deaths take place weeks to months after the acute symptoms have subsided. Such numbers emphasize the importance of continuous monitoring of the mother's behavior, well beyond the initial psychotic episode. The capacity for the psychosis to recur after lucid periods must always be kept in mind.

7. Are there specific risk factors for postpartum psychosis?

Hereditary factors and **prior history of affective episodes** confer the greatest risk. A woman with a history of depression unrelated to pregnancy has a 20–25% risk of developing postpartum psychosis. This risk is higher for women with bipolar mood disorders than for women with a history of unipolar depression. If a bipolar woman develops postpartum psychosis, she carries a 50% risk for recurrence with subsequent deliveries. Women with a history of postpartum psychosis have a 1 in 3 chance of recurrence with future deliveries. The same women have a 38% risk for developing nonpsychotic postpartum depression. The need for careful prenatal screening and counseling is obvious. Other risk factors include single or primiparous women, cesarean section, or perinatal death. Postpartum psychosis peaks between ages 25–29 and 30–34 years, which coincide with vulnerable times for the development of PMS. A relationship between the two disorders has yet to be established.

8. What is the cause of postpartum psychosis?

Postpartum psychosis is regarded as an **organic syndrome**. Psychological and social variables are considered secondary to organic factors. After delivery of the placenta, a large source of hormone production is lost. As with maternity blues, the sudden and dramatic decline in serum estrogen may initiate a sequence of neuroendocrine events that produce serious psychiatric symptoms in susceptible women. Estrogen has antidopaminergic properties. It is hypothesized that the abrupt **with-**

drawal of estrogen exposes sensitive postsynaptic receptors in the brain; this may be the triggering event for development of psychosis. The propensity for relapse at the time of menses further implicates sex hormones in development of this disorder.

A decline in serum estrogen also leads to a fall in serum binding proteins, including transcortin. **Cortisol levels** are elevated during pregnancy. A surge of cortisol at labor is followed by an accelerated decline to second trimester levels within 72 hours. Acute psychotic reactions have been reported with adrenal insufficiency and/or steroid withdrawal. Small doses of the cortisol analog given to women with postpartum illness appear to decrease the severity and duration of symptoms. Unfortunately, no controlled studies of this regimen have been conducted.

Finally, women with postpartum illness have a high incidence of **thyroid abnormalities**. T3 levels are significantly lowered in women with postpartum psychosis compared with controls. The absolute values often fall within the normal range, with no overt physical signs of hypothyroidism. Perhaps it is the slope of the T3 decline rather than the specific serum concentration that influences the development of psychosis.

9. Describe postpartum depression.

Between the extremes of maternity blues and postpartum psychosis lies postpartum depression, which develops in 10–20% of women after delivery. Unlike the blues or psychosis, postpartum depression tends to develop insidiously 3 or more weeks after delivery. The mood symptoms are more sustained, and the course of the illness is typically prolonged. Symptoms include crying spells, poor concentration, indecisiveness, and profound sadness. Thoughts are characterized by themes of failure and inadequacy. Suicidal ideation is common. Postpartum depression is characterized by physical signs and symptoms resembling moderate-to-severe hypothyroidism. Cold intolerance, fatigue, dry skin, slowed mentation, constipation, and fluid retention are commonly reported.

10. What are the risk factors for postpartum depression?

As with the blues and psychosis, **hereditary factors** and a **history of previous psychiatric illness** are identified as significant risk factors for postpartum depression. Women with previous episodes of depression unrelated to reproduction have a 10–40% chance of developing postpartum depression. Women with a history of postpartum depression have a 50% rate of recurrence with subsequent pregnancies. Several psychosocial risk factors have been identified, including marital discord, stressful life events during pregnancy, ambivalence about motherhood, low socioeconomic status, isolation from extended family or friends, and single status. Unrealistic expectations or romanticized ideas about motherhood, which inevitably clash with reality, may predispose a woman to depression. High prenatal scores on neuroticism scales are associated with postpartum depression.

11. Is postpartum depression considered to be primarily a biologic illness?

Not entirely. Ethnographic literature about childbirth suggests that the depressive reaction is at least partly attributable to cultural patterning of the postpartum period. Postpartum depression is not expressed globally; it appears rarely in non-Western cultures in which a new mother is absolved of all responsibilities beyond self-care and feeding her infant. Rituals practiced in third-world countries include provisions of social support for the new mother and clearly define her role. With modern birthing practices in Western society, there is less social structuring of postpartum events and a lack of clear role definition and social support for new mothers.

12. Are there endocrine or biologic correlates for postpartum depression?

Postpartum depression often is accompanied by symptoms related to hypothyroidism, and research points to varying degrees of pituitary dysfunction and related thyroid abnormalities as contributing factors in development of the illness.

After normal delivery, blood supply to the pituitary gland wanes. Trophic hormone secretion is reduced to prepregnancy quantities. If the delivery is complicated by shock (e.g., massive hemorrhage), the anterior pituitary may be damaged by infarction. In this scenario, secretion of trophic hormones ceases. Targeted endocrine glands fail. The patient develops profound apathy, cold sensitivity, loss of libido, memory impairment, lethargy, and thinning of axillary and pubic hair. Psychosis and eventually coma develop in untreated cases. This is known as **Sheehan's syndrome**.

It is hypothesized that postpartum depression is an intermediate condition. A sluggish pituitary may compromise endocrine functioning. After delivery thyroxine levels tend to decline and remain at values below the nonpregnant average for up to 1 year. Although depressed, the thyroxine level tends to overlap with the normal range, possibly masking hypothyroidism. The level of thyroid-stimulating hormone (TSH) usually is normal in **hypothyroidism of pituitary origin (secondary hypothyroidism)**.

Case studies support the link between subclinical hypothyroidism of pituitary origin and postpartum illness. Antidepressant and antipsychotic medications, alone or in combination, frequently fail to treat adequately the symptoms of postpartum depression. With the addition of thyroid hormone, some patients experience rapid alleviation of psychiatric symptoms.

Further support for partial pituitary dysfunction or damage is suggested by the heightened sensitivity to sunburn or diminished capacity to tan reported by several postpartum women. This finding suggests reduced or absent melanin production by the pituitary gland. Finally, 5–30% of postpartum cases become chronic, implying some degree of residual damage.

Primary hypothyroidism, which originates in the **thyroid gland**, is also diagnosed in the postpartum period. Painless autoimmune thyroiditis, characterized by positive thyroid antibodies, occurs in 2–9% of postpartum women, surpassing the number observed in nonpregnant controls. Thyroxine may rise briefly with the inflammation. This rise is followed by a reduction in thyroid hormone and a corresponding rise in TSH. One study revealed persistent thyroid abnormalities 3 years after delivery in 50% of women.

In summary, postpartum depression often includes symptoms identical to moderate-to-severe hypothyroidism. Routine laboratory screening may fail to identify the abnormality if it is of pituitary origin. Such subclinical hypothyroidism may render postpartum depression refractory to treatment.

13. Can postpartum disorders be prevented?

Postpartum illnesses are notoriously difficult to treat. For this reason, efforts should be made to prevent their onset by eliminating or at least reducing known risk factors. High-risk patients can be identified early in the course of pregnancy through the use of **risk assessment checklists**, ideally at the first prenatal visit. When significant vulnerability is identified, interventions may include reducing environmental stress, enlisting the aid of family members, and mobilizing additional sources of support. Prenatal anticipatory guidance prepares a new mother for maternity blues and helps her to distinguish the blues from more ominous symptoms that warrant professional attention. Women with past histories of depression or psychosis should be followed more closely. The earlier a postpartum illness is identified, the greater the opportunity for secondary prevention.

14. What are the barriers to diagnosis?

Early detection of postpartum illness is rare, in part as a result of modern obstetric practices. In the United States, postpartum women are discharged from the hospital within 48 hours. The symptoms of postpartum illnesses are usually manifest after the third postpartum day, when the expert observation of nursing staff and physicians is no longer available. Six weeks pass before the next professional contact is made, resulting in a window of extreme vulnerability for new mothers.

The stigma placed by American culture on mental illness creates another barrier to early diagnosis. Patients and their families may conceal the severity of the problem out of shame, guilt, or embarrassment. Furthermore, depression after delivery contradicts the cultural expectation of "parental bliss."

The prodrome for serious postpartum pathology often mimics the blues. Women who voice concerns about such symptoms may be reassured without further investigation. Finally, the focus of the first postnatal visit is the reproductive health of the mother; her emotional well-being is not routinely addressed.

15. What biologic treatment strategies are available?

Maternity blues is a mild, transitory mood syndrome that typically resolves within a few days.

Reassurance, observation, and occasionally a short-acting sedative are the primary interventions. It is important, however, to take the patient's complaints seriously. This increases the likelihood of her reporting symptoms that linger or become more severe.

Postpartum psychosis usually merits hospitalization because of the level of dysfunction and grave risk for both infanticide and suicide. The symptoms of postpartum psychosis are predominantly affective. Lithium or other mood-stabilizing medications are often helpful. Antipsychotic doses are typically lower than those required for other psychotic disorders. Electroconvulsive therapy (ECT) is indicated for severe, pharmacologically refractory cases.

For **postpartum depression** antidepressants, especially those that are selective for serotonin, appear to have some efficacy in targeting symptoms. Low doses of antipsychotic medications should be included if symptoms of psychosis are present. As with postpartum psychosis, some women may respond preferentially to ECT.

Thyroid screening should be performed routinely. For all postpartum cases, levels of serum thyroxine, TSH, and autoimmune antibodies should be assessed. Weekly thyroxine levels should be obtained. If a downward trend is identified, thyroxine replacement therapy should be initiated. A typical starting dose is 0.05 mg per day.

In women at **risk for recurrence**, psychotropic drugs to prevent or mitigate serious psychiatric symptoms should be given serious consideration. Women with histories of postpartum psychosis should receive lithium immediately after delivery. Rapid achievement of therapeutic blood levels is the goal. Care must be exercised to prevent toxicity. Lithium excretion may be impaired by fluid and electrolyte changes in the immediate postpartum period. Low-dose antipsychotic medications are also recommended for at least 2–3 weeks after delivery. In women with previous nonpsychotic postpartum depressions, antidepressant medication may be initiated somewhat earlier than onset of the previous episode.

Postpartum disorders that develop a more **chronic course** warrant endocrinology consultation to rule out more subtle disorders of the hypothalamic–pituitary–thyroid axis.

16. Which psychosocial interventions are effective?

Psychotherapy is crucial for preventing psychological scarring. Most patients have not experienced prior mental illness and may have difficulty with accepting the need to participate in treatment. It is often helpful to emphasize the biologic aspects of postpartum illness, which should be considered a complication of pregnancy—a medical illness with psychiatric symptoms related to physiologic changes after childbirth. Opportunities for eliminating feelings of failure and guilt become obvious. Group therapy is particularly helpful for postpartum women. It is important to convey that postpartum illness has an excellent prognosis.

New fathers are often the silent victims of postpartum disorders. They benefit from supportive outreach and education. Studies demonstrate that a father's support positively influences his partner's recovery.

Extended family must be recruited to support a postpartum woman during recovery. Providing literature and directing them to local support groups are often helpful.

17. How may the infant be affected?

Aggressive treatment of the mother's depression may prevent complications in the newborn. Studies show that depressed mothers demonstrate less positive attunement to their infants. They tend to be less affectionate and misread cues. Infants of depressed mothers are at risk for poorer mental and motor development, as well as emotional disturbances in childhood.

18. What areas are the focus of current research?

Depressed levels of **tryptophan** and a slower than normal rise in tryptophan levels after delivery predict the blues. Attempts to avert the blues through tryptophan loading have failed, leading to speculation that a defect in metabolism rather than an absolute deficiency in tryptophan may be causally related to maternity blues.

Pyridoxine is a cofactor required for neuronal utilization of tryptophan. With oral administration for 28 days after delivery, an experimental group of high-risk women demonstrated a recurrence rate of the blues several times lower than the rate in a control group receiving placebo. A tryptophan study including pyridoxine supplementation may yield valuable information.

Another highly experimental strategy for preventing more severe postpartum disorders involves administering **long-acting estrogen** to high-risk women at delivery. It is theorized that the supplementation of estrogen cushions the fall of the hormone after the placenta is delivered. In a series of 50 high-risk women receiving estrogen at delivery, none had recurrences. Because of concerns about the risk of thromboembolic phenomena, this strategy is not currently recommended for routine prophylactic treatment in women with histories of postpartum disorders.

BIBLIOGRAPHY

1. Barnett B, Morgan M: Postpartum psychiatric disorder: Who should be admitted and to which hospital? (Review) Aust N Z J Psychiatry 30(6):709–714, 1996.
2. Button JH, Reivich RS: Obsessions of infanticide. Arch Gen Psychiatry 27:235–240, 1972.
3. Cox JL, Murray D, Chapman G: A controlled study of the onset, duration, and prevalence of postnatal depression. Br J Psychol 163:27–31, 1993.
4. Fossey L, Papiernik E, Bydlowski M: Postpartum blues: A clinical syndrome and predictor of postnatal depression? J Psychosom Obstet Gynecol 18(1):17–21, 1997.
5. Hamilton JA, Harberger PN (eds): Postpartum Psychiatric Illness: A Picture Puzzle. Philadelphia, University of Pennsylvania Press, 1992.
6. Hamilton JA: Postpartum psychiatric syndromes. Psychiatr Clin North Am 12:89–102, 1989.
7. Leathers SJ, Kelley MA, Richman JA: Postpartum depressive symptomatology in new mothers and fathers: Parenting, work and support. J Nerv Ment Dis 185(3):129–137, 1997.
8. Martell LK: Postpartum depression as a family problem. Am J Matern Child nurs 15(2):90–93, 1990.
9. McGory P, Connell S: The nosology and prognosis of puerperal psychosis: A review. Compr Psychiatry 31(6):519–534, 1990.
10. Meager I, Milgrom J: Group treatment for postpartum depression: A pilot study. Aust N Z J Psychiatry 30(6):852–860, 1996.
11. O'Hara MW, Schlechte JA, Lewis DA, Wright EJ: Prospective study of postpartum blues. Arch Gen Psychiatry 48:801–806, 1991.
12. Parry BL (ed): Women's disorders. Psychiatr Clin North Am 12:207–220, 1989.
13. Rosenblatt JE, Rosenblatt NC (ed): Currents in Affective Illness, vol. 11. Bethesda, MD, Currents Publications, Ltd.., 1992, pp 5–11.
14. Rosenblatt JE, Rosenblatt NC (eds): Currents in Affective Illness, vol. 12. Bethesda, MD, Currents Publications, Ltd.., 1993, pp 1–2.
15. Sholomskas DE, Wickamarathe PJ, Dogolo L, et al: Postpartum onset of panic disorder. A coincidental event? J Clin Psychiatry 54(12):476–480, 1993.
16. Stamp GE, Williams AS, Crowther CA: Predicting postnatal depression among pregnant women. Birth 23(4):218–223, 1996.
17. Steiner M: Postpartum psychiatric disorders. Can J Psychiatry 35:89–95, 1990.
18. Stewart DE, Addison AM:Thyroid function in psychosis following childbirth. Am J Psychiatry 145:1579–1581, 1988.

IX. Geriatric Psychiatry

65. DEVELOPMENTAL ISSUES IN LATE LIFE

Roberta M. Richardson, M.D.

1. What are some of the central themes of development in the later years of adulthood?

According to Nemiroff and Colarusso,[9] a central theme of adult development is "the normative crisis precipitated by a growing awareness of the finiteness of time and the inevitability of personal death." This normative crisis leads to thoughts and questions about the meaning of one's life, accomplishments, and mark on the world and may underlie such psychiatric presentations as the depression that sometimes accompanies retirement and anxiety about a decline in personal health, or illness and death of friends and loved ones.

Erikson defines the developmental task of late life as integrity vs. despair. He refers to the task of reviewing life and integrating experiences into a value system that leads to a feeling of fulfillment and satisfaction. If this task is not accomplished, the emotion associated with this stage of life is most likely to be despair, caused by the conclusion that one did not accomplish what is perceived as necessary—and no longer has the time to do so.

Jung noted that in the second half of life, men become more aware of their "feminine" side and women of their "masculine" side.

Another central theme of late life involves repeated injury to self-esteem as the older adult is displaced at work, loses physical and possibly sexual prowess, and must accept a degree of dependence on others. The realities of aging undermine defenses in some individuals, leading to intense feelings of envy, rivalry, rage, and, subsequently, loneliness. Psychotherapy may be especially useful in such patients by assisting them to accept the changes of aging and refocusing their attention on positive feelings about themselves.

2. How can changes in relationships stimulate developmental crises in older adults?

The aging and death of one's parents are major events in life. If parents become feeble, roles often are reversed. This reversal involves at least some degree of difficulty for most adult children. Psychologically, adult children can no longer maintain the fantasy that their parents will take care of them. This may be particularly difficult if psychological separation has not fully occurred and feelings about the adequacy of parenting received in childhood remain ambivalent. Thoughts of mortality are strongly stimulated by the death of parents, which brings the realization that one's own generation is the next to pass.

Changes in relationships with grown children also may precipitate developmental crises in parents. The classic "empty nest" syndrome occurs later in life as childbearing is delayed and adult children stay longer in the home. Some parents may be reluctant to lose the parenting role as they face other losses and changes in their bodies. They may feel envy of their own children as they watch them start out with "their whole lives ahead of them."

3. Discuss the compensating aspects of relationships with grandchildren.

In most cases, relationships with grandchildren are idealized and mutually gratifying. Through grandchildren the displaced parent may recapture unqualified love and admiration. The grandparent may identify with the grandchild and act out frustrated, self-indulgent impulses through "spoiling" of the child. This process also may compensate for possible envious feelings toward adult children, the parents of the grandchild.

Grandchildren also represent immortality. It may be tremendously gratifying and reassuring to notice inherited genetic features in a grandchild when one is struggling with questions about one's legacy and asking, "Will I be remembered when I'm gone?"

4. How does late life development affect psychotherapy?

The older patient's experience of the therapist may be influenced by any number of important relationships in life, such as parent, spouse, sibling, or child. When the therapist is young, a transference related to the patient's relationship with his or her own children is more easily stimulated. Themes of unresolved expectations and disappointments with children may arise early. The therapist may be idealized as the "good" child who offers what the patient's own children do not, or may become the focus of angry feelings about abandonment.

The therapist's reactions to the psychotherapeutic relationship with an elderly patient may color which themes and reactions emerge. The therapist may be uncomfortable, for example, with sexuality in an older person or with the patient's dependency needs. If the patient is experienced as a parent, the therapist's unresolved wishes to control the parent or fears of domination may interfere with the therapy. Ongoing problems with parents in real life may make it particularly difficult for some therapists to work with older patients.

5. Do sex and sexuality continue to be a concern for people over the age of 60 years?

In 1974 the Duke Longitudinal Study on Aging found that 70% of men at age 63 and 25% of men at age 78 were still sexually active. Pearlman[10] found that 25% of men in their 60s and 10% of men over 70 reported sexual intercourse at least once a week. Data for older women are fewer. Christenson and Gagnon[4] found that 50% of married women over age 65 reported regular coitus. For women the availability of a socially sanctioned partner is a significant factor in the frequency of sexual activity, whereas for men this factor is not as important. For example, it is culturally more acceptable for an elderly man than an elderly woman to date a younger partner. Single women in their later years, however, remain interested in sex, and many compensate for the lack of a partner by masturbation.

Many doctors do not recognize the importance of sex and the prevalence of sexual dysfunction in older patients, because they do not ask. Doctors who routinely ask about sex estimate that 50% of geriatric patients have sexual complaints, whereas doctors who do not routinely ask place the estimate at less than 10%.

6. What normal changes in sexual functioning occur with aging?

For men aging brings fewer spontaneous erections. Direct stimulation is usually required to obtain full erection, and the process takes longer. The force of ejaculation is decreased, along with the volume of seminal fluid. Ejaculatory control is improved, but the refractory period is longer (i.e., a longer period is necessary before another erection is possible).

For women late middle age often brings an increase in sexual desire, which gradually declines with old age. Lubrication decreases postmenopausally, and a longer period is required to achieve adequate lubrication. The vaginal vault decreases in size, with thinning walls. The orgasmic phase is shorter, and orgasmic uterine contractions may cause pain in the lower abdomen.

7. Discuss the causes of male impotence.

According to Hackett,[6] "Achieving a normal erection is a complex event requiring an adequate blood and nerve supply to the penile area and appropriate psychological conditions." Although it used to be thought that psychological factors were primarily responsible for the great majority of cases of male impotence, it is now believed that at least 50% have an organic basis. As would be expected, the incidence of organic factors increases with age.

Vasculogenic impotence is probably the most common organic type. It usually appears around age 50 and is characterized by partial erections and retained ability to achieve orgasm, which is neurologically controlled. **Neurologic impotence** occurs when diseases such as Parkinson's disease, multiple sclerosis, spinal cord injury, diabetes, alcoholism, or tumor interfere with the functioning of the nerves involved in developing and maintaining an erection. **Endocrinologic impotence** occurs when testosterone levels are low. Finally, many **prescription drugs** may decrease libido, reduce potency, or interfere with the ability to ejaculate, particularly antihypertensives and antidepressants.

Psychological factors are the primary cause in about one-half of the cases of male impotence. Depression, both as a primary major affective disorder and as a mood associated with bereavement or other losses, is by far the most common psychological cause of impotence and other sexual dysfunction. Another major category of psychological impotence involves medical illnesses unrelated biologically to sexual function, including common fears of sexual activity after myocardial infarction and fears of hurting oneself or one's partner when diseases such as arthritis or chronic lung disease are present.

Psychological factors often play a significant role in cases of impotence in which an organic cause is primary. Low self-esteem and performance anxiety may result from recognition of diminished sexual prowess.

8. What are the common complaints and causes of sexual dysfunction in elderly women?

Dyspareunia (painful intercourse) is a common complaint after menopause because of decreased lubrication and/or narrowing of the vagina. The vaginal mucosa also atrophy. Such problems can be overcome with systemic estrogen or estrogen creams applied to the vagina. Nonhormonal vaginal lubricants also may be helpful.

Psychological factors are equally important in the sexual functioning of older women and older men. Women may suffer from feelings of unattractiveness that makes them recoil from sexual activity. Such feelings may be caused or compounded by an apparent decrease in interest on the part of a spouse or partner who is having his own difficulties with sexual functioning. Often partners do not discuss the problem with each other, and the woman may assume that the cause is her loss of attractiveness.

Mastectomy often leaves many women feeling disfigured and reluctant to pursue sexual activity. Fortunately, more and more hospitals anticipate this problem and address it immediately after or even before surgery. The partner often needs to be involved in the counseling. Involving the partner in surgical aftercare and rehabilitation is a good way to desensitize and address such issues. Wearing of a prosthesis during intercourse is *not* a good solution, because it tends to perpetuate denial and self-doubt.

9. How can the physician assist older patients with problems related to sex and sexuality?

The most important intervention is to incorporate questions about sexual functioning into the routine history. Many people are uncomfortable bringing up such issues, even to the doctor. Often allowing the patient to air concerns and educating the patient about normal changes in sexual functioning with aging make all the difference.

Once sexual difficulties are described, the physician first should consider the patient's medical history, including medications, to see whether a physical factor is involved, especially one that can be corrected. Inquiries about alcohol and over-the-counter medications are also important. Referral to a urologist or gynecologist may be appropriate for further evaluation of specific problems.

The patient also should be screened for depression, and inquiries should be made about relationship difficulties and sexual functioning of the partner. Pharmacologic treatment for depression may be appropriate, but the high incidence of sexual dysfunction caused by antidepressants should be kept in mind. A mental health referral may be appropriate.

10. Discuss grief and its role in the evaluation and treatment of older adults.

Grief is the emotional suffering experienced in reaction to loss. Late life is characterized by increasing numbers and severity of losses. The death of a spouse is perhaps the best known cause for grief in older people—and one of the most devastating. However, many other major losses also are common. Parents, siblings, and, as more people live to a more advanced age, children also die. Friends may die in fairly quick succession.

Death of loved ones is not the only cause of grief. Older people lose relationships through retirement, changes in residence (by themselves or others), and inability to congregate for social activities because of loss of transportation or failing health. Grief also may be triggered by material loss, such as loss of home and possessions (when one must move to a smaller place). A move also may necessitate loss of a beloved pet. Finally, one may grieve for loss of body parts or functions, such as eyesight, hearing, or mobility. Avid readers, for example, may feel desperate when they no longer can see. Loss of hearing isolates one from others as communication becomes more and more difficult.

The symptoms of grief are varied. Loss is often instrumental in precipitating major depressive episodes. Although antidepressant medications are often helpful and may be necessary, psychotherapy may be at least as important. Sometimes a depressive episode represents the culmination of a series of losses so close together that one is not dealt with before the next comes along, overwhelming individual coping capacity.

Anger and resentment are also common reactions to loss, especially losses that undermine the sense of self-esteem, such as loss of physical function and opportunities. Anxiety and fear may underlie the anger or be frank expressions of loss. Suicide may be considered or threatened as a way of gaining a feeling of control over one's body and life.

The **deficit model** of loss and grief is helpful in guiding intervention. A loss leads to deficits in the sufferer's life. Grief will not be eased until other resources are found to compensate for such deficits. For example, loss of a spouse leads to loss of help with basic activities of living (e.g., "he always balanced the checkbook"), validating responses that enhance self-esteem, and emotional supports. It also leaves a deficit in social identity. Older people with a greater number of social contacts and a diversity of roles fare better than those who functioned mainly as a spouse, with few outside contacts.

11. What are the tasks of the therapist in assisting grief-stricken older patients?

The therapist helps patients by encouraging them to talk about the loss of the loved one. Although **listening** may seem like a cliché, the therapist may be the only person who is willing to sit quietly with patients while they cry, express their feelings, and repeat painful stories. Some therapists may be too quick to jump in with reassurances, platitudes, or distractions, giving the message that they do not want to hear the pain. *The therapist must tolerate intense affect* and let patients know that avoiding the pain often only prolongs grief or causes it to remain unresolved.

Education about grief and loss is important, because many people had abnormal models or were taught myths about the grieving process. Grieving alone, keeping a "stiff upper lip," and not feeling sorry for oneself are among the myths that many people have learned. Validating feelings of all kinds, including anger, relief, and guilt, is important.

Assistance with **problem solving** also helps to replace the deficits left by loss. In the case of bereavement, the survivor must adjust to an environment from which the deceased is missing and reinvest emotional energy in other relationships. The bereaved may need concrete guidance and instructions for moving on to other people and activities.

According to Taylor, effective work with grief must involve a search for meaning in the experience, an attempt to regain mastery over one's life, and an effort to enhance self-esteem. These guidelines are particularly helpful in assisting with losses of function and role that are almost inevitable in the elderly. For example, the man who is forced to retire at age 65 may not feel ready to leave his job, which may be his primary source of self-esteem and the area in which he feels most capable and in control. He may feel helpless and frustrated. The therapist's task is to help the man look beyond his job for meaningful activity, self-esteem, and fulfillment.

12. Discuss the common fears older adults have about death and dying.

Attitudes toward death are grounded in culture. North American culture tends to deny death and to stigmatize the notion of vulnerability. Independence, self-control, and autonomy are highly valued. Thus many adults come to old age with fears and conflicts about death with which they must struggle alone.

Most people in North America do not die suddenly, but become progressively ill with one or more diseases that eventually kill them. Most of these diseases are chronic and ambiguous.

Increasingly, even cancer is a diagnosis that may or may not be terminal. Thus, older people are fated to ponder the circumstances of their death.

The most common fears center on the dying process, specifically on **isolation** or **abandonment** and **loss of dignity and control**. Fortunately, we seem to have passed the heyday of high-tech death, but many people still have fears of dying alone in a hospital room with tubes in every orifice and hisses and beeps for company. Many fear humiliating exposure in the presence of strangers as they struggle with terrible physical suffering and possible loss of mental capacities.

Older people must have the opportunity to discuss such issues with their loved ones and doctors. They need assurances that they will be cared for with courtesy, concern for their dignity, and attention to alleviation of suffering. Most people also want reassurance that every effort will be made not to allow them to die alone. In addition, efforts should be made to clarify specific wishes for medical interventions near the end of life, before circumstances render the individual incompetent to choose. Such efforts should include choosing and executing some form of formal advance directive for health care, according to various state laws.

13. Discuss common characteristics of people most likely to have a debilitating fear of death.

People who have unresolved religious questions about death and dying may develop severe anxiety in late life. They may fear that they will die before resolving their doubts and suffer after death as a consequence; for example, by spending eternity in hell. Or they may have been raised in a tradition that promises a blissful afterlife but fear they instead will find an eternal unbearable nothingness.

For some, the realization of personal death arouses intense separation anxiety. Such individuals have struggled with separation anxiety in their relationships throughout life. They may envision death as an agonizing aloneness. A resurgence of clinging, regressive behavior may be the manifestation of this unspoken fear.

People with lingering guilt for hostile or impulsive acts and an immature ego structure may view death as a punishment and thus develop debilitating fears in late life. Such people continue to struggle with anger over their lot, feelings of mistreatment, and subsequent guilt over having and/or expressing such feelings. They present with mixed emotions of hostility, depression, and anxiety.

On a more concrete level, people who live alone are more likely to develop debilitating fear of death, because they are afraid they will become ill or injured and die alone before they are able to get help. Additionally, an individual may fear leaving a disabled spouse alone.

14. What interventions are helpful to older people facing death?

Assistance in clarifying beliefs and feelings about death and end-of-life issues may be helpful. Such issues may be discussed with the physician, a religious leader, family and friends, or a counselor or psychotherapist. The family may need assistance in knowing how to help a dying relative. The quality of close relationships strongly influences the reactions to dying.

If problems are sufficiently debilitating to require professional therapy, the therapist can help the person to develop a "fantasy of immortality." It is soothing for most people to feel that they will continue to live in a positive way through their children, creations, or even possessions. A **life review** also is therapeutic at this stage. The therapist guides the person through a review of the facts and accomplishments of his or her life to assist in developing a feeling that life has had meaning and purpose. *Note that this technique is not advisable for patients suffering from major depression.* The nature of depression leads patients to recall selectively and to dwell on negative life events and deeds, which is more harmful than helpful.

BIBLIOGRAPHY

1. Adams SG Jr, Dubbert PM, Chupurdia KM, et al: Assessment of sexual beliefs and information in aging couples with sexual dysfunction. Arch Sex Behav 25:249–260, 1996.
1a. Atchley RC: The aging self. Psychother Theory Res Pract 19:388–396, 1982.
2. Baum N, Sakauye K: What's causing your patient's impotence? Senior Patient Oct:21–26, 1990.
3. Butler RN: The life-review: An unrecognized bonanza. Intl J Aging Hum Dev 12:35–38, 1980.
4. Christenson CV, Gagnon JG: Sexual behavior in a group of older women. J Gerontol 20:351–356, 1965.

5. Fry PS: Depression, Stress, and Adaptations in the Elderly. Rockville, MD, Aspen, 1986, pp 323–347.
6. Hackett TP: Sexual activity in the elderly. In Jenicke MA (ed): Clinical Perspectives on Aging. Philadelphia, Wyeth-Ayerst Laboratories, 1985.
7. James JW, Cherry F: The Grief Recovery Handbook. New York, Harper & Row, 1988.
8. Meston CM: Aging and sexuality. West J Med 167:285–290, 1997.
9. Nemiroff RA, Colarusso CA: The Race Against Time. New York, Plenum Press, 1985.
10. Pearlman CK: Frequency of intercourse in males at different ages. Med Aspects Hum Sex 6:92, 1972.
11. Pipher M: Another Country: Navigating the Emotional Terrain of Our Elders. Riverhead Books, 1999.
12. Weisman A: On Dying and Denying. Behavioral Publications, 1972, pp 137–157.
13. Zarit SH, Knight BG (eds): A Guide to Psychotherapy and Aging: Effective Clinical Interventions in a Life State Context. Washington, DC, American Psychological Association, Oct 1997.

66. PSYCHOPHARMACOLOGY FOR ELDERLY PATIENTS

Roberta M. Richardson, M.D.

1. How do changes in body composition that occur with aging affect your choice of psychotropic medication?

The aging body shows a significant **decrease in lean body mass**, corresponding **increase in total body fat**, and **decrease in total body water**. Thus, water-soluble drugs have a greater concentration per unit dose because of the apparent decrease in the size of the reservoir. The blood alcohol level per drink rises with age, and the usual two martinis a day can't be tolerated at age 70.

Fat-soluble drugs have a greater volume of distribution. They are stored in fat and released gradually, and therefore show a longer half-life in the elderly. The highly fat-soluble benzodiazepines, such as diazepam, have a greatly increased half-life in older individuals, and typical antipsychotics are affected by this phenomenon as well. Remember, too, that the brain is a very fatty organ.

2. Why is it essential to know the route of metabolism of any drug prescribed?

Most drugs are metabolized primarily in the liver. In general, hepatic blood flow and size decrease significantly with aging. However, individual variation in activity of liver enzymes is vast. For this reason, there can be a 20-fold difference in appropriate dose of some antidepressants among patients of the same advanced age.

Ignorance of this fact leads to two common prescribing mistakes: **overdosing and underdosing**. Remember to start low, go slow—but don't stop too soon. Also take into account metabolic interactions with other medications. This is especially crucial for older patients who may be taking a number of different medications, and who are more vulnerable to adverse effects of blood levels that climb too high, or drop too low.

Medications with renal metabolism are more predictable. Creatinine clearance decreases steadily and predictably with age. Age and body weight are factors, such that the older and smaller a person is, the lower his or her creatinine clearance will be. Lithium is the psychotropic medication most influenced by this phenomenon. Dosages must be drastically reduced in the elderly to avoid toxicity. Some of the benzodiazepines also are metabolized renally and have a slower clearance in elderly patients.

3. How are changes in receptor sensitivity and neurotransmitters relevant?

Aging brings reduced sensitivity to some pharmacologic agents and increased sensitivity to others. The most important consideration in prescribing psychotropics, however, is the **cholinergic neurotransmitter system**. Several of the commonly used psychotropic agents have significant anticholinergic properties. But in the aging brain, cholinergic binding sites are decreased; choline acetyltransferase, vital for making acetylcholine, is decreased; and acetylcholine is even more decreased in the brains of patients with Alzheimer's disease. Therefore, the elderly are predisposed to central anticholinergic toxicity in the form of confusion, delirium, and psychosis.

Whenever prescribing psychotropic medications for the elderly, therefore, choose the least anticholinergic agent in each class and avoid combining two or more highly anticholinergic medications. For example, among the tricyclic antidepressants (TCAs), the secondary amines nortriptyline and desipramine are preferred. Amitriptyline is highly anticholinergic and should be avoided. Among the antipsychotics, the high-potency agents such as haloperidol are preferred over the more anticholinergic thioridazine or chlorpromazine. Clozapine also is highly anticholinergic. Avoid over-the-counter sleep medications and antihistamines.

Note: Central anticholinergic toxicity may occur without peripheral manifestations in older patients.

Summary of Changes in the Aging Body and Their Effect on Psychotropic Drugs

CHANGE	EFFECT	EXAMPLE
Increased body fat	Fat-soluble drugs stored longer, releasing slowly	Diazepam
Decreased body water	Water-soluble drugs show higher concentration	Ethanol
Decreased liver size and blood flow	Drugs metabolized in liver cleared more slowly, but individual variation is great	Antidepressants
Decreased creatinine clearance	Drugs metabolized renally cleared more slowly; predictable	Lithium, gabapentin
Decreased acetylcholine in brain	Anticholinergic drugs more likely to cause central toxicity	Amitriptyline Chlorpromazine

4. What are the major considerations in choosing an antidepressant for older patients?

All treatments for depression are potentially useful for elderly patients (see Chapter 47). As in any patient, the many available agents carry various risks, side effects, and costs. Consider the individual patient's health, other medications, tolerance of particular side effects, cognitive abilities, social resources, and financial means. Comorbid psychiatric conditions such as anxiety, psychosis, and substance abuse also may affect the choice. Most importantly, be thoroughly familiar with **contraindications** to specific agents, **major drug interactions**, and common **side effects** of agents being prescribed.

5. Why should I always check the electrocardiogram before prescribing a TCA in patients over the age of 40?

The TCAs have quinidine-like effects on cardiac conduction; they slow conduction across the atrioventricular node. Clinically relevant problems at therapeutic blood levels are limited to patients with preexisting conduction disease. However, only severe disease absolutely contraindicates use of TCAs. Stoudamire and Atkinson reported that "asymptomatic patients with right bundle branch block, isolated left anterior fascicular block, and left posterior fascicular block usually can be treated safely with TCAs if dosage is increased gradually and ECGs obtained following each dosage increase."[11] Note the word *asymptomatic*. Syncopal attacks suggest an intermittently higher degree of block, and TCAs should not be used unless a pacemaker is in place. The same applies to patients with bifascicular or trifascicular block.

TCAs also are contraindicated for at least 6 weeks after an acute myocardial infarction. In patients who develop persistently long Q-Tc intervals, the risk for fatal ventricular fibrillation is increased. If TCAs must be used, they should be used cautiously, in association with ECG monitoring and consultation with a cardiologist about the acceptable upper limit of Q-Tc intervals for the particular patient.

6. List other contraindications to the use of TCAs.

Other contraindications to TCAs are due to their anticholinergic effects and include: (1) narrow-angle glaucoma, (2) significantly enlarged prostate, (3) marginally compensated congestive heart failure (because tachycardia may precipitate failure). Also consider the possibility of (4) orthostatic hypotension, which increases the risk of falling.

7. Is it safe to prescribe monoamine oxidase inhibitors (MAOIs) to elderly patients?

MAOIs can be tricky in elderly patients. The biggest concern is the need for **compliance with dietary restrictions**, because ingestion of foods high in tyramine may cause a hypertensive crisis. MAOIs should not be prescribed for patients who cannot be relied on to understand and follow this diet. Certain concurrent medications also must be avoided. Most significant are the sympathomimetics, which include medications used to treat asthma; therefore, patients with asthma should not receive MAOIs. The same applies to patients with a history of anaphylaxis, because the epinephrine required for treatment may precipitate a hypertensive crisis in the presence of MAOIs. Orthostatic hypotension also is a common side effect.

8. Aren't the newer antidepressants preferable?

To date, the selective serotonin reuptake inhibitors (SSRIs) appear to be the safest of the antidepressants. There are no data to suggest that nefazodone, venlafaxine, or mirtazapine are unsafe, but fewer data have been collected about the use of these relatively newer agents in the geriatric population.

SSRIs should be started at low doses, and increased more gradually in the elderly. In rare instances, they can cause parkinsonism and, less rarely, an akathisia-like syndrome. Therefore, use them cautiously in those with Parkinson's disease. Older patients frequently experience postural instability early in the course of treatment with SSRIs; although this resolves within a few weeks, it may cause falls, with serious consequences for an older person. Other significant and common side effects include nausea, anorexia, diarrhea, headache, tremor, insomnia, and sedation. Because of the extraordinarily long half-life of fluoxetine, the shorter acting ones might be preferable. Sertraline and citalopram also are less likely to interfere with the metabolism of commonly prescribed medications such as coumadin, phenytoin, and cimetadine.

9. How can the other, newer antidepressants be used?

Bupropion is a useful antidepressant in a class by itself. It can be used safely and effectively in the elderly, always with a consideration toward seizure risk. It should not be used in anyone with a history of seizures, or significant brain lesions that might predispose to seizures. Dosing guidelines must be strictly followed. An advantage over other antidepressants is its mildly stimulating effect, rather than sedation which accompanies most of the others. A disadvantage is that two to three times a day dosing is necessary, increasing the likelihood of mistakes, missed dosages, and noncompliance.

Nefazodone and mirtazapine may be especially helpful for the person with high anxiety and/or insomnia. Vanlafaxine has many similarities to the SSRIs, but may be effective when an SSRI is not. It also has been approved recently for the treatment of generalized anxiety disorder, based on controlled studies of its effectiveness.

10. What are the treatment options if none of the above antidepressants is safe, tolerated, and/or effective?

Psychostimulants, such as methylphenidate, may be helpful in very old, frail patients with apathetic depression; for example, medically ill patients who are not participating in their care or rehabilitation or not eating. In spite of their reputation for suppressing appetite, in this setting the stimulants generally increase appetite, energy, and interest. The stimulants are rarely contraindicated; even patients with heart disease usually tolerate them. A careful approach, beginning with a low dose and monitoring vital signs after each dose until stabilized, is recommended.

Electroconvulsive therapy is another possibility for frail elderly persons who are depressed. Despite its scary reputation, ECT is one of the safest treatments for certain older people. Intracranial masses should be ruled out, and consultation with a cardiologist is necessary for patients with significant heart disease. In addition, patients with a history of retinal detachment should have a consultation with a knowledgeable ophthalmologist, because the sudden increase in blood pressure may cause problems.

11. How should I approach the treatment of anxiety in elderly patients?

First, make a careful diagnosis. In many older people who present with anxiety as their chief complaint, the actual diagnosis is major depression. Anxiolytics do not treat such patients adequately. In fact, the sedative-hypnotics may worsen depression. The appropriate response is to **prescribe an antidepressant**, which often provides sufficient treatment even in the short term while waiting for the antidepressant to take full effect. Venlafaxine may be a good choice, as it has recently obtained FDA approval for treatment of generalized anxiety disorder.

If an anxiolytic medication is needed, consider low doses of the **benzodiazepines lorazepam and oxazepam**, both of which are metabolized in the blood through oxidation. Because this process does not change appreciably with aging, lorazepam and oxazepam, unlike other anxiolytic agents, do not accumulate in the aging body as a result of slowed metabolism. This unique method of metabolism, however, does not mean that older people should receive the same dosages as younger people. Older people are much more susceptible to postural instability and memory loss. In all cases, the lowest possible dosage should be used, and signs of toxicity should be monitored carefully.

Buspirone is *not* a substitute for benzodiazepines, because the patient will feel no immediate relief. Buspirone may be helpful with generalized anxiety over time, and some evidence suggests that it may have antidepressant effects. However, it is not very helpful as an early treatment of depression nor as treatment for situational anxiety.

Do not neglect nonpharmacologic means of anxiety control, such as relaxation exercises, deep breathing, and manipulation of the environment.

12. Which agents are preferred in the treatment of psychosis in elderly patients?

As always, the first consideration is diagnosis. Elderly schizophrenics need and usually tolerate higher doses than demented or delirious patients. Patients with affective illness show a wide range of need and tolerance.

The **high-potency agents** are preferred for geriatric patients because of their side-effect profile. The minimal advantage of increased sedation with the low-potency medications, such as chlorpromazine and thioridazine, is far outweighed by the disadvantages of increased anticholinergic side effects and higher incidence of orthostatic hypotension. The second-generation antipsychotics risperidone, olanzapine, and perhaps quetiapine are preferred because of their lower risk of extrapyramidal symptoms. Olanzapine, especially, combines the benefits of sedation with low risk of EPS. The high cost of these agents should be considered, however.

13. What is the main problem with high-potency antipsychotics?

The main problem with haloperidol and other high-potency antipsychotics is the likely occurrence of **extrapyramidal symptoms**. Acute dystonia is extremely uncommon in the elderly. Parkinsonism, however, is quite common and contributes significantly to the risk for falling. Its onset may be insidious. One month after hospital discharge, for example, the patient may be found to be stooped, shuffling, stiff, and possibly tremulous. For these reasons, the physician must be very cautious, using the lowest effective dose and monitoring the patient closely for a few months if he or she is to stay on the antipsychotic medication. Prophylactic anticholinergic medications such as benztropine are no substitute; they increase the risk of mental confusion and other side effects of anticholinergics.

Evaluate elderly patients for symptoms of parkinsonism *before* starting an antipsychotic. Patients with Parkinson's disease or similar syndromes may deteriorate clinically, and antipsychotics should be avoided in such patients if at all possible. The only currently available antipsychotic that has definitely been proven not to worsen Parkinson's disease symptoms is clozapine, which is quite useful in treating psychosis associated with Parkinson's disease. The required dosages are much lower than those used to treat schizophrenia—25–50 mg/day is often sufficient. Weekly blood counts are needed because of the risk of agranulocytosis. Quetiapine, the newest antipsychotic at this writing, also looks quite promising for use in Parkinson's patients.

14. What is the risk of tardive dyskinesia in antipsychotic treatment?

The risk of tardive dyskinesia increases with age. A recent study showed that among those over age 65 treated with a typical antipsychotic, one-third developed tardive dyskinesia at 12 months; one-half at 2 years; and two-thirds at 3 years. The incidence is higher in women and in patients with mood disorders. Thus elderly women with psychotic depression are at particular risk for developing tardive dyskinesia; antipsychotic medications should be prescribed only with informed consent and close follow-up. Use newer agents if at all possible. With frequent and careful examination for early signs, tardive dyskinesia can be detected and the offending agent stopped before a debilitating condition develops.

15. Name one of the most common and serious, yet overlooked, complications of psychotropic medication in elderly patients.

Most of the psychotropics in current use increase the risk of falling in older patients. Osteoporosis is endemic among elderly women; thus, it does not take much to cause serious fractures. A fractured hip may lead to all of the morbidity and mortality associated with prolonged immobility and possible surgery, including pulmonary embolus, pneumonia, urosepsis, decubitus ulcers, and lengthy and expensive rehabilitation efforts after the bone has healed. Subdural hematomas may result from relatively minor blows to the head in older people. The elder who lives alone and cannot get up after a fall may develop muscular necrosis and even dehydration if not found for some time.

For many elderly people the prospect of falling is so frightening that, especially after one fall has occurred, activity may be significantly limited. Such limitation may lead to increasing depression and declining health.

Psychotropic medications can contribute to falling through various mechanisms, and the physician must be alert for symptoms in several areas. TCAs, MAOIs, and some of the antipsychotics commonly cause orthostatic hypotension. Patients must be warned and then asked about a feeling of faintness upon rising from a lying or sitting position. If the reply is positive, blood pressure should be measured in recumbent and standing positions. A drop of 20 points or more in systolic pressure usually is considered significant. Asymptomatic findings may be tolerated; symptomatic findings should not. Fainting is one of the most dangerous reasons for a fall, because the victim has no control over the landing.

16. True or false: The SSRIs do not cause risk of falling.

False. Unfortunately, the SSRIs are not foolproof in this regard. SSRIs can cause significant postural instability in many older people early in the course of treatment. Fortunately, this symptom seems to resolve within a few weeks, and the risk may be minimized by more gradual titration of the dose. Dizziness is a relatively common side effect of the new antidepressant venlafaxine at all ages. Elderly patients taking these medications should be asked if they feel dizzy or unsteady on their feet. If so, the dosage should be lowered or special precautions taken to increase safety, depending on the frailty and dependability of the patient as well as the severity of the depression and dizziness.

17. Discuss the effects of benzodiazepines on fall risk in the elderly.

Benzodiazepines also cause postural instability. The effect may be subtle, but the risks are not. When geriatric patients are prescribed doses that are too high or a long-acting agent that accumulates over time, frank intoxication may lead to a fall as long as 2 weeks after the drug is started. The classic example is the patient who is prescribed flurazepam in the hospital and discharged with instructions to continue the drug at home. Two weeks later, when this particularly long-acting medication reaches peak blood level, the patient falls—or falls asleep at the wheel of a car! Nystagmus is a sign of excessive levels of benzodiazepine and indicates cerebellar dysfunction.

18. How might antipsychotics cause falls?

Antipsychotics also are commonly associated with falls among elderly persons because of the induction of parkinsonism. One of the cardinal features of this syndrome is postural instability. If the more obvious signs of parkinsonism are present (i.e., pill-rolling tremor, cogwheel rigidity, shuffling gait, masked facies, inhibited arm swing), postural instability is present too. Steps should be taken either to decrease, discontinue, or change the medication or to treat the parkinsonism with anticholinergic agents (with attention to possible attendant complications).

BIBLIOGRAPHY

1. Blazer DG: Generalized anxiety disorder and panic disorder in the elderly: A review. Harv Rev Psychiatry 5:18–27, 1997.
2. Finkel SI: Efficacy and tolerability of antidepressant therapy in the old-old. J Clin Psychiatry 57:23–28, 1996.
3. Friedman JH: A role for clozapine in Parkinson's disease. Neurol For 3:3–15, 1992.
4. Jenike MA: Geriatric Psychiatry and Psychopharmacology: A Clinical Approach. Chicago, Year Book, 1989.
5. Jeste DV, Rockwell E, Harris MJ, et al: Conventional vs. newer antipsychotics in elderly patients. Am J Geriat Psychiatry 7:70–76, 1999.
6. Liu B, Anderson G, et al: Use of selective serotonin-reuptake inhibitors or tricyclic antidepressants and risk of hip fractures in elderly people. Lancet 351:1303–1307, 1998.
7. Nakra BRS, Grossberg GT: Lithium use in the elderly. J Geriatr Drug Ther 2:47–63, 1987.
8. Salzman C: Recent advances in geriatric psychopharmacology. In Tasman A, Goldfinger SM, Kaufmann CA (eds): American Psychiatric Press Review of Psychiatry, vol 9. Washington, DC, American Psychiatric Press, 1990, pp 279–293.
9. Schneider L: Clues to Psychotropic Prescribing Practices in Geriatric Medicine. Primary Psychiatry 5:23–26, 1998.
10. Stanislav SW, Fabre T, Crismon ML, et al: Buspirone's efficacy in organic-induced aggression. J Clin Psychopharmacol 14:126–130, 1994.
11. Stoudemire A, Fogel BS, Gulley LR, et al: Psychopharmacology in the medical patient. In Stoudemire A, Fogel BS (eds): Psychiatric Care of the Medical Patient. New York, Oxford University Press, 1993, pp 155–206.
12. Tune LE, Steele C, Cooper T: Neuroleptic drugs in the management of behavioral symptoms of Alzheimer's disease. Psychiatr Clin North Am 14:353–373, 1991.
13. Yudofsky SC, Silver JM, Hales RE: Pharmacologic management of aggression in the elderly. J Clin Psychiatry 51:22–32, 1990.

X. Consultation–Liaison Psychiatry

67. PSYCHIATRIC CONSULTATION IN THE GENERAL HOSPITAL

Michael K. Popkin, M.D.

1. When is psychiatric consultation indicated or advisable?

Most general hospital psychiatric consultation services see 3–5% of all admissions to the medical-surgical units of the hospital. Consultation is requested for many reasons: disturbances in behavior; changes in cognition, thinking, or mood; maladaptive responses to the physical illness process or hospitalization; legal issues, such as competency, informed consent, desire to leave against medical advice; and problems in the doctor-patient relationship.

Psychiatric disorders are common in the general hospital population: 20–30% of of medical-surgical inpatients have current depressive disturbances; an equal or higher percentage manifest symptoms of anxiety; and 5–10% experience an episode of delirium during hospitalization. Collectively these data suggest high rates of psychiatric disorders in the general hospital, but only select patients are referred for psychiatric consultation.

Consultation is prompted routinely by issues such as violence or profound noncompliance. Frequently, difficulties in the interaction between the patient and physician are crucial to the decision to seek consultation. Hard and fast rules do not apply here, but consultation is advisable when:

- First-line or standard psychiatric remedies have not resolved the issue
- Diagnostic expertise is required
- The primary physician is "at bay" in the engagement and management of the patient
- An objective, external review is needed to weigh a proposed course of action.

2. What are the consulting psychiatrist's goals in the initial dialogue with the referring physician or nurse?

Direct dialogue with the referring physician is crucial to the consultation process; seldom does a written request suffice. In this first exchange, the consultant's principal task is to identify a *specific* question or questions. The consultant's ability to assist is largely a function of pinpointing the concern or issues generating the referral. Surprisingly, physicians often are reluctant to explain their reasons for consulting a psychiatrist. The consultant may need to ask, "What would you like to have done?" The more precise the answer, the better the chance that the consultant may render a service. (The phrase "Please evaluate" is unlikely to yield the desired endpoint.)

Next, the consultant must ensure that the request for psychiatric consultation has been discussed with the patient. The unexpected arrival of a psychiatrist usually is met with hostility.

Finally, the consultant should inform the referring physician of the proposed consultative steps, including when impressions and recommendations will be conveyed and how further communication will be achieved.

3. How should the consultation interview be conducted?

At the outset, the consultant should inquire whether the patient has been advised of the consultation and its purpose. A negative answer usually requires postponing of the interview. Once the primary physician has informed the patient of the request for consultation and the objectives in this step, the consultant may proceed.

Begin the interview with basic questions concerning age, place of origin, family, education, marital status, and number of children, to obtain important background information. The answers, along with the details of the medical situation, offer nonthreatening topics with which to develop rapport. In the first meeting, the goal is to facilitate an alliance and maintain neutrality (see Chapter 1). Encourage the patient to tell his or her own story, and pay attention to the style of presentation. Generally the consultant should be friendly and tolerant, but also should signal clearly if the patient's interpersonal conduct is inappropriate or "out-of-bounds."

The interview must be flexible in timing and format, less formal than that conducted in the office or clinic setting. Strive to maintain privacy; this may require asking a roommate to depart for a time or herding away direct care personnel. Advise the patient at the start how much time will be needed; similarly, at the close, the patient deserves a summary statement regarding observations and the plan of action. It is important that followup be specified.

Although its goal is largely investigatory, the initial interview can, and should, be therapeutic as well. Even humor can have its place in the sometimes all-too-serious medical setting.

4. Any suggestions for interacting with a reticent patient?

Often in conducting the consultation interview, pursuit of specific content or data is frustrated. Either intentionally or unwittingly, the patient obstructs or blockades the consultant's efforts to secure information. When this occurs repeatedly and threatens to disrupt the sequence, consider "changing gears" by addressing the process of the interview. For example, "I'm here to try to be of assistance, but for the last 10 minutes you've refused to allow me to understand what you are feeling or experiencing. How will this be helpful to you?" The theme is *not* necessarily confrontation; rather, it is shifting focus to the *process* unfolding between the consultant and the patient (as opposed to the pursuit of *data*).

5. What is the role of corroborative history in the consultation setting?

The elderly and cognitively impaired comprise a significant percentage of patients referred for psychiatric consultation. Histories and accounts provided by these patients may be marred or jeopardized by questionable reliability, altered levels of consciousness, and cognitive dysfunction (in an otherwise clear sensorium). Accordingly, corroborative or alternative histories often are vitally important in the consultation-liaison setting. The consultant is obligated to review carefully the available medical records and to elicit the input of direct care personnel familiar with the patient. Corroborative reports from family members and significant others should be gathered after the patient is interviewed; contact before engaging the patient can make the consultant an agent of the family and disrupt the consultant's link to the patient.

6. What should be included in the consultation report?

The consultation report is a legal document which should concisely address (and, hopefully, answer) the original consultation questions. Lengthy reports typically are not read by consultees; the tendency is to skip to the conclusions and recommendations. One strategy, now common with psychiatric consultation services, is to present resultant diagnoses and recommended actions first, followed by the case synopsis or summary and mental status examination (MSE). The consultant must convey an awareness of the patient's medical/surgical issues, but it is not necessary to reiterate the full chronology of the medical situation. Psychiatrically, the focus should be on the history of the present illness, rather than a lengthy reconstruction of early childhood or adolescent trauma. In most cases, no more than a page-long synopsis of the problem is indicated, in addition to the MSE, differential diagnosis, and recommendations.

Elements of the Consultation Report and Suggested Sequence of Presentation

---

- Resultant psychiatric diagnosis (per DSM-IV) in order of reason for the consultation
- Recommendations, prioritized and specific
- One page synopsis of the psychiatric problem
    History of presenting complaint(s)
    Pertinent psychiatric history, including familial and medical history
    Mental status examination
    Psychiatric differential diagnosis

---

7. What psychiatric disorders are most commonly encountered by the consulting psychiatrist?

Formal studies of the distribution of psychiatric diagnoses assigned by psychiatric consultation services show clustering into a relatively brief list.

• Affective disorders (primary, or secondary to medical condition)	25%
• Delirium, dementia, amnesia, other cognitive disorders	25%
• Adjustment disorder (maladaptive response to identified stressors, including medical illness)	15%
• Somatoform disorders, anxiety disorders, personality disorders	each < 10%

Data on the the distribution of Axis II disorders in consultation-liaison are limited. The interface of psychiatry and medicine has long posed problems with regard to psychiatric diagnosis and nosology. This is most readily exemplified in the problem of depression emerging in the context of medical illness. The usual guideposts for the diagnosis of major depression are sleep, appetite, energy, libido, and the like; such "vegetative" parameters often are confounded in the medical-surgical patient with a disseminated malignancy or poorly controlled diabetes. Substitute criteria and guidelines for judgments regarding the relative contributions of the medical illness have not achieved strong consensus to date. In DSM-IV, clinicians can identify depressions as well as psychotic and anxiety disorders due to medical conditions, putting Axis III directly in the Axis I diagnosis.

8. To what extent are the recommendations of consulting psychiatrists followed?

Studies with specific concordance criteria indicate a hierarchy in which more than two thirds of consultants' recommendations for psychotropic medications are implemented, but only half the directives for diagnostic steps are instituted. Referring physicians also are unlikely to demonstrate an interest in, or an appreciation for, the consultant's psychiatric diagnoses: fewer than 50% of these diagnoses are accurately represented in discharge summaries of the hospitalization.

Thus, the psychiatric consultant can expect heightened receptivity to management suggestions, but less concern for proposals that involve further assessment and matters of diagnostic classification. The data suggest that consultees are largely concerned with practical or empiric steps to control behavior or improve mood. In the busy medical-surgical setting, the pursuit of psychiatric diagnosis or clarification of psychiatric factors often is overlooked or set aside. Most strikingly, some data suggest that medical work-up and management frequently are abbreviated in patients with comorbid psychiatric conditions, compared to patients without psychiatric issues.

9. What factors govern concordance with consultants' recommendations?

When concordance studies were first initiated, investigators expected that a major factor in achieving concordance would be the individual consultants. As some consultants are more skilled, articulate, and compelling than others, it seemed logical that consultants' identities and the particular pairings with referring physicians would be crucial to the outcomes achieved. However, concordance is *not* a function of the identities of the consultants or consultees. Concordance rates are surprisingly consistent no matter who performs the two roles. Additionally, concordance with recommendations for psychotropic drugs or diagnostic actions is not a function of which class of drug (antipsychotic, anxiolytic, or antidepressant) or which diagnostic measure (laboratory test, procedure, or consultation) is advised.

What explains concordance? There is no single or simple answer. However, best concordance rates are achieved when recommendations are *brief, prioritized,* and *unequivocal.* Conditional recommendations (i.e., do "A" if the following things happen) often are perceived as a sign of an indecisive or uncertain consultant. Most consultees want a pragmatic set of directives, not a lengthy academic discussion of possibilities.

10. Describe the primary characteristics of consultant work.

The main task of the psychiatric consultant is to help the medical-surgical patient cope with the demands of hospitalization. Consultation work is pragmatic. It is based in the present. Its objectives are to identify and strengthen the patient's own defensive constellation and proclivities in the short-term; consultation-liaison (CL) is seldom confrontational. CL work favors an active approach in which establishing a direct personal linkage with the patient is vital.

11. What are the usual interventions provided by the consulting psychiatrist?

Many regard supportive intervention as the psychiatric consultant's primary function: reassuring, comforting, listening, and coordinating. At the heart of the intervention are genuine concern for the patient's plight and a willingness and ability to empathize. The psychiatrist must be attuned to themes of uncertainty, fear, and abandonment. The repertoire must include skills in grief work, engaging the spouse or significant other and family, and anticipating the likely progression of events in the hospitalization and medical course.

In addition, the CL psychiatrist must be conversant with a range of psychopharmacologic interventions to manage agitation, delirium, depression, anxiety, drug-induced psychotic disorders, and psychiatric presentations "due to a general medical condition." Regrettably, the use of psychotropics in the medically ill has had limited systematic study. Thus, the consultant often assumes liaison or educational functions with referring physicians and nursing staff.

Psychosocial interventions are emphasized by some clinicians (especially in Europe). Cognitive and behavioral interventions occasionally are employed.

Note that 5–10% of CL interventions result in a psychiatric hospitalization/transfer. The number of patients referred for outpatient treatment or followup is presently undefined but is growing.

12. Is medical depression the same as primary depression?

The idea that depression arising in the patient with a medical illness might differ from depression found in patients without physical disease has only lately gained a measure of acceptance. Because physical illness confounds many of the vegetative signs by which depression is routinely diagnosed, investigators generally have avoided the nosologic and diagnostic complexities of "medical depression." Many have found it simpler to assume that medical depression is the same as primary depression. However, some data suggest that this is not so:

• The prevalence of primary depression in women is twice that of men, but medical depression is equally prevalent in both genders.

• Primary depression has strong genetic loading; medical depression appears independently of of familial affective history.

• A shortened REM latency is a useful biologic marker of primary depression, but REM latency has been shown to be "normal" in medical depression.

• Depression in the medically ill (predominantly pathophysiologic rather than reactive) responds less favorably to antidepressant medication than does primary depression.

13. List some prevalence rates of major depression in medical illness.

In several major neurologic illnesses (Parkinson's disease, Huntington's disease, stroke, Alzheimer's), lifetime prevalence rates of major depression are surprisingly consistent (30–50%). Multiple sclerosis is an exception. In multiple sclerosis, the prevalence of depression in patients with only spinal involvement is less than 10%; for those with cortical disease, the rate of occurrence of depression exceeds 30%. Lifetime prevalence rates of depression in systemic medical illnesses are more variable, ranging from 20–30% in diabetes mellitus and coronary artery disease, and 33–67% in Cushing's disease.

14. Is depression in the medically ill a discrete entity?
Collectively, evidence argues that depression occurring in the medically ill *is* a discrete entity, with features all its own. Rather than the old construct that depression is best understood in these patients as a reactive response to the stress of medical illness, it is increasingly appreciated that depression may constitute an independent risk factor in the progression of an Axis III condition. This has been most sharply demonstrated in recent studies concerning cardiovascular disease.[7] The critical question is whether intervention aimed at the psychiatric condition arrests or retards the progression of the Axis III condition.

15. Are these depressions generic, or specific to the physical illness?
Unknown.

16. How should a *medical* depression be treated by the psychiatric consultant?
This remains an area of controversy. Literature indicates that electroconvulsive therapy may be the intervention most likely to benefit the patient with marked medical depression. However, such data are retrospective rather than prospective. In the medically ill, some traditional tricyclic antidepressants have questionable efficacy and carry substantial side effects.[6,8]

Selective serotonin reuptake inhibitors (SSRIs) await further study in populations of medically ill patients, but hold some potential (benefits include single daily dosing without increments and a more tolerable side effect profile). The combination of an SSRI and supportive psychotherapy is a reasonable first step in the face of medical depression. Subsequent steps may be necessary as the medical illness waxes and wanes, hospitalization concludes, and additional stressors emerge.

BIBLIOGRAPHY

1. Fava GA, Sonino N, Wise TN: Management of depression in medical patients. Psychother Psychosom 49:81, 1988.
2. Hackett TP, Cassem NH: Handbook of General Hospital Psychiatry. Littleton, MA, PSG Publishing, 1987.
3. Hales RE: The benefits of a psychiatric consultation-liaison service in a general hospital. General Hosp Psychiatry 7:214–218, 1985.
4. Huyse F: Systematic Interventions in CL. Amsterdam, Free University Press, 1989.
5. Levenson JL, Hammer RM, Rossiter LF: Relation of psychopathology in general medical inpatients to use and cost of services. Am J Psychiatry 147:1498, 1990.
6. Lustman PJ, Griffith LS, Clouse RE, et al: Effects of nortriptyline on depression and glycemic control in diabetes. Results of a double blind placebo-controlled trial. Psychosom Med 59:241–250, 1997.
7. Musselman DC, Evans DL, Nemeroff CB: The relationship of depression to cardiovascular disease: Epidemiology, biology, and treatment. Arch Gen Psychiatry 55(7):580–592, 1998.
8. Nelson JC, Kennedy JS, Pollock BG, et al: Treatment of major depression with nortriptyline and paroxetine in patients with ischemic heart disease. Am J Psychiatry 156:1024–1028, 1999.
9. Pasnau RO: Consultation-liaison psychiatry: Progress, problems and prospects. Psychosomatics 29:1, 1988.
10. Popkin MK, Mackenzie TB, Callies AL: Consultation-liaison outcome evaluation system: Consultation-consultee interaction. Arch Gen Psychiatry 40:125, 1983.
11. Popkin MK, Tucker GJ: "Secondary" and drug-induced mood, anxiety, psychotic, catatonic, and personality disorders: A review of the literature. J Neuropsychiatry Clin Neurosci 4:369–385, 1992.
12. Seward LN, Smith GC, Stuart GW: Concordance with recommendations in a consultation-liaison psychiatry service. Aust N Z J Psychiatry 25:243–254, 1991.
13. Stoudemire A, Fogel BS: Psychiatric Care of the Medical Patient. Oxford, Oxford University Press, 1993.
14. Thompson T (ed): Research advances in consultation-liaison psychiatry. Psychiatr Med 9:506–648, 1991.
15. Wells KB, Golding JM, Burnham MD: Psychiatric disorder in a sample of the general population with and without chronic medical conditions. Am J Psychiatry 145:976, 1988.

68. PSYCHIATRIC DISORDERS IN PRIMARY CARE SETTINGS

Steven Kick, M.D., M.S.P.H.

1. How common are psychiatric disorders in primary care settings?

The primary care sector has been labeled a de facto mental healthcare system because almost two-thirds of all patients with psychiatric illnesses in the U.S. are seen exclusively in primary care settings. Prevalence studies in primary care clinics have consistently shown rates of up to 30% for psychiatric disorders meeting DSM-IV criteria. It is probable, however, that significant psychiatric illness exceeds this rate because of so-called mixed or minor disorders that do not meet full diagnostic criteria. In any case, primary healthcare settings carry the burden of patients with psychiatric disorders in the U.S.

2. Which disorders are seen most frequently in primary care settings?

Anxiety, mood disturbance, and psychoactive substance abuse are the most common disorders in primary care settings. The following table lists the disorders by decreasing lifetime prevalence rates:

Disorder	%
Major depression	17.1
Alcohol dependence	14.1
Social phobia	13.3
Simple phobia	11.3
Alcohol abuse	9.4
Drug dependence	7.5
Dysthymia	6.4
Agoraphobia	5.3
Generalized anxiety disorder	5.1
Panic disorder	3.5
Manic episode	1.6
Nonaffective psychosis	0.7

3. How do persons with psychiatric disorders present to the clinician?

Patients with psychiatric disorders often present to primary care providers with somatic complaints referable to their underlying disorder. For mood disorders, the most frequent complaints are fatigue, alteration in sleep, and chronic pain. Among anxiety disorders, panic disorder has been the most thoroughly studied for association with medically unexplained symptoms. The following table lists the prevalence of panic disorder among patients with medically unexplained symptoms:

Symptoms	Prevalence of Panic Disorder (%)
Chest pain with negative angiogram	33–43
Irritable bowel	29–38
Unexplained dizziness	13
Migraine headache	4.9 (panic) 1.6 (agoraphobia)
Chronic fatigue	13–30
Chest pain in emergency department	18

In patients with 5 or more medically unexplained symptoms, the odds of having panic disorder are 204 to 1.

Frequently, patients have a number of nonspecific symptoms that frustrate both patient and provider. For example, a young man with lightheadedness and atypical chest pain underwent magnetic resonance imaging (MRI) scan of the brain, electroencephalogram, Holter monitor testing, exercise treadmill, echocardiogram, cerebral angiography, and numerous blood tests. A careful history revealed that he had panic disorder. In this case, a good history may have saved thousands of unnecessary dollars in testing.

4. What medical conditions are associated with psychiatric disorders?

A number of medical conditions are associated with symptoms that may mimic psychiatric disorders. Illnesses with significant functional impairment or mortality may be associated with anxious or depressed moods. Usually, medical conditions can be diagnosed with a careful history, physical exam, and prudent laboratory tests, as demonstrated with the differentiation between panic disorder and pheochromocytomas. **Panic disorder** is associated with intense fear, apprehension, and, often, avoidant behavior, whereas pheochromocytomas present with recurrent bouts of hypertension, palpitations, and sweating; fear and apprehension develop later in the episode.

Establishing causal relationships between medical and psychiatric disorders can be difficult, especially when the prevalence of both is high. Such is the case with **depression** and hypothyroidism. Although it is popular to do a variety of tests, the history and physical exam should guide the clinician. For example, computed tomography or MRI scanning of the brain generally is helpful only if the patient has a dementia or focal neurologic findings; brain scans are not helpful for the diagnosis of other psychiatric disorders.

Medications also can result in symptoms that mimic psychiatric disorders. In particular, sedative-hypnotics and centrally acting antihypertensive agents, such as reserpine and clonidine, may produce a depressed mood. Contrary to popular belief, beta-adrenergic blocking agents do not generally cause depressive symptoms. Several agents can cause sleep disturbances and agitation or anorexia, such as pseudoephedrine and thyroxine. A careful medication history with diminution or cessation of the drug may reveal the cause and treat the apparent psychiatric disorder.

5. How common are substance abuse problems in primary care?

Substance abuse and dependence are quite common in primary care settings and carry significant morbidity and mortality. It is estimated that 10% of the adult population and **30–50% of persons** in primary care may have alcohol abuse or dependence. The cost to society for medical care and lost productivity was estimated to be $246 billion in 1992. Alcohol abuse and dependence, the most common disorder, may aggravate a number of medical problems, including sleep disturbances, hypertension, diabetes, peptic ulcer disease, anemia, and mood disorders. Often such aggravations or laboratory abnormalities (elevated aspartate aminotransferase, alanine aminotransferase, gamma glutamyl transpeptidase, mean corpuscular volume) may alert the clinician to the possibility of alcohol use. Similarly, alteration in daily activities such as work delinquency and/or legal problems may suggest alcoholism.

Screening instruments such as the CAGE questionnaire are easy to use and may have diagnostic sensitivities of 85–89%:
1. Are you Concerned about your drinking?
2. Have others Angered you about your drinking?
3. Have you felt Guilty about your drinking?
4. Have you ever had an Eye-opener (e.g., morning drink)?

Unfortunately, clinicians often do not inquire about a history of substance use or use readily available screening tools.

Finally, alcohol and other psychoactive substances are strongly correlated with other psychiatric disorders, particularly major depression, bipolar disorder, panic disorder, social phobia, and post-traumatic stress disorder.

6. Which psychiatric disorders can the primary care provider treat?

The type of psychiatric disorder that a primary care physician can treat varies with the severity of the disorder, expertise of the physician, availability of treatment options, and desires of the patient. Disorders marked by psychosis, severe behavioral changes (such as avoidant behavior), and lethality (suicide or homicide) should be treated by or with a mental health professional. Because psychiatric disorders occur so commonly in general medical settings, the primary care provider must be confident in assessing such patients. Indeed, patients tend to feel more comfortable and less stigmatized with primary care physicians. Often, treatment may be initiated and the patient closely followed. If improvement in symptoms does not occur in 6–8 weeks, the patient may then be referred.

7. Why should the primary care provider not treat every depressed patient with the newer antidepressants such as fluoxetine, which appear safe?

It is certainly easy for the primary care physician to prescribe the newer antidepressants, as evidenced by the overwhelming increase in the number of prescriptions. Such drugs are attractive because they are simple to dose, do not require monitoring of serum levels, and generally are well-tolerated. Nonetheless, *ease of prescription does not warrant their use outside approved indications.* It is not known whether such agents are effective for mixed or minor disorders. In addition, they may precipitate agitation or mania and are therefore to be used cautiously or not at all in persons with a history of hypomania, mania, or agitation. Likewise, they are not free from side effects, may have adverse interactions with nonpsychotropic medications, and are not inexpensive. Therefore they should be used prudently by the primary care provider.

In addition, research demonstrates the need for psychotherapy in many depressed patients. Combining psychotherapy with pharmacologic treatment is likely to provide better results. Hence, providing medication alone may treat a depressive illness only partially.

8. How useful are screening instruments for psychiatric case-finding?

Currently, several screening instruments are available to the primary care provider, ranging from self-administered questionnaires to more formal interviewer-rated instruments. All have the advantage of suggesting a disorder when the provider faces times constraints. However, even the best instruments have predictive value of only 70–85%, and, unfortunately, few have been adequately validated against standard structured interviews. Such instruments should be used only for case-finding and not for definitive diagnosis.

Commonly Used Screening Instruments

DISORDER	PATIENT-RATED	INTERVIEWER-RATED
Depression		
CES-D	X	
Beck	X	
Hamilton		X
MOS	X	
HADS	X	
Anxiety		
Zung	X	
Hamilton	X	
Sheehan	X	X
Beck Cognition	X	
HADS	X	
Both		
SDDS-PC	X	X
Prime-MD	X	X

CES-D = Center for Epidemiologic Studies—Depression, MOS = Medical Outcomes Study, HADS = Hospital Anxiety and Depression Scale. SDDS-PC = Symptom-Driven Diagnostic Schedule—Primary Care

BIBLIOGRAPHY

1. Brody DS, Hahn SR, Spitzer RL, et al: Identifying patients with depression in the primary care setting: A more efficient method. Arch Intern Med 158(22):2469–2975, 1998.
2. Katon WJ, Walker EA: Medically unexplained symptoms in primary care. J Clin Psychiatry 59 Suppl 20:15–21, 1998.
3. Kessler RC, McGonagle KA, Zhao S, et al: Lifetime and 12-month prevalence of DSM-III-R psychiatric disorders in the United States: Results from the National Comorbidity Survey. Arch Gen Psychiatry 51:8–19, 1994.
4. Kessler LG, Cleary PD, Burke JD: Psychiatric disorders in primary care. Arch Gen Psychiatry 42:583–587, 1985.
5. Lustman PJ: Anxiety disorders in adults with diabetes mellitus. Psychiatr Clin North Am 11(2):419–431, 1988.
6. Von Korff M, Shapiro S, Burke JD: Anxiety and depression in a primary care clinic. Arch Gen Psychiatry 44:152–156, 1987.
7. Walker EA, Katon WJ, Jemelka RP: Psychiatric disorders and medical care utilization among people in the general population who report fatigue. J Gen Intern Med 8:436–440, 1993.
8. Yingling KW, Wulsin LR, Arnold LM, Rouan GW: Estimated prevalences of panic disorder and depression among consecutive patients seen in an emergency department with acute chest pain. J Gen Intern Med 8:231–235, 1993.

69. THE MANAGEMENT OF CHRONIC PAIN

Robert N. Jamison, Ph.D.

1. What is the difference between acute and chronic pain?

Acute pain generally is associated with tissue damage and represents a *warning of injury* to the individual. It is expected to be directly proportional to the sensory input of the tissue damage and to continue until the damaged tissue and/or afferent pathways have returned to normal functioning. Chronic noncancer pain, in contrast, is a persistent condition often associated with an initial episode of acute pain but continuing long past the time when healing would normally take place. Chronic noncancer pain serves *no beneficial purpose* and is resistant to medical intervention.

2. What are the different categories of pain?

Pain syndromes may be categorized according to the character and history of the symptom:
- **Acute pain** is self-limiting, usually of less than 6-month duration, and generally adaptive in nature (e.g., postsurgical pain, dental pain, pain following injury).
- **Recurrent acute pain** consists of a series of intermittent episodes of pain that are acute in character but chronic insofar as the condition persists for more than 6 months (e.g., migraine headaches, trigeminal neuralgia, temporomandibular disorder).
- **Chronic nonmalignant pain** persists beyond 6 months and is intractable. Pain severity varies over time and may or may not have a known relationship to active pathophysiologic or pathoanatomic process (e.g., chronic mechanical low back pain, diffuse myofascial pain syndrome).
- **Chronic progressive pain** increases in severity over time and often is associated with malignancies and degenerative disorders (e.g., skeletal metastatic disease, rheumatoid arthritis).

3. How do psychogenic and organic pain differ?

Chronic pain represents a complex interaction of factors. The pain typically is related to an initial somatic event but, over time, is increasingly influenced by the patient's personality, beliefs, and environment. Attempts to reliably distinguish between organic and psychogenic pain have been largely unsuccessful. Many practitioners incorrectly believe that chronic pain reflects either organic pathology or psychogenic symptoms. If physical findings are inadequate to account for a patient's report of chronic pain, then the pain often is perceived to be mostly psychological. It generally is unwarranted, however, to assume that psychological factors are the primary cause of pain.

4. Which measures are useful in assessing pain intensity?

Pain intensity can be measured by subjective numerical pain ratings (scales from 0–10 or 0–100), visual analogue scales, verbal rating scales, pain drawings, and combined standardized questionnaires.

5. What is a visual analogue scale?

A popular means of measuring pain intensity is the visual analogue scale (VAS), which uses a straight line, usually 10 cm long, with the extreme limits of pain on either end of the line. The patient is instructed to place a mark on the line to best indicate pain severity. Scores are obtained by measuring the distance from the end labeled "no pain" to the mark made by the patient. Although frequently used to measure chronic pain, the VAS is time-consuming to score and has questionable validity for older patients.

6. What are verbal ratings of pain?

A verbal pain-rating scale consists of 4–15 words that are ranked according to expression of pain (from "no pain" to "excruciating pain"). The patient chooses the words that best describe the pain. Verbal scales not only measure *pain intensity* but also assess *sensory and affective dimensions* of the pain experience. Verbal scales also can be used to measure pain description. The patient chooses words from a list of words, such as piercing, stabbing, shooting, burning, and throbbing, that best describe the pain experience.

7. What is the McGill Pain Questionnaire?

The McGill Pain Questionnaire (MPQ) is a popular, comprehensive questionnaire that includes 20 subclasses of descriptors as well as a numerical pain-intensity scale and a dermatomal pain drawing. It is a frequently employed clinical tool in the subjective measurement of pain. A short form also is popular. The MPQ allows for measurement of different aspects of the pain experience and is sensitive to treatment effects and the differential diagnosis.

8. What tools best evaluate psychopathology in chronic pain patients?

There is ongoing debate among mental health professionals about the best ways to measure psychopathology in chronic pain patients. Most chronic pain patients do not have a history of premorbid psychiatric disturbance, but show reactive emotional distress in response to their pain. However, when present, major psychopathology is indicative of a poor prognosis for pain therapy. Pain patients frequently endorse somatic complaints in response to their condition. Thus, caution is necessary in interpreting psychological tests in which somatic complaints are considered indicative of psychopathology in pain patients.

The measures most commonly used to evaluate psychopathology and emotional distress in chronic pain patients include the Minnesota Multiphasic Personality Inventory (MMPI), the Symptom Checklist 90 (SCL-90-R), the Millon Behavior Health Inventory (MBHI), the Illness Behavior Questionnaire (IBQ), and the Beck Depression Inventory (BDI).

Assessment Categories and Frequently Used Psychometric Measures

PSYCHOSOCIAL HISTORY
    CAGE Questionnaire
    Comprehensive Pain Questionnaire
    Michigan Alcoholism Screening Test (MAST)
    Self-Administered Alcoholism Screening Test (SAAST)
    Structured Clinical Interview for DSM-IV (SCID)

Table continued on following page

Assessment Categories and Frequently Used Psychometric Measures (Cont.)

PAIN INTENSITY
  Numerical rating scales
  Pain drawings
  Verbal rating scales (VRS)
  Visual analog scales (VAS)

MOOD AND PERSONALITY
  Beck Depression Inventory (BDI)
  Center for Epidemiologic Studies Depression Scale (CES-D)
  Illness Behavior Questionnaire (IBQ)
  Millon Behavior Health Inventory (MBHI)
  Minnesota Multiphasic Personality Inventory (MMPI-2)
  Symptom Checklist 90-R (SCL-90)

PAIN BELIEFS AND COPING
  Coping Strategies Questionnaire (CSQ)
  Inventory of Negative Thoughts in Response to Pain (INTRP)
  Pain Management Inventory (PMI)
  Pain Self-Efficacy Questionnaire (PSEQ)
  Survey of Pain Attitudes (SOPA)

FUNCTIONAL CAPACITY
  Multidimensional Pain Inventory (MPI)
  Oswestry Disability Questionnaire (ODQ)
  Pain Disability Index (PDI)
  Short-Form Health Survey (SF-36)
  Sickness Impact Profile (SIP)

9. How is the MMPI used in assessing chronic pain patients?

The MMPI, which consists of 561 true-or-false items, produces distinct profiles of pain patients. Studies have shown that profile patterns allow prediction of return to work and response to surgical treatment in males. A revised version, MMPI-2, replicates the profile patterns of the original MMPI. Again, despite this test's popularity in measuring the presence of psychopathology, remember that profiles of chronic pain patients can be misinterpreted because these patients frequently endorse physical symptoms.

10. Describe the Beck Depression Inventory.

The BDI is a 21-item, self-report questionnaire that provides a measure of severity of depression. It is commonly used to assess depressive symptomatology in chronic pain patients and determine treatment outcome. It is easy to administer and score.

11. What other tools are valuable in assessing depression?

Other valuable measures include the Center for Epidemiologic Studies Depression Scale and the Hamilton and the Zung Depression Scales. Regardless of the tool used, a shared limitation is the possible misinterpretation of an elevated score: chronic pain patients frequently report fatigue, sleep disturbances, and loss of sexual interest, which can be interpreted as signs of clinical depression.

12. Describe the SCL-90-R, the MBHI, and the IBQ.

The SCL-90-R is a 90-item checklist that uses a five-point scale. It offers a global index score as well as nine subscale scores to provide a general assessment of emotional distress. The SCL-90-R is a relatively brief measure and offers some validity for pain patients (the items make sense to them). It is easy to inspect individual items that may pertain specifically to persons with chronic pain. The disadvantages of this measure are that all subscales are highly correlated and there are no validity scales to determine the presence of subtle inconsistencies in responses.

The MBHI contains 150 true-or-false items to assess mood and personality, and offers 20 subscales that measure styles relating to providers, psychosocial stressors, and response to illness. The advantage of the MBHI is that the scales are not subject to misinterpretation due to physical symptoms. Unlike the other measures, the MBHI emphasizes medical rather than emotional concerns.

The IBQ determines emotionality and illness behavior in chronic pain patients. It contains 62 true-or-false items and comprises seven subscales measuring symptom complaints and abnormal illness behavior. Patients who are not known to have organic pathology that would account for their pain tend to produce higher IBQ scores. The IBQ also is correlated with anxiety measures.

13. How are pain-related beliefs measured?

A person's beliefs about pain are important in predicting the outcome of treatment. Negative thoughts about an ongoing pain problem may contribute to increased pain and emotional distress, decreased functioning, and greater reliance on medication. Certain chronic pain patients are prone to maladaptive beliefs about their condition that may not be compatible with its physical nature (e.g., "This pain will make me lose my mind." "Soon I will become an invalid."). The tests most frequently used to measure maladaptive beliefs include the Coping Strategies Questionnaire, the Pain Management Inventory, the Pain Self-Efficacy Questionnaire, the Survey of Pain Attitudes, and the Inventory of Negative Thoughts in Response to Pain.

14. What are the best ways to measure functional capacity?

The assessment of functional capacity and interference with activity is important since third-party payers frequently judge treatment outcome as successful on the basis of improved function and return to work. Reliable instruments for measuring function include the Sickness Impact Profile, the Short-Form Health Survey, the Multidimensional Pain Inventory, the Pain Disability Index, and the Oswestry Disability Questionnaire.

Other functional measures, which are not as popular, include The Chronic Illness Problem Inventory, The Waddell Disability Instrument, and The Functional Rating Scale. Automated devices such as the portable up-time calculator and the pedometer are useful ways to obtain accurate measures of activity. These devices should be used in conjunction with self-monitoring assessment techniques.

15. List the options for treating chronic pain.

Hot and cold packs	Psychotherapy
Massage therapy	Acupuncture
Physical therapy	Medication
Didactic instruction	Nerve block therapy
Relaxation training	Implantable devices
Hypnosis	Surgical treatments
Biofeedback	

16. What is an interdisciplinary pain treatment program?

Chronic pain involves a complex interaction of physiological and psychosocial factors, and successful intervention requires the coordinated effort of a treatment team with expertise in a variety of therapeutic disciplines. Although some pain centers offer a unimodal treatment approach, most programs blend medical, psychological, vocational, and educational techniques. The interdisciplinary core staff typically includes one or more physicians, a clinical psychologist, and a physical therapist. Other health professionals who may play important roles include clinical nurse specialists, occupational therapists, vocational rehabilitation counselors, and acupuncturists.

17. How are outpatient pain programs typically structured?

Multidisciplinary pain programs administered on an outpatient basis often are highly structured, time limited, and organized along a specific treatment schedule. The patient is expected to attend clinic sessions and to participate actively in all aspects of the program. These expectations must be made clear.

To this end, patients frequently sign a **treatment contract** that spells out the general program require-ments as well as individual treatment goals. In addition to helping patients understand exactly what is expected of them, such a contract provides a mechanism for identifying those patients who, prior to treatment, lack motivation or may have difficulty conforming to the structure of the program. Patients are asked to keep a daily written record of their pain intensity, medication use, and activity levels.

18. What are the desired outcomes of interdisciplinary treatment?

The therapeutic aims of interdisciplinary interventions for chronic noncancer pain include de-creased pain intensity, increased physical activity, decreased reliance on pain medication, a return to work, improved psychosocial functioning, and reduced use of healthcare services.

19. List the main objectives of cognitive/behavioral therapy for chronic pain patients.

• Help patients view their problem as manageable, instead of overwhelming. Patients who are prone to "catastrophize" benefit from examining the way they view their situation. What could be perceived as a hopeless condition can be reframed as a difficult yet manageable condition over which they can exercise some control.

• Help convince patients that the treatment is relevant to their problem and that they need to be actively involved in their treatment and rehabilitation.

• Teach patients to monitor maladaptive thoughts and substitute positive thoughts. Persons with chronic pain are plagued, either consciously or unconsciously, by negative thoughts related to their condition. These negative thoughts perpetuate pain behaviors and feelings of hopelessness. Adaptive management techniques for chronic pain are an important component of cognitive restructuring.

20. What is the role of group therapy for pain patients?

Pain patients frequently show signs of emotional distress, with evidence of depression, anxiety, and irritability. Group therapy with a cognitive/behavioral orientation is designed to help patients gain control of the emotional reactions associated with chronic pain. Specific problem-solving strategies can be offered, including: identifying maladaptive and negative thoughts, disrupting irrational thinking, constructing and repeating positive self-statements, learning distraction techniques, working to prevent future "catastrophizing," and examining ways to increase social support. In addition, group therapy presents an opportunity to discuss any concerns or problems that patients may have in common.

21. How important is family involvement in therapy?

Chronic pain significantly impacts all members of a family. Family members need to be edu-cated about the goals of therapy and should have an opportunity to share their worries and concerns. Moreover, active involvement of family members helps ensure the patient's long-term success. Therefore, both patients and members of their families should be invited to attend family therapy sessions. Besides enhanced communication, important outcomes of these sessions are that family members learn how to help the patient achieve and maintain goals, and they come to understand that they are not alone in their dealings with the person in pain.

22. What are the benefits of relaxation training for chronic pain patients?

Chronic pain patients tend to experience substantial residual muscle tension as a function of the bracing, posturing, and emotional arousal often associated with pain. Such responses, maintained over a long period, can exacerbate pain in injured areas of the body and increase muscular discom-fort. For example, patients with low back pain or limb injuries commonly experience neck stiffness and tension-type headaches. Relaxation training can lead to pain reduction by relaxing tense muscle groups, reducing anxiety, distracting the patient from the pain, and enhancing self-efficacy. In addi-tion, this training can increase the patient's sense of control over physiological responses.

In a pain management program, patients are taught and encouraged to practice a variety of re-laxation strategies, including diaphragmatic breathing, progressive muscle relaxation, autogenic re-laxation, guided imagery, and cue-controlled relaxation. Hypnosis and biofeedback training also are commonly employed.

23. Which variables predict a low probability of return to work?

The most relevant predictor of return to work is the duration of unemployment. After 6 months of unemployment due to chronic pain, the probability of return of work is 50%; the likelihood decreases to 10% after 1 year. Other factors negatively impacting the likelihood of return to work include limited formal education, limited transferable skills, poor perceived social support, ongoing litigation, a poor relationship with the employer, and job dissatisfaction.

24. How can vocational rehabilitation help chronic pain patients?

The goal of vocational rehabilitation is to return a patient with chronic pain to work. After an extended period out of work, patients become both physically and psychologically deconditioned to the demands and stresses of the workplace. A vocational rehabilitation counselor helps the patient develop a plan that incorporates long-range employment goals and short-term objectives based on medical, psychological, social, and vocational information. These counselors are specialists in the assessment of aptitudes and interests, transferable skills, physical capacity, modifications in the workplace, skills training, and job readiness.

25. What is the role of activity and exercise for persons with chronic pain?

Most patients lose physical stamina and flexibility because of reluctance to exercise and a perceived need to protect themselves from additional physical injury. Some patients have been medically advised to restrict activity when pain increases. Patients with chronic pain need to know that exercise is important. Getting back to usual activities as soon as possible after an injury helps to prevent disability. Some stretching, cardiovascular activity, and weight training should be considered.

26. Under what circumstances should opioid therapy be prescribed?

The use of opioid analgesics for chronic noncancer pain is controversial, due to concerns about efficacy, adverse effects, tolerance, and addiction. Opioid therapy is contraindicated by a history of substance abuse, a major psychiatric diagnosis, the seeking of drugs from multiple physicians, uncontrolled dose escalation, and/or evidence of lack of compliance. Patients with significant adverse reactions to low-dose opioid therapy also are poor candidates. The decision to use opioid therapy often rests on clinical judgment and treatment orientation.

27. What are the roles of invasive procedures and implantable devices in pain management?

There are many types of invasive interventions for pain. They range from trigger point injections to spinal cord stimulation and deep brain surgery. Patients are attracted to any treatment that is designed to decrease their pain. However, careful assessment and evaluation of the patients prior to the procedures, including a thorough psychological evaluation, helps to identify those patients who are poor candidates and improves the chances for a positive outcome. Many insurance carriers require a comprehensive psychological evaluation prior to approval of an implantable device for pain.

28. How can relapse be avoided?

Most chronic pain patients need support after completing a pain treatment program, to maintain the gains they have achieved. Patients should be encouraged to identify and anticipate situations that place them at risk for returning to previous maladaptive behavior patterns. They also should be encouraged to rehearse problem-solving techniques and behavioral responses that enable them to avoid a relapse. The goals of relapse prevention are to help the patient (1) maintain a steady level of activity, emotional stability, and appropriate medication use; (2) anticipate and deal with situations that cause setbacks; and (3) acquire skills that decrease reliance on the healthcare system. Followup has been shown to be vital in helping to prevent relapse. A specific followup plan should be written out for each patient.

29. What criteria are important in the evaluation of a pain treatment program?

An important component of any group-based pain program is its ability to measure its own effectiveness and determine which services are most beneficial in the treatment of chronic pain patients. A number of recommendations for effective program evaluation have been put forward by the Commission on the Accreditation of Rehabilitation Facilities (CARF).

• A system should be in place for obtaining followup information from patients on the use of medications, use of healthcare services, return to gainful employment, functional activities, ability to manage pain, and subjective pain intensity.

• Provisions should also be made for periodic contact after discharge.

• Program evaluation should encompass goals and objectives that are achievable and end results that are measurable.

• A program evaluation report should include primary objectives, measures, time of measurement, source of information, and expectancies as well as outcome.

BIBLIOGRAPHY

1. Accident Rehabilitation and Compensation Insurance Corporation and the National Health Committee: New Zealand Acute Low Back Pain Guide. Wellington, New Zealand, AAC and NHC, 1997.
2. American Academy of Pain Medicine and American Pain Society Consensus Statement: The use of opioids for the treatment of chronic pain. Pain Forum 6:77–79, 1997.
3. Cicala RS, Wright H: Outpatient treatment of patients with chronic pain: An analysis of cost savings. Clin J Pain 5:223–226, 1989.
4. Commission on the Accreditation of Rehabilitation Facilities: Standards Manual for Organizations Servicing People with Disabilities, Tucson, Arizona, CARF, 1999.
5. Fishbain DA, Cutler R, Rosomoff HL, Rosomoff RS: Chronic pain-associated depression: Antecedent or consequence of chronic pain? A review. Clin J Pain 13:116–137, 1997.
6. Follick MJ, Ahern DK, Aberger EW: Behavioral treatment of chronic pain. In Blumenthal JA, McKee DC (eds): Applications in Behavioral Medicine and Health Psychology: A Clinician's Source Book. Sarasota, Florida, Professional Resource Exchange, Inc., 1987, pp 237–270.
7. Fordyce WE (ed): Back Pain in the Workplace: Management of Disability in Nonspecific Conditions. Seattle, International Association for the Study of Pain Press, 1995.
8. Gatchel RJ, Turk DC (eds): Psychological Approaches to Pain Management: A Practitioner's Handbook. New York, The Guilford Press, 1996.
9. Jamison RN: Learning to Master Your Chronic Pain. Sarasota, FL, Professional Resource Press, 1996.
10. Jamison RN: Mastering Chronic Pain: A Professional's Guide to Behavioral Treatment. Sarasota, FL, Professional Resource Press, 1996.
11. Karoly P, Jensen MP: Multimethod Assessment of Chronic Pain. New York, Pergamon Press, 1987.
12. Nigl AJ: Biofeedback and Behavioral Strategies in Pain Treatment. New York, Spectrum Publications, Inc., 1984.
13. Turk DC, Melzack R (eds): Handbook of Pain Assessment. New York, The Guilford Press, 1992.

70. THE ASSESSMENT AND TREATMENT OF SEXUAL DYSFUNCTION

Thomas D. Stewart, M.D.

1. Can sexual dysfunction be a symptom of medical illness?

Yes. Sexual dysfunction is a neglected vital sign in medical history taking. It can be the first presenting symptom for conditions as diverse as diabetes mellitus, temporal lobe epilepsy, multiple sclerosis, and thyroid dysfunction.

2. Describe a framework for the clinical evaluation of sexual dysfunction.

Masters and Johnson's well-known sexual response cycle provides a paradigm for understanding and treating sexual dysfunction:

Appetitive phase—involves noticing attractive people and having an intact libido. There are no specific physiologic responses.

Excitement—is marked by vascular engorgement and lubrication in women and erection in men. These responses, associated with flushed skin, intensify and reach a plateau phase before orgasm.

Orgasm—is associated with pelvic muscle contraction and pleasure and is accompanied by ejaculation in men.

Resolution—genital vascular engorgement gradually abates. The exercise involved in sex can cause perspiration in all phases, but only in the resolution phase is sweating a specific, associated finding, regardless of exercise levels.

All sexual dysfunctions are connected with one or more phases of this response cycle.

3. Name medical conditions that disrupt the appetitive phase. Which medications are corrective?

Hypoactive sexual desire disorder can be caused by temporal lobe epilepsy, hyperprolactinemia, and hypogonadotropic hypogonadism. **Carbamazepine** can stabilize temporal lobe input to the anterior pituitary gland, which has been disrupted by the complex partial seizures of temporal lobe epilepsy. This stabilized input allows the anterior pituitary to increase luteinizing hormone (LH) release, leading to increased production of testosterone from Leydig cells found in the testicles. Testosterone regulates libido in both sexes.

Bromocriptine, a D agonist, can reduce prolactin levels coming from pituitary microadenomas. Intramuscular testosterone offsets the low testosterone levels resulting from low LH production in hypogonadotropic hypogonadism. These medications can restore sexual desire by correcting the underlying medical problem. Medications (e.g., alpha methyl dopa) also can impair libido. Libido is reduced in psychiatric conditions such as depression, anxiety, and post-traumatic stress disorder. Psychotropic medications can restore libido lost through mental illness. Proper use of psychotropics helps improve mood and reduce apprehension that underlies loss of desire.

4. What are the analogies between the excitement phase in men and women?

Erections, vaginal engorgement, and lubrication are analogous. They are similar from both embryologic and physiologic perspectives. The work-up for disorders of the excitement phase in men and women (see Questions 7–9) is virtually identical.

5. Which factors in the medical history might contribute to an impaired excitement phase?

Here is a rule of thumb: if something is bad for the heart, it is bad for erections, lubrication, and engorgement. For example, smoking, diabetes, alcohol abuse, hypertension, and hyperlipidemia are associated with excitement phase dysfunction.

6. Name physical findings connected with erectile dysfunction.

Gynecomastia, hypogonadism, hyperreflexia, reduced peripheral pulses, and loss of sensation.

7. What constitutes an endocrine work-up for impairment of the sexual excitement phase?

Thyroid function, liver function, and glucose tolerance tests. Also serum testosterone and prolactin levels.

8. What are some vascular studies that shed light on the etiology of sexual arousal impairment?

There are several, including Doppler determination of penile blood flow, and penile blood pressure compared to brachial blood pressure. Penile angiography can spot arterial occlusion. Venous cavernoscopy can pinpoint venous valvular incompetence that leads to impotence. Internal iliac angiography can identify arterial occlusions that impair erections or lubrication.

9. List some medication categories that can disrupt the excitement phase.

Beta blockers, such as inderal; anticholinergics like tricyclic antidepressants, low-potency phenothiazines, and selective serotonin reuptake inhibitors (SSRIs); and diuretics such as hydrochlorothiazide.

10. What is a nocturnal penile tumescence (NPT) study?

The NPT is a sleep study usually done over at least two nights. A donut-shaped plethysmographic device is placed over the penis. It transduces erectile pressure changes into graphic data. The sleep EEG records rapid eye movement sleep that is associated with firm erections in healthy subjects. This study can demonstrate physiologically intact erectile function, which may be undermined by psychogenic factors such as anxiety in the waking state.

11. Is the NPT really the gold standard for separating organic from psychogenic sexual dysfunction?

The NPT is subject to false-positives. Consider the format for this study: a man sleeps in a strange bed with electrodes glued to his hair. He has a gel-filled donut around his penis. Should he have the good fortune to achieve an erection while sleeping in the EEG lab, a technician emerges and checks the buckling pressure. Is it any surprise that there are false positives? In addition, clinical anxiety and depressive disorders cause abnormal results in men known to be physiologically intact. Furthermore, results of the NPT may not correlate with known functional capabilities. While the NPT is sometimes a helpful diagnostic tool, it is not a gold standard.

12. Name some antihypertensive medication categories that do not appear to cause excitement-phase dysfunction.

ACE inhibitors (enalapril, captopril), calcium channel blockers (verapamil, diltiazem), and alpha antagonists (terazosin, prazosin). The latter category may help potency and lubrication.

13. What are some practical techniques for improving sexual functioning in the excitement phase?

Water-soluble lubricants can help women with problems in arousal. These lubricants do not linger and dissolve diaphragms and condoms as oils do. Men can enhance their erections by pushing down their index and third finger at the base of the penis, thus partially occluding venous return. This method requires females to be in a superior position for intercourse, with their bodies at a 45° angle to their partners and their weight on their arms.

14. Which medications restore erectile function?

Intraurethral application of **alprostadil**, a prostaglandin E derivative vasodilator, can enhance erections for previously impotent men with relatively intact vasculature. These erections occur in the absence of sexual stimulation, but are enhanced by it. The dosage range is 500–1000 mcg.

Sildenafil is an oral medication that enhances erection by inhibiting the metabolism of cyclic guanosine monophosphate, which relaxes genital arteriolar smooth muscle, producing vasodilatation and erection. Sildenafil has no effect in the absence of sexual stimulation. Studies are underway to assess its possible beneficial effects for enhancing female arousal states. Side effects include flushing, dyspepsia, and headache. Priapism has not been reported. Sildenafil is contraindicated in patients receiving nitrates used to treat chest pain. The dosing range is 50–100 mg.

15. Does sildenafil have benefits beyond enhanced erections?

Yes. There is evidence that overall sexual satisfaction and quality of climaxes are improved. There is an open-label trial that demonstrates improvement in orgasmic function in those with SRI-induced orgasmic dysfunction.

16. What is a vacuum constriction device?

It is a plastic tube, closed at one end, that is placed over the penis. Vaseline forms a seal between the device and the mons pubis. Air is pumped out of the tube, creating a partial vacuum. Within 5–10 minutes an erection develops. A constriction band is then placed at the base of the penis, and the vacuum is released, allowing removal of the tube. This erection allows vaginal penetration for 20–30 minutes. The erections produced by these devices are wider and shorter than those that occur naturally. They are light blue and cool to touch. Complications include pain and bruises. Several studies have demonstrated their safety and effectiveness.

17. What does a psychodynamic approach to excitement disorders involve?

Psychodynamic psychotherapy can help resolve unconscious conflicts over sexual expression, leading to restored responsiveness. This method explores the meaning of potency and arousal, along with fears avoided by not having intercourse.

18. Give an example of a behavioral approach to arousal dysfunction.

Masters and Johnson have described a behavioral approach that emphasizes **deconditioning** stress-related responses that impair sexual functioning. Couples are encouraged to stop attempting relations and to start sensate focus explorations of how to please each other without genital contact. As they become more comfortable, they progress to more overtly sexual contact according to a protocol designed to enhance feelings of safety and control.

Helen Singer Kaplan modified this technique to include more exploration of individual and couple dynamics and patterns of communication. Kaplan uses deconditioning techniques to treat sexual dysfunction similar to those emphasized by Masters and Johnson. Her method includes more evaluation and treatment of maladaptive patterns of communication that interfere with a couple's relationship in and out of bed. It also considers the individual, psychodynamic, conflictual issues germane to sexual dysfunction. Couples benefit from understanding each other's irrational fears of sexual activity as uncovered with Kaplan's approach.

19. What are some vascular interventions to restore excitement phase function?

• Balloon angioplasty can open the internal iliac arteries leading to restored potency or lubrication.

• Repair of incompetent venous valves, the most common vascular cause of impotence, can restore erectile function.

20. Describe penile intracavernosal injections used to restore erectile function.

A vasodilator, such as phentolamine and yohimbine, or prostaglandin E is injected through 29-gauge needles into the corpora cavernosum at 3 o'clock and 9 o'clock. The urethra is at 6 o'clock, and the dorsal artery of the penis at 12. Injection at 12 or 6 would cause injury, whereas injection at 3 or 9 allows safe entry into the corpora cavernosa.

Prostaglandin E is locally metabolized in the corpora cavernosa and thus less apt to cause priapism than the other agents, which must enter systemic blood flow to be metabolized in the liver. Prostaglandin E also can be dose adjusted to control the duration of erection, but it may cause a burning sensation at the injection site.

21. What are complications of these injections?

There is a low risk of priapism. There can be painful bruising and the development of fibrosis, leading to adhesions with Peyronie's disease, a condition characterized by painful curvature of the penis during erections.

22. Describe penile prostheses.

Penile prostheses are now in widespread use; well over 100,000 have been installed. Implants vary in design. Some have wire inside silastic to allow the penis to be moved into position. Others are inflatable to allow a more normal appearance. Surgical complications following the insertion of prostheses are remarkably rare, even in diabetics. Postoperative infection and erosion through the skin are the main complications. Several studies indicate that patient and partner satisfaction with these devices exceeds 80%.

23. What are some expectations men may have about these devices that lead to disappointment?

"It will make her respond."

"I will regain my self-esteem."

"I will now have something to offer her."

Should a urologist recommend placement of a phallic prosthesis, the consulting psychiatrist should carefully explore the patient's expectations regarding this operation. These expectations are likely to lead to disappointment if not combined with a concern for the quality of relationship which these men want to achieve with their partners. Patients should be strongly encouraged to discuss the prosthesis with their partners so as to gather their feelings about this device. One woman surprised her partner by saying, "Your message is more important than your method." She was clear that she wanted him and not a prosthetic device.

24. Are there sexual dysfunctions specific to the plateau phase?
No, disruptions of this phase are secondary to malfunctions in other phases. Disorders of excitement undermine the evolution of the plateau phase. Orgasmic dysfunction prolongs the plateau phase in both genders, leading to discomfort and irritability secondary to lack of release of sexual tension and genital engorgement.

25. What are some causes of orgasmic phase dysfunction?
Peripheral neuropathy, psychodynamic conflict, and medications.

26. What are some medications that cause orgasmic dysfunction?
SSRIs (fluoxetine, paroxetine, and sertraline), monoamine oxidase inhibitors (phenelzine, tranylcypromine), and anticholinergic agents (low-potency neuroleptics, tricyclic antidepressants), can inhibit orgasm. Alpha 2 blockers such as trazadone, prazosin, and thioridazine can impair sperm emission by paralyzing the vas deferens.

27. What helps restore orgasm in patients on SSRIs?
Four milligrams of cyproheptadine, a serotonin antagonist, taken 30 minutes before sexual activity has been reported to help.

28. Are there other antidepressants with few autonomic side effects that are less apt to impact sexual function than SSRIs?
Yes. Examples are nefazadone and bupropion.

29. What are some treatments for premature ejaculation?
SSRIs have been reported to help. Masters and Johnson describe a behavioral method designed to help a couple achieve mastery over ejaculation timing. This technique features deconditioning the anxiety that leads to premature ejaculation. The male communicates to his partner that he is close to ejaculation, and the partner then stops the stimulation, squeezes the glans with the index and third fingers, and presses the urethra with the thumb. The couple can gradually prolong sexual activity before orgasm with this method.

30. Is there a disorder of the resolution phase?
Yes, priapism is an erection that does not go away. It can be caused by alpha blockers, such as trazodone, and penile injections (described in Questions 19 and 20).

CONTROVERSY

31. Is sildenafil safe for treatment of erectile dysfunction?
No: There have been several reports of sudden death following the use of sildenafil. The fatal scenario often involves a man with coronary artery disease (CAD) and poor physical fitness. He becomes sexually active with the aid of sildenafil and suffers a myocardial infarction (MI) as a result of this activity. Emergency medical professionals give intravenous nitrates to this man as part of routine management. The man does not tell them he just took sildenafil. He then becomes hypotensive with an acutely damaged heart. He dies in cardiovascular shock.
Yes: Properly used, sildenafil is a safe medication, even for those with hypertension and CAD. It was developed initially to treat angina, and it was shown to be safe *as long as it was not used in conjunction with nitrates*. In phase II placebo-controlled studies of 2722 patients taking nonnitrate

antihypertensive medications, the discontinuation rate for adverse cardiovascular events for sildenafil was equal to that for placebo.

In these same studies, the incidence of MI for those using sildenafil was 1.7 per 100 man years of treatment, versus 1.4 for those on placebo—yielding no statistically significant difference between the two groups. Open-label sildenafil studies provided an even lower rate of MI: 1 infarction per 100 man years.

Sildenafil clearly is safe as long as it is properly prescribed. Patients receiving sildenafil must be able to tolerate moderate exercise and must not receive nitrate agonists.

BIBLIOGRAPHY

1. Condra M, Morales A, Surridge D, et al: The unreliability of nocturnal penile tumescence recording as an outcome measurement in the treatment of organic impotence. J Urol 135:280–282, 1986.
2. Drugs that cause sexual dysfunction. Med Lett 34:73–78, 1992.
3. Fava M, Rankin M, Alpert J, et al: An open trial of oral sildenafil in antidepressant-induced sexual dysfunction. Psychother Psychosom 67:328–331, 1998.
4. Goldstein I, Lue TF, Nathan-Padma H, et al: Oral sildenafil in the treatment of erectile dysfunction. N Engl J Med 338:1397–1404, 1998.
5. Kaplan HS: The New Sex Therapy. Active Treatment of Sexual Dysfunction. New York, Bruner/Mazel, 1974.
6. Masters W, Johnson V: Human Sexual Inadequacy. Boston, Little Brown, 1970.
7. Morales A, Gingell C, Collins M, et al: Clinical safety of oral sildenafil citrate in the treatment of erectile dysfunction. Int J Impot Res 10:69–74, 1998.
8. Nadig PW: Vacuum constriction devices in patients with neurogenic impotence. Sexuality Disability 12:99–105, 1994.
9. Nathan-Padma H, Hellstrom WJ, Kaiser FE, et al: Treatment of men with erectile dysfunction with transurethral alprostadil. N Engl J Med 336:1–7, 1997.
10. Rendell M, Rajfer J, Wicker P: Sildenafil for treatment of erectile dysfunction in men with diabetes. JAMA 281:421–425, 1999.

71. PSYCHIATRIC ASPECTS OF AIDS

Carl Clark, MD.

1. What are HIV and AIDS?

Human immunodeficiency virus (HIV) is a retrovirus that infects humans and causes various clinical problems ranging from an asymptomatic carrier state to fatal immune deficiency. Acquired immunodeficiency syndrome (AIDS), the most serious form of HIV infection, results from progressive destruction of the immune system.

2. How does HIV act in the body?

HIV propagates best in lymphocytes and leads to the destruction of its host cell, primarily the CD4 helper-inducer cells. Destruction of CD4 helper-inducer cells impairs the body's ability to mount an effective immune response. HIV also infects the central nervous system cells and leads to dysfunctions such as peripheral neuropathies and encephalopathies. Current treatments attempt to stop viral replication and maintain viral suppression in order to assist immune system functioning.

3. How is HIV detected?

HIV antibodies, which develop in most people in response to HIV infection, can be detected by two standard laboratory tests, the enzyme immunoassay (EIA, formerly ELISA, or enzyme-linked immunosorbent assay) and the Western Blot. The EIA uses a reactive serum and is regarded as positive if measured absorbance is equal or greater than a defined cut-off value. The EIA has a sensitivity of 99.7%, but a specificity of only 98.5% (for double-reactive EIAs). Therefore, the EIA is used as a screening test for HIV antibodies. A positive EIA result is confirmed with the Western Blot test, an immunoblot test that detects antibody to specific viral proteins and glycoproteins. The Western Blot is highly specific.

In general, patients are diagnosed with AIDS if they are positive for HIV antibodies and have an opportunistic infection or cancer, HIV encephalopathy, or a helper T-cell (CD4) count < 200 cells/mm^3. The Centers for Disease Control (CDC) developed the original case definition for AIDS in 1981 before understanding of its etiology or pathophysiology.

4. How is HIV transmitted?

HIV is transmitted by three routes: sexual, parenteral, and perinatal.

Sexual transmission of HIV. Get an accurate sexual history to assess a patient's risk of HIV transmission or infection. Sexual transmission may occur when genital secretions and blood are transferred from one partner to another. Risk is decreased by using latex protective barriers (e.g., condoms). Lubricants must be water-based; petroleum or oil-based lubricants damage latex condoms. Note that use of condoms alone will not decrease transmission. Attitudes and feeling about safe sexual practices must be explored and discussed before meaningful and lasting changes occur. Sexual behaviors considered to contribute to HIV transmission include the following (by order of risk):

- Unprotected anal intercourse. HIV transmission may occur when the virus comes in contact with the rectal mucosa. The rectal mucosa may sustain small rectal tears that allow HIV direct entry into the blood stream. Activities that increase the risk of damaging the rectal mucosa prior to intercourse may increase the risk of HIV transmission (e.g., enemas, manual rectal manipulation or "fisting"). Unprotected receptive anal intercourse is more risky than unprotected insertive anal intercourse.
- Oral ingestion of semen. HIV may enter the blood stream through breaks in oral or gastrointestinal mucosa. Epidemiologic studies of homosexual men do not support the ingestion of semen as a risk for HIV infection.
- Oral contact with feces.

Parenteral transmission.

- Before it was possible to screen the blood supply for HIV, transmission occurred through blood products. The primary route of parenteral transmission currently is through the sharing of needles by intravenous drug users. Needle exchange programs are effective in reducing HIV transmission. Cleaning needles also reduces risk for drug users who share needles. The additional step of cleaning a needle before injecting a drug is unreliable because of the intensity of addiction and difficulty in delaying the desired drug effect.

Perinatal transmission. In the United States less than 30% of HIV-infected mothers transmit the virus to their infants. The primary prevention for HIV transmission to infants is to prevent infection in women. Breast feeding may result in HIV transmission to the infant. HIV-infected mothers reduce the risk of transmission by using safe alternatives to breast feeding. The U.S. Public Health Service Task Force recommends the use of zidovudine (AZT) to reduce perinatal transmission of HIV.

5. Which interventions decrease transmission?

Mode of Transmission	Interventions to Decrease Risk
Sexual transmission	Education regarding safe sex practices Latex condoms (with water-soluble lubricants)
Parenteral	Screening of blood products prior to transfusion Needle exchange programs for IV drug users
Perinatal	Primary HIV prevention (see above) ? Avoid breast feeding ? Pharmacologic treatment during pregnancy of HIV-infected mother

6. Describe the epidemiology of HIV infection and AIDS.

In the United States the AIDS epidemic has occurred in all social groups. The largest number of AIDS cases have been in homosexual and bisexual men, followed by intravenous drug users. HIV disease occurs disproportionately in certain racial and ethnic groups. Three-fourths of pediatric cases and fourth-fifths of cases associated with IV drug use occur in minorities. The AIDS epidemic has paralleled the drug epidemic. Primary prevention efforts have resulted in a decrease in new cases of HIV infection in homosexual men; however, prevention efforts have been less successful in reducing transmission rates in other populations. Knowledge of the sociocultural aspects of each group is important if primary prevention efforts are to be successful.

7. Describe the psychological and emotional impact of HIV infection.

Patients should receive education about HIV and AIDS before being tested for HIV antibodies. Nevertheless, a patient can never be fully prepared for the emotional impact of learning that he or she is HIV-positive. This information disrupts the psychological state of the patient and may lead to a stress response that includes a process of denial (refusal to believe or hear the information about being HIV-positive), disorganization (being flooded with thoughts, fantasies, and feelings about being HIV-positive), symptom formation (e.g., anxiety, sadness, depression, anger), and an adaptive or maladaptive response. Examples of *adaptive responses* include incorporation of the information into personal lifestyle and active attempts to promote well-being and health. Examples of *maladaptive responses* include denial, avoidance of medical care, impulsive behaviors, suicidal behavior, and other behaviors that do not help patients to attend to their health needs, including continued high-risk sexual behavior. Symptoms are assessed for severity and for their impact on the person's ability to deal with the current situation.

8. How might anxiety affect the HIV-positive patient?

Anxiety may produce somatic symptoms, nervousness, sweating, tremors, gastrointestinal disturbances (diarrhea, nausea), or visual impairments. Such symptoms can result from HIV illness, anxiety, or both; elicit a careful history to determine the cause of the dysfunction. Reactions to being HIV-positive rarely result in specific anxiety disorders such as phobias, generalized anxiety disorder, or panic disorder. A form of posttraumatic stress disorder has been described.

Treatment interventions include supportive therapy and referral to community support groups and agencies that can assist with both the physical and emotional impacts of the illness. Family members (both biologic and chosen) should receive education about the disorder and supportive counseling.

9. Is treatment of depression advisable in the HIV-positive patient?

Depression ranges from mild symptoms with little interference in the person's functioning to major depression. Treatment is indicated if the depression interferes with the person's functioning and does not depend on the underlying medical condition. The psychiatric consultant should differentiate between major depression and the cognitive deficits that may accompany early signs of dementia.

Treatment interventions include cognitive therapy, group therapy, and antidepressant medications or psychostimulants. People with HIV infection can be especially vulnerable to the memory impairments caused by the anticholinergic side effects of antidepressants. Therefore, selection of antidepressants with the least anticholinergic side effects is recommended (e.g., venlafaxine, fluoxetine). People in support groups may become demoralized when members of the group die. In general, groups are more effective if the members of the group have a similar stage of HIV infection (e.g., grouping individuals who are asymptomatic or individuals with AIDS).

10. Is psychosis a possible response?

Psychosis may result from the direct effect of HIV infection in the brain. The differential diagnosis includes acute CNS infections, drug reactions, untreated psychiatric disorders (e.g., bipolar disorder or psychotic depression), and continued effects of drug abuse in the drug-using population.

Treatment includes antipsychotic medications with minimal anticholinergic side effects (e.g., risperidone, haloperidol), in the lowest effective dose; behavior management; and, in severe cases, electroconvulsive therapy.

11. When does a patient need a psychiatric evaluation?

Patients who experience a disturbance in mood, cognition, or behavior that interferes with their ability to care adequately for themselves or to keep themselves safe warrant a psychiatric consultation. Emergency intervention is necessary when patients are suicidal, homicidal, or unable to care for themselves. Suicide rates are higher for people with chronic illnesses than for the general population. People with AIDS have a 7.4-fold higher rate of suicide than the general population; people who are HIV-positive also have higher rates of suicide. HIV seropositivity may be a significant risk factor for suicide in general hospital patient populations. Some communities of people living with AIDS consider suicide a legitimate response to the debilitation of the disease and dementia. This view was supported by the Hemlock Society in *Final Exit* (1991). Patients with suicidal ideation must be carefully evaluated for major depression, dementia, and/or delirium.

12. Describe HIV dementia.

HIV dementia is a syndrome of progressive dementia that results from direct infection of the brain with HIV. The diagnosis is difficult to make and requires documentation of HIV infection accompanied by decrements in abstract reasoning, difficulties in learning and memory, self-reports of changes in cognition and motor functioning, and observations of such changes by friends and family. The differential diagnosis includes other neurologic diseases associated with HIV (such as CNS infection, neoplasms), medication-induced cognitive impairments, alcohol- and drug-induced impairments, and malnutrition or other metabolic imbalances.

Clinical Manifestations of HIV-Related Dementia

Early Stages

• Cognitive impairments	• Psychotic symptoms
Short-term memory deficit; forgetfulness rather than amnesia	Hallucinations
Decreased concentration and attention	Suspiciousness and delusions
Confusion and disorientation	Agitation and inappropriate behavior
Overall intellectual ability generally well preserved until late in the disease	• Motor symptoms
Visuospatial perception deficits	Ataxia, loss of coordination, weakness
• Changes in personality or behavior	Tremors
Apathy, decreased interest	• Generalized systemic symptoms
Impaired judgment, erratic behavior	Fatigue, sleep changes (hypersomnia)
Social withdrawal	Anorexia, weight loss
Rigidity of thought	Enuresis
Speech impairment: slow dysarthria, hypophonia, difficulty in following other speakers	Hypersensitivity to medications and alcohol

Advanced Stages

• Cognitive symptoms	• Motor symptoms
Global cognitive impairment	Ataxia
Rudimentary or impaired social relationship	Spastic weakness
Disorientation	Paraplegia, quadriparesis
Psychomotor retardation, decreased spontaneity	Hyperreflexia, myoclonus, seizures
Agitation, "sundowning" (e.g., nighttime delusions)	Bladder and bowel incontinence
Coma	

13. What is a critical factor to consider when HIV dementia is present?

Safety is a concern for demented patients and their caregivers. Caring for a patient with dementia is physically and emotionally demanding. Often, significant others try to care for the severely demented patient for longer than they can reasonably do so. Hospice and nursing home care should be considered. The patient and family may struggle with such options, feeling that they represent surrender to the disease. Work is needed to help them to understand that getting assistance with the symptoms of the illness is not the same as giving up on the patient.

14. What is the risk of acquiring HIV infection in a health care setting?

The fear of infection is a complex response based on personal history and development, including cultural and emotional components. Health care workers should educate themselves about the risk of acquiring an infection from blood-borne pathogens. Universal blood and body fluid precautions protect health care workers from the probability of infection with HIV, hepatitis B, or other blood-borne pathogens. HIV is not acquired through casual contact such as hand shaking or physical examination.

15. What is safe sex?

Safe-sex practices decrease the risk of acquiring HIV infection through sexual transmission. The goal is to modify behavior. Most educators currently use a risk reduction model when working with sexually active adults who want to decrease unsafe sexual behaviors. This model encourages people to continue attempts at behavior modification, even if they have an episode of unsafe sex. Safe-sex education has been successful in decreasing transmission rates of HIV in the homosexual community; recent reports, however, show that some gay men have begun to disregard safe-sex practices.

Safe sex may be difficult for some women to negotiate if they feel that discussions with their partner may threaten other aspects of the relationship or influence self-perception. This issue may be particularly difficult for adolescents.

Note that alcohol and drug use decreases adherence to safe-sex guidelines and has been associated with behaviors that transmit HIV.

Safe Sex Guidelines

SAFE	POSSIBLY SAFE	UNSAFE
Mutual masturbation	Anal or vaginal intercourse with a condom	Receptive anal intercourse without a condom
Social (dry) kissing		
Body massage, hugging	Fellatio (sucking; stopping before climax)	Insertive anal intercourse without a condom
Body-to-body rubbing (frottage)	Mouth-to-mouth kissing (French kissing, wet kissing)	Manual-anal intercourse (fisting)
Light S & M activities (without bruising or bleeding)	Urine contact (water sports)	Fellatio (sucking to climax)
Using one's own sex toys	Cunnilingus (oral-vaginal contact)	Oral-anal contact (rimming)
		Any activities involving bruising or bleeding (heavy S & M)
		Using someone else's sex toys

16. How should the clinician teach patients about prevention of HIV transmission?

Patients must understand that they cannot be given absolute assurance that their sexual activities are safe; they must assess the relative risk of their sexual behaviors. Although HIV has been detected in saliva, there are no documented cases of transmission through saliva. Patients must assess whether they will alter their kissing behaviors based on this information and how they judge the relative risk of each behavior. Safe-sex education addresses the emotional impact of changing sexual behaviors (for example, the need to eroticise the use of condoms). Many communities offer courses on safe-sex practices through public health departments or community-based AIDS organizations. Questions from physicians or medical personnel about sexual practices may be the first opportunity for patients to discuss openly their concerns about HIV infection.

17. How does HIV infection affect the patient's sexual self-image?

Some HIV-infected patients come to view themselves as pariahs who no longer deserve sexual feelings or expression. Fear of transmitting the virus may stop all sexual activities. Fear of rejection by a sex partner may interfere with self-disclosure about HIV status. Issues of sexuality need to be addressed to help HIV-positive patients make informed decisions about future sexual activities. *Risk assessment should be based on current knowledge*, not on uninformed fears and misconceptions.

18. How does discrimination interfere with the treatment of a person with AIDS?

HIV and AIDS have affected large numbers of gay and bisexual men. Especially in the earlier years of the epidemic, discrimination against people with AIDS was based on homophobia, prejudice, and fear of contagion. Discrimination also occurs because people fear transmission of HIV. Homophobia is the fear and rejection of homosexuality and homosexuals; the attitude that homosexuality is undesirable, hateful, or evil; and a condensation of various negative cultural stereotypes about gay men and lesbians. As the epidemic has continued, education about homosexuality in the U.S. has helped to decrease the negative stereotypes of gay people.

Gay men and lesbians may be reticent to disclose their sexual orientation to healthcare providers for fear of receiving inferior care. Healthcare providers may be uncomfortable treating them because of strong cultural beliefs, feelings, or views about homosexuals. Healthcare providers must address such issues so that patient care is not compromised. HIV-infected people may be concerned about confidentiality and fear discrimination in the workplace, from both employers and employees.

Each state has its own statutes concerning the reporting of HIV status to the health department. In confidential reporting of HIV status, a person's name is kept on record at the health department in confidential files. Health departments with such approaches try to assure the public that records are safe from public disclosure. In states with anonymous testing for HIV, information about the number of HIV positive tests is known, but no record of the HIV-positive person is kept.

The largest rise in new cases of HIV infection is among minority groups. Racism and culturally inappropriate educational materials contribute to the ineffective preventive efforts among ethnic populations.

19. How should the clinician teach intravenous drug users about prevention of HIV transmission?

Needle exchange programs have been shown to be effective in decreasing HIV transmission. Complex social barriers prevent real implementation of this intervention. Clean needles must be used to decrease transmission of HIV and hepatitis. Some states have programs that teach drug users to clean needles with bleach and/or water. Cleaning of needles is somewhat effective. Bleach may cause blood to clot in needles, and clots may lead to transmission of HIV. Addicts may have difficulties in taking time to clean needles, especially when they are withdrawing from their drug of choice.

20. How can the clinician introduce the topic of HIV and AIDS in history taking?

The mnemonic AIDS facilitates interviewing and identifies patients at risk for HIV infection. The mnemonic begins with a general and less threatening question before moving to more specific questions that deal with sensitive areas.

A = **A**re you afraid you may have been exposed to AIDS?
I = **I**ntravenous drug use
D = **D**iagnostic signs and symptoms of HIV infection
S = **S**exual behaviors

A "yes" answer to any question signals the need for further exploration and consideration of serologic testing for HIV.

21. What are the particular issues of discrimination for families?

Children with AIDS frequently come from families in which multiple members may be infected with HIV. Complex social problems often face such families, including drug addiction, poverty, and social ostracism. Communication among family members may be thwarted by the need to keep HIV infection a secret. This need often is a result of the family's fear of discrimination for the child in nursery or school settings. HIV-positive children are confronted with the deterioration of developmental skills, social isolation, and the possibility of imminent death. HIV-infected mothers are confronted with the question of how their child became infected. They must cope with illness, motherhood, disclosure of information about the illness to their children, and the effect of HIV infection on their reproductive choices.

BIBLIOGRAPHY

1. Alfonso CA, Cohen MA, Aladjem AD, et al: HIV seropositivity as a major risk factor for suicide in the general hospital. Psychosomatics 35:368–373, 1994.
2. Chung JY, Magraw MM: A group approach to psychosocial issues faced by HIV-positive women. Hosp Community Psychiatry 43:891–894, 1992.
3. Cote TR, Biggar RJ, Dannenberg AL: Risk of suicide among persons with AIDS—a national assessment. JAMA 268:2066–2068, 1992.
4. Mahler J, Stebinger A, Yi D, et al: Reliability of admission history in predicting HIV infection among alcoholic inpatients. Am J Addictions 3:222–226, 1994.
5. Mueller TL, Swift RM: Screening for risk of HIV exposure using the A-I-D-S mnemonic. Am J Addictions 1:203–209, 1992.

72. PSYCHIATRIC CONSULTATION IN PATIENTS WITH CARDIOVASCULAR DISEASE

Andrew B. Littman, M.D.

1. Describe type A behavior.

The best known psychosocial risk factor for the development of coronary artery disease (CAD) is the type A behavior pattern. Type A behavior is defined as the habitual response to perceived demands with impatience and easily provoked aggravation, anger, and/or aggression. The global type A concept includes components of hard-driving nature, perfectionism, and low self-esteem. These global factors have waned in importance as **hostility** repeatedly has been found to be the toxic element of the type A syndrome. Hostility is linked to poor CAD outcomes by numerous mechanisms: increased atherosclerosis and sudden cardiac death, precipitation of myocardial ischemia and coronary vasospasm, and persistent cigarette smoking.

2. What other psychosocial factors are associated with poor outcomes in CAD?

Lack of social support	Phobic anxiety
Social isolation and/or alienation	Anxiety disorders
Low socioeconomic status	Vital exhaustion
Lack of economic resources	Depressive symptoms
Job strain (low control and high demand)	Major depressive disorder

3. What is the impact of major depressive disorder and depressive symptoms in patients with CAD?

The impact is profound. Major depressive disorder is common in patients with CAD, and 20% have depressive disorder before their cardiac diagnosis. Only around 30% of these depressed patients and virtually none of the patients with depressive symptoms alone are diagnosed or treated. In a recent study, 18% of patients hospitalized for myocardial infarction (MI) had major depressive disorder, and depression predicted mortality at 6 months with a relative risk of 4.3, equivalent to left ventricular dysfunction and history of previous MI, the most potent prognostic measures known.

In the past, in the absence of full-blown major depressive disorder, depressive symptoms were considered to be self-limited and of minimal importance. However, depressive symptoms also are common in coronary patients (18–40%). Like major depressive disorder, depressive symptoms commonly predate the onset of the initial clinical manifestations of CAD.

The impact of depressive symptoms and disorder on functional status and quality of life equals that of organic cardiac factors, such as left ventricular function. In addition, depressive syndromes are related to poorer adherence to medical treatment, lack of improvement of exercise functioning in coronary patients undergoing an exercise program, and increased risk of coronary atherosclerotic morbidity and mortality in studies of patients with pre-existing coronary disease as well as in population-based studies.

4. Is the behavioral treatment of stress effective in patients with CAD?

A number of treatments can be effective in reducing type A behavior and anger in patients with CAD, including yoga, emotional support, and group therapy. The most effective techniques are comprehensive in their scope, involving education, training in coping methods with either a relaxation or cognitive focus, and frequent training with behavioral techniques.

The earliest studies of stress modification in patients having had an MI employed group cognitive behavioral therapy and showed a reduction of 50% in 3-year combined mortality and recurrent MI. A more recent study by Frasure-Smith of patients with MI evaluated the impact of stress monitoring and reduction. The mortality rate was three times higher for highly stressed patients who did not receive treatment than for highly stressed patients who received stress-reduction treatment.

5. Are special diets beneficial?

Ornish used a multi-modal treatment of comprehensive lifestyle change, low-fat vegetarian diet (less than 8% total calories from fat), stress management, and moderate exercise in an attempt to reverse coronary atherosclerosis without lipid-lowering drugs. Both 1- and 4-year followups showed continued progression of atherosclerosis in the usual care group compared with regression of atherosclerosis in the comprehensive intervention group.

The Mediterranean diet, which is not as fat-restrictive as Ornish's approach but does feature sharp reductions in saturated and animal fat as well as increases in monosaturated fat (olive oil) and omega-3 fatty acid (fish oils and some nuts), was used in cardiac patients in the Lyon Heart Study. Dramatic (85%) reductions in recurrent cardiac events and cardiac and all-cause mortality were seen. Moreover, several preliminary controlled trials of omega-3 fatty acid supplementation demonstrate its efficacy in reducing anger and stress reactivity and stabilizing mood.

Note that the efficacy of these dietary interventions does not negate the impact of behavior change in this population.

6. Can pharmacotherapy of type A behavior, anger, and hostility improve CAD morbidity and mortality rates?

This treatment is still in its infancy. In contrast to behavioral treatment, there are no studies currently available evaluating the impact of psychopharmacology on CAD morbidity and mortality. Beta-blockers are effective in reducing mortality in coronary patients with MI. In addition, beta-blockers have been shown to be effective in reducing aggression in the elderly and those with organic brain syndromes. However, trials of beta-blockers have not been successful in reducing type A behavior or hostility in patients with CAD. Benzodiazepines do not alter type A behavior or hostility, but have reduced duration of silent ischemia in a minority of CAD patients.

7. What is the role of serotonin in this risky behavior?

The prevailing hypothesis about the neurobiology of the hostility syndrome suggests that it is produced by low levels of central serotonin. An increasingly large body of literature demonstrates that patients with mood and personality disorders as well as normal volunteers with low levels of central serotonin have a lower threshold for aggressive responses or urges to act angrily.

Serotonergic agents have been used to treat anger in patients with comorbid mood disorders as well as in patients without a current diagnosable psychiatric condition. Anger attacks are common (44%) in individuals with major depressive disorder. Treatment with fluoxetine reduced such expressions of anger by 70%. In addition, in patients with CAD and hostility but with no axis I psychiatric condition, hostility was reduced by treatment with buspirone, a serotonin 1A partial agonist. Thus, serotonergic agents may have a special role in treating type A behavior.

8. What effects do tricyclic antidepressants (TCAs) have on depressed patients with CAD?

TCAs have widespread cardiovascular effects, including tachycardia, orthostatic hypotension, conduction delays, and cardiac rhythm. Desipramine is the least anticholinergic tricyclic compound and thus produces the least tachycardia. Orthostatic hypotension is most common (up to 50%) in patients with congestive heart failure, and nortriptyline produces orthostatic hypotension less frequently than any other tricyclic. Pre-existing defects of the His-Purkinje conduction system, such as bundle branch blocks, put patients placed on TCAs at risk for serious second- or third-degree blocks. Tricyclics also increase the P-R and Q-T intervals and the QRS segment, and shorten T-wave height.

9. Describe the cardiovascular effects of some other antidepressants.

Antidepressants such as amoxapine produce conduction abnormalities and atrial arrhythmias. Maprotiline has caused torsade de pointes, a characteristic malignant ventricular arrhythmia, at the high end of the therapeutic range. Trazodone has little effect on cardiac conduction, produces beneficial hemodynamics, and rarely exacerbates ventricular ectopy. Venlafaxine appears safe in CAD patients, except for an infrequent tendency to produce hypertension at higher doses. Bupropion has no cardiotoxicity or anticholinergic effects. Fluoxetine, sertraline, paroxetine, nefazodone, and citalopram appear to have little cardotoxicity, no anticholinergic effects, no effect on the electrocardiogram, and in initial studies, no effect on cardiac function. Thus, these selective serotonin reuptake inhibitors (SSRIs) may be especially safe among patients with CAD. However, each SSRI affects the P450 cytochrome metabolic pathway differently, and drug-drug interactions are increasingly commonplace.

10. Which treatment of depression is best in post-MI patients?

Several studies are now underway to determine which treatment of depression in post-MI patients is safe, effective, and associated with a reduction in morbidity and mortality. ENRICHD is an NIH study evaluating the use of cognitive behavioral therapy and SSRIs in post-MI patients. SADHART is a strictly psychopharmacologic intervention study of depressed post-MI patients. Both of these studies will be completed shortly.

11. How does patient denial affect cardiac illness?

Many patients with CAD deny their emotional reactions, characteristically during the acute phases of a hospitalization for cardiac illness. They also deny the presence of cardiac symptoms, such as angina. In fact, recent studies demonstrate that emotional denial leads to symptom denial and **delay seeking treatment**.

Early research evaluating the effect of emotional denial on morbidity and mortality during acutely stressful hospitalizations for cardiac disease suggested that denial is adaptive. However, followup studies show that emotional denial is deleterious to patients' health over time. One mechanism appears to be that patients with emotional denial have a greater difficulty modifying cardiac risk factors and resume deleterious health behaviors, especially smoking.

12. Does serum cholesterol have an impact on behavior?

Lowering serum cholesterol reduces mortality from coronary atherosclerosis, but may not improve overall survival because of an increase in deaths due to accidents, suicide, and violence. One study demonstrated that lowering dietary fat **increased aggression** and lowered levels of central serotonin in monkeys. Other studies of cholesterol lowering suggested an increased risk of violent death only for patients using medications to lower cholesterol; depressive symptoms were more common in coronary patients treated for hyperlipidemia than in untreated patients. The possible effect of lipid lowering on behavior currently is receiving a great deal of attention. Case reports of hyperlipidemic patients developing depression on lipid-lowering agents are not uncommon. No firm recommendations can be given, except to be observant for behavioral changes in individuals being treated for hyperlipidemia.

13. What is the effect of physical activity on patients with CAD?

Regular aerobic exercise appears to reduce mortality from CAD by 25%. Less recognized is the fact that lower levels of everyday exertion also can be beneficial for coronary patients. Moderate levels of leisure physical activity (30–69 minutes of light-to-moderate activities per day) are enough to **reduce CAD mortality by 63%**; increased levels of leisure activity do not provide more risk reduction.

Aerobic exercise appears to reduce both the cardiovascular and sympathoadrenal responses to mental stress. Yet despite such benefits, adherence to regular exercise is poor; over one-half of patients who initiate an exercise program drop out of the program after several months. Two-thirds of Americans do not exercise regularly. For patients with pre-existing CAD, entry into a comprehensive, structured cardiac rehabilitation program with a credible psychosocial component can help with long-term adherence. Structured, long-term maintenance programs with active social support are now a common feature of many cardiac rehabilitation programs. For patients who do not have a chronic medical illness, adherence to an exercise regimen is enhanced by joining employer-sponsored and conveniently located exercise programs.

14. What is the impact of obesity?

Obesity has a negative impact on hypertension, diabetes mellitus, lipid abnormalities, and physical activity, and is an independent risk for development of coronary atherosclerosis. Approximately one-third of overweight individuals who attempt to lose weight maintain the loss; two-thirds regain the weight. Successful weight-reduction programs focus on long-term change in dietary behavior, with restriction of dietary fat intake and behavioral modification of eating habits and dietary urges. Exercise four times per week is also a critical element. If weight loss cannot be maintained or initiated, a small (10–15%) reduction in weight in addition to a regular exercise program may help minimize the medical risks of obesity.

15. Can obesity be treated pharmacologically?

Since amphetamines were a common tool of weight loss 20 years ago, until recently, pharmacologic interventions to reduce weight were not used. The frequent application of a combination of dexfenfluramine, an indirect and direct serotonergic agent, and phentermine, sometimes called fen/phen, was halted with the finding of heart valve thickening in a subgroup of patients taking this drug combination. Currently, many clinical research programs are evaluating novel drugs, which work by a host of different mechanisms, for efficacy in weight loss. See Chapter 79 for a fuller discussion of obesity treatment.

16. Can systemic arterial hypertension be treated with behavioral techniques?

Many studies have shown that psychosocial stress is associated with elevated arterial blood pressure (BP). Although relaxation training and biofeedback can significantly reduce both systolic and diastolic BPs, and apparently generalize this effect to nontraining periods for some time, only one study demonstrated the effectiveness of these stress management tools in reducing BP. Nine other studies demonstrated only a minimal (2 mmHG) drop in diastolic BP in nonmedicated patients. Recent research comparing the effects of dietary sodium restriction, stress management, nutritional supplementation, and weight reduction showed beneficial effects only from weight reduction and, secondarily, sodium restriction. Thus, the behavioral technique of choice for reducing BP appears to be **weight reduction**—in conjunction with antihypertensive medication.

17. How can I assist compliance with antihypertensive treatment?

There are several components to successful treatment of noncompliance in patients with hypertension or medical illness:

• A drug profile with minimal negative effect on **quality of life** is critical. The selection process involves matching the drug's side effects to the patient's physiologic state (e.g., congestive heart failure, persistent tachycardia, sleep disturbance) and to the patient's priorities and values concerning physical and mental functioning. In studies of quality of life among patients receiving antihypertensive drugs, captopril was shown to be superior to other agents. However, the advent of numerous new antihypertensive agents with even better side-effect profiles has increased the clinician's options.

• The **dosing regimen** should match the current one or minimize the number of doses a day.

• **Patient education** should provide information about their illness and medication, so that they recognize the risks and benefits.

• Psychiatric elements such as subtle mood, anxiety, post-traumatic stress, substance abuse, or organic cognitive disorders, may impair compliance. Often the patient's past personal experiences with illness, dependency, or loss help explain the lack of compliance. **Treatment of disorders** and recognition of the coping style of the patient may dramatically improve compliance.

18. How can I help my patients stop smoking?

If you are working in a primary care setting, track your patients' smoking status, briefly discuss the hazards of smoking in a personalized way, and work with them to agree on a specific date for attempting to quit. This approach doubles the quit rate, from 4% to around 8% per year. For patients who require additional help, standard behaviorally based smoking cessation programs have long-term quit rates of approximately 30%. These programs are psychoeducational, providing didactic information about nicotine addiction and the process of quitting; specific behavioral coping techniques for withdrawal symptoms and relapse prevention; assertiveness and relaxation training; and group social support. The effectiveness of smoking cessation programs is maximized when behavioral skills are taught, in contrast to a strictly didactic approach.

19. What are some products that are helpful in smoking cessation?

Nicotine chewing gum improves long-term quit rates, but its effectiveness depends on several elements. It appears to have minimal effect if used outside specialized smoking cessation programs, without clear instructions about use, or without adequate social support. Transdermal nicotine patches are commonly used and effective, especially in a structured program. In addition, nicotine now can be delivered therapeutically as a nasal spray or inhaled into the lungs.

20. How are depression and other mood states related to smoking?

New findings link depressive and impulsive disorders with cigarette smoking. Individuals with higher smoking rates, a history of regular smoking, or difficulty quitting smoking have a history of major depressive disorder or impulsivity more frequently than those who find it relatively easy to quit smoking. In addition, when patients with a history of depression quit smoking, depressive symptoms or disorder commonly recurs. Thus, such individuals are much less likely to mount a successful quit attempt. Other mood states, such as anger, impatience, and tension, as well as sleep disturbance are predictive of inability to quit smoking.

21. What is the role of medication in smoking cessation?

First, try behavioral treatment for smokers who have high baseline levels of mood disturbance or develop such symptoms in the process of quitting. If the symptoms do not improve with behavioral treatment, undertake psychopharmacologic treatment. **Doxepin** and **nortriptyline** improve quit rates in depressed smokers, and **SSRIs** improve the quit rate to the rates seen in nondepressed smokers. **Buspirone** reduces craving, irritability, restlessness, and dysphoria during nicotine withdrawal, and smokers with high anxiety have significantly improved quit rates compared to placebo. **Bupropion**, usually prescribed in slow-release form, improves quit rates in nondepressed smokers. Bupropion especially helps smokers who have difficulty controlling their nicotine cravings. In addition, use of bupropion for up to 1 year after quitting smoking improves the 1-year quit rate compared to those smokers who only use bupropion for 8 weeks to assist in smoking cessation.

22. What are the causes of disability in patients with CAD?

The physical manifestations of CAD have a profoundly negative effect on functional status and quality of life. It is less recognized that depressive symptoms and depressive disorder have a similar effect, in an independent manner. This additional negative effect can be ameliorated by direct treatment of the depressive disorder. In addition, approximately 25% of patients with CAD do not return to work after an MI. Work disability is predicted by low educational level, number of previous MIs, and degree of depression. Level of depression is the best predictor of job loss after an MI.

Current clinical practice dictates referral to a cardiac rehabilitation program for patients whose functional or work status is impaired, and further psychiatric evaluation for patients who fail to improve to a level clearly explained by their physiologic status during the rehabilitation program.

23. How is sexual function altered in patients with CAD?

The majority of patients with CAD have diminished sexual desire and frequency of sexual activity; impotence is not uncommon. There are numerous causes for sexual dysfunction, but cardiac function alone is a relatively rare cause. Physiologic capacity to resume sexual activity has been reached when the patient can climb two flights of stairs at a brisk pace. The occasional patient experiences angina during sex; prophylactic nitroglycerine or changing positions so that there is less isometric muscular tension is helpful. *Permission to resume sexual activity and unambiguous responses to the patient's and partner's concerns and fears are critical to successful recovery of sexual function.* Patients with CAD also may have medication-related, neurogenic, or vascular causes for sexual dysfunction. Beta-blockers frequently are the culprit. Often overlooked are marital conflicts after a serious cardiac event; they are common when convalescence includes poor sexual adjustment.

24. What are important psychiatric causes of noncardiac chest pain?

A common presenting symptom of patients in general medical as well as specialty cardiology settings is chest pain without objective organic findings to explain the symptoms. Historically such patients have been labeled as having neurocirculatory asthenia, syndrome X, or hyperventilation syndrome. They frequently have demonstrated psychiatric symptoms, such as anxiety, mood, and somatization disorders. Some series have demonstrated a 50% incidence of panic disorder in patients in cardiology clinics with noncardiac chest pain. Controlled trials of cognitive-behavioral therapy and antidepressants, such as imipramine, have shown persistent reduction of pain, psychosocial limitations, and distress for patients with atypical noncardiac chest pain, even in the absence of panic disorder.

BIBLIOGRAPHY

1. Beitman BD, Basha I, Flaker G, et al: Atypical or nonanginal chest pain, panic disorder, or coronary artery disease? Arch Int Med 147:1548–1552, 1987.
2. Fava M, Rosenbaum JF, Pava JA, et al: Anger attacks in unipolar depression. Part 1: Clinical correlates and response to fluoxetine treatment. Am J Psychiatry 150(8):1158–1163, 1993.
3. Frasure-Smith N, Lesperance F, Talajic M: Depression following myocardial infarction: Impact on 6-month survival. J Am Med Assoc 270:1819–1825, 1993.
4. Hlatky MA, Haney T, Barefoot C, et al: Medical, psychological, and social correlates of work disability among men with coronary artery disease. Am J Cardiol 58:911–915, 1986.
5. Littman AB: Prevention of disability due to cardiovascular disease. Heart Dis Stroke 2:274–277, 1993.
6. Littman AB, Fava M, McKool K, et al: The use of buspirone in the treatment of stress, hostility, and type A behavior in cardiac patients: An open trial. Psychother Psychosom 59:107–110, 1993.
7. Littman AB: A review of psychosomatic aspects of cardiovascular disease. In Fava GA, Freyberger H (eds): Handbook of Psychosomatic Medicine. Madison, CT, International Universities Press, 1998, pp 261–294.
8. Littman AB, Ketterer MW: Behavioral medicine in consultation-liaison psychiatry. In Rundell J, Wise M (eds): American Psychiatric Press Textbook of Consultation-Liaison Psychiatry, 1st ed. Washington, D.C., American Psychiatric Press, Inc., 1996, pp 1080–1109.
9. Milani RV, Littman AB, Lavie CJ: Depressive symptoms predict functional improvement following cardiac rehabilitation and exercise program. J Cardiopul Rehab 13:406–411, 1993.
10. Milani RV, Littman AB, Lavie CJ: Psychological adaptation to cardiovascular disease. In Messerli FH (ed): Cardiovascular Disease in the Elderly, 3rd ed. Boston, Kluwer Academic Publishers, 1993, pp 401–412.
11. Ornish D, Brown SE, Scherwitz LW, et al: Can lifestyle changes reverse coronary heart disease? Lancet 336:129–133, 1990.
12. Rosal M, Downing J, Littman AB, Ahern DK: Sexual functioning post-myocardial infarction: Effects of beta-blockers, psychological status, and safety information. J Psychosom Res 38(7):655–667, 1994.
13. Wells KB, Stewart A, Hays RD, et al: The functioning and well-being of depressed patients: Results from the medical outcome study. J Am Med Assoc 262:914–919, 1989.

73. CONSULTATION FOR THE CANCER PATIENT

Andrew Roth, M.D., Mary Jane Massie, M.D., and William H. Redd, Ph.D.

1. What are the most stressful times for cancer patients and their families?
- Learning of the diagnosis of cancer
- Beginning any new treatment (surgery, radiation, chemotherapy)
- Waiting for test results
- Learning that treatment efforts have failed or of disease recurrence
- Undergoing painful medical procedures
- Struggling with uncontrolled pain

Psychiatrists and psychologists often are asked to bolster patients' and families' coping skills during these crisis points. Issues of dying, palliative care, and end-of-life decisions (such as health care proxies and "do not resuscitate" orders) also must be dealt with. Patients' families have to manage their own fatigue, put much of the rest of their lives on hold, and tolerate frequent interruptions in work, parenting, social, and school schedules while providing support and practical services for their loved one.

2. Do all cancer patients get depressed?
No. Reported rates of major depression in patients with cancer vary widely (1–53%), depending on the measures used and the population studied. Increased rates are noted in patients with more advanced disease. Most patients experience a brief period of denial or despair followed by distress with a mixture of symptoms of depressed mood, anxiety, insomnia, anorexia, and irritability. They have difficulty carrying out daily activities and lingering thoughts about the uncertain future. These symptoms last for days to several weeks, after which usual patterns of adaptation return. During crisis points, distress typically recurs.

This normal response is highly variable and is modulated by medical factors, such as extent of disease, physical symptoms, degree of debilitation, and prognosis. About 25% of cancer patients continue to have high levels of anxiety and depression persisting for weeks to months. These disorders are called **adjustment disorders** with depressed, anxious, or mixed moods depending on the major symptoms.

Of course, before making any diagnosis of depression or anxiety, the clinician must first consider whether uncontrolled pain or other cancer symptoms are causative.

3. Given that many cancer patients are distressed, how is depression diagnosed in patients with cancer?
When a patient's depressed mood is persistent or worsening and is accompanied by hopelessness, despondency, guilty feelings, and suicidal ideation, major depression is the likely diagnosis. Depression is treatable and is not "normal" in most patients with cancer. The patient's mood, physical symptoms (vegetative or somatic) of depression, and the severity of depression, including suicide risk, must be assessed. Carefully evaluate whether physical symptoms such as fatigue, insomnia, and decreased libido are caused by depression, cancer, or the treatment. Doctors often underestimate the morbidity caused by depression, because they tend to believe that they would feel depressed, even suicidal, if the roles were reversed.

The biologic correlates of depression, or neurovegetative symptoms (e.g., decreased appetite, insomnia, fatigue, loss of energy, loss of libido, and psychomotor slowing), are the best measures for depression in physically healthy adults. They are, however, unreliable in cancer patients who often have no appetite because of chemotherapy, sleep poorly due to pain or because they are hospitalized, and are fatigued by the cancer and the radiation therapy or chemotherapy.

Note that when both depression and debilitation are present in patients with advanced cancer, it is difficult to decide which condition is primary, and a trial of antidepressants is warranted.

Questions Used to Assess Depressive Symptoms in Cancer Patients

QUESTION	SYMPTOM
Mood	
How well are you coping with your cancer? Well? Poorly?	Difficulty coping
How are your spirits since diagnosis? Down? Blue? During treatment? Depressed? Sad? Do you cry sometimes? How often? Only alone?	Depression
Are there things you still enjoy doing or have you lost pleasure in things you used to do before you had cancer?	Anhedonia
How does the future look to you? Bright? Black?	Hopelessness
Do you feel you can influence your care or is your care totally under others' control?	Helplessness
Do you worry about being a burden to family and friends during treatment for cancer?	Worthlessness
Feel others might be better off without you?	Guilt
Physical Symptoms (Evaluate in the context of cancer-related symptoms)	
Do you have pain that isn't controlled?	Pain
How much time do you spend in bed? Weak? Fatigue easily? Rested after sleep? Any relationship to change in treatment or how you feel otherwise physically?	Fatigue
How is your sleeping? Trouble going to sleep? Awake early? Often?	Insomnia
How is your appetite? Food tastes good? Weight loss or gain?	Decreased appetite
How is your interest in sex? Extent of sexual activity?	Decreased libido
Do you think or move more slowly?	Psychomotor slowing

4. What medical conditions and medications cause depression in cancer patients?

- Uncontrolled Pain
- Metabolic Abnormalities
  - Hypercalcemia
  - Sodium, potassium imbalance
  - Anemia
  - Deficient vitamin B_{12} or folate
- Endocrinologic Abnormalities
  - Hyper- or hypothyroidism
  - Adrenal insufficiency

- Medications
  - Steroids
  - Interferon and interleukin-2
  - Methyldopa
  - Reserpine
  - Barbiturates
  - Propranolol
  - Some antibiotics (amphotericin B)
  - Some chemotherapeutic agents (vincristine, vinblastine, procarbazine, L-asparaginase)

Uncontrolled pain is a common cause of depressed mood in cancer patients. It is accompanied by symptoms of anxiety and a sense of anguish that life is intolerable unless pain is relieved. Patients interpret a new or increasingly severe pain as a sign that the cancer has progressed, resulting in greater depression and hopelessness. Suicide is a real risk in these patients, especially if they do not believe that efforts are being made to control the pain or that pain relief is possible. Suicidal ideation and major depressive symptoms usually abate when the pain is controlled.

When medical conditions are the cause of depressed mood, the mood can usually be reversed when the condition is reversed, or with antidepressant medication.

5. How is depression treated in patients with cancer?

Treatment is directed at helping patients adapt to the stresses they are undergoing and strengthening coping abilities. Individual or group psychotherapy may help clarify the medical situation and the meaning of illness, and support and encourage positive coping strategies. Cognitive therapy, which focuses on inaccurate perceptions and assessments that lead to anxious and depressed feelings, can help patients develop an adaptive perspective.

The use of psychotropic medication is determined by level of distress, inability to carry out daily activities, and response to psychotherapeutic interventions. Antidepressants are used in conjunction with psychotherapeutic interventions for some severe adjustment disorders with depression, as well as major depressive disorders.

6. Which antidepressants are most useful for patients with cancer?

Dosages in Cancer Patients

MEDICATION	START/DAILY DOSE (MG)*	PRIMARY SIDE EFFECTS/COMMENTS
Selective Serotonin Reuptake Inhibitors (SSRIs)		SSRIs have few anticholinergic or cardiovascular side effects
Fluoxetine (Prozac)	10/20–40	Sexual dysfunction including anorgasmia. Headache nausea, anxiety, insomnia. Has a very long half life; may be even longer in debilitated patient.
Sertraline (Zoloft)	25/50–150	Nausea, insomnia
Paroxetine (Paxil)	10/20–50	Nausea, somnolence, asthenia; no active metabolites
Citalopram (Celexa)	20/20–40	Reportedly fewer GI and sexual side effects; fewer problematic interactions with other medications.
Second Generation		
Bupropion (Wellbutrin)	75/200–450	May cause seizures in those with low seizure threshold/brain tumors; initially activating. Fewer sexual side effects. Useful for smoking cessation.
Trazodone (Desyrel)	50/150–200	Sedating; not anticholinergic; risk of priapism
Tricyclics (TCAs)		All TCAs can cause cardiac arrhythmias; blood levels are available for all but doxepin. Get baseline ECG.
Amitriptyline (Elavil)	10–25/50–100	Sedation; anticholinergic; orthostasis
Imipramine (Tofranil)	10–25/50–150	Intermediate sedation; anticholinergic; orthostasis
Desipramine (Norpramin)	25/75–150	Little sedation or orthostasis; moderate anticholinergic
Nortriptyline (Pamelor)	10–25/75–150	Little anticholinergic or orthostatic; intermediate sedation; therapeutic window
Doxepin (Sinequan)	25/75–150	Very sedating; orthostatic hypotension, intermediate anticholinergic effects; potent antihistamine
Psychostimulants		All psychostimulants may cause nightmares, insomnia, psychosis, anorexia, agitation, and restlessness.
d-Amphetamine (Dexedrine)	2.5/5–30	
Methylphenidate (Ritalin)	2.5/5–30	Possible cardiac complications. Give in two divided doses at 8 AM and noon; can be used as analgesic adjuvant and to counter sedation of opiates
Pemoline (Cylert)	18.75/37.5–150	Follow liver tests
Other		
Venlafaxine (Effexor)	75/225–375	Inhibits reuptake of both serotonin and norepinephrine. Achieves steady state in 3 days. May increase blood pressure. Fewer sexual side effects.
Nefazodone (Serzone)	100/200–500	Affects serotonin, $5HT_2$, and norepinephrine; sedating; decreased cardiotoxicity; less reported sexual dysfunction than SSRIs.
Mirtazipine (Remeron)	15/15–45	Sedating at lower doses, useful for agitated depression, insomnia. Less reported GI problems; may cause weight gain. Fewer sexual side effects.

* Starting doses used in cancer patients differ from those prescribed for physically healthy depressed patients.

7. How do I choose an antidepressant?

It is important to consider secondary effects, which may be of positive value. For example, a sedating antidepressant (such as amitriptyline, trazodone, nefazodone, or mirtazipine) is useful for an agitated patient who has difficulty sleeping, because it has both calming and sedating effects. A patient's earlier response to a particular medication, or a family member's experience with an antidepressant, can help predict the response.

An energizing antidepressant or psychostimulant is useful for people experiencing fatigue, either from their disease or medications. Bupropion, nefazodone, and mirtazipine reportedly have fewer sexual side effects than most of the SSRIs. Mirtazipine has fewer GI side effects and may cause weight gain, perhaps a desirable result in a patient having difficulty eating due to the cancer.

8. Describe the selective serotonin reuptake inhibitors.

In the last few years, the SSRIs have become widely used because of their efficacy and low risk of significant side effects.

- **Fluoxetine** side effects: gastric distress and nausea, brief periods of anxiety, headache, insomnia (less common, hypersomnia), and anorgasmia (troubling).
- **Sertraline** side effects: nausea, diarrhea, dyspepsia, tremor, dizziness, ejaculatory delay in men, and insomnia.
- **Paroxetine** side effects: nausea, somnolence, and asthenia.
- **Citalopram** side effects: somnolence.

Sertraline's shorter half-life allows for more rapid hepatic clearance or renal excretion than fluoxetine, often a useful effect in the medically ill. Paroxetine has no active metabolites and therefore also is excreted relatively quickly upon discontinuation. Because all these drugs are strongly protein-bound, consider their ability to increase blood levels of other medications such as coumadin, digoxin, some anticonvulsants, and cisplatin. Citalopram, the newest SSRI available in the U.S., reportedly has fewer GI and sexual side effects and fewer problematic drug-drug interactions than other SSRIs.

9. Describe the tricyclic antidepressants.

In the past, tricyclic antidepressants, or TCAs (amitriptyline, doxepin, imipramine, nortriptyline, and desipramine), were the most commonly used drugs for depression and for the treatment of neuropathic pain. They are started at a low dose (10–25 mg at bedtime), especially in debilitated patients, and increased slowly (by 10–25 mg every few days) until symptoms improve. For reasons that are unclear, depressed cancer patients often show a therapeutic response to a tricyclic at much lower doses (75–125 mg daily) than are usually required in physically healthy depressed patients (150–300 mg daily). Blood levels should be obtained for amitriptyline, imipramine, desipramine, and nortriptyline 5 days after initiating a new dose to prevent toxicity, verify compliance with treatment, and, in the case of nortriptyline, target the therapeutic window of 50–150 ng/ml.

10. How do I know if a tricyclic antidepressant is appropriate?

The choice of a TCA also depends on the nature of the depressive symptoms, medical problems present, and side effects. The depressed patient with psychomotor slowing will benefit from the use of the compounds with the fewest sedating effects, such as desipramine. Patients with stomatitis secondary to chemotherapy or radiotherapy, or with slow intestinal motility or urinary retention, should receive an antidepressant with the fewest anticholinergic side effects. These might include bupropion, trazodone, desipramine, nortriptyline, or an SSRI. Bupropion is less cardiotoxic than TCAs and has an activating effect in withdrawn, medically ill patients. It should be used with caution in patients at risk for seizures or those with brain metastases or primary brain tumors, however, because it is reported to lower the seizure threshold more than other antidepressants.

11. What options are available for the cancer patient having difficulty with oral administration of medication?

Patients who are unable to swallow pills may be able to take an antidepressant in an elixir (amitriptyline, nortriptyline, doxepin, fluoxetine, or paroxetine). Parenteral administration of TCAs can be considered for the cancer patient unable to tolerate oral administration (because of absence of swallowing reflex, presence of gastric or jejunal drainage tubes, or intestinal obstruction). Three TCAs are available in injectable form: amitriptyline, imipramine, and clomipramine. All three have been given intravenously; however, only imipramine and amitriptyline are available for IM injection. The IM route may cause excessive bleeding in the cancer patient with low platelet levels. It also causes discomfort because of the volume of the vehicle; hence 50 mg is usually the maximum dosage that can be delivered per IM injection. Close monitoring of cardiac conduction by electrocardiogram is recommended when these medications are used intravenously.

Hospital pharmacies can prepare some TCAs (e.g., amitriptyline) in rectal suppository form, but absorption by this route has not been studied in cancer patients.

12. Are TCAs useful in the management of neuropathic pain?

Yes. Imipramine, doxepin, amitriptyline, desipramine, and nortriptyline frequently are used in the management of neuropathic pain in cancer patients. Dosing is similar to the treatment of depression, and analgesic efficacy, if it occurs, usually is observed at a dose of 50–150 mg daily; higher doses are needed occasionally. Although the initial assumption was that analgesic effect resulted indirectly from the effect on depression, it is now clear that these tricyclics have a separate specific analgesic action, probably mediated through several neurotransmitters, most prominently norepinephrine and serotonin. TCAs may be used as adjuncts to opioids, as well.

13. What role do psychostimulants play in fighting depression in cancer patients?

The psychostimulants are useful in low doses for patients who are suffering from depressed mood, apathy, depressed energy, poor concentration, and weakness. They promote a sense of well-being, decrease fatigue, and stimulate appetite. They are helpful in countering the sedating effects of morphine, and they produce a rapid effect in comparison to the other antidepressants. Side effects include insomnia, euphoria, and mood lability. High doses and long-term use may produce anorexia, nightmares, insomnia, euphoria, or paranoid thinking.

Treatment with **dextroamphetamine** and **methylphenidate** usually is initiated at a dose of 2.5 mg at 8:00 AM and noon, and increased by 2.5 mg as needed. Typically, patients are maintained on the medication for 1–2 months, after which approximately two thirds can be withdrawn without a recurrence of depressive symptoms. **Pemoline**, a less potent psychostimulant, comes in a chewable tablet so patients who have difficulty swallowing can absorb the drug through the buccal mucosa. Pemoline should be used with caution in patients with renal impairment; liver function tests should be monitored periodically with longer term treatment.

14. How common is anxiety in patients with cancer?

More than two thirds of cancer patients who have a psychiatric disorder have reactive depression or anxiety (adjustment disorder with depressed or anxious mood). About 4–5% have pre-existing anxiety disorders. These disorders can cause severe suffering and compromise clinical care. Early recognition and treatment and a careful search for etiology are essential to optimize patient care.

Reactive anxiety—an exaggerated form of normal anxious response—is the most common type of anxiety in cancer patients. It is distinguished from typical fears of cancer by the duration and intensity of symptoms and the degree of functional impairment, especially noncompliance with treatment. Fearfulness, accompanied by symptoms of anxiety, is expected and *normal* before painful or stressful procedures (e.g., bone marrow aspiration, chemotherapy, radiation therapy, wound debridement); before surgery; and while awaiting test results.

Many anxious patients respond to reassurance and support; some require aggressive treatment. Patients who are extremely fearful may be unable to absorb information or cooperate with procedures; these individuals usually require psychotherapy, medication, and/or behavioral interventions to reduce symptoms to a manageable level.

15. What are the medical causes of anxiety in cancer patients?

Another frequent cause of anxiety in the cancer patient is a set of medical factors: uncontrolled pain, abnormal metabolic states, medications that produce withdrawal states, and, less frequently, hormone-producing tumors. These types of anxiety are classified as anxiety disorders of medical origin.

The acute onset of anxiety may herald a **change in metabolic state** or an **impending cata-strophic event**. Sudden anxiety accompanied by chest pain or respiratory distress suggests a pulmonary embolus. Patients who are hypoxic are anxious and fearful that they are suffocating or dying. Sepsis and delirium also can cause anxiety symptoms.

Many **drugs** can precipitate anxiety in the medically ill. Corticosteroids can produce motor restlessness and agitation, as well as depression and suicidal ideation. Symptoms tend to develop on high doses or during rapid tapering-off. Bronchodilators and beta-adrenergic receptor stimulants used for chronic respiratory conditions can cause anxiety, irritability, and tremulousness.

Akathisia—motor restlessness accompanied by subjective feelings of distress and hyperactivity—is a side effect of several neuroleptic drugs (e.g., prochlorperazine, metoclopramide) used to control emesis. Metoclopramide also causes depression and suicidal ideation in some patients. Ondansetron and granisetron produce few side effects of this kind.

Withdrawal from narcotics, benzodiazepines, barbiturates, and alcohol results in anxiety, agitation, and behaviors which may be problematic in the patient being treated for cancer. Withdrawal after hospital admission often occurs in patients with cancers of the head and neck, because they frequently have histories of heavy alcohol use.

Questions to Ask about Symptoms of Anxiety

• Have you experienced any of the following symptoms since your cancer diagnosis or treatment?

Nervous, shaky, or jittery	Unjustified sweating or trembling
Fearful, apprehensive, and tense	A knot in the pit of your stomach
Avoiding certain places or activities because of fear	A lump in your throat when getting upset
	Pacing back and forth
Heart pounding or racing	Afraid to close your eyes at night for
Trouble catching your breath when nervous	fear of dying in your sleep

• If yes, when do they occur (days before treatment, during procedures, at night, no specific time)?

• How long do the symptoms last?

---

16. List some additional symptoms of anxiety.

Nervousness	Diaphoresis
Tremulousness	Numbness and tingling of extremities
Palpitations	Feelings of imminent death
Shortness of breath	Phobias
Diarrhea	Derealization or depersonalization

17. How would you manage the anxiety associated with pain syndromes?

Patients in severe pain appear anxious and agitated and usually respond to adequate pain control with analgesics. Note that analgesics should never be ordered on an as-needed basis for significant pain because such dosing generates anxiety about control of the pain. Analgesics ordered around-the-clock reach a steady state, which allows the patient to relax and trust that the pain will not return between doses, though rescue doses should be made available. Anxiolytics may be added to pain regimens to control secondary anxiety; however, pain treatment should be the primary focus.

18. What are some other anxiety syndromes seen in cancer patients?

The stress of cancer may reactivate a pre-existing phobia, panic disorder, generalized anxiety disorder, or post-traumatic stress disorder. Some patients become very anxious before surgery, chemotherapy, and painful procedures or dressing changes (anticipatory anxiety), which can be a conditioned anxiety response.

19. How is anxiety treated in cancer patients?

The initial management of anxiety entails providing adequate information and support to the patient. **Psychological approaches** include combinations of cognitive-behavioral therapeutic techniques, brief supportive therapy and crisis intervention, insight-oriented psychotherapy, and behavioral interventions. **Behavioral approaches** such as progressive relaxation, guided imagery, meditation, biofeedback, and hypnosis can be used to treat anxiety symptoms associated with painful procedures, pain syndromes, waiting for results of tests (e.g., prostate specific antigen levels), and anticipatory fears of chemotherapy and radiation therapy or other cancer treatments.

20. What forms of drug therapy are appropriate?

An anxiolytic medication usually is combined with a psychological approach. Choice of a benzodiazepine depends on the duration of action best suited to the patient, desired rapidity of onset, route of administration available, presence or absence of active metabolites, and metabolic problems to be considered. The benzodiazepines most commonly used for the treatment of anxiety in the oncology setting are **clonazepam, lorazepam,** and **alprazolam.** The dosing schedule depends on the patient's tolerance and requires individual titration.

The short-acting benzodiazepines (i.e., alprazolam and lorazepam) are given three to four times per day. They have become widely used with medically ill patients. Alprazolam can be absorbed sublingually for patients who have difficulty swallowing. Clonazepam, a longer-acting drug with antiseizure properties, is useful for panic symptoms and associated insomnia. A drug with a rapid onset of effect (e.g., lorazepam, diazepam) is effective for high levels of distress. Benzodiazepines decrease daytime anxiety and reduce insomnia. The most common side effects of benzodiazepines are dose-dependent and are controlled by titrating the dose to avoid drowsiness, confusion, motor incoordination, and sedation.

All benzodiazepines can cause **respiratory depression** and must be used cautiously (or not at all) in the presence of respiratory impairment. The depressant effects are additive or even synergistic in the presence of other drugs such as antidepressants, antiemetics, and analgesics. Low doses of the antihistamine hydroxyzine, or of the neuroleptic chlorpromazine, are safe and relatively effective when concern exists.

In patients with **hepatic dysfunction**, use short-acting benzodiazepines that are metabolized primarily by conjugation and excreted by the kidney (e.g., oxazepam and lorazepam) or those that lack active metabolites (e.g., lorazepam).

21. What are some alternatives to benzodiazepines?

Buspirone, a nonbenzodiazepine anxiolytic, is useful for elderly patients, for those who have not previously been treated with a benzodiazepine, and for those at risk of habituation with benzodiazepines. It is started at 5 mg t.i.d. and can be increased to 15 mg t.i.d. Low-dose neuroleptics (e.g., thioridazine 10–25 mg t.i.d.) are used to treat severe anxiety when an adequate dose of a benzodiazepine cannot be reached or is not helpful, or when the patient has a mild confusional state accompanied by symptoms of anxiety.

22. What are some medical causes of anxiety in cancer patients?

Akathisia can be quickly controlled by stopping or changing the causative drug (if possible) or by the addition of a benzodiazepine, a beta-blocker such as propranolol, or an antiparkinsonian agent such as benztropine. Treatment of withdrawal states depends on the particular agent. Sometimes the goal is to stabilize the patient on the agent (i.e., a benzodiazepine) and sometimes a suitable substitute can be given (i.e., a benzodiazepine for ethanol or for a barbiturate). Anxiety before chemotherapy or painful procedures and dressing changes is controlled by a short-acting benzodiazepine such as lorazepam, which also provides anterograde amnesia. Given intravenously, lorazepam also reduces vomiting in patients receiving emetogenic chemotherapy. Both oral lorazepam and alprazolam reduce nausea and vomiting related to chemotherapy.

23. Are these patients at risk of addiction?

In general, cancer patients should be encouraged to take sufficient amounts of medication to relieve anxiety and pain. Medications are readily discontinued when symptoms subside; concerns about addiction in cancer patients with no history of drug abuse are exaggerated (see Question 45).

24. What is the most likely psychiatric diagnosis of a patient who was disoriented and agitated when his family was visiting an hour ago, but now is calm?

The most likely diagnosis is **delirium** (also called encephalopathy).Psychiatric consultations frequently are requested for patients who appear depressed, angry, psychotic, or anxious, but on further evaluation are found to be delirious. The distinctions are important, because treatment recommendations are quite different for these disorders. Untreated delirium can lead to death. Delirium, dementia, and other cognitive disorders caused by medical conditions or substances occur in roughly 15–20% of hospitalized cancer patients and in more than 75% of terminally ill cancer patients.

Delirium is an etiologically nonspecific, global, cerebral dysfunction characterized by an inability to maintain or shift attention properly. Other symptoms include decreased levels of consciousness; disturbance in the sleep-wake cycle; disorientation to person, place, or time; abnormal perceptions such as visual or auditory (less frequent) hallucinations; and problems with cognition, such as memory impairment and language disturbance (i.e., dysnomia or dysgraphia). An important diagnostic feature of a delirium is the waxing and waning of these symptoms.

Delirium is distinguished from dementia by more rapid onset, fluctuation in symptoms, potential for reversibility, and less severe memory problems.

25. Which metabolic disorders may cause confusional states and other psychiatric symptoms?

ABNORMALITY	MOOD DISORDER	MANIA	DELIRIUM	DEMENTIA	PSYCHOTIC DISORDER	ANXIETY DISORDER	PERSONALITY CHANGES
Hypercortisolism	+++	++	++	+	+++	+	+
Hypocortisolism	++	—	+	+	+	—	+
Hyperthyroidism	+	+	++	+	++	+++	+
Hypothyroidism	+++	—	++	+	++	—	—
Hypercalcemia	++	—	++	++	++	—	—
Hypoglycemia	++	+	+++	++	++	+++	+
Hyponatremia (SIADH)	++	—	++	++	+	—	—
Hypokalemia	++	—	++	++	+	+	—
Hypophosphatemia	+	—	++	+	—	++	++
Pheochromocytoma	—	—	—	—	—	+++	++

+++ = Frequent; ++ = Common; + = rare; SIADH = sustained inappropriate antidiuretic hormone.
Adapted from Breitbart WB: Endocrine-related psychiatric disorders. In Holland JC, Rowland JH (eds): Handbook of Psycho-oncology: Psychological Care of the Patient with Cancer. New York, Oxford University Press, 1989, pp 356–366; and Breitbart W, Holland JC: Psychiatric Aspects of Symptom Management in Cancer Patients. Washington, APA Press, 1993, p 29.

26. Which chemotherapeutic agents may cause confusional states and other psychiatric symptoms?

AGENTS	DEL	LET	HALL	DEM	DEP	PER	MAN	PSY	EPS	COG
Aminoglutethimide										x
L-Asparaginase	x	x	x							x
5-Azacytidine										x
Bleomycin	x									
Carmustine	x			x						
Cisplatin	x									
Cytosine arabinoside	x	x								x
Dacarbazine				x						

Table continued on following page

AGENTS	DEL	LET	HALL	DEM	DEP	PER	MAN	PSY	EPS	COG
Fludarabine	x		x							x
Fluorouracil	x								x	
Hexylmethylamine			x							
Hydroxyurea			x							
Imidazolecarboxamide (DITC)										x
Interferon	x	x	x		x			x		
Interleukin	x	x	x							x
Isophosphamide	x	x	x							
Methotrexate	x	x		x		x				
Prednisone	x		x		x	x	x	x		x
Procarbazine	x	x	x		x		x			
Vinblastine	x	x	x		x					
Vincristine	x	x	x							

Del = delirium; Let = lethargy; Hall = hallucination; Dem = dementia; Dep = depression; Per = personality change; Man = mania; Psy = psychosis; EPS = extrapyramidal symptoms; Cog = cognitive dysfunction.
Adapted from Breitbart W, Holland JC: Psychiatric Aspects of Symptom Management in Cancer Patients. Washington, DC, APA Press, 1993, p 33.

27. How is delirium diagnosed?

The underlying etiology must be determined, and if possible, reversed. Work-up should include metabolic studies (sodium, potassium, calcium, magnesium, renal functions, liver functions), B12 and folate levels, thyroid function tests, medication review, and, if a CNS infection or hemorrhage is suspected, lumbar puncture. Brain imaging may be necessary.

28. What is the treatment for delirium?

Treatment of delirium includes maintenance of the patient's safety and symptomatic therapy. In drug-induced delirium, the drug (e.g., steroids) often cannot be discontinued or tapered, and the clinical syndrome must be managed with psychotropic medication. Environmental manipulation and a low dose of a neuroleptic are useful for a patient who has a mild delirium without agitation. Frequent reminders by staff or family of location, day, time, and outside events help distract patients from their thoughts, hallucinations, or delusions, and can afford them appropriate orientation.

Haloperidol, a high-potency neuroleptic, used in low dose orally, is the preferred drug for treatment of mild organic mental disorders in patients with cancer. It also can be used safely parenterally. The usual starting dose is 0.5 mg once or twice daily (PO, IV, IM, SC), with doses repeated every 45–60 minutes and titrated against symptoms. Haloperidol provides mild sedation and amelioration of behavioral problems.

Lower potency **neuroleptics** such as thioridazine and chlorpromazine are used in low doses when a more sedating medication is desired; however, they carry increased risk of postural hypotension and anticholinergic effects. Newer atypical neuroleptic agents such as risperidone (Risperdal) and olanzapine (Zyprexa) have not been studied in cancer patients. They show promise because of improved side-effect profiles, particularly less extrapyramidal symptoms. However, their use in delirious patients is limited by lack of parenteral administration.

Benzodiazepines and barbiturates should be avoided because they paradoxically worsen the patient's confusion as active metabolites accumulate.

29. Discuss methods for addressing severely agitated delirium.

When delirium is accompanied by agitation, combativeness, and paranoid thinking, immediate recognition and rapid collaborative intervention by oncologic, psychiatric, nursing, and security staffs is required. Move the patient to a quiet, but visible, area on the unit with a companion, away from potentially dangerous objects, such as scissors, needles, glassware, knives, and other sharp objects. Neuroleptics may be given in oral concentrate form or parenterally, for faster absorption and to assure administration. The minimal effective dose should be used and titrated to achieve sedation but minimal autonomic and extrapyramidal effects. Relatively low doses of haloperidol (1–3 mg/day) are usually effective in treating agitation, paranoia, and fear. Parenteral doses are roughly twice as potent as oral doses. The addition of intravenous lorazepam, 0.5–1 mg every 1–2 hours PO or IV, adds to the sedation produced by haloperidol and may reduce the risk of extrapyramidal effects.

Once stabilized, the patient can be maintained on an oral or intravenous dose of haloperidol that is equivalent to half to two-thirds of the dose required to calm the patient over the initial 24 hours. This may be given two to three times per day.

30. How is terminal delirium controlled?

Methotrimeprazine (IV or SC) often is used to control confusion and agitation in terminal delirium. Dosages range from 12.5–50 mg every 4–8 hours up to 300 mg per 24 hours for most patients. Hypotension and excessive sedation are limitations of this drug. **Midazolam**, given by subcutaneous or intravenous infusion in doses ranging from 30–100 mg over 24 hours, also is used to control agitation related to delirium in terminal stages. The goal of treatment with midazolam and methotrimeprazine is quiet sedation only.

31. What should you do if a patient tells you that he or she has suffered enough and now wants to commit suicide?

Sit down and talk with the patient. Determine whether the suicidal statement is an off-hand comment resulting from frustration or disgust (such as, "If I have to have one more MRI this year, I'll jump out the window") or whether the patient is communicating despair ("I can no longer bear what this disease is doing to all of us"). Does the patient have a plan? Is the patient stockpiling medication? Does the patient own or have access to a weapon?

Note also whether there are psychological predictors (e.g., prior psychiatric disorder, particularly depression or substance abuse; recent bereavement; few social supports) or medical predictors (e.g., poorly controlled pain, advanced stage of disease with debilitation, mild delirium with poor impulse control, or hopelessness or helplessness in the context of depression) that may be contributory. Resolution of these issues facilitates resolution of the suicidal ideation.

Assessing Risk of Suicide

Opening statement: "Most patients with cancer have passing thoughts about suicide, such as 'I might do something if it gets bad enough.'"*

Questions	Issue Addressed
Have you ever had thoughts like that? Any thoughts of not wanting to live or that it would be easier if you died?	Acknowledgment
Do you have thoughts of suicide? Plan? Have you thought about how you would do it?	Seriousness
Have you ever been depressed or made a suicide attempt?	Prior history
Have you ever been treated for other psychiatric problems or have you been psychiatrically hospitalized before getting diagnosed with cancer?	
Have you had a problem with alcohol or drugs?	Substance abuse
Have you lost anyone close to you recently? (family, friends, co-patients)	Bereavement

* Note: statement does not enhance risk.

32. How is the suicidal patient managed?

Management of the suicidal patient includes maintaining a supportive relationship, giving the patient a sense of control by helping him or her to focus on that which can still be controlled, and conveying the attitude that much can be done to improve the quality, if not the quantity, of life. Aggressively treat symptoms such as pain, nausea, insomnia, anxiety, and depression. If the patient is actively suicidal, a 24-hour companion must be provided to establish constant observation, monitor the suicidal risk, and reassure the patient.

33. What if the patient wants your help committing suicide?

Often we say, "We have failed you if suicide seems to be your only alternative." Explore medical and psychological issues that can be reversed. For instance, continuous uncontrolled pain can lead to a desire to be "put out of my misery." Aggressive treatment of pain, depression, insomnia, and anxiety, or at least making an alliance to try to resolve these problems, can help turn the tide for a patient. Patients who are thinking about dying often have specific issues that are frustrating them, and clinicians must help them regain some hope. Perhaps a patient would be more comfortable at home than in the hospital. Staff sometimes arrange for weddings to be moved to the hospital so that a patient can participate in an important family event. The patient's call for help is also an opportunity for clinicians to help mobilize support systems (i.e., family, colleagues, and religious community members). Volunteers can visit patients who are lonely and have no family in the hospital or at home, providing welcome distraction from medical issues.

The issue of physician-assisted suicide is controversial for legal as well as ethical reasons. Discussion of these issues and realistic alternatives for the patient with attending physicians, hospital clergy, and the psychiatrist is strongly encouraged.

34. If a patient wants to join a support group, what should the physician's attitude be?

Supportive and encouraging! Support groups for cancer patients are present in a variety of locales and settings. They often are distinguished by site of disease, professional nature of those running the group, and different schools of therapeutic theory. Note that not all patients want therapy (either individual or group), and not all patients benefit from it. Variables include a person's previous involvement in therapy, psychological mindedness, current social supports, extent of physical disease or limitations, and cognitive deficits. However, two studies have shown that participation in cancer therapy groups improves the quality of patients' lives, and some data suggests they also may increase longevity.

Patients can find out about existing support groups by contacting their local American Cancer Society Chapter, The National Coalition of Cancer Survivors, Cancer Care, Cansurmount, or their local hospital or oncologist.

35. A patient wants to try an alternative cancer therapy. What is your response?

As long as it doesn't interfere with the ongoing traditional therapy and is not harmful, you can be supportive. Many alternative cancer treatments are available both in the United States and abroad. Their respectability has increased in recent years: the National Institutes of Health developed an Office of Alternative Medicine in 1992, and major cancer centers are developing complementary/integrative care programs. Treatments range from outright frauds that can be lethal, to valid modalities aimed at improving well-being. The latter are assumed to enhance the body's ability to fight the cancer. These treatments include nutritional approaches, psychological-spiritual approaches, and immunotherapeutic approaches, or some combination of all of these.

As individuals assume more responsibility for their own health and hold more holistic health beliefs, interest will continue. Physicians are increasingly informed about alternative treatments, and staff should respect patients' consideration of them. Clinicians should encourage questions and offer information on risks and benefits.

36. What can you tell a patient who wants to know more about guided imagery and how it can help?

Guided imagery is a technique that facilitates and deepens relaxation. It adds a component of distraction to other methods of symptom control, e.g., medication. Some patients use guided imagery with the expectation of treating their cancers and controlling tumor growth. They visualize the body's own physiologic defenses fighting cancer cells. For example, the patient may visualize his or her white blood cells as "pac-men" ingesting cancer cells in a particular part of the body.

Note that at this time no compelling scientific evidence indicates that any specific visualization technique has anticancer effects. Patients should discuss these issues with their primary physician. Generally, you can support patients' attempts to cope with their disease, as long as they do not compromise ongoing medical care.

37. Cancer in a child is overwhelming. How does the family react?

Cancer in a child is difficult for the patient and devastating for the family and the healthcare professional. Parents question their competence as caregivers when illness strikes their children. Older siblings are likely to feel guilty, angry, sad, and neglected. A child treated for cancer before age 3 will have virtually no recollection of the experience; his parents will never forget.

38. What is important to understand about how a child copes with cancer?

Specific developmental stages affect a child's understanding and acceptance of various medical procedures, adjustment to strangers, and comfort with machines for advanced medical treatment.

From birth to 2 years of age, important developmental milestones include an appreciation that people will respond in a certain fashion, and that they will meet all needs. Typically the mother is the primary caretaker, from whom the child develops a basic sense of trust and hope. The child also learns an ability to interact with and explore the environment. By the end of this phase children are beginning to master a sense of autonomy and independence.

When parental ties are disrupted by hospitalization during this phase, the effect is profound. Inconsistent parenting, painful procedures, and handling by strangers often lead to helpless feelings, fears, mistrust, and exaggerated stranger anxiety.

39. Does the child react differently at 3 years?

From 3 to 5 years of age, children are experimenting with their autonomy and interacting in the world. A transition to symbolic thought evolves with language development. Fantasy and imaginative play are possible. Cognitive and affective aspects of development predominate. Health and illness are seen as two separate states, not on a continuum, as viewed by older children and adults. Separation from both parents and siblings by hospitalization and other time-occupying treatments is felt acutely. The sick child may show jealousy of healthy siblings and friends.

Play is the primary form of intervention in this period, because of its link with normal growth activity. Rehearsal of procedures, such as pretending to take blood pressures or blood with a play kit, also is helpful. Information given to a child should be concrete, nontechnical, and at the appropriate developmental level for the child, such as: "We need to take a picture of your head while you lie on a table. There will be a great big doughnut surrounding your head, and you'll need to lie very still," rather than, "You are going for an MRI scan of your brain."

40. As treatment of a child progresses, how is the family involved?

Parents are tempted to protect their children and reassert a level of control more appropriate to earlier periods of life. Having parents "room in" during hospitalizations can be useful, but exhausting, which leads to decreased parenting ability.

Cancer in a child of any age often causes parental conflicts over caretaking and difficult emotions for siblings.

Parents' level of distress plays a large role in modulating children's expressions of emotional distress. Therefore, support and education of parents is crucial to treatment of children.

41. How can you help a child between the ages of 6 and 11 handle cancer treatment?

The middle childhood and latency years (ages 6 to 11) are characterized by **entry into school**, a major socializing force in children's lives. Children compare themselves with others and master important developmental tasks. School disruption and isolation of the sick child from peers can have a major impact on the child's sense of competence and self-esteem. At this age, children are aware of the gravity of their disease even if they do not yet have a full appreciation of the irreversibility of death.

The child's reintegration into school can be aided by discussions with the hospital social worker or nurse clinician and workshops for teachers and classmates. Help the patient master various tasks by setting realistic and attainable goals, increasing caretakers' flexibility, modifying tasks, and providing additional support and encouragement.

Treatment for cancer in children can be extremely aggressive and, for many, can be more painful than the disease itself. Repeated infusions of highly emetic chemotherapeutic agents, bone marrow aspirations, lumbar punctures, and venipunctures can be painful and frightening to a child who may not be able to understand their purpose. Some children believe that they can die from procedures. As with younger children, those who are experiencing hair loss or loss of limbs because of their cancer treatment may think that doctors or nurses are punishing them for some wrong deed. Ask the child about such thoughts, and determine if the child understands what is happening. Try to **correct misperceptions**.

Anxiolytic medications can be useful in children; however, many children do not like being sedated and will resist this type of intervention on a regular basis. **Behavioral interventions** such as breathing exercises, attentional distraction, reinforcement, imagery, and behavioral rehearsal are useful for a variety of problems facing children and their parents, including pain, anxiety, and nausea.

42. Adolescence can be a difficult time for a *healthy* teenager. What are some things to know that can help a teenager deal with cancer?

In adolescence, major changes are occurring in the physical, cognitive, social, mood, and sexual spheres simultaneously. Each of these areas must be acknowledged when designing interventions to help a teenager cope better. Dramatic physical and physiologic changes occur in puberty, accompanied by significant psychological changes. Adolescents try to achieve a stable self-identity, enter into mature relationships with peers of both sexes, and gain independence from their parents and family. Illness or treatment during this period leads to disturbances in some of these areas of functioning. Hospitalizations and prolonged separations from friends may lead to feelings of isolation and of missing out on important life activities.

Support from peers is crucial to the adolescent. It usually is desired from other sick adolescents, rather than from "well friends," who are perceived by patients as not being able to understand what they are going through. Because support groups are popular in this age group, encourage participation. "Veteran patients" can demonstrate effective coping strategies.

The more independence and control of treatment decisions and responsibilities that can be given to the adolescent patient, the better the long-term adjustment to illness. For instance, patients should be encouraged to participate in self-care. Parents still can provide an important source of support, though they may appear less important in the communication process than at earlier ages.

43. You find a staff member getting teary while talking with a patient, crying openly when leaving the room, and visiting the patient on a day off. What is going on?

One explanation is that this patient is having a difficult time, and the staff member is extremely empathetic. However, this behavior likely has more to do with the staff member's life and overinvolvement with the patient than with the patient's life. For instance, memories of a family member who was in a situation similar to the patient's or recollection of losses experienced by a clinician at an earlier time may be triggered by an interaction with a patient.

These types of feelings also may be related to the staff person's current mood state; for instance, he or she may be feeling depressed or overwhelmed by work issues (e.g., many recent deaths on a particular ward) or may be having difficulty at home. Medical students, house staff, and nurses usually do not want to admit that they are having a hard time. Yet support can be made available by administrative and counseling staffs and peers.

44. What are some signals of a problematic patient-staff relationship?

- The need to try to save the patient, resulting in adversarial relationships with other health professionals involved in a patient's care.

• Overinvolvement with, or avoidance of, a patient and angry feelings toward a patient whose condition is deteriorating or toward other staff involved in the care of the patient.
• The need to protect the patient, which involves not bringing up for discussion, even when appropriate, topics that may be painful or emotionally distressing for the patient (e.g., healthcare proxies, resuscitation orders, failed treatments, worsening prognosis).

Recognition of our limitations and vulnerabilities is as important as being aware of these common reactions. If similar circumstances are occurring to you or an associate, talk to an advisor or supervisor to get help with the situation.

45. Is cancer always associated with pain?

Unfortunately, almost always. Pain can be related to the disease, to treatment for the disease, and to procedures. Psychological variables such as the meaning of pain, perceptions of control, fear of death, depressed mood, and hopelessness are recognized as contributing to the cancer pain experience and may increase the likelihood of a patient reporting pain. It is estimated that about 15% of patients with localized disease and 60–90% of those with advanced cancer report debilitating pain.

Today, more attention is being given to alleviating and preventing pain. In cancer patients, however, pain often is undertreated. Factors contributing to the undertreatment of pain include lack of proper assessment of the pain, the assumption that psychological rather than medical variables are the cause of pain, lack of knowledge of current therapeutic approaches, focus on prolonging life and cure versus alleviating suffering, the belief that opioids should be "saved in case you need them later," inadequate physician-patient relationship, and fear of respiratory depression.

Fear of addiction also is a factor in undertreatment of pain. Both patients and physicians share this fear. Although tolerance and physical dependence commonly occur, addiction (i.e., psychological dependence) is rare and almost never occurs in individuals who do not have a history of substance abuse before cancer.

46. What is a useful approach to treatment of cancer pain?

The step ladder approach advocated by the World Health Organization. Mild pain is treated with nonopioids, such as nonsteroidal anti-inflammatories, and doses are increased to dose-limiting toxicity or relief. Moderate pain is treated with weak opioids (codeine or oxycodone), and severe pain is treated with strong opioids (morphine) regardless of stage of disease. Adjuvant analgesics (i.e., tricyclic antidepressants, phenothiazines, psychostimulants, and benzodiazepines) can be used with any of these choices, when therapy is limited by dose-related side effects.

Adjuncts to the treatment of pain include the provision of support, knowledge, and skills using a crisis intervention model. Cognitive-behavioral therapy techniques, such as relaxation, distraction, and desensitization also are useful.

BIBLIOGRAPHY

1. American Psychiatric Association: Practice guideline for treatment of patients with delirium. Am J Psychiatry (Suppl) 156:1–20, 1999.
2. Breitbart W, Holland JC: Aspects of Symptom Management in Cancer Patients. Washington, DC, American Psychiatric Press, 1993.
3. DeFlorio ML, Massie MJ: Review of depression in cancer: Gender differences. Depression 3:66–80, 1995.
4. Derogatis LR, Morrow GR, Fetting J, et al: Prevalence of psychiatric disorders among cancer patients. JAMA 249:751–757, 1983.
5. Holland JC (ed): Psycho-Oncology. New York, Oxford University Press, 1998.
6. Roth AJ, Massie MJ: Psychiatric complications in cancer patients. In Hall L (ed): American Cancer Society Textbook of Clinical Oncology. Atlanta, Georgia, American Cancer Society, In Press.
7. Roth AJ, McClear KZ, Massie MJ: Oncology. In Stoudemire A, Fogel B, Greenberg D (eds): Psychiatric Care of teh Medical Patient. New York, Oxford University Press, In Press.
8. Shuster JL, Stern TA, Greenberg DB: Pros and cons of fluoxetine for depressed cancer patients. Oncology 6:45–55, 1993.
9. U.S. Department of Health, Management of Cancer Pain, Clinical Practice Guidelines. Washington, DC, U.S. Government Printing Office, 1994.

74. PSYCHOLOGICAL PERSPECTIVES IN THE CARE OF PATIENTS WITH DIABETES MELLITUS

Alan M. Jacobson, M.D.

1. Why are psychological perspectives so important for the treatment of diabetes mellitus?

Both type I and type II diabetes demand considerable change in lifestyle and learning of complex information, pose threats of future complications, and may lead to premature death. Diabetes also involves enforced role change, potential for suffering pain, and numerous insults to the person and family, including bias in hiring, problems in getting insurance, embarrassment, and living with fear of the future. Treatment rests on a strong foundation of **knowledge** on the part of the physician, other health care professionals, and the patient and his or her family.

Patients with type I diabetes must learn the complex task of using insulin. Patients with type II diabetes are forced to make major lifestyle changes well after they have developed consistent habits. Patients with type II diabetes often are obese and must take a new approach to diet in the face of well-ingrained behaviors. Furthermore, later in the course of type II diabetes patients may need to take insulin at the very time when it is more difficult to see and manipulate small objects.

For these reasons—especially because of the need for behavior change—the psychological management of the patient and the identification of emotional problems may be critical for successful treatment of diabetes mellitus.

2. What is the starting point for a psychological approach to care?

Successful treatment of a complex chronic condition such as diabetes mellitus rests on the therapeutic relationship between the patient and his or her healthcare provider(s), including physicians, dietitians, psychologists, and nurse educators. The **therapeutic alliance** refers to the underlying level of agreement about the goals of and approaches to treatment. The nature and strength of the alliance often go unaddressed during the course of most treatment. Indeed, the exact strength of the therapeutic alliance may remain entirely hidden to the clinician. Yet it may have important positive and negative effects on the course of treatment.

3. Give an example of a therapeutic alliance.

A therapy group for patients with diabetes had been meeting for several weeks when a new member entered treatment. The group therapist had been concerned in previous meetings that the patients had not developed clear understanding of the objectives and methods of treatment. The new patient posed immediate problems because he was suspicious and frightened of the patients and therapist. In his first session the other patients spontaneously responded to these feelings by explaining carefully and repetitively the purpose of the group therapy, the style of approach that would be taken, and their own hopes for benefit. The new patient, relieved and reassured by the other patients' explicit and thoughtful explanations that addressed his worries, went on to use the group treatment effectively. The explanations were given with such accuracy that they virtually mirrored what the therapist herself might have said, thus reflecting a strong but previously latent alliance that was firmly in place during treatment.

As in medical treatment, the strength of the relationship or alliance may not be readily apparent to the physician.

4. True or false: The therapeutic alliance, once created, is static.

False. Temporary breaches in the alliance may mask underlying strengths that can be shored up over time. Such breaks typically are noticeable when patients fail to follow through with treatment recommendations, e.g., repeatedly forgetting to bring the results of metabolic monitoring to a medical appointment. The same patient may follow through at other times with other requests, reflecting clear agreement and comfort with treatment objectives. Such variations represent the **fluidity** of the therapeutic alliance. From visit to visit the strength of the alliance may vary, depending on the task.

For example, the patient failing to bring home glucose testing records may have particular discomfort with this aspect of treatment. Such discomfort suggests that the strength of the alliance may not be sufficient to work on an especially upsetting problem. In a sense, the additional stress temporarily overwhelms the working alliance.

This fluidity suggests an important principle of treatment: *The therapeutic alliance should not be taken for granted.* Continual attention is required to buttress the alliance and address provocative treatment issues over the course of follow-up. Indeed, treatment often moves in a direction from easier to more difficult tasks.

The alliance may be sufficiently strong for the patient to learn the basic technique of insulin treatment, but not sufficiently strong to address the more difficult challenges of decreasing fat and carbohydrate intake or beginning to make changes in an otherwise erratic lifestyle to establish metabolic control.

5. How important is "transactional expertise"?

The patient pays for a service that the clinician with special expertise provides. Equally essential to the physician's technical expertise is knowledge of how to engage patients in a joint exercise of decision making and treatment. Whereas technical and medical expertise bring the patient to the clinician, transactional expertise builds an effective alliance and facilitates behavior change.

6. Are there specific ways to improve patient compliance?

Some patients may want and even demand, directly and/or indirectly, shared responsibility for setting the agenda for each medical appointment. Other patients may prefer that the physician assume complete responsibility. Recent studies from typical clinical practices in the U.S. suggest that encouraging patients to take an active role in setting the agenda for the meeting may improve adherence to the clinician's recommendations. For example, one study of a group of patients with diabetes demonstrated that an intervention designed to activate patients to take more responsibility for directing the medical interview led to better glycemic control and improved adherence. Sharing control appears to enhance respect for the clinician's advice. Note, however, that encouraging patient activity does not mean abrogating responsibility for providing clear, coherent direction.

This shift in orientation mirrors a widely espoused change in the workplace, wherein added responsibility for decision making is given to employees. In factories, for example, teams of workers on the assembly line are given more opportunity to suggest and implement ideas about improving efficiency and quality.

7. What can the physician do to strengthen the therapeutic alliance?

One approach, conceptualized by Lazare and colleagues, focuses on the identification of hidden patient requests and negotiation between patient and clinician. Asking questions not only gives patients the opportunity to help set the agenda of the meeting, but also uncovers new information (e.g., patient concerns and goals) that can be used in planning treatment.

Clinicians typically select an intervention and have clear, predetermined goals. Changes in the treatment regimen may be involved. For example, recognizing that the patient with type II diabetes has not been able to maintain adequate glycemic control on diet plus an oral agent may lead to a recommendation for insulin. However, *the patient may come to the same appointment with entirely different requests and goals*—and these may remain unexpressed.

In many transactions it is sufficient for the clinician to make recommendations that the patient will follow. This does not imply inadequate attention to the needs of the patient; it means simply that the therapeutic alliance is strong and that the patient is comfortable and ready to follow the recommendations of the expert.

8. Give an example of a weak period in the fluid therapeutic alliance.

The therapeutic alliance can be weakened by patient distress about a particular aspect of treatment, prior problems in the relationship, inadequate communication between clinician and patient, or psychological problems on the part of either. In such instances, physician recommendations may not be acceptable, and the patient's concerns and goals must be identified. However, even after discussion, the patient may not be ready to begin insulin. He or she may want to try again a previously failed diet. How should the clinician react? The clinician knows that on past occasions the patient has tried to lose weight to decrease insulin resistance and improve the likelihood of better glycemic control. The patient is terrified of insulin injections. If the clinician insists by making a strong recommendation, the patient often will not follow through.

At this juncture, after identifying the patient's hidden concerns and requests, the clinician has the opportunity to **negotiate a settlement**.

9. What are the benefits of negotiation with a patient who is rejecting treatment advice?

First, negotiation strengthens the therapeutic alliance by reassuring the patient that he or she retains some sense of control over the future. Second, and of even greater importance, the patient knows that the clinician has listened and comprehended the underlying concerns. This recognition can be a remarkably reassuring and comforting experience for patients. Being heard may calm anxiety to the point that the patient accepts the original recommendation.

Some patients will insist on trying again the failed diet before beginning insulin. Such interactions can be frustrating, because the patient may wish to try many times something that obviously is no longer working. However, each attempt provides an opportunity for rediscussion as well as strengthening the bond that, eventually, will allow the patient to begin something that is terrifying.

10. True or false: The formation of a therapeutic alliance begins with negotiation.

False. Uncovering hidden concerns is the first step in forming a strong alliance.The uncovered concerns may seem indirectly related to treatment. Examples include requests to write a letter to support an application for special housing, wishes to discuss work problems, or demands for apparently unwarranted treatment.

Negotiation may be necessary when the relationship between the patient and clinician is not at its strongest (see Questions 8 and 9).

11. Should I always make time for negotiation?

Not always. Certainly there may be emergency situations in which something must be done. For example, the patient's glycemic control is so poor that ketoacidosis has led to hospitalization. A change must be made. Previous identification of hidden requests and negotiation of settlements let the patient know that he or she can be heard. When a crisis is reached, forceful direction based on fundamental trust can lead to acceptance of a confronting recommendation that "it is now time; we can't wait any longer."

12. How may a therapeutic alliance be weakened?

If patient and clinician have not agreed on a **model for interaction**, the therapeutic alliance may be weakened. Patients have implicit models for the way in which clinicians should act. For example, some patients may not value a treatment recommendation unless it includes a prescription. Furthermore, underlying beliefs about the value of certain types of treatments may be derived from traditional views of medicine and treatment. Cultural factors typically play an important role in determining such assumptions. The clinician may anticipate such differences when patients from distinct cultures come for help, but important variations in attitude exist even among different groups in the same country. In addition, personality, family upbringing, and past experiences with illness may engender different views of the nature of therapeutics.

13. Describe the roles of the treatment team members.

The nurse educator's job is to educate or train the patient about injection techniques and handling insulin; the dietitian must teach the patient how to select appropriate foods; the physician makes the diagnosis, addresses intercurrent problems, and directs treatment (e.g., insulin regimen and dosage).

14. What role can the psychiatrist play in the care of patients with diabetes?

In the most difficult of situations, when the physician has difficulty maintaining objectivity and a comfortable relationship with the patient, psychological consultation and conjoint treatment approaches can be extremely helpful. The psychiatrist can provide the patient a time and place to consider the expectations of the physician, and can help negotiate between patient and physician the steps of treatment. Sometimes such consultations are initiated by the patient, but more often they are initiated by the physician who feels loss of control. This may occur early in treatment when the therapeutic alliance usually is weak.

15. Give an example of a psychiatrist's participation in caring for a diabetic patient.

A 25-year-old man was hospitalized in diabetic ketoacidosis with previously undiagnosed type I diabetes mellitus. After initial stabilization in the intensive care unit, he was transferred to a medical floor, where the first steps of teaching and diabetes treatment were instituted. The patient was terrified of taking insulin by injection and refused all but two injections over the first few day on the unit. A psychiatric consultation was requested, because the physician believed that the patient was not ready to accept treatment recommendations and required immediate transfer to an inpatient psychiatric unit. The patient, according to the medical team, had recognizable signs of diabetes for several months but had been avoiding contact with a physician. He had a history of hospitalization for an apparent psychotic disorder and had remained marginally functional in the community. He had a supportive family, but was unable to maintain independent living.

The psychiatrist found that the patient was guarded and frightened, but not overtly psychotic or clinically depressed. He had denied the possibility of diabetes until transfer to the medical unit, where he made the first struggling attempts to accept the notion of taking insulin. During the consultation he asked questions about the course of diabetes and its treatment and expressed some optimism because he had given himself one injection. The patient wanted the staff to give him more time to get used to shots. The psychiatrist answered each question, suggested further discussions with the nursing staff, and indicated to the staff that the patient was beginning to acknowledge his need for insulin. He stated that transfer to a psychiatric unit was not needed, and suggested that the team give the patient another few days to grapple with the reality of his new diagnosis. During followup sessions, the psychiatrist allowed the patient to vent feelings about his new medical condition.

Over the next few days, the patient accepted twice-daily injections and started to learn self-injection and self-monitoring techniques. When he was discharged, he was taking his own injections. The patient's fears decreased as he came to experience the actuality of diabetes care. In turn he gradually accepted treatment without forced change through confrontations. In essence, the illness did the confronting and the staff—once comfortable with the patient's participation in decisions to start treatment in a less than optimal manner—provided expert support.

16. What role does the family play in the treatment of diabetes?

Many studies have addressed the effects of diabetes on patients and their families, with specific focus on child and adolescent patients. Consistent effects on personality and psychological maturation in children with diabetes have not been shown; however, there is little doubt that diabetes increases stress in both parents and patients. It is not clear whether there are distinct changes in families of patients with diabetes, but evidence suggests that children of families that adapt more successfully are more likely to cope effectively with their illness. Well-adapted families are organized and cohesive, and maintain a warm, nurturing environment. Thus, family factors are critical influences on the course of illness, and involvement of the family is an important feature of the care of patients with diabetes.

The consciousness-raising process is entered jointly by the medical professional and appropriate loved ones. For example, a spouse may contact the physician about her husband, who tests infrequently, because he feels "okay," even though he has had periodic hypoglycemic episodes that required assistance. In all instances, confrontations must be carried out nonjudgmentally and with great care, to avoid backlash that may lead to even greater problems with self-care.

17. Is there an important link between depression and diabetes?

Yes. Major depression is more common among adult patients with type I diabetes than in the general population; this increased prevalence is greatest among men. The relationship of diabetes and depression is not unique. It has been widely recognized that depressive disorders are more common in many groups with chronic illness than in community samples. The link is important because depression can have a profound influence on functional health status—perhaps to even greater extent than chronic medical illness. Furthermore, depression in diabetic patients is associated with problems with glycemic control. The magnitude of the effect of depression on glycemic control suggests that depression places diabetic patients at risk for chronic hyperglycemia and more rapid progression of microvascular complications.

18. Does diabetes influence the diagnosis and treatment of depression?

The diagnosis and treatment of depressive disorders in patients with diabetes should follow the same general principles as in patients without a concomitant medical condition. However, certain issues deserve special consideration. The diagnosis of clinical depression rests on identification of a specific set of symptoms that may involve physical, cognitive, affective, and attitudinal changes. Attitudinal changes include pessimism about the future and a sense that actions cannot lead to positive consequences.

Symptoms of Depression

PHYSICAL	COGNITIVE	AFFECTIVE
Fatigue	Decreased concentration	Depressed mood
Psychomotor retardation	Poor recent memory	Loss of interest in activities
Insomnia or excessive sleeping		Increased guilt, shame, fear,
Weight loss		or anxiety

Most patients present with only a few such symptoms. If the presentation consists predominantly of physical symptoms, the diagnosis of depression in a patient with diabetes may be difficult. Physical symptoms are similar in poorly controlled diabetes with persistent hyperglycemia and ketonuria, and depression. Thus it may be important to evaluate the patient's status after a short period of improved glycemic control. If after 2 weeks of improved control physical symptoms persist, a diagnosis of depression may be warranted. If physical symptoms are accompanied by depressive attitudes and affective symptoms, it is unlikely that poorly controlled diabetes accounts for the problem. In such instances, earlier treatment for depression should be considered.

19. What special considerations pertain to the pharmacologic treatment of depression in patients with diabetes?

Despite suggestions that antidepressants and lithium carbonate may affect blood glucose levels, in practice this is rarely a significant clinical problem. Patients starting antidepressants should be alerted to the possibility of more irregular control of blood glucose levels. Because lithium carbonate appears to have an insulin-like action, lower blood glucose levels may be anticipated. Possible long-term effects of lithium (e.g., renal toxicity and hypothyroidism) should not be considered an absolute contraindication to its use in patients with diabetes. As with all patients treated with lithium, regular follow-up of medical status is necessary.

The commonly used antidepressants have side effects that may be especially problematic in patients with diabetes. For example, tricyclic antidepressants (TCAs) may cause orthostatic hypotension. In patients with autonomic neuropathy such side effects may be exacerbated. The possible cardiac side effects of TCAs may increase the risk for arrhythmias in diabetic patients with advanced coronary vessel disease. The newer antidepressants, such as the selective serotonin reuptake inhibitors

(SSRIs), have fewer cardiovascular side effects. However, their use may pose specific problems in patients with gastroparesis; one of the common side effects of SSRIs, nausea and vomiting, may be especially problematic. Moreover, impotence secondary to diabetes may be compounded by TCAs and SSRIs.

Patients with diabetes may require several trials of antidepressants because of such complexities. Moreover, slow titration to optimal doses may be needed to initiate successful treatment. As with all depressed patients, it is important to recognize that the most common reasons for treatment failure are inadequate length of treatment and inadequate dosing. Patients presenting with side effects at low doses may be able to tolerate the medication if the dose is increased slowly.

20. Why is self-care particularly concerning in depressed, diabetic patients?

Patients with depression may have symptoms that limit learning ability and confidence in self-treatment. Thus, treatment of depression in patients who have problems with glycemic control or other aspects of self-care should be accompanied by appropriate counseling. For example, pessimistic attitudes may inhibit willingness or ability to care for diabetes and patients may need reeducation about material that was either not learned or forgotten during the depressed period.

21. Are eating disorders common in patients with diabetes?

Available studies do not answer this question clearly. Given its considerable requirements for changes in diet, diabetes mellitus, especially type I, may pose a special risk for the development of eating disorders. Diabetes in the population at greatest risk of eating disorders—women aged 15–35 years—may precipitate eating disturbances. Some evidence suggests increased rates of anorexia nervosa and bulimia in young women with diabetes. Ideals of body weight, which lead women to strive for weight loss, have problematic consequences in patients with diabetes. Polonsky and colleagues have shown that 30% of women with type I diabetes across the adolescent and adult age range acknowledged at least some omission of insulin and that 9% of all women acknowledged frequent omission of insulin. As expected, omission occurred even more commonly in women aged 15–30, but was found even in older women.

Binging and purging typically are experienced as shameful and may be hidden. Because of the likelihood of underreporting, current rates may underestimate the frequency of insulin omission. A significant minority of women who acknowledge omitting insulin do so explicitly to lose weight. Omission of insulin to lose weight is associated with a high level of psychopathology and is linked to significant problems with glycemic control. A history of eating disorder is also predictive of early development of retinopathy. Such findings underline the importance of identifying possible problems with body weight ideals and their association with habits of self-care.

Many patients with diabetes do not fully develop an eating disorder, although they discover the "merits" of occasional insulin underuse to control weight. Such patients, who do not meet threshold for diagnosis, may be the most difficult to identify, yet they represent an important high-risk group.

22. What are special considerations for the treatment of diabetic patients with eating disorders?

The treatment of eating disorders and associated conceptions of body weight often is difficult and time-consuming. Physician and patient may find themselves struggling to agree on goals for treatment. Thus, eating-related problems are particularly fruitful areas for collaborative models of treatment and for identifying specific areas of change that the patient is prepared to address.

The main problem is **underuse of self-administered insulin** as a method of "purging." These patients fear weight gain, and underdosing with insulin becomes the preferred method of regulating weight. Underdosing may be present without other methods of purging. The identification of this form of eating disorder may require repeated questioning in a nonjudgmental manner. The clinician may uncover such problems only when the patient is sufficiently comfortable and senses that she will not be chastised.

The **water-retaining effects** of insulin complicate the problem. Reinsulinization may require considerable negotiation between patient and physician. The patient often does not differentiate between sources of weight gain or body size change. A 10-pound weight loss is a 10-pound weight loss, and a 10-pound weight gain is a 10-pound weight gain, whether due to changes in water volume, fat stores, or muscle mass. Thus reinsulinization accompanied by rapid weight gain and overt edema may be a terrifying experience for patients with intense beliefs about excessive weight.

23. Give an example of how a diabetic patient with an eating disorder may require special management.

A 23-year-old woman presented with bulimia that included binge eating and extensive underdosing with insulin. When hospitalized because of diabetic ketoacidosis and restarted on insulin, she rapidly regained the weight lost through dehydration and experienced pitting edema of the ankles. She became increasingly depressed and panicked by the weight gain to the extent that she requested a lower dose of insulin to control the terrifying spiral of weight. Despite careful explanation about the source of added weight, the patient could not differentiate between water gain and gain in fat stores. Thus, as part of the treatment plan, the dose of insulin was lowered and gradually increased to an optimal level. Hospitalization was extended until her weight stabilized; patient compliance could be relied on only after the threat of continuing weight gain from fluid retention disappeared.

24. Discuss how gastroparesis can be confused with anorexia in diabetic patients.

In rare instances, gastroparesis that causes vomiting and weight loss may mimic or complicate anorexia and bulimia. Among young women with relatively short durations of diabetes and complicated family histories, eating disorders and gastroparesis may be difficult to differentiate. Functional gastrointestinal investigations suggesting slowed gastric emptying may be used to identify the gastroparetic component, but effective treatment usually requires intervention at family, individual, and medical levels. In some instances, symptoms may be secondary to psychological and family conflicts; in others, psychological and family conflicts may stem in part from the severe, early onset of the confusing and frightening diabetic complication of gastroparesis.

25. Are anxiety disorders readily diagnosable in patients with diabetes?

As with affective disorders, anxiety syndromes may be confused with diabetes-related symptoms. Most commonly, patients are unable to differentiate between symptoms of panic anxiety and hypoglycemic states. Anxiety syndromes may include physical symptoms such as palpitations, sweats, and headaches, as well as physical and emotional feelings of trembling, foreboding, and panic. In most instances, repeated self-testing of blood glucose levels can help the patient discriminate between hypoglycemic and anxiety-related symptoms.

When emotional symptoms predominate, the patient probably is experiencing a form of anxiety disorder. Thus patients whose presentation includes increased obsessive thoughts, compulsive acts, fear, or obsessive worry are more likely to have an underlying anxiety disorder.

Treatment with currently available antianxiety agents usually poses no special problems in patients with diabetes. As in patients with depression, treatment should incorporate counseling to help patients deal with underlying concerns that may be important causes of the anxiety syndrome. In some instances such concerns are diabetes-related; however, the problem may relate only partially to the patient's illness.

26. Give an example of management of anxiety in a diabetic patient.

A 45-year-old patient with type I diabetes presented with increased fear, obsessional thoughts, and panic anxiety. Initially the symptoms were associated with worries about future complications that began soon after the patient increased his frequency of home glucose testing and insulin injections. Heightened awareness of diabetes appeared to be the critical trigger for the psychological reaction. On further inquiry, it became clear that the patient also was experiencing considerable marital difficulties, which played an important role in causing the anxiety disorder. Therefore, treatment that addressed both diabetic and marital issues was instituted.

27. Can psychological screening measures be useful in the care of patients with diabetes?

Given the practical problems of caring for patients in busy clinical practices, psychosocial screening can help clinicians identify problems for further assessment. Three measures may be of some use in identifying at-risk patients:

• **The Beck Depression Inventory** is a widely used, brief, self-report inquiry into symptoms of depression. It may be used by the primary care physician and/or the diabetologist to identify areas for further inquiry as well as to document the level of depressive symptoms. Many other screening measures also have been developed for assessing anxiety and depression.

• **The Diabetes Quality of Life Measure** developed for the Diabetes Control and Complications Trial may be useful in identifying the impact of illness on the patient's perception of well-being. Assessment can identify the overall level of quality of life as well as particular areas of patient concern. Prior studies suggest a high degree of reliability and validity. Quality-of-life measures can be augmented by specific questions that the practitioner finds helpful, or shortened by selection of a subset of especially relevant questions from the scale. This measure includes particular questions oriented toward adolescents and young adults with diabetes; although designed for type I patients, it also may be used in older patients with type II diabetes.

• **The Problem Areas in Diabetes Scale** scrutinizes specific concerns about diabetes and the distress level associated with their presence. The measure is designed as a screen and covers multiple issues. It may be used to identify particular problem areas in the emotional experience of diabetes and behavioral problem areas that can be targeted for special attention and intervention. Practitioners are encouraged to add to the list for clinical use.

These screening measures are guides for the clinician. They can be used to stimulate discussion, identify hidden patient concerns, and provide an improved understanding of the patient's emotional life.

28. Summarize key features of the psychological care of patients with diabetes.

• Development of **new attitudes and behaviors** in the patient. Maintenance of such behaviors requires repeated effort from patients, family members, and healthcare providers.

• A strong, close **working relationship** between healthcare provider and patient. The psychological management of patient problems begins with recognition of the importance of this relationship.

• Clinician understanding of the **psychological themes** embedded in the life of the patient. The more that the clinician integrates these themes into the treatment process, the more likely that care will succeed.

The doctor's office must be what Hemingway described as a "clean, well-lighted place"; that is, a place that appeals in the darkest of night and at the moment of greatest despair. Even if behavior change has been minimal, the patient seeing that light will be comforted throughout the process of adaptation to diabetes.

BIBLIOGRAPHY

1. Beck AT: The Beck Depression Inventory. Psychological Corporation, Harcourt-Brace Jovanovich, 1978.
2. Curry S: Commentary: In search of how people change. Diabetes Spect 6:34–35, 1993.
3. DCCT Research Group: The effect of intensive treatment of diabetes on the development and progression of long-term complications in insulin-dependent diabetes mellitus. N Engl J Med 329:886–977, 1993.
4. Dunn SM, Turtle JR: The myth of the diabetic personality. Diabetes Care 4:640–646, 1982.
5. Gavard JA, Lustman PJ, Clouse RE: Prevalence of depression in adults with diabetes: An epidemiological evaluation. Diabetes Care 16:1167–1178, 1993.
6. Hemingway E: The Complete Short Stories. New York, Scribners, 1987.
7. Jacobson AM: Psychological care of patients with insulin-dependent diabetes mellitus. N Engl J Med 334: 1249–1253, 1996.
8. Jacobson AM, de Groot M, Samson JA: The evaluation of two measures of quality of life in patients with type I and type II diabetes mellitus. Diabetes Care 17:267–274, 1994.
9. Jacobson AM, Hauser S, Anderson B, Polonsky W: Psychosocial aspects of diabetes. In Kahn C, Weir G (eds): Joslin's Diabetes Mellitus, 13th ed. Philadelphia, Lea & Febiger, 1994.

10. Kaplan S, Greenfield S, Ware J: Assessing the effects of physician-patient interactions on the outcome of chronic disease. Med Care 27(Suppl):S110–S127, 1989.
11. Lazare A, Cohen F, Jacobson AM, et al: The walk-in patient as a customer: A key dimension in evaluation and treatment. Am J Orthopsychiatry 42:872–873, 1972.
12. Lustman PJ, Griffith LA, Clouse RE, Cryer PE: Psychiatric illness in diabetes mellitus. Relationship to symptoms and glucose control. J Nerv Ment Dis 174:736–742, 1986.
13. Polonsky W, Anderson B, Lohrer P, et al: Insulin omission in women with IDDM. Diabetes Care 17:1178–1185, 1994.
14. Rodin GM, Daneman D: Eating disorders and IDDM: A problematic association. Diabetes Care 14:1402–1411, 1992.
15. Rodin G, Rydall A, Olmstead M, et al: A four-year follow-up study of eating disorders and medical complications in young women with insulin-dependent diabetes mellitus. Psychosom Med 56:179, 1994.
16. Welch G, Jacobson A, Polonksy W: The problem areas in diabetes (PAID) scale. An examination of its clinical utility. Diabetes Care 20:760–766, 1997.

XI. Special Treatment Populations

75. SUICIDE: RISK FACTORS AND MANAGEMENT
Randall D. Buzan, M.D., and Lester Butt, Ph.D.

1. Define suicide.

Suicide is the act of intentionally killing oneself, but patients often use the term differently. For instance, patients who repeatedly cut themselves superficially to assuage severe anxiety may describe themselves as "suicidal," but with further questioning they often can distinguish these acts from more ominous injuries inflicted with the intent to kill. It is thus important to clarify what patients mean when they say they are feeling "suicidal."

2. How common is suicide?

One percent of Americans die by suicide, and over 30,000 people take their own lives each year in the United States, making suicide the eighth leading cause of death. Eight to 10 people attempt suicide for every one who completes it. The U.S. suicide rate has averaged 12.5 per 100,000 over the past century; it peaked at 17.4 during the Depression in 1932, dipped to a nadir of 9.8 in 1957, and has hovered at 12.4 over the past decade.

Adolescent rates have tripled over the past 40 years, from 4 per 100,000 to 13.2 per 100,000, making suicide the third leading cause of death in this group. Almost twice as many adolescents die from suicide as die from all other natural causes combined. Although suicide in preadolescent children is rare, more than 12,000 children under the age of 13 years are hospitalized each year for self-destructive acts.

3. Name four demographic risk factors for suicide.

Age. Among Caucasians, the suicide rate has correlated with age for the past 40 years; Caucasians aged 75–84 kill themselves twice as often as those aged 15–24. Among African-Americans, rates are highest in men aged 25–34, but still lower than the rate of their white same-age counterparts.

Race. Overall, whites complete suicide twice as frequently as do African-Americans or Hispanics. Suicide rates in American Indians and Alaskan Natives are 1.7 times higher than in whites, occurring predominantly in the young.

Sex. Although the relationship between age and suicide varies among races, male rates consistently exceed female rates across races, with an overall male/female ratio of 3:1 to 4:1. On the other hand, women make 60–70% of suicide *attempts*, which exceed completed suicides by a ratio of 23:1.

Marital status. Divorced or widowed people clearly have the highest rates, followed by single people and finally by married people. Among women, the more children they have, the lower the suicide rate.

4. List the most commonly used suicide methods in order of frequency.

Men: Firearms, hanging, gases-vapors, drug ingestion
Women: Drug ingestion, firearms, gases-vapors, hanging

5. Which psychiatric patients are at risk?

Ninety to 95% of suicide victims suffer from a psychiatric illness at the time they die; therefore, defining subgroups at risk may help to focus prevention efforts. Whereas 45–70% of victims suffer from **clinical depression** at the time of death, making depression an important risk factor, several studies demonstrate that the **degree of hopelessness** is even more predictive of future suicidal behavior than the severity of depression. Others at increased risk include those with a previous suicide attempt, depression accompanied by severe anxiety or panic attacks, anorexia nervosa, and a history of child abuse or incest.

Up to 60% of psychiatric inpatients who kill themselves do so within 6 months of hospital discharge, and the month immediately after discharge is a particularly high-risk period. Therefore, *careful planning of discharge for suicidal inpatients is essential.*

Diagnosis	Suicide Rate (%)
Major depression	15*
Bipolar disorder	10–15*
Schizophrenia	10*
Alcohol dependence	2
Borderline personality disorder	4–9.5
Antisocial personality	5

* Note that these percentages are well-established and widely cited, but based on older studies that disproportionately included patients with a recently diagnosed psychiatric illness (patients are at substantially elevated suicide risk in the first months following diagnosis of a major mental disorder). Recent reanalyses suggest that the actual lifetime risk of suicide in depression and bipolar disorder is 6%, and in schizophrenia is 4%.

6. What medical illnesses are associated with an increased suicide risk?

In spite of empirical design and assessment differences, the following reflect diagnoses with heightened suicide risk*:

Acquired immunodeficiency syndrome (21 to 36 times [×] higher risk)
Gastrointestinal cancers (5×)
Head injury (5×)
Epilepsy (5×)
Temporal lobe epilepsy (25×)
Huntington's chorea (5×)
Klinefelter's syndrome (?)
Multiple sclerosis (5×)
Porphyria (5×)
Delirium tremens (?)
Cushing's disease (5×)
Renal failure on hemodialysis (40×)
Peptic ulcer disease (5×)
Spinal cord injuries (5–10×)

Most studies do not describe the mental status of the patients; thus it is unclear whether the increased suicide risk is due to comorbid depression, organic brain disease, or some specific factor from the medical condition itself.

* over the age-adjusted risk in the general population

7. Describe the biological findings in suicide victims.

The most compelling data thus far indicate a relative **deficiency of serotonin** (5-hydroxytyramine [5-HT]) in the central nervous system (CNS) of suicide victims. Postmortem studies reveal decreased presynaptic inhibitory 5-HT receptors and increased postsynaptic 5-HT receptors in the prefrontal cortex. 5-hydroxyindoleacetic acid (5-HIAA), the major metabolite of serotonin, is reduced in the cerebrospinal fluid of depressed patients and is even further reduced in depressed patients who are suicidal or have attempted suicide. This finding is particularly robust in patients who have attempted suicide by violent means (such as with firearms).

Compared with those who have died by other causes, suicide victims have: (1) increased beta and decreased alpha-1 adrenoreceptors, and (2) reduced numbers of corticotropin-releasing–factor receptors in the frontal cortex. These findings suggest dysregulation of CNS adrenergic function and the hypothalamic-pituitary-adrenal axis, respectively, but they may represent the neurophysiology of depression and may not be specific to suicidal behavior.

Studies of the dexamethasone suppression test, thyrotropin-releasing hormone stimulation test, and platelet monoamine oxidase levels in suicidal patients have yielded mixed results. While some studies of cholesterol-lowering agents have found a decrease in mortality from cardiovascular disease that is partially offset by an increase in suicide, other trials have not, and the role of cholesterol in mood regulation continues to be debated.

8. Is suicide hereditary?

Partly. Adoption studies demonstrate a suicide incidence of roughly 4% in the biological relatives of adoptees who killed themselves, significantly different than the less than 1% observed in adoptive relatives and in biologic relatives of matched nonsuicidal adoptees. Twin studies show a nineteen-fold greater concordance for suicide in monozygotic than in dizygotic twins (13.2% vs. 0.7%). Such findings may represent inheritance of predisposing psychiatric illnesses rather than a specific genetic susceptibility for suicide, although an Australian study of 5995 twins that controlled for psychopathology still found a significant association between twins' suicidal thoughts and behavior, stronger in monozygotic than dizygotic pairs.

A related issue is the finding that patients may copy the behavior of a loved one who has committed suicide; knowing a suicide victim is, in fact, a risk factor for suicidal behavior. This element of family history is important to elicit when evaluating a suicidal patient.

9. Why do people kill themselves?

Suicide has many determinants, but it is always an attempt to solve a problem, albeit in a maladaptive way. Wondering with the patient why he or she is feeling suicidal helps to define the problem. Asking patients to describe what they think would happen if they killed themselves may elicit wishes for revenge, power, control, punishment, atonement, sacrifice, restitution, escape, sleep, rescue, rebirth, reunion with the dead, or a new life.

10. Which psychiatric medications have been shown to decrease suicide risk?

In several large, recent studies, **lithium** decreased the rate of suicidal acts seven-fold in bipolar patients. The suicide risk of patients who stop their lithium is 4.8 times higher during periods off of this drug, and a whopping 20-fold higher during the first year off of the drug. Antipsychotic drugs, and particularly the atypical antipsychotic **clozapine**, appear to reduce the risk of suicide in schizophrenic patients.

While clinicians routinely see improvement of suicidal feelings and self-destructive behaviors in patients treated with **antidepressants**, studies of antidepressants do not show a dramatic reduction of suicide risk with treatment. The reasons for this are unclear, but a well-replicated finding is that depressed patients are grossly under-treated by their doctors, with only 8–25% ever receiving adequate doses of an antidepressant for a sufficient period of time to be effective. Thus even those patients "treated" with antidepressants in naturalistic studies generally were not getting enough medication to adequately treat their depression and diminish their suicidality. Institution of a depression education program for all primary care physicians in Gotland, Sweden was followed by a significant decrease in suicide rates. The message here is clear: *we need to to a better job of identifying and aggressively treating depressed patients to impact suicide rates.*

11. What is important to remember when prescribing antidepressants?

Antidepressants are the most commonly used drugs in fatal overdoses. They must be prescribed carefully. Dividing the dose that is lethal to 50% of subjects (LD50) by the dose that is effective for 50% of subjects (ED50) derives the therapeutic index of a drug. In laboratory animals, the therapeutic indices of neuroleptics, tricyclic antidepressants, and lithium are 100, 10, and 3, respectively. In humans, neuroleptics alone rarely kill in overdose, but it may take only a 10-day supply of an antidepressant or a 3-day supply of lithium to kill 50% of patients. Thus, when a patient is in the midst of a suicidal crisis, it is sensible to prescribe no more than a week's worth of medication, and often less. Perhaps because of their effects of cardiac conduction, tricyclic antidepressants are more lethal in overdose than fluoxetine and the newer antidepressants. Some clinicians therefore prefer to use the newer drugs in suicidal patients.

12. Does asking patients about suicidal feelings "put the idea into their heads"?

No. No evidence supports this common misconception. Suicidal patients typically are relieved to find someone who wants to help.

13. How do I ask a patient about suicidal feelings?

Communicating a genuine interest in the patient's feelings is far more important than the exact wording used to find out about suicide potential. The following list of questions proceeds from general to more specific queries:

- Have you ever wished you (weren't here) were dead?
- Have you ever thought about hurting or killing yourself?
- Have you ever acted on those feelings? (When, how, what precipitated each attempt? Was there an actual intent to die? Who rescued/found you? What treatment was obtained?).
- When is the last time you felt suicidal?
- Have you been feeling suicidal lately?
- How have you thought you might go about killing yourself?
- Do you currently have the means to carry out this plan (e.g., rope, pills, gun)?
- Do you have easy access to a gun? Is it at home? Is it loaded? (Always discuss guns with suicidal patients, even if they are not part of the divulged plan, because of their high lethality and frequent use in suicide.)
- How close have you come to actually carrying out this plan?
- Do you wish you were dead now?
- Have you thought about killing anyone else? (Homicidal and suicidal feelings often coexist, and homicidal thoughts can be explored much like suicidal thoughts.)

14. Describe the next steps in the evaluation of the suicidal patient.

Once the suicidal patient has been identified and the issues above have been explored, the evaluation proceeds as follows:

Answer the question "Why now?" That is, try to understand what recent experience gave rise to the patient's suicidal feelings and what problem the patient is trying to "solve."

Make a diagnosis. Psychological factors aside, suicide is an indication of an underlying disorder. Most patients are depressed, alcoholic, or character-disordered, and diagnosis of the underlying condition guides arrangement of appropriate treatment.

Perform a mental status examination. The presence of delirium or psychosis may make the history unreliable and predispose the patient to impulsive and unpredictable behavior, thus increasing suicide risk. The presence of "command hallucinations" (i.e., hearing voices telling the individual to kill themselves) may be especially ominous.

Meet the family (or most important social support/best friend). Evaluating the patient's resources for support and contacting collateral sources (such as the patient's therapist or physician) are the key steps in deciding how reliable the patient may be and in corroborating the patient's account of his or her circumstances. Collateral contacts often are instrumental in discerning the actual problem the patient is trying to solve and in designing alternative sensible solutions.

15. List five immediate treatment objectives in the management of acutely suicidal patients.

1. Protect the patient from self-abuse until the suicide crisis has passed. Suicidal feelings are always episodic, and the task is to keep the patient safe while helping to defuse the crisis.
2. Anticipate and treat any medical complications of a suicide attempt.
3. Define and solve, if possible, the acute problem that precipitated the crisis.
4. Diagnose and arrange treatment of the underlying problem that predisposes the patient to suicidal behavior.
5. Deal with the acute grief reactions of bereaved family members of the suicide victim.

16. List criteria that should be fulfilled before considering discharge of the suicidal patient from the emergency department or doctor's office.
- The patient is medically stable.
- The patient is able to promise believably to return to the emergency department or doctor's office before harming him- or herself if suicidal thoughts recur.
- The patient is not intoxicated, delirious, demented, or psychotic.
- All firearms at home have been removed.
- The acute precipitants to the crisis have been identified, addressed, and in some way resolved.
- Treatment for the underlying psychiatric illness has been arranged.
- The physician believes that the patient will follow through on the treatment plan.
- The patient's social supports have been contacted and agree with the discharge plan.

Patients who do not meet these criteria generally must either (1) remain in the emergency room or doctor's office until the issue in question is resolved, or (2) be admitted to a psychiatric facility.

17. Upon what legal foundations are malpractice claims based?
- Failure to properly diagnose
- Failure to properly take adequate protective measures
- Premature inpatient hospital discharge
- Failure to commit
- Hospital liability for lack of appropriate safety
- Abandonment

18. What are the primary risk management measures that best protect the mental health practitioner?
1. Document meticulously.
2. Garner information regarding previous psychological treatment.
3. Involve significant others and family members.
4. Obtain psychiatric consultation from a more experienced clinician in this area.
5. Consider comorbid medical conditions that may heighten risk.
6. Possess a knowledge of community resources.
7. Regularly document suicide assessment(s).

CONTROVERSY

19. Do patients have a right to kill themselves?
For: People have a fundamental right to self-determination as long as exercising that right does not impinge on anyone else's rights. Prevention of suicide represents misguided paternalism that inappropriately violates individual rights.

Against: In all but terminally ill patients, suicide is *symptomatic of treatable mental illness.* Evidence for this position is commonplace in that almost all suicide attempters are subsequently grateful that they did not succeed. Even in one study of terminally ill patients, the few patients who wished for death to come early suffered from clinical depression.

Opinions that suicide is an act of free will sometimes derive more from antipathy toward these frequently provocative and covertly furious patients than from an objective, well-considered desire to further their best interests.

Religious and moral objections (e.g., suicide is against God's will) abound.

BIBLIOGRAPHY

1. Baldessarini RJ, Tondo L, Hennen J: Effects of lithium treatment and its discontinuation on suicidal behavior in bipolar manic-depressive disorders. J Clin Psychiatry 60(suppl 2):77–84, 1999.
2. Blumenthal SJ, Kupfer DJ (eds): Suicide over the Life Cycle: Risk Factors, Assessment, and Treatment of Suicidal Patients. Washington, DC, American Psychiatric Press, 1990.

3. Brown JH, Hentelff P, Barakat S, Rowe CJ: Is it normal for terminally ill patients to desire death? Am J Psychiatry 143:208–211, 1986.
4. Buzan RD, Weissberg MP: Suicide: Risk factors and therapeutic considerations in the emergency department. J Emerg Med 10:335–343, 1992.
5. Mann JJ, Oquendo M, Underwood MD, Arango V: The neurobiology of suicide risk: A review for the clinician. J Clin Psychiatry 60(suppl 2):7–11, 1999.
6. Oquendo MA, Malone KM, Ellis SP, et al: Inadequacy of antidepressant treatment for patients with major depression who are at risk for suicidal behavior. Am J Psychiatry 156:190–194, 1999.
7. Palmer DD, Henter ID, Wyatt RJ: Do antipsychotic medications decrease the risk of suicide in patients with schizophrenia? J Clin Psychiatry 60(suppl 2):100–103, 1999.
8. Roy A, Nielsen D, Rylander G, et al: Genetics of suicide in depression. J Clin Psychiatry 60(suppl 2):12–17, 1999.
9. Simpson SG, Jamison KR: The risk of suicide in patients with bipolar disorders. J Clin Psychiatry 60(suppl 2):53–56, 1999.
10. Bongar B: The Suicidal Patient: Clinical and Legal Standards of Care. Washington, DC, American Psychological Association, 1991.

76. ASSESSMENT AND MANAGEMENT OF THE VIOLENT PATIENT

Jane L. Erb, M.D.

1. How common is violent behavior in the health care setting?

Up to 60% of patients have been reported to exhibit physically aggressive behavior at some time. The rate depends on a number of variables, including the clinical site of the study, how one defines "violent" behavior, and the manner in which the incidence of such behavior is tracked. Although extrapolation from these studies to a specific clinical populations is difficult, violence is clearly common and probably increasing. Most acts of aggression fortunately do not result in serious injury, yet an understanding by the clinician of their causes and management is imperative.

2. What causes violent behavior?

It is generally believed that an act of violence implies a psychiatric disturbance. Although numerous studies, including studies of violent offenders, support this relationship, not all acts of aggression occur in conjunction with psychiatric or medical disease. Premeditated acts of violence, particularly those that are not recurrent, may occur in the absence of definable illness. Conversely, not all psychiatric illness has the same potential for violence. Violent behavior, therefore, is a nonspecific symptom that may or may not reflect underlying medical or psychiatric illness.

3. Which specific disorders are more likely to be associated with violent behavior?

Schizophrenia	Intermittent explosive disorder
Manic phase, bipolar disorders	Mental disorders due to general medical condition
Substance and alcohol abuse	Personality change
Personality disorders	Dementia
Antisocial personality disorder	Delirium
Borderline personality disorder	Mood and psychotic disorders
Childhood disorders	
Conduct disorder	
Oppositional disorder	
Mental retardation	

4. Which major mental disorder is associated most frequently with violent behavior?

Schizophrenia. Whether in response to command hallucinations or to paranoid delusions, schizophrenia is aggravated by disorganization of thought and behavior and may manifest with aggressive behavior. Signs of impending violence may or may not be present: violent behavior may occur precipitously, without warning, in response to internal stimuli. This awareness is essential for clinicians evaluating and treating schizophrenic patients.

5. What causes violent behavior in manic patients?

The combination of agitation, impulsivity, and delusional ideation or hallucinations puts manic patients at risk for violent behavior. Their violence often is markedly sudden because of the lack of inhibitions. An inadvertent challenge to their control, especially in light of their grandiosity, typically provokes such an outburst.

6. How do alcohol and drugs impact violent behavior?

Substance abuse poses a far greater risk of violence than mental illness, per se. The risk further increases with comorbid psychiatric disorders. **Alcohol** appears to heighten the risk through the disinhibition of intoxication and the agitation, delirium, or hallucinations of withdrawal. Both **stimulants** and **hallucinogens** frequently are incriminated in acts of violence. **Cocaine** and **amphetamines** may lead to agitation, emotional lability, and psychosis, particularly once the initial euphoria dissipates or with chronic use. **Amphetamines**, in particular, are known to affect mental status up to 2 weeks after use. **Phencyclidine** (PCP) is probably the hallucinogen most often associated with severe violence because of its effect on thinking, judgment, and perception. The presence of horizontal or vertical nystagmus in association with agitation should alert the clinician to the possibility of PCP intoxication. **Barbiturates** and **benzodiazepines** may cause aggression in two instances: (1) during the withdrawal phase agitation may be associated with violent behavior and (2) elderly, mentally retarded, and certain other persons with central nervous system dysfunction may respond paradoxically to sedatives with agitation and violence. The mechanisms are presumed to be similar to those of alcohol withdrawal and pathologic intoxication, respectively. **Opiates** are associated indirectly with violence, probably through behaviors related to drug acquisition rather than psychogenic effect.

7. Describe the relationship between personality disorders and violence.

In **borderline personality disorders**, traits of intense anger, impulsivity, and turbulent relationships often occur in conjunction with substance abuse and other self-destructive behaviors. Such patients are especially at risk for both suicidal and assaultive behaviors. Given their tendency toward affective instability, **mood disorders** are inevitably an important part of the differential diagnosis. In **antisocial personality disorder**, the patient violates many societal norms; violence is but one manifestation.

8. Describe the relationship between childhood disorders and violence.

Conduct disorder, by definition, is the childhood antecedent to adult antisocial personality disorder, although not all children with conduct disorder later develop the adult counterpart. Children with **oppositional disorder** display frequent temper outbursts, anger, and defiant behavior; physical aggression is not a prominent problem but may occur. Finally, **mentally retarded children** and adults are at risk for violent behavior. Their threshold for aggression appears to be lower because of (1) a tendency toward impulsivity and (2) difficulty in communicating their needs effectively.

9. Define intermittent explosive disorder.

Intermittent explosive disorder, formerly called episodic dyscontrol, is a disturbance of impulse in which acts of aggression occur out of proportion to the stimulus. Interepisode behavior is not marked by impulsivity. The diagnosis requires that all other potential causes and disorders associated with violence be ruled out. Although some authors suggest that the incidence of such dyscontrol may be higher among patients with seizure disorders, no evidence indicates that ictal or postictal states cause such behavior.

10. Which neurologic and medical illnesses can lead to violence?

A host of general medical conditions can lead to violence by altering personality or mood, or causing delirium or dementia.

Neurologic diseases:
   Dementias (e.g., Alzheimer's, Pick's, normal pressure hydrocephalus)
   Stroke syndromes
   Anoxic encephalopathy
   Wilson's disease
   Infections of the central nervous system (syphilis, human immunodeficiency virus, herpes
      simplex virus, other encephalitides, and meningitis)
   Ictal, postictal, and interictal states
   Tumors, especially of temporal and frontal lobes
   Multiple sclerosis
   Huntington's disease
   Head trauma
   Parkinson's disease

Systemic disorders affecting CNS function
   Metabolic disease (e.g., hypoglycemia, electrolyte disturbance)
   Toxic agents (e.g., drug, alcohol, heavy metal, poisons)
   Infectious disease
   Vitamin deficiencies (B12, folate, thiamine)
   Endocrine disturbances (thyroid, Cushing's disease)
   Hepatic and uremic encephalopathy
   Acute intermittent porphyria
   Lupus erythematosus

11. What are the risk factors for violence?

Obviously, any disorder associated with an increased incidence of violence is a risk factor, particularly when there is medication noncompliance. In addition, studies of violent behavior have revealed other specific risk factors, many of which occur in conjunction with the disorders listed in Question 10:

• A **history of physical abuse** as a child or witnessing such abuse is an increasingly publicized correlate of adult violence.

• **Present environment** also should be considered; for example, subcultures in which physical aggression is an accepted expression of anger or frustration may place a person at higher risk for aggressive behavior. Such cultures often are associated with an increased rate of unemployment, physical crowding, and poverty, all of which are independent risk factors. Ethnicity has *not* been found to be among the risk factors of violence.

• **Men** generally are involved more often in aggression than women, although the sex ratio equalizes in inpatient settings, perhaps because of the diversion of violent men into the prison system.

• **Young age** groups consistently are found to be more apt to display aggression. However, an examination of the full spectrum of the population reveals that the incidence of violence increases in the elderly, presumably because of the aggression associated with dementia and delirium.

• As is the case with suicide, a **history of violence or impulsivity** or an articulated plan with access to a weapon increases the risk of violence immensely. These are critical elements in the history (see Questions 15 and 16).

12. What is the relationship between seizures and violence?

While individuals with epilepsy demonstrate an increased incidence of psychiatric disorders, they are otherwise *not* at increased risk for violent behavior. Aggression displayed during an ictal event is not directed at an individual nor focused within the environment. However, goal-directed violence has been described during post-ictal states. These states are marked by psychosis, and the violence does not appear to be attributable to any post-ictal confusion. This aggression is similar to that seen in psychotic disorders due to other medical conditions.

13. What is the neurobiologic substrate of aggression?

Although there is no strict correlation between aggression and site of lesion, experiments of nature and animal studies support an association of such behavior with lesions of the medial temporal lobe, hypothalamus, and septum. The disinhibition that may occur with frontal lobe pathology also may result in violent and other impulsive behaviors.

Numerous researchers have attempted to identify the neurochemical substrate of violence. Although testosterone, norepinephrine, and dopamine have a putative role, probably the largest body of consistent data implicates serotonin. Decreased levels of serotonin metabolites in the cerebrospinal fluid appear to relate to violent behavior, particularly when committed impulsively.

14. What are the subtle cues to potential violence?

Impending violence is not always preceded by warning signs. However, clinicians should be familiar with certain common indicators. The diagnostic groups in Question 3 and the risk factors in Question 11 should be considered, particularly in conjunction with the following:

- In the emergency room, staff refusal of medications or services sought by the patient is a common precipitant of aggression.
- The first days in the hospital, a time during which the patient is unclear about acceptable limits on behavior or treatment plans, involve a higher risk.
- A sudden change in behavior, evidence of intoxication, or use of sunglasses indoors should serve as potential warning signs of impending violence or at least draw attention to potential paranoia or possible use of drugs.
- Agitation, pacing, loud or pressured speech, and anger should be monitored closely.
- Above all, verbal threats of violence must always be taken seriously and followed up with further questioning.

15. What is the work-up of violent behavior?

Violence is a symptom and therefore should be evaluated like any other presenting symptom:

- Thorough history of violent behavior
  - Present and past behavior
  - Other impulsive behaviors
- Detailed questioning of violent threats
  - Onset, duration, frequency
  - Specific methods
  - Intent
- Access to weapons
- Mental status and cognitive examinations
  - Agitation
  - Signs of psychosis, mania, or intoxication
  - Attentional and memory functioning
- Physical and neurologic examination
- Laboratory studies
  - Screening chemistries and hematologic tests
  - Thyroid function studies
  - Assessment of B_{12}, folate, calcium, magnesium, PO4, rapid plasmin reagin
  - Serum and urine toxicology
  - Other studies as clinically indicated (e.g., imaging study of brain, specialized studies of cerebrospinal fluid, serum, or urine)
- Imaging studies of brain
- Electroencephalogram
- Documentation
  - Direct quotations from patient
  - Detailed rationale for treatment or referral
  - Conversations with third parties

16. How do you facilitate a thorough history?

A thorough history of the behavior by the patient as well as by other informants is essential. It is often helpful to begin by eliciting the history of the patient's chief complaint and to shift into the history of the violent behavior later in the interview, when a rapport is established.

17. How should you respond _verbally_ to violent behavior?

Try to maintain a calm, controlled demeanor. Anger is a common response to a threat, but such expression by the clinician inevitably leads to escalation by the patient. Escalation is also the likely result if the clinician challenges the patient through any display of condescension or counterattack. Remain as conscious as possible of inappropriate responses and maintain restraint. You can gain the upper hand in such situations by assuming the submissive position. Admit that you feel frightened by the patient's behavior; this admission usually leads to a de-escalation of rage and provides a useful reality check for the patient. Also useful is identifying the emotion that the patient appears to be experiencing in the form of an inquiry (e.g., "You seem quite upset?"). Encourage the patient to talk about what is upsetting him or her.

If threats of violence continue, tell the patient that you are going to call for help—_and do so immediately_. If violence appears imminent, the clinician should leave the room, mobilize staff, and arrange for the safety of staff and other patients.

18. Describe the appropriate _behavioral_ response to a violent patient.

Verbal management usually should be attempted first, but it is not always sufficient, especially with patients who have organic or psychotic disorders. Hence, the clinician should have a well-organized behavioral strategy established with associated staff that can be implemented efficiently when necessary. In high-risk settings, such as emergency rooms or psychiatric outpatient clinics, offices should be set up with an emergency buzzer, code word, or signal that can discreetly alert other staff of a potentially volatile patient. Staff should be clear on how to respond, including whom to call (e.g., security, police) and how to provide for the safety of other staff or patients in the area. Occasional drills to practice such responses may be life-saving. Whenever violent behavior is a concern, the patient should be seen with staff (clinical or security) located either nearby or in the same room.

Clinicians who work in high-risk settings should set up their interviewing space so that both the clinician and the patient have easy, unobstructed access to the door. Never sit behind a desk, and remove heavy or sharp objects. Consider avoiding jewelry and neckties when working with such patients.

In the event the patient escapes, do not run after him or her. If a weapon is revealed, do not attempt to retrieve it; instead, attempt to engage the patient in conversation, signal for help, and encourage the patient to place the weapon in a neutral place.

19. What is the appropriate role of seclusion and restraint?

This is a specific form of behavioral management that provides for the safety of the patient and staff when all else fails. Implementation requires access to staff who undergo regular inservice training in the application and monitoring of restraints or seclusion. A restraint team typically has a designated leader who directs the application of restraints and talks to the patient as they are applied. The staff must understand the experience of the patient; in some states, staff are required by law to be personally placed in restraints as part of their training.

Whether physical or chemical restraint is preferred continues to be controversial; in general, the choice depends on the individual case and availability of resources in the treatment setting. When the cause of the aggression is unclear or when frank delirium is present, consider minimizing exposure to psychotropic medications, because they may confuse or exacerbate the clinical picture.

20. Describe the proper use of drugs and chemical restraint in treating violent behavior.

First and foremost, the underlying disorder should be treated pharmacologically whenever possible. The use of chemical restraints in controlling acutely violent behavior is another form of therapeutic intervention. Pharmacologic restraint may be used after verbal and behavioral interventions have failed, either alone or in combination with physical restraint. Medication is an ideal intervention when it has been determined that the underlying cause of the aggression in a psychiatric disturbance that is pharmacologically responsive. *All patients should be given an opportunity to take the medication voluntarily,* in either the oral or intramuscular form.

21. Which psychotropic agents should be considered for chemical restraint?

Benzodiazepines. Through their sedative action, benzodiazepines usually have a calming effect and may provide a speedy and effective response, particularly when administered intramuscularly (IM). Close observation of the patient is essential, with frequent monitoring of vital signs, because of the potential for respiratory depression. Paradoxical responses, including increased anger and agitation, also may occur, particularly in mentally retarded, elderly, and personality-disordered patients. Organic brain syndromes also are thought to increase the risk of paradoxical response.

Neuroleptics. Although neuroleptics may be especially beneficial for treating psychotic patients who are assaultive, the antipsychotic effects may not occur for 7–10 days. It is more likely that the tranquilizing properties of the neuroleptics are responsible for the sedating effects. Again, close observation of the patient is necessary, including monitoring for extrapyramidal side effects, dystonic reactions, and akathisia. A pattern of increasing agitation should immediately trigger the question of whether the clinician is ensnared in a vicious cycle of chasing akathisia, which may manifest as mounting agitation, with increasing doses of neuroleptics. If akathisia is suspected, first try lowering the dose of the neuroleptic. If this leads to a further increase in agitation, try benzodiazepines or beta blockers, because they often are more effective against akathisia than are anticholinergics.

Barbiturates. Respiratory depression and risk of laryngospasm precludes the use of barbiturates in most instances, given the relative advantages of benzodiazepines and neuroleptics.

22. What are the recommended doses of benzodiazepines and neuroleptics for emergency treatment of assaultive behavior?

Benzodiazepines

Lorazepam: 0.5–2 mg PO or IM every 1–4 hr

Use lower doses for elderly or medically ill patients.

Watch for respiratory depression or laryngospasm (rare).

Watch for paradoxical agitation.

Neuroleptics

Haloperidol: 0.5–5 mg PO or IM every 1–4 hr

Droperidol: 5 mg IM or slow intravenous push every 15 min until sedated, not to exceed 50 mg/24 hr

Chlorpromazine: 10–25 mg every 1–4 hr

Watch for orthostatic hypotension, especially with chlorpromazine.

Monitor regularly for extrapyramidal signs; treat with anticholinergics (e.g., benztropine, 1–2 mg PO or IM every 4 hr)

Be especially attentive to signs of akathisia; treat with dose reduction or propranolol, 10–20 mg PO every 4 hr, lorazepam, 0.5–2 mg every 4 hr

23. What should be done if a staff member or another patient is hurt?

If there is any question of physical contact, an immediate physical examination should be performed by the physician on call if the victim is a patient. If the victim is a staff member or visitor, the nearest emergency department or employee health office is usually appropriate. Documentation of any findings or the absence of injury is important both in the examining physician's medical report and in an incident report form, which is available in most institutions.

Once physical injuries are clarified and treated, the victim must be supported emotionally—not only at the time of the incident but also during the following weeks. Emotional sequelae may take several weeks to surface and may be quite severe. Symptoms often take the form of a posttraumatic stress reaction, with easy startle, autonomic hyperactivity, sleep disturbances, and even avoidance behaviors. In addition, a tremendous amount of self-blame, anger, and guilt often emerge as the sense of vulnerability intensifies.

Complicating matters is the response, or lack thereof, of the institution. The dynamics of institutional systems may involve, in part, a contagious spread of fear and unconscious threat; peers as well as administrators may inadvertently pathologize the victim. Such a reaction further entrenches the self-blame. Because of this potential, some hospitals establish a committee that routinely interviews and offers limited support services to staff who are assaulted. Such committees are equipped to refer for more intensive counseling, if necessary.

24. Is long-term treatment available for violent patients?

Yes. If a definable underlying medical or psychiatric condition causes the aggression, it should be identified and treated. When addressing the underlying condition fails to fully control the violent behavior, the following strategies, though not FDA-approved for the treatment of violence, may be considered:

Pharmacologic strategies.

• Mood stabilizers. Lithium, in particular, as well as carbamazepine and valproate have been shown effective in some violent patients. Newer agents such as gabapentin and lamotrigine also may prove useful, but have not yet been formally studied.

• Beta blockers. Propranolol has long been used in the treatment of aggressive behavior. It must be titrated gradually starting with 10–20 mg tid so as to minimize cardiovascular side effects. Latency to response may be 1–2 months. Other beta-blockers such as pindolol may be less prone to causing orthostasis and lethargy due to its partial agonist effect.

• Neuroleptics. The atypical antipsychotics may be a valuable addition to our armamentarium, perhaps in part due to their serotonergic activity. Clozapine has been demonstrated to reduce aggressive behavior in chronically psychotic individuals. Risperdal appears to share this benefit and, in a comparative study with haloperidol, was superior in reducing hostility scores.

• Antidepressants. Fluoxetine is probably the antidepressant most frequently cited in reducing aggression and impulsivity. While a report of heightened suicidality in association with fluoxetine stirred much public attention, subsequent analyses of this potential association suggest a minimal risk for heightened aggression, including that directed towards oneself. Nonetheless, it is most prudent to provide close monitoring, especially for manifestations of akathisia and heightened agitation, when using these agents.

• Anxiolytics. Benzodiazepines are not a long-term solution for managing aggression, and may in fact heighten the risk for aggression through their disinhibiting effects. However, buspirone may provide a long-term solution through its antiaggressive effects.

Behavioral strategies. Modification of aggression through behavioral strategies is particularly successful in institutional settings with the potential for structure. Treatment may include the use of rewards in exchange for self-control of aggression. Note that excess attention to the patient can reinforce negative behaviors. Of course, chemical or physical restraints are imperative if physical danger is imminent or assault has occurred. However, staff members should be conscious of the attention that they pay to the patient in the process of restraining him or her, because such attention may serve as a reinforcer. An important addition to the behavioral strategy is social skills training, particularly for regressed, psychotic, or retarded individuals who may be aggressive out of frustration at not getting their needs met. Such individuals need to be educated about more socially appropriate ways of meeting their needs.

Psychotherapy. Individual, family, and/or group psychotherapy may be beneficial for individuals who are genuinely invested in trying to change their violent behavior and who can maintain sufficient control of their impulses to allow the therapist and others involved in the therapy to feel safe. It is critical that the therapist monitor accurately both his or her emotional responses to the patient and shifts in the affective expression of the patient. Dealing with mounting fear is crucial (see Questions 17 and 18). The therapist also must be aware of the potential for his or her anger toward the patient as an expression of vulnerability. Unattended anger may directly influence the therapy in destructive ways.

BIBLIOGRAPHY

1. Beck JC: The potentially violent patient: Legal duties, clinical practice, and risk management. Psychiatr Ann 17:695–699, 1987.
2. Birkett DP: Violence in geropsychiatry. Psychiatr Ann 27(11):752–756, 1997.
3. Blair DT: Assaultive behavior. Does provocation begin in the front office? J Psychosoc Nurs 29(5):21–26, 1991.
4. Citrome L, Volauka J: Psychopharmacology of violence. Part II: Beyond the acute episode. Psychiatr Ann 27(10):696–703, 1997.
5. Davis S: Violence by psychiatric inpatients: A review. Hosp Community Psychiatry 42:585–590, 1991.
6. Eichelman B: Aggressive behavior: From laboratory to clinic. Quo vadit? Arch Gen Psychiatry 49:488–492, 1992.
7. Elliot FA: Violence. The neurologic contribution: An overview. Arch Neurol 49:595–603, 1992.
8. Franzen MD, Lovell MR: Behavioral treatments of aggressive sequelae of brain injury. Psychiatr Ann 17: 389– 396, 1989.
8a. Kanemoto K, Kawasaki J, Mori E: Violence and epilepsy: A close relation between violence and postictal psychosis. Epilepsia 40(1):107–109, 1999.
9. Lanza ML: The reactions of nursing staff to physical assault by a patient. Hosp Community Psychiatry 34: 44–47, 1983.
10. McNiel DE: Correlates of violence in psychotic patients. Psychiatr Ann 27(10):683–690, 1997.
11. McNiel DE, Myers RS, Zeiner HK, et al: The role of violence in decisions about hospitalization from the psychiatric emergency room. Am J Psychiatry 149:207–212, 1992.
12. Miller RJ, Zadolinnyi K, Hafner RJ: Profiles and predictors of assaultiveness for different psychiatric ward populations. Am J Psychiatry 150:1368–1373, 1993.
13. Randolph LB: When a patient becomes violent. Psychiatr Resident, May/June 1992, pp 18–22.
14. Stevenson S: Heading off violence with verbal de-escalation. J Psychosoc Nurs 29(9):6–10, 1991.
15. Swartz M, Swanson J, et al: Violence and severe mental illness: The effects of substance abuse and nonadherence to medication. Am J Psych 155(2):226–231, 1998.
16. Tardiff K: Concise Guide to Assessment and Management of Violent Patients. Washington, DC, American Psychiatric Press, 1989.
17. Tardiff K: The current state of psychiatry in the treatment of violent patients. Arch Gen Psychiatry 49:493–499, 1992.

77. NEUROLEPTIC MALIGNANT SYNDROME

James L. Jacobson, M.D.

1. Describe neuroleptic malignant syndrome.

Neuroleptic malignant syndrome (NMS) is an acute, potentially fatal, idiosyncratic reaction to neuroleptic medications (which primarily are antipsychotic medications). The principal manifestations are due to disorders of thermoregulation and skeletal muscle metabolism mediated via central mechanisms. The usual presentation consists of four primary features: (1) hyperthermia, (2) extreme generalized rigidity, (3) autonomic instability, and (4) altered mental status. The overall appearance is of a profoundly ill individual with an alert, frightened stare.

2. What are the specific criteria for diagnosis of NMS?

The diagnosis of NMS requires the presence of specific historical information, physical signs, symptoms, and exclusionary criteria. There must be a **recent history of exposure** to neuroleptic medication. Usually this exposure is acute and occurs within 7–10 days of onset of the syndrome. However, NMS can occur in chronic usage. **Temperature elevation** can be mild or severe, early or late in the progression of NMS. **Autonomic instability** is indicated by labile hypertension (less often hypotension) and tachycardia. **Mental status** is always **altered**, typically in the form of delirium, which may progress to stupor, obtundation, and coma. Extreme **muscular rigidity** has been characterized as "lead-pipe rigidity" and is present in all skeletal muscle. **Diaphoresis** is nearly always present. **Sialorrhea** is often present, as is **dysphagia**. Alternative etiologies for these symptoms must be excluded by history, examination, and laboratory studies. (See also DSM-IV, pp 739–742.)

3. Are there specific laboratory findings for NMS?

No laboratory findings are pathognomonic for NMS, but certain studies are important both to support the diagnosis of NMS and to exclude other systemic illnesses. Common laboratory abnormalities include elevation of creatinine phosphokinase (muscle fraction often massively elevated) and leukocytosis. Electrolyte disturbances may occur secondarily, as well as hypocalcemia, hypomagnesemia, and hypophosphatemia. Urinalysis often reveals proteinuria and myoglobinuria from rhabdomyolysis. Elevated BUN and creatinine may occur, indicating renal compromise due to rhabdomyolysis and/or dehydration. Cerebrospinal fluid (CSF) studies should be normal. An EEG may show diffuse slowing without focal abnormalities. When evaluating a patient with suspected NMS, perform the following studies to exclude a systemic illness: CBC with a differential WBC; serum electrolytes; creatinine and BUN; muscle and hepatic enzymes; thyroid function tests; urinalysis; EKG; appropriate cultures for infection; and brain imaging, EEG, CSF studies (when indicated).

4. What is the differential diagnosis of NMS?

The differential diagnosis includes several processes that can cause increased temperature due to abnormal thermoregulation. These are divided into primary CNS disorders and systemic disorders.

Differential Diagnosis of NMS

PRIMARY CNS DISORDERS	SYSTEMIC DISORDERS
Infections (viral encephalitis, post-infectious encephalitis, HIV)	Infections
Tumors	Metabolic conditions
Cerebrovascular disease	Endocrinopathies (thyrotoxicosis, pheochromocytoma)
Head trauma	Autoimmune disease (SLE)
Seizures	Heat stroke
Major psychoses (lethal catatonia)	Toxins (CO, phenols, strychnine, tetanus)
	Drugs (salicylates, dopamine inhibitors and antagonists, stimulants, psychedelics, MAOIs, anesthetics, anticholinergics, alcohol or sedative withdrawal)

From Caroff SN, et al: Neuroleptic malignant syndrome: Diagnostic issues. Psychiatr Ann 21:130–147, 1991, with permission.

5. What causes NMS?

The specific antidopaminergic activity of antipsychotic medications appears to be the predominant cause of NMS, particularly D_2 receptor antagonism. Central dopaminergic systems are involved in thermoregulation as well as regulation of muscle tone and movement. Defects in hypothalamic sympathetic nervous system regulation also have been postulated. The relatively infrequent occurrence of NMS, however, suggests the concurrence of other factors. Speculations have included imbalances with other neurotransmitter systems, abnormalities in second messenger systems, and the presentation of particular risk factors. Currently, all of the antipsychotic medications, including the atypical antipsychotic medications, have been reported to cause NMS. NMS also has been reported with some antiemetic medications such as prochlorperazine maleate and metoclopramide, which are also neuroleptics.

6. Which risk factors predispose to the development of NMS?

Suggested risk factors include dehydration, a primary diagnosis of affective disorder (especially bipolar disorder and psychotic depression), concurrent presence of dementia, use of other neuroactive medications, higher relative doses and parenteral administration of neuroleptics, prior history of

NMS, electrolyte disturbances, any medical or neurologic illness, and a recent history of substance abuse or dependence.

7. How common is NMS?

Rates as low as 0.02% and as high as 2.5% have been reported, but overall the rate appears to be just under 1%.

8. What is the mortality rate associated with NMS?

Mortality from NMS has been declining since its original description in 1968. The earliest reports suggested mortality rates as high as 75%. In the early 1980s mortality rates declined to 20–30%. Current studies suggest that the mortality rate declined further, probably to less than 15%. Early recognition and familiarity with the syndrome are the most likely reasons for this hopeful trend.

9. Discuss the treatments for NMS.

Early recognition is crucial. Increased temperature, elevated blood pressure, tachycardia, muscle stiffness not responsive to antiparkinsonian agents, clustering of risk factors, dysphagia, and severe diaphoresis early in the course of treatment with neuroleptic medication should alert the physician to the possible emergence of NMS. Neuroleptic and other potentially neurotoxic medications must be stopped. Supportive measures to lower temperature and ensure good fluid intake are essential. Electrolyte disturbances must be corrected. Closely monitor the patient for signs of impending respiratory failure secondary to severe muscle rigidity and inability to handle oral secretions. Carefully watch renal function. Although there is no evidence that osmotic diuresis hastens recovery from NMS, it may help to maintain renal function. Often, treatment in a medical intensive care unit is necessary.

Pharmacologic intervention has tended to be reserved for severe cases. **Dopamine agonists** (bromocriptine and amantadine) and/or **direct muscle relaxants** (dantrolene) have been used: decreased mortality rates have been reported with both types. Dosages vary widely, but doses of bromocriptine have been documented between 2.5 and 35 mg/day. Generally bromocriptine has been started at 2.5 to 5 mg three times daily given orally (or via nasogastric tube in patients with dysphagia or severely compromised mental status). Dopamine agonists, particularly in higher doses, can cause psychosis and/or vomiting, which clearly can complicate the picture and compromise the patient. The only data available on direct-acting muscle relaxants are for dantrolene. Doses of up to 10 mg/kg have been used. The goal is to decrease muscular rigidity in order to decrease the hypermetabolic state in skeletal muscle, which is partially responsible for the hyperthermia in NMS. Dantrolene can cause hepatoxicity, which can lead to overt hepatitis and death. Combinations of dantrolene and dopamine agonists have been used, although there is no clear evidence that they further decrease mortality when used in combination.

Anticholinergic medications commonly used to treat pseudoparkinsonism have little benefit and may further impair heat dissipation mechanisms. Treatment with carbamazapine recently has been reported, with rapid symptom resolution in a few cases. Although there is no clear evidence to support the use of benzodiazepines in the treatment of NMS, they can be useful in managing an agitated hyperactive patient once NMS has begun to resolve.

10. Will NMS recur with subsequent use of neuroleptic medication?

The risk of recurrence decreases with time. Of patients rechallenged with neuroleptics prior to 2 weeks after resolution of NMS, there is a high recurrence rate. Those cautiously rechallenged 2 weeks or longer after resolution of NMS often tolerated neuroleptics without difficulty. A low-potency neuroleptic agent is chosen for the rechallenge. In addition, atypical antipsychotic medications with lower D_2 receptor affinity may offer a particular advantage. Dosing should be conservative and increased gradually. Recent interest in the concurrent use of the calcium channel blocker nifedipine has also shown promise in prevention of recurrence, although the data are still incomplete. Some individuals are prone to NMS and, of course, close attention to early symptoms is crucial.

Guidelines for Managing Patients with NMS

---

1. History of a previous episode of NMS confirmed?
   Yes: Go to (2)
   No: Speak with patient, family, and treating physician(s). Retrieve pertinent medical records to confirm the diagnosis of NMS.
2. Based on careful review of the psychiatric history and previous response to treatment, is neuroleptic therapy essential?
   Yes: Go to (3)
   No: Treat accordingly, without neuroleptics
3. Two or more episodes of NMS with more than one neuroleptic?
   Yes: Go to (4)
   No: Wait 2 weeks after recovery from NMS. Rechallenge with a low-potency neuroleptic. If a low-potency neuroleptic originally caused NMS, rechallenge with a low-potency neuroleptic from a different chemical class.
4. Have prophylactic agents—bromocriptine, dantrolene, or nifedipine—been used in conjunction with neuroleptics?
   Yes: Go to (5)
   No: Consider such a trial, or go to (5)
5. Alternatives to conventional neuroleptic therapy:
   (a) clozapine, (b) benzodiazepines, (c) electroconvulsive therapy, (d) anticonvulsants, and (e) lithium.

From Lazarus et al: Beyond NMS: Management after the acute episode. Psychiatr Ann 21:165–174, 1991; with permission.

11. Is there any way to prevent NMS?
   No. Early recognition and, when clinically warranted, lower dosing, avoidance of parenteral neuroleptic medication, avoidance of rapid increases in dosages, and minimization of the other risk factors (e.g., good hydration) may decrease the incidence of NMS.

12. Are there alternatives to neuroleptic treatment for the acutely psychotic patient?
   There are a number of treatment options. Benzodiazepines may help in the management of the hyperactive psychotic patient and lower the absolute dose of neuroleptic needed. When the primary diagnosis is affective disorder (as in a significant percentage of patients developing NMS), aggressive treatment of mania with valproate, lithium carbonate, or carbamazepine and of depression with antidepressants is indicated. It is usually necessary to administer neuroleptic medications concomitantly when psychotic symptoms are present. Electroconvulsive therapy is a viable alternative for manic psychosis and depressive psychosis, and may alleviate catatonia.
   In chronic psychotic disorders (e.g., schizophrenia, schizoaffective disorder, delusional disorder) there may be no alternative to the use of neuroleptic medications. Hence, cautious rechallenging with different classes of neuroleptics (with special attention to atypical antipsychotic agents and treatment of reversible risk factors) is virtually always necessary.

ACKNOWLEDGMENT

   This chapter is modified with permission from Critical Care Secrets, Philadelphia, Hanley & Belfus, 1991.

BIBLIOGRAPHY

1. Addonizio G, Susman VL: Neuroleptic Malignant Syndrome: A Clinical Approach. St. Louis, Mosby, 1991.
2. Caroff SN (ed): Neuroleptic malignant syndrome. Psychiatr Ann 21:128–180, 1991.
3. Castillo E, Rubin R, Holsboer-Truacster E: Clinical differentiation between lethal catatonia and neuroleptic malignant syndrome. Am J Psychiatry 145:324–328, 1989.
4. Fink M: Neuroleptic malignant syndrome and catatonia: One entity or two? Biol Psychiatry 39:1–4, 1996.
5. Gurrera RJ: Sympathoadrenal hyperactivity and the etiology of neuroleptic malignant syndrome. Am J Psychiatry 156(2): 169–180, 1999.

6. Gurrera RJ, Chang SS: Thermoregulatory dysfunction in neuroleptic malignant syndrome. Biol Psychiatry 39:207–212, 1996.
7. Keck PE, Caroff SN, McElroy SL: Neuroleptic malignant syndrome and malignant hyperthermia. End of a controversy? J Neuropsychiatry Clin Neurosci 7:135–144, 1995.
8. Levenson JL: Neuroleptic malignant syndrome. Am J Psychiatry 142:1137–1145, 1985.
9. Pelonero AL, Levenson JL, Pandurangi AK: Neuroleptic malignant syndrome: A review. Psychiatric Services 49(9):1163–1172, 1998.
10. Pope JG Jr, Aizley HG, Keck PE, McElroy SL: Neuroleptic malignant syndrome: Long-term follow-up of 20 cases. J Clin Psychiatry 42:208–212, 1991.
11. Pope HG Jr, Keck Jr, McElroy SL: Frequency and presentation of neuroleptic malignant syndrome in a large psychiatric hospital. Am J Psychiatry 143:1227–1232, 1986.
12. Rosenberg MR, Green M: Neuroleptic malignant syndrome: A review of response to therapy. Arch Intern Med 149:1927–1931, 1989.
13. Rosebush P, Stewart T: A prospective analysis of 24 episodes of neuroleptic malignant syndrome. Am J Psychiatry 146:717–725, 1989.
14. Rosebush PI, Stewart TD, Gelenberg AJ: Twenty neuroleptic rechallenges after neuroleptic malignant syndrome in 15 patients. J Clin Psychiatry 50:295–298, 1989.
15. Shalev A, Heresh H, Munitz H: Mortality from neuroleptic malignant syndrome. Clin Psychiatry 50:18–22, 1989.
16. Susman VL, Addonizio G: Recurrence of neuroleptic malignant syndrome. J Nerv Ment Dis 176:234–241, 1988.
17. Zubenko G, Pope HG: Management of a case of neuroleptic malignant syndrome with bromocriptine. Am J Psychiatry 140:1619–1629, 1983.

78. TREATMENT-RESISTANT DEPRESSION

Marshall R. Thomas, M.D., and Christopher Schneck, M.D.

1. How is treatment-resistant depression defined?

Treatment resistance is a relative term. A frequently used definition is failure to respond to an adequate trial of at least two standard antidepressants. However, even this seemingly straightforward definition presents several problems. What constitutes an adequate drug trial in terms of dose and duration is still debated. Moreover, the definition of "treatment response" also varies: one commonly used definition—a greater than 50% reduction in the Hamilton Depression Rating Scale—defines as responders some patients with significant residual depression.

The time required for an adequate trial is now considered in the 6–10 week range, in light of studies showing a high rate of response conversion in the second month of treatment. The notion of "adequate dosage" of an antidepressant has been complicated by the introduction of many new agents for which antidepressant blood levels are either unavailable or uninterpretable. Given that patients taking tricyclic antidepressants (TCAs) can demonstrate a 10–40 fold interindividual variability of blood levels for a given dose of drug, many clinicians became convinced of the importance of serum drug levels for TCAs when faced with treatment-resistant conditions.

2. How are patients with treatment-resistant depression different from other depressives?

Patients with treatment-resistant depression are likely to have a past history of relapsing depression or chronic depression. They are likely to have an older age at onset of their illness and to show decreased cortical mass and ventricular enlargement on neuroimaging studies. They often fail to normalize a nonsuppressed dexamethasone suppression test (DST). They typically have comorbid psychiatric and medical illnesses.

3. What psychiatric conditions are commonly comorbid with treatment resistance?

Substance abuse, panic disorder, eating disorders, and personality disorders are associated with treatment resistance. Depressed substance abusers are less likely to respond to treatment, more likely to relapse, and more likely to attempt suicide. Patients with comorbid panic have more severe depressions and a poorer response to standard treatments. Patients with bulimia and especially anorexia can show a poor response to treatment. Comorbid personality disorders are seen in 40–60% of depressives. These patients typically demonstrate depressions with a younger age of onset, more lifetime episodes, more suicidal ideation, and a decreased response to treatment.

4. How do medical disorders affect treatment resistance?

Medical disorders can cause, worsen, or potentially complicate the course of depression. Some conditions, such as undiagnosed hypothyroidism, can cause a seemingly "refractory depression." Other conditions, such as chronic pain, may interact reciprocally: worsening or improving one may lead to parallel worsening or improving the other. Still other conditions, such as cardiac disease, may limit choices in antidepressants. Seek and treat underlying medical illness in any patient who is considered treatment-refractory.

5. What is the most common cause of supposed "treatment-refractory" depression?

Inadequate treatment is probably the most common cause of chronicity and relapse. An estimated two-thirds of the patients treated in the community receive treatment that is inadequate in terms of dosage or duration (i.e., at least 4–6 weeks).

6. What is the importance of depressive subtypes?

Psychotic, atypical, bipolar, and geriatric depressions are important subtypes of depressive illness, in that each may require specific treatment strategies.

Depressive Subtypes

Psychotic-nonpsychotic	Atypical-typical
Bipolar-unipolar	Geriatric-late onset

Unrecognized **psychotic depression** is a common cause of treatment resistance. Often, psychotic symptoms are subtle and revealed only with careful and specific questions. Patients with psychotic depression respond poorly to antidepressants and antipsychotic drugs when either is used alone. However, these patients respond well to combinations of the two drugs, or to electroconvulsive therapy (ECT).

Atypical depression is characterized by mood reactivity (i.e., mood varies with the nature of interpersonal interactions), leaden fatigue (the patient's arms and legs feel extremely heavy), rejection sensitivity (overly sensitive to slight criticism), and the reversed vegetative signs of increased sleep and appetite. Such patients respond poorly to TCAs and show a superior response to selective serotonin reuptake inhibitors (SSRIs) and monoamine oxidase inhibitors (MAOIs). These patients may respond to newer agents such as buproprion, venlafaxine, mirtazapine, or nefazodone, but further studies are needed.

Treatment of **bipolar depression** is discussed elsewhere (see Chapters 12 and 49). Failure to recognize a depression as bipolar may lead to mood cycling, mania, or mixed states. Improper choices in medications can fail to treat the underlying illness and worsen the long-term course of the disease.

Geriatric depressives are more likely to experience masked depression and to have symptoms of anxiety, memory problems, and bodily complaints. Late-onset depression, defined as having an onset after age 65, is more likely to be associated with a dementing illness, delusions, and complicating medical conditions. Many elderly depressives have difficulty in tolerating medication trials and respond preferentially to ECT.

7. How do I assess a treatment-resistant patient?

The patient presenting as "treatment resistant" warrants a careful review of his/her psychiatric and medical condition. First, clarify whether the patient has a depressive subtype that requires a specific treatment. Next, review dosage and duration of past medication trials in detail to determine the adequacy of past treatment strategies. If TCAs were used, ascertain whether blood levels were obtained and, if so, whether therapeutic levels were achieved.

Review of the patient's physical condition may reveal an untreated medical problem that needs attention. Attempt to detect undiagnosed comorbid psychiatric conditions such as substance abuse, anxiety, and eating or obsessive-compulsive disorders. Lastly, assess personality factors, coping style, social supports, psychosocial stressors, and response to any previous psychotherapy.

Common Causes of Treatment Resistance

Inadequate dosages	Comorbid conditions
Inadequate duration	Medication noncompliance
Inaccurate subtype	Medical causation

8. What role do psychosocial issues play in treatment resistance?

Several studies indicate that a nonsupportive spouse correlates with treatment refractoriness, especially for women. Unemployment is associated with increased rates of depression for men; having a job outside of the home appears protective against depression for both sexes. Financial impoverishment, in general, is associated with an increase in severity and chronicity for a variety of psychiatric conditions for both men and women, including depression.

Premorbid personality traits, such as chronically low self-esteem, are associated with longer-term treatment resistance, although such symptoms may represent subsyndromal or prodromal expressions of a depressive illness. Patients with borderline personality disorder may present a special challenge to clinicians, as often these patients have histories of physical, sexual, and emotional abuse. How a history of abuse or neglect affects treatment is a subject of some debate and probably varies from patient to patient.

9. How do I proceed if the previous antidepressant trials appear to have been adequate?

Once genuine treatment resistance is established, a variety of treatment options exist, with no one option clearly proven to be "the best" choice. Given the large number of options and the fact that serial drug trials often are required, it is important to develop a **collaborative and supportive relationship** with the patient, who thereby becomes an active partner in the decision-making process. The clinician's role in providing an ongoing sense of hopefulness is extremely important. In general, interventions involve switching medications, augmentation strategies, and/or psychosocial therapy.

Intervention Strategies for Treatment-Resistant Depression

Switching
  TCAs (with blood levels)
  SSRIs
  MAOIs
  Mixed reuptake inhibitors (nefazodone, mirtazapine, venlafaxine, buproprion)
  ECT
Augmentation
  Lithium
  Thyroid (T$_3$)
  Combinations (TCA + SSRI, venlafaxine + mirtazapine, SSRIs + buproprion, etc.)
  Buspirone
  Stimulants
  Pindolol
  Phototherapy
Psychosocial
  Reassess therapeutic strategy
  Couples/family therapy
  Substance abuse treatment
  Cognitive, behavioral, and interpersonal techniques

10. What is a switching strategy?

Switching strategies involve abandoning one medication or treatment strategy and replacing it with another. The literature concerning switches to a drug in the same class is mixed. There is little evidence to support a switch from one TCA to another unless it is a matter of changing side-effect profiles. There is some evidence that changing from one SSRI to another may provide a more robust antidepressant response in some patients. Switching to a new class of antidepressants has the best support in the literature; some studies show 50–65% response rates to a subsequent trial of a new class of antidepressant or ECT. Previously it was thought that 70% of treatment refractory cases would respond to adequate trials of either a TCA, MAOI, or ECT. The addition of SSRIs, buproprion, venlafaxine, mirtazapine, and nefazodone (though not to an MAOI due to the risk of hypertensive crisis) should increase these numbers even further.

11. What is an augmentation strategy?

Augmentation strategies involve adding a new intervention to ongoing treatment. They are most frequently used when the patient has had a partial response to the current medication. An augmentation strategy is an attempt to augment and improve antidepressant response by adding to an existing treatment, rather than risk losing current gains by using a switching strategy.

Lithium augmentation has the most support from research. Lithium augmentation is effective in the treatment of unipolar as well as bipolar depression, with response rates of 30–75% in previously refractory patients. With thyroid augmentation, there is more data supporting the effectiveness of triiodothyronine (T3) compared to thyroxine (T4). In one well-designed study, T3 in the dose range of 25–50 µg/day was found to be as effective as lithium as an augmenting agent.

Other augmenting strategies involving buspirone, stimulants, anticonvulsants, pindolol, risperidone, and alpha-2 antagonists are less proven or have not been systematically studied. Combination strategies, such as TCAs + SSRIs, mirtazapine + venlafaxine, and SSRIs + buproprion, are becoming more popular, but lack systematic research as to their effectiveness in refractory illnesses.

12. What is the role of ECT?

ECT is still the single most potent treatment for severe depression. ECT may be the treatment of first choice in patients with:

• Severe depression with suicidal intent
• Depression associated with life-threatening medical debilitation
• Patients with a history of nonresponse to medication and a positive response to ECT.

Overall the 85–90% response rates to ECT drop to 50% if rigid criteria for previous treatment resistance are applied. As with medication nonresponse, some patients with a history of ECT nonresponse have had inadequate dose (inadequate electrical stimuli or unilateral stimulation only) or duration (inadequate number of treatments). In patients who do not respond, bilateral treatment with a stimulus intensity 150% greater than seizure threshold is warranted.

One problem with ECT is the high rate of relapse (50–60%) in the year after treatment, even if a supposedly adequate medication regimen is resumed. This finding suggests that either novel pharmacologic strategies or maintenance ECT are needed to prevent relapse in previously treatment-resistant patients who respond to ECT.

CONTROVERSY

13. What is the role of psychostimulants in treating treatment-refractory depression?

Psychostimulants, such as methylphenidate and dextroamphetamine, appear to be effective antidepressants for some patients. However, clinicians remain hesitant to use them because of concerns about abuse, tolerance, and side effects. The majority of controlled studies using stimulants as antidepressants show them to be no more effective than placebo.

Patients with a history of depression and attention-deficit hyperactivity disorder may be particularly good candidates for the use of stimulants. Medically ill patients also may be good candidates, particularly those who are excessively fatigued or lacking motivation. However, the advent of SSRIs and newer antidepressants (e.g., buproprion, venlafaxine) has expanded the range of antidepressants and provided alternatives with fewer liabilities compared to stimulants.

In patients with a history of treatment refractoriness as opposed to antidepressant intolerance, controlled trials of stimulant drugs are lacking, although clinicians note significantly positive effects in some patients. In terms of side effects, stimulants may worsen hypertension in adults and cause tics in children. Another concern is that chronic use of high-dose stimulants may worsen psychosis in psychosis-prone individuals.

BIBLIOGRAPHY

1. American Psychiatric Association: Diagnostic and Statistical Manual of Mental Disorders, 4th ed. Washington, DC, American Psychiatric Association, 1994.
2. Amsterdam JD (ed): Pharmacotherapy of Depression. New York, Marcel Dekker, 1990.
3. Clayton PJ: Bipolar illness. In Winokur G, Clayton PJ (eds): The Medical Basis of Psychiatry, 2nd ed. Philadelphia, W.B. Saunders, 1994, pp 47–67.
3a. Fava M: New approaches to the treatment of refractory depression. J Clin Psychiatry 61(Suppl):26, 2000.
4. Nelson JC: Overcoming treatment resistance in depression. J Clin Psychiatry 59(suppl 16):13–19, 1998.
5. Nierenberg AA, White K: What next? A review of pharmacologic strategies in treatment resistant depression. Psychopharmacol Bull 26:429, 1990.
6. Phillips KA, Nierenberg AA: The assessment and treatment of refractory depression. J Clin Psychiatry 55(Suppl):20, 1994.
7. Thase ME, Rush AJ: Treatment-resistant depression. In Bloom FE, Kupfer DJ (eds): Psychopharmacology: The Fourth Generation of Progress. New York, Raven Press, 1995, pp 1081–1097.
8. Winokur G: Unipolar depression. In Winokur G (ed): The Medical Basis of Psychiatry, 2nd ed. Philadelphia, W.B. Saunders, 1994, pp 69–86.

79. OBESITY

Rena R. Wing, Ph.D., and Mary Lou Klem, Ph.D.

1. What is body mass index?

Body mass index (BMI) is the currently recommended method of determining a patient's weight status. BMI is calculated by the following formula:

$$\frac{\text{weight in kg}}{(\text{height in meters})^2}$$

BMI correlates well with other measures of body fatness, such as hydrostatic weighing. Patients with a BMI of 19–24 are typically defined as within the optimal weight range; those with BMI of 25–29 are considered overweight (approximately 15–30% above ideal body weight), and those with a BMI $\geq$ 30 are considered obese.

2. How is body fat distribution a factor?

Body fat distribution is an important measure. Recent studies show that the risk of disease (including diabetes and heart disease) and mortality are related to the *location* of body fat in addition to the total amount. Patients with greater **abdominal obesity** appear to be at significantly increased risk for medical problems. Total abdominal fat is most accurately measured with computed tomography or magnetic resonance imaging, but such methods are expensive and not readily available in many clinics. Waist circumference has been shown to provide an accurate measure of abdominal fatness, and can be obtained easily in a clinical or office setting. Waist circumferences of greater than 102 cm (40 in) for men and 88 cm (35 in) for women are associated with increased risk of morbidity and mortality.

3. When should a patient be encouraged to lose weight?

In determining when to encourage weight loss, the patient's BMI and body fat distribution, other risk factors for coronary heart disease (CHD), and family history of obesity-related disease should be considered.

4. How common is obesity?

According to typical definitions (see Question 1), 59.4% of men and 50% of women in the United States are overweight or obese. Ethnic minority and socioeconomic status, as well as older age, are associated with higher prevalence rates; a striking example is found in African-American women, among whom a prevalence rate of 66% has been observed.

Whereas prevalence rates provide a clear picture of who is currently obese, incidence rates are helpful in understanding when a patient may be at risk for becoming overweight. A recent prospective study of adults aged 25–74 years concluded that the risk of major weight gain (defined as an increase of 5 kg/m^2, or about 14 kg within a 10-year period) was highest in adults aged 25–34 years; women were twice as likely as men to experience a major weight gain. Thus, although the greatest number of currently overweight adults is found among individuals aged 45 and above, the process of becoming overweight is likely to have begun years earlier.

5. Are social and cultural pressures increasing the prevalence of dieting and concerns about being overweight?

Yes. Every period of history develops its own standards of beauty and attractiveness. American society places a strong emphasis on thinness as beauty, and the ideal body weight has become increasingly lower. For example, researchers who followed the body weights of Miss America contestants over time found significant decreases in contestants' body weights and measurements in a 20-year period. Concomitant with changes in ideal body weight are rising levels of discontent with body size among the general public. At any one time, 20% of Americans report that they are dieting to lose weight.

Given the enormous social pressures to lose weight and individuals' sometimes unrealistic beliefs about weight loss (e.g., that a "perfect body" is achievable), it is important to discuss the *purpose* of weight loss (to prevent future health problems or to avoid exacerbation of existing problems) and healthy methods of achieving *reasonable weight loss goals* with all patients seeking to lose weight.

6. What causes obesity?

Obesity results from the combination of genetic predisposition and environmental influences. Studies of twins and adoption studies have shown a strong **genetic component** to obesity. The body weight of adults who were adopted as infants has been found to resemble the weight of their biologic parents, rather than the weight of their adoptive parents. Moreover, the ability to gain weight is under genetic control. When pairs of monozygote twins were overfed by 1000 kcal/day for 84 days, the amount of weight gain differed among the pairs (range 4.3–13.3 kg), but was extremely similar within a pair.

Environmental factors, particularly the amount of food available, the fat content of the food, and the amount of exercise, also contribute to the development of obesity. Migration studies have shown clearly that weight increases as people move from rural to urban environments or from non-westernized to westernized lifestyles. For example, Japanese living in Japan are thinner than Japanese who migrate to Hawaii, who in turn are thinner than Japanese living in the continental U.S.

In discussing with a patient the cause of his or her obesity, the practitioner should explain that a genetic predisposition for obesity is an inherited tendency to become overweight and does *not* mean that the patient is doomed to be obese. This genetic tendency probably can be blunted by regular physical activity and a low-fat diet.

7. What are the medical and psychological consequences of obesity?

Obesity is one of the most serious health problems in the U.S. Among adults aged 20–75 years, excessive weight increases the relative risk of hypertension three-fold, the risk of hypercholesterolemia

1.5-fold, and the risk of diabetes three-fold. The increased risks associated with obesity are particularly pronounced in people aged 20–45 years.

Psychosocial studies of overweight people suggest that obesity also has significant social and economic consequences. For example, overweight women are less likely to marry than normal-weight peers and have lower annual incomes and higher rates of household poverty. Overweight men are also less likely to marry than their normal-weight peers.

8. What are the financial costs of obesity?

The association of obesity with hypertension, diabetes, cardiovascular disease (CVD), gallbladder disease, cancer, and other illnesses has been estimated to cost a total of $99.2 billion per year. Direct medical costs (those associated with diseases attributable to obesity) amount to $51.6 billion of total costs, or approximately 5.7% of the yearly national health expenditure in the U.S. The remaining $47.6 billion reflects indirect costs attributable to obesity, and includes the value of excess physician visits, lost work-days, and restricted activity.

9. Is weight gain a risk even in individuals who are not obese?

Yes. Recent studies show that modest weight gain in young adults is associated with increases in systolic and diastolic blood pressure (BP), triglyceride levels, and fasting insulin and glucose levels. Weight gain in young women appears to increase their risk of disease in later life, including CHD, diabetes, hypertension, and post-menopausal breast cancer. Thus, all patients, regardless of their current weight status, should be encouraged to avoid future weight gain by developing healthy eating and exercise habits.

10. Are there psychological differences between obese and lean people?

Although overweight people clearly face a number of social and economic disadvantages, current research does not support the hypothesis that in general they exhibit higher levels of psychopathology than normal-weight counterparts. The earliest studies used highly select (and thus unrepresentative) samples of obese patients who were seeking treatment for weight and psychological problems; not surprisingly, the studies found that such patients indeed showed high levels of psychological distress. Later studies that used nonclinical samples found no such differences between obese and normal-weight people on measures of depressive symptoms, general psychopathology, assertiveness, and self-consciousness.

There is, however, a subset of overweight patients who report frequent episodes of **binge eating** and increased levels of psychological distress. Such patients typically consume large amounts of food in a short period, during which they feel that they are unable to stop eating. They experience marked distress over these episodes, and display elevated scores on measures of depressive symptoms. Such patients may require individualized treatment or a program specifically designed for obese binge-eaters.

11. What are the benefits of weight loss?

Weight loss significantly reduces many of the health risks associated with obesity, including diabetes, hypertension, dyslipidemia, CVD, and postoperative complications. In obese people who develop diabetes, weight loss is associated with increased insulin sensitivity and improved serum glucose levels; in many cases, weight loss may allow reduction or elimination of oral medication or insulin. Weight loss also may lead to significant improvements in hypertension, with a 10% decrease in systolic BP among men who achieve a 15% decrease in body weight. Obesity often is associated with elevations in serum triglycerides and decreases in high-density lipoprotein (HDL) levels. A significant weight loss may reverse both lipid abnormalities and thus reduce atherogenic risk.

Other health-related benefits of weight loss include improved pulmonary function, lower surgical risk and risk of postoperative complications, and improved functional capacity in patients experiencing low back pain and osteoarthritis of the knee. Weight loss also has been shown to decrease the level of self-reported depressive symptoms.

12. How much does the patient need to lose to achieve benefits?

In discussing with patients the role of weight loss in treatment of their medical problems, it is important to emphasize that many improvements in health can be achieved with relatively small losses. For example, a decrease in body weight of as little as 10% has been reported to normalize BP in overweight patients, and improvement in HDL levels has been observed in people losing only 5–10% of initial body weight. Modest weight losses also produce long-term benefits in obese patients with type II diabetes. Thus, even severely overweight patients or patients with a history of unsuccessful attempts to lose weight should be encouraged to achieve modest losses.

13. What are the main components of an effective weight loss program?

The most successful weight loss programs involve a combination of diet, exercise, and behavior modification. The **diet** typically is set at 1000–1500 kcal/day, depending on initial body weight. Weight loss programs increasingly emphasize low fat intake, with 20–30% of calories consumed as fat. Walking usually is recommended as the form of **exercise**, with gradually increasing goals until the patient is walking 2 miles per day 5 days per week. **Behavior modification** strategies generally are taught in a group format with weekly meetings for about 6 months, followed by periodic booster sessions. The goal of behavioral programs is to teach patients to modify eating and exercise behaviors by changing the environmental stimuli (cues) and reinforcers that control such behaviors.

Obesity is a chronic disease that requires chronic, ongoing treatment. Thus, it is important to identify programs that provide ongoing care and combine diet, exercise, and behavior modification. Initially such programs produce weight losses of 10 kg, and approximately 60% of this loss is maintained 1 year after the program.

14. Give some examples of behavioral modification strategies.

Examples of Strategies Used in Behavioral Treatment Programs

STRATEGIES FOCUSING ON BEHAVIOR	
Self monitoring	Patients record eating and exercise in a daily diary: calories and fat grams in each food; calories expended through physical activity.
Goal setting	Patients are given short- and long-term goals for intake, exercise, and weight loss (e.g., to lose 2 lb/week). Goals are attainable, but challenging.
STRATEGIES FOCUSING ON CHANGING ANTECEDENTS (CUES)	
Stimulus control	Patients are taught to remove cues for inappropriate behaviors and to increase cues for appropriate behavior (e.g., to refrain from bringing ice cream into the house, to put the exercise bike where it can be more easily seen and used).
Cognitive restructuring	Patients learn to counter negative self-statements with positive ones (e.g., instead of "I ate that candy; now I might as well eat the whole box," patients learn to say to themselves, "Eating candy is no big deal. I'll just make sure I follow my meal plan closely for the rest of the day.")
STRATEGIES FOCUSING ON CHANGING CONSEQUENCES (REINFORCERS)	
Self-reinforcement	Patients are taught to reward themselves for behavior changes (e.g., putting aside $1.00 each time they take a walk to save for a new blouse).
Contingency contracts	Patients sign a written statement with a therapist or friend, indicating a specific behavior or short-term weight loss and and a specific reward if and only if they achieve their goal.

15. What is the role of very low calorie diets?

Very low calorie diets (VLCDs) allow < 800 kcal/day and are given as liquid formula or as lean meat, fish, and fowl with appropriate vitamin and mineral supplements. Intake of 1 g/kg ideal body weight of protein of high biologic value is important in VLCDs to help preserve lean body mass. VLCDs appear to be safe when used with proper medical supervision in carefully selected patients who are moderately to severely overweight (BMI $\geq$ 30). Moreover, they are effective in producing **substantial initial weight losses** and concomitant improvements in obesity-related conditions. Patients find the **rigid structure** of VLCDs helpful and on average lose 20 kg in 12 weeks. Such diets may be helpful to patients who require immediate weight loss and **amelioration of medical conditions**; they also may be highly motivating in patients who feel that they cannot succeed at weight loss.

The long-term outcome of VLCDs is no better than what can be achieved with balanced low calorie diets of 1000–1500 kcal/day. To limit weight regain, which may be rapid, a gradual refeeding program must be implemented after the VLCD, and all participants must receive behavior therapy and guidance on increasing physical activity. Although such approaches limit weight regain, they do not prevent it; at 1-year followup, there are no significant differences in weight loss with VLCDs versus other dietary regimens.

16. Are any drugs useful in the treatment of obesity?

The primary treatment for obesity is diet, exercise, and behavior modification. For patients who have tried these approaches unsuccessfully and have either a BMI > 30 or a BMI > 27 plus obesity-related comorbidities, adding medication to this regimen may be helpful. Currently there are two FDA-approved medications for weight loss—sibutramine and orlistat. These drugs produce weight loss via different mechanisms.

Sibutramine (Meridia) inhibits the reuptake of norepinephrine and serotonin. Patients report reduced appetite and increased satiety. After 1 year of treatment, sibutramine patients lost 6.1 kg versus 1.8 kg in placebo-treated patients; the maximum benefits were achieved at 6 months, followed by slight regain. Marked increases in BP (15 mmHg) have occurred in 1 of 8 patients treated with sibutramine; thus BP and pulse must be monitored regularly.

Orlistat (Xenical) is a lipase inhibitor that acts in the gastrointestinal tract to reduce absorption of fat by 30%. This medication has no apparent effect on appetite. In a year-long study, Xenical-treated patients lost 8.7 kg versus 5.8 kg in a placebo group. The maximum benefit was at week 32. Because orlistat blocks fat absorption, it has a positive effect on lipids over and above the benefits of weight loss. The most common side effects of orlistat are gastrointestinal, including oily stools and spotting. Since this medication may affect absorption of fat-soluble vitamins, vitamin supplementation is recommended.

17. What are key points to remember about drug treatment?

• Most drug regimens have modest effects on weight loss.

• Drug treatments for obesity work only if the drugs are continued over time; once treatment stops, the weight is regained. Thus, a patient probably will need to be maintained on drug treatment for life.

• The most effective way to use any drug is in combination with education about diet and exercise and behavior modification training.

18. How important is exercise for weight loss and maintenance?

Exercise alone (e.g., without diet) appears to produce only minor weight losses. However, in conjunction with modest caloric restriction, exercise produces a greater loss of body weight and body fat and greater improvements in abdominal obesity than either technique alone.

Several randomized controlled trials also have shown that the combination of diet and exercise produces better long-term maintenance of weight losses than diet only. Moreover, the single best predictor of long-term maintenance of weight loss is habitual exercise.

Given such data, as well as data indicating that regular exercise (independent of weight loss) decreases the incidence of noninsulin-dependent diabetes mellitus and coronary disease in overweight persons and has a positive effect on mood, it is reasonable for physicians to recommend moderate physical activity for *all* overweight patients.

19. Which types of exercise should be recommended?

While traditional gym-based activities are suitable for some patients, individuals also should be encouraged to engage in lifestyle exercise, or activities that they can perform as part of their daily routine. One such exercise is walking. A 150-pound individual expends 100 calories by walking 1 mile. A reasonable exercise goal for an overweight individual is to walk 2 miles per day 5 days per week. To increase adherence and prevent injury, the patient may wish to start exercising in short bouts (e.g., a half-mile walk twice a day) and gradually increase his/her activity level over time.

20. What do we know about successful weight loss maintainers?

Consumption of a low-fat diet and regular physical activity seem to be characteristic of successful weight loss maintainers. In a recent study, a sample of 784 successful weight loss maintainers reported consuming low-fat, low-calorie diets and expending an average of 2800 kcals per week in exercise (the equivalent of walking 4 miles per day, 7 days per week). The behavioral skill of self-monitoring also was widely used by this sample: 75% reported weighing themselves at least once a week, and 50% reported they still keep track of their calorie or fat intake. While these successful weight loss maintainers are clearly devoting a significant amount of time to their weight maintenance efforts, they report that it is time well spent: at least 85% reported that weight loss and maintenance had a positive impact on their quality of life, level of energy, physical mobility, general mood, self-confidence, and physical health.

21. What are the risks of weight cycling?

Repeated episodes of weight loss followed by weight regain have been said to decrease metabolic rate and to alter body composition, thus making subsequent efforts at weight loss more difficult. However, the majority of animal and human studies do not support such statements. In general, weight cycling appears to have no consistent negative effects on body composition, energy expenditure, or future attempts at weight loss.

Another concern has been that weight-cycling may affect cardiovascular morbidity and mortality, because people with marked variability in body weight have greater morbidity and mortality than people whose weight remains stable. Such data come mainly from large epidemiologic studies that were not originally designed to analyze this issue: few provide information about whether the weight cycles involved voluntary or involuntary weight loss (i.e., was the cycling due to prior illness or to voluntary effort?), and many do not address the question separately for obese and normal-weight people. Weight cycling may have negative effects in thinner people (in whom it is likely to be unintentional), but little or no effect in overweight people. Moreover, no evidence suggests that weight cycling has negative effects on cardiovascular risk factors, such as BP, lipids, or body fat distribution.

22. What advice is appropriate regarding weight cycling?

On the basis of present findings about weight cycling, physicians should encourage nonobese patients to maintain a stable weight. Obese patients should be encouraged to lose modest amounts of weight and to use strategies that promote long-term weight control (namely, diet, exercise, and behavior modification). Fear of weight cycling, however, should not deter efforts at weight loss among obese people, because the risks of remaining obese are greater than the risks of weight cycling.

23. Is obesity a major problem in children?

The prevalence of obesity among children is increasing at alarming rates in the U.S., and many overweight children become overweight adults. The chances that an overweight child will remain overweight are increased in families with overweight parents and in children who remain overweight through adolescence.

Treatment of obesity in children appears to be far more effective than treatment of obesity in adults. A behavioral treatment program in which both the overweight child (age 8–12 years) and his or her overweight parent are treated together and taught to modify diet and exercise habits has been shown to be successful in reducing obesity in overweight children through a 10-year followup interval.

BIBLIOGRAPHY

1. Expert Panel on the Identification, Evaluation, and Treatment of Overweight in Adults: Clinical guidelines on the identification, evaluation, and treatment of overweight and obesity in adults. Am J Clin Nutr 68:899–917, 1998.
2. Flegal KM, Carroll MD, Kuczmarski RJ, Johnson CL: Overweight and obesity in the United States: Prevalence and trends. Int J Obes 22:39–47, 1998.
3. Klem WL, Wing RR, McGuire MT, et al: A descriptive study of individuals successful at long-term maintenance of substantial weight loss. Am J Clin Nutr 66:239–246, 1997.
4. Van Itallie TB: Waist circumference: A useful index in clinical care and health promotion. Nutr Rev 56:300–302, 1998.
5. Wing RR: Behavioral approaches to the treatment of obesity. In Bray G, Bouchard C, James PT (eds): Handbook of Obesity. New York, Marcel Dekker, Inc., 1997, pp 855–873.
6. Wolf AM, Colditz GA: Current estimates of the economic cost of obesity in the United States. Obes Res 6:97–106, 1998.

XII. Ethical and Legal Issues in Psychiatry

80. CONFIDENTIALITY AND PRIVILEGE

Jeffrey L. Metzner, M.D.

1. What is confidentiality?

Confidentiality refers to the ethical duty of the physician not to disclose information learned from the patient to any other person or organization without the consent of the patient or under proper legal compulsion. The Hippocratic Oath describes the duty of confidentiality as follows:

Whatsoever I shall see or hear in the course of my profession as well as outside my profession in my intercourse with men, if it be what should not be published abroad, I will never divulge, holding such things to be holy secrets.

This duty is described by the American Medical Association in Section 4 of the *Principles of Medical Ethics:*[5]

A physician shall respect the rights of patients, of colleagues, and of other health professionals, and shall safeguard patient confidences within the constraints of law.

The *Principles of Medical Ethics with Annotations Especially Applicable to Psychiatry* elaborates in Section 4, Annotation 1, that:

Confidentiality is essential to psychiatric treatment. This is based in part on the special nature of psychiatric therapy as well as on the traditional ethical relationship between physician and patient. Growing concern between the civil rights of patients and the possible adverse effects of computerization, duplication equipment, and data banks makes the dissemination of confidential information an increasing hazard.[5]

2. Does the psychiatrist have a legal duty of confidentiality?

The existence of a legal obligation to protect the confidentiality of communications arising from the physician-patient relationship has evolved primarily through court decisions, although statutory regulations also may be pertinent. Successful lawsuits against physicians for breach of confidentiality have been based on the following legal theories:

• Implied contract to keep information confidential
• Invasion of privacy
• Tortious breach of duty of confidentiality
• Statutory regulations.

Courts have awarded damages for breach of confidentiality based on the **contractual relationship** between the physician and patient, which was determined to include an implied agreement that the physician would keep confidential any information received from the patient. Recovery also has been based on **invasion of privacy**, which has been defined as an unjustified disclosure of a person's private affairs with which the public has no legitimate concern in such a fashion as to cause humiliation and/or emotional suffering to ordinary persons. The nature of the physician-patient relationship has been determined to create for the physician a **fiduciary duty** (i.e., to act primarily for the benefit of another) to keep information obtained through such a relationship confidential. Therefore, a tort action can be used to recover damages. A tort is a civil wrong, other than breach of contract, for which the court will provide a remedy in the form of an action for damages. Finally, courts occasionally have allowed recovery based on **licensing statutes** that focus on issues of privileged communications.[12]

3. When are physician's disclosures legally justified?

A **valid consent** for a release of information protects the psychiatrist ethically and legally. State law and/or relevant rules and regulations often specify the requirements for such a release. A valid consent minimally means that the patient was competent to provide such authorization and did so knowingly and voluntarily. It is recommended that *written* consent be obtained, specifying the purpose and scope of information to be released. Written consent often provides more clarity to the patient regarding the nature of the disclosure and provides documentation—a useful risk-management measure—for the physician.

Many **evaluations for medical/legal (i.e., forensic) purposes**, performed at the request of third parties to address issues such as impairment ratings for worker's compensation, disability insurance payments, and appropriateness of treatment, are not confidential. The *Ethical Guidelines for the Practice of Forensic Psychiatry*, developed by the American Academy of Psychiatry and the Law, state that

> *[t]he psychiatrist maintains confidentiality to the extent possible given the legal context. Special attention is paid to any limitations on the usual precepts of medical confidentiality. An evaluation for forensic purposes begins with notice to the evaluee of any limitations on confidentiality. Information or reports derived from the forensic evaluation are subject to the rules of confidentiality as apply to the evaluation and any disclosure is restricted accordingly.*[2]

Reports and/or information obtained from such examinations can be disclosed to the third party that requested the examination without risk of a successful lawsuit by the evaluee concerning breach of confidentiality. Consent is implied when the person proceeds with the evaluation after having been provided appropriate information concerning the nature of the evaluation and lack of or limits of confidentiality.

Disclosures without consent from the patient have been found to be permissible by courts when an **overriding public interest** (e.g., public safety) was at issue. However, a careful risk-benefit analysis needs to be made prior to such disclosures. Consultation with a colleague and/or attorney should be part of the risk-benefit analysis process. Information released under such circumstances should be relevant to the potential public harm and provided only to those in need of the information.

Many state court decisions and/or statutes have adopted a psychotherapist's **duty to protect principle**, as described in the *Tarasoff II (Tarasoff v. Regents of the University of California*, 551 P.2d 334 [1976]) decision. This duty may, in certain circumstances, be legally discharged by warning of the patient's intended victim (whether or not the patient consents to releasing such information). However, jurisdictions differ concerning recognition and discharge of such a duty, and it is important for the clinician to be familiar with the law in his/her state concerning this issue. A physician could be liable for breach of confidentiality if a warning to a third party is provided without obtaining valid consent from the patient in states without such a duty.

State statutes often require physicians to report to various governmental agencies certain conditions such as **infectious diseases** (e.g., sexually transmitted diseases, tuberculosis), **suspected child abuse**, and **gunshot wounds**. States have taken very different approaches regarding confidentiality and reporting issues relevant to **HIV/AIDS infection**. Physicians need to be familiar with pertinent statutes in their own states concerning both the conditions that are to be reported and the threshold criteria for making such reports.

4. Are there any reporting requirements concerning patients who may have a medical or psychiatric condition that could cause impairments in their driving ability?

Most states clearly indicate in their statutes, and in the information they provide to motorists licensed in their state, that the driver is primarily responsible for his or her own safety and the safety of others. Ten states have clearly written guidelines under which drivers must inform their state of their medical conditions. However, few states have written criteria for determining driver safety, and physician reporting of unsafe drivers generally is not required by state law.[13] There generally has not been a great impetus to interfere with the physician-patient relationship, although physicians are encouraged to report individuals who they feel would be unsafe behind the wheel to the Department of

Motor Vehicles. Physicians generally are granted some form of immunity from liability when making such reports in good faith.

Physicians in Pennsylvania appear to have the strictest reporting requirements. Judicial decisions have held physicians liable for injuries in motor vehicle accidents involving their patients who drive. Several significant duty to warn and/or to protect third party cases involving psychiatrists arose from driving cases. Physicians should be familiar with pertinent statutes and case law within their jurisdiction concerning these issues.

5. Are there statutes pertinent to confidentiality other than the reporting statutes?

A number of states have enacted **mental health confidentiality statutes** that establish a rule of confidentiality and describe exceptions. For example, the Colorado statute which establishes procedures for involuntary commitment provides that "all information obtained and records prepared in the course of providing any services [for the care and treatment of the mentally ill] . . . shall be confidential and privileged matter" (C.R.S. 27-10-120). This law specifies a variety of exceptions such as peer review, communications between qualified professional personnel in the provision of services or appropriate referrals, releasing information to the courts as necessary to the administration of the provisions of this article, certain circumstances for releasing confidential information to family member(s) of an adult with mental illness, and appropriate research (C.R.S. 27-10-101, 102, 116, 120, 120.5 as amended).

Legislation often requires that rules and regulations be promulgated by the state's Division of Mental Health or equivalent agency concerning confidentiality. Physicians should be familiar with these rules and regulations within their own jurisdiction, because they vary significantly among states. There also are Federal rules and regulations regarding confidentiality applicable to **substance abuse treatment programs** that receive federal funds (42 C.F.R. Part 2). Records and information from such programs can be released only under conditions as specified in the regulations. These regulations provide detailed information concerning the nature of the written release required. Access to information concerning patients and records in the **Veterans Administration Hospitals** is determined by a variety of Federal laws and regulations, such as the Freedom of Information Act and Privacy Act.

6. How do the ethical guidelines address issues relevant to confidentiality?

The American Psychiatric Association (APA) has emphasized that:

[t]he continuing duty of the psychiatrist to protect the patient includes fully apprising him/her of the connotations of waiving the privilege of privacy . . . Ethically the psychiatrist may disclose only that information which is relevant to a given situation. He/she should avoid offering speculation as fact . . .[5]

It is good practice, both clinically and from a risk-management perspective, to provide the patient with a copy of the information (e.g., report, completed insurance form) to be disclosed *prior to releasing the information*. Generating the report in the presence of the patient and/or with direct input from the patient often can be therapeutic and contribute to good treatment planning. The most frequent request for information comes from insurance companies related to diagnosis, treatment progress, and planning, or issues relevant to disability and/or insurability.

Confidentiality may be breached ethically in the interest of **protecting the patient:**

Psychiatrists at times may find it necessary, in order to protect the patient or the community from imminent danger, to reveal confidential information disclosed by the patient.[5]

Thus, it often is clinically and ethically appropriate for the physician to inform a patient's relative or roommate about a depressed patient's suicide risk. The physician's legal liability under such circumstances is low if his/her assessment was reasonable. Physicians do not have a legal duty to warn others of a potential suicide attempt, although the physician does have a duty to provide reasonable care to his/her patients (which would include implementing appropriate steps to decrease the risk of suicide). Without patient authorization, a psychiatrist should not release information to family members or others, unless there is an overriding interest of protecting the patient. For example, do not give confidential information to a spouse who is requesting help concerning problems that may impact on the marriage unless the patient provides appropriate authorization.

7. How does confidentiality apply to the treatment of minors?

Until the 1990s, the general and forensic psychiatric literature was sparse concerning issues specific to confidentiality with children and adolescents. From a legal perspective, the psychiatrist generally can assume that a parent has a legal right to full information about the treatment of a minor if the parent is legally entitled to authorize treatment for a minor child. However, full implementation of such a legal principle often causes significant clinical problems. Such problems can be minimized by establishing **ground rules of confidentiality and exceptions** with patients and parents prior to beginning the treatment process. The ground rules generally are different for adolescents as compared to young minors due to both developmental differences and an increased right to privacy enjoyed by the older adolescent population.

State statutes often provide some guidance regarding issues of confidentiality in the treatment of minors. The American Academy of Child and Adolescent Psychiatry Code of Ethics[1] and chapters by Macbeth,[11] Benedek,[7] and Weintrob[14] provide detailed discussions concerning legal, clinical, and ethical considerations relevant to confidentiality and the treatment of minors. For example, the AACAP's Code of Ethics indicates that "it is necessary that the child or adolescent, within his/her capacity for understanding, be clearly apprised of confidentiality in regard both to his/her own communication and those of parents or guardians. He/she should also be informed of the limits to the general principle of confidentiality that the sharing of care-taking responsibility requires."

The AMA's Council on Ethical and Judicial Affairs indicated that "when the law does not require otherwise, physicians should permit a competent minor to consent to medical care and should not notify parents without the patient's consent . . . for minors who are mature enough to be unaccompanied by their parents for their examination, confidentiality of information disclosed during an exam, interview, or in counseling, should be maintained. Such information may be disclosed to parents when the patient consents to disclosure . . . confidentiality may be justifiably breached in situations for which confidentiality for adults may be breached . . . or when such a breach is necessary to overt serious harm to the minor. . . ."

8. What is the physician-patient privilege?

Most state legislatures have created a testimonial privilege that prohibits a physician from disclosing in a judicial or quasi-judicial proceeding, with certain exceptions, any confidential information learned during the course of treatment with a patient. Thus, **testimonial privilege** is an evidentiary rule, applicable to judicial settings and limited in scope, that is created by statute. The privilege belongs to the patient—not to the physician. A breach of privileged communication can result in a lawsuit against the physician. Physician-patient privilege statutes have enacted due to the recognition that confidentiality is needed to maintain the therapeutic relationship, which also may have benefits for the community (e.g., people receive necessary treatment for illness). The recognition of the importance of a patient's privacy interests also has been a justification for such statutes.

In 1996, the U.S. Supreme Court in its *Jaffee v. Redmond*, 116 S.Ct. 1923 (1996), decision held that federal law recognizes privilege protecting confidential communications between a psychotherapist and his/her patient.

9. What exceptions to privilege exist?

Exceptions to the privilege generally include:
- When a valid waiver of privilege is executed by a competent adult patient or his/her legal guardian
- The patient-litigant exception, in which the patient has initiated litigation when his/her mental or emotional condition is an element of a claim or defense in a legal proceeding
- Most court-ordered examinations involving a wide range of legal issues
- Malpractice proceedings initiated by the patient against the physician
- Involuntary civil commitment proceedings
- Will contest
- Certain criminal proceedings
- Reports required by various mandatory reporting statutes.

The above list is not inclusive, and the type of exceptions differs from state to state. For example, some state statutes allow for the waiver of a physician-patient privilege, at the discretion of the judge, in child custody disputes. Familiarize yourself with the appropriate law in your state.

Disclosures made to the physician for purposes other than obtaining treatment are not covered by the privilege. States vary regarding the presence of privilege if disclosure occurs when third parties (e.g., family members) are present during the course of the communication. Jurisdictions also differ whether communications arising in the course of couple's and/or group psychotherapy are privileged. Nonphysician providers supervised by physicians generally are not covered by the patient-physician privilege statute, although they may be covered by a statute specific to their profession.

10. How should the psychiatrist respond to a subpoena?

A **subpoena duces tecum** is a subpoena issued by a court, at the request of one of the parties to a lawsuit, to require a physician to bring (i.e., produce) pertinent medical records. A **subpoena ad testificandum** requires the attendance of the physician for testimony purposes. Neither subpoena *compels* the physician; ethical and legal principles may properly prevent the psychiatrist from testifying and/or disclosing the subpoenaed medical records.

The psychiatrist may release medical records and/or testify when the subpoena is accompanied by a valid consent form signed by the patient. Reasonable attempts should be made to **inform the patient** or his/her attorney about the subpoena, to verify the validity of the consent and discuss relevant issues.

The psychiatrist should contact the patient or the patient's attorney when a signed consent form is not attached to the subpoena, to determine whether the patient has consented, explicitly or implicitly, to waive the privilege. Remember that *the privilege belongs to the patient*, and not to the physician. However, the physician has an ethical and legal obligation to withhold information obtained during the course of treatment as privileged from disclosure in a legal context unless it is clear that an exception exists (e.g., signed consent obtained) or a court directs the physician to testify and/or release the record.

The psychiatrist should discuss with the attorney, when appropriate, issues concerning disclosure of very sensitive information that appears not to be pertinent to the issues being litigated. The patient's attorney or the psychiatrist have the option of filing a motion to **quash the subpoena** or **limit the nature of the information** to be disclosed, based on protection under the physician-patient privilege and the duty to maintain confidentiality, when the patient has not consented to waive the privilege. A hearing will be held in which the judge will rule on the motion. The psychiatrist can ethically testify and/or release medical records when ordered to do so by the court, despite lack of consent from the patient. The psychiatrist should not rely on the statements or opinions of the attorney who has requested the subpoena concerning issues relevant to waiver of the privilege.

11. What are the principles of confidentiality following a patient's death?

The U.S. Supreme Court decision in *Swidler § Berlin v. United States*, 118 S.Ct. 2081 (1998), which held that the attorney-client privilege survives the death of the client, provides support that the physician-patient privilege also generally is maintained following a patient's death. The ethics committee of the APA has written that confidentiality ethically survives a patient's death unless disclosures are required by statute or case law. Some state statutes allow the executor or administrator of the deceased patient's estate or certain relatives to have access to the patient's medical record. Additionally, the physician-patient privilege may be waived in certain states following the patient's death. The psychiatrist should obtain guidance from legal counsel or the court concerning this issue when questions exist concerning the waiver of the privilege.

Similar issues arise which are not addressed by statute or case law. The psychiatrist may be questioned by the police during the course of an investigation involving the death of a patient, or may be asked specific questions by grieving family members. The psychiatrist should not disclose specific information obtained from the patient, although answering questions in terms of general psychiatric principles is appropriate. The psychiatrist's liability for breach of confidentiality is minimized by obtaining authorization from the patient's legal representative and close family members.[12]

12. Is it a breach of confidentiality to use a collection agency or attorney in an attempt to collect unpaid bills?

There are no ethical principles that preclude psychiatrists from using the legal system or collection agencies for bill collection. The physician-patient privilege does not prevent a doctor from suing to collect proper fees. However, the legal and ethical obligations of the psychiatrist to protect the patient's confidentiality continue despite the breach of the treatment contract by the patient caused by not paying the bill. Patients may sue for breach of confidentiality when the psychiatrist discloses their *status* as patients to an attorney or collection agency. In general, the only information that needs to be disclosed to the collection agency or attorney is the patient's name, balance due, and dates of services. Confidentiality is best preserved by describing the dates of services as office visits in contrast to psychotherapy or medication management visits.

Due to issues of confidentiality and risk management, the psychiatrist should first use other methods of recovering fees. A matter-of-fact letter to the patient requesting either payment in full within a specified time frame or a proposal for a payment schedule is a useful alternative. If there is not a response to such letter within a reasonable period of time, another letter should be sent which requests a similar response within a specified time period and informs the patient that referral will be made to an attorney or collection agency for initiation of appropriate legal action if the patient does not respond.

Select a *responsible* collection agency or attorney—for professional reasons and to minimize the risk that the patient will retaliate by filing a counterclaim for malpractice, ethical complaint, or a complaint to the Board of Medical Examiners or equivalent agency. Learn about any pertinent laws within your state that specify procedures that must be followed before using a collection agency or attorney to recover unpaid bills.

13. What confidentiality issues are involved with new technology?

The availability of voicemail, cellular telephones, and fax machines can lead to unintentional breaches of confidentiality. **Voicemail messages** may be played back by persons other than the patient; cellular telephone conversations may be heard by other parties; and records sent via fax machines may be sent to the wrong number. Therefore, detailed voicemail messages should not be left for patients unless assurances have been given by them that other persons do not have access to their voicemail box. Patients should be told when a **cellular telephone** is being used and reminded that confidentiality is not guaranteed under such circumstances. **Fax machines** should not be used for routine transmission of confidential information, and procedures should be implemented to ensure safeguarding of confidential information that needs to be sent promptly.

The use of **computerized medical records** by healthcare providers and systems has increased rapidly. Medical data are being used for nontraditional purposes (i.e., other than clinical assessment or treatment) that are not governed by regulations, laws, or professional practices. The rapidly emerging infrastructure of healthcare information and its relation to patient privacy have been described in the literature.[6,10] The advantage of these information systems for the organization, delivery, and financing of health care is attractive to policymakers. Future electronic databases will contain a vast amount of personal information, including demographic, financial, medical, genomic, and social data. Unfortunately, there is significant potential for erosion of patient privacy in such systems.

The APA has developed resource documents for preserving patient confidentiality in the era of information technology and a guide to security relevant to computerized records.[3] These documents provide direction to policymakers, as they establish ground rules for the management of patient records in electronic form in new healthcare systems. A complete **medical record security program** should include policies, standards, training, technical and procedural controls, risk assessment, auditing and monitoring, sanctions for violations, and assigned responsibility for management of the program. Extra levels of security should be developed for information generally regarded as sensitive by tradition, or by agreement between the physician and patient.

The genetic revolution has taken a markedly clinical turn as evidenced by the work of the **Human Genome Project**, which soon will map the entire genetic code embedded in human DNA. This project and other research in molecular genetics raise new ethical and legal issues for physicians, who eventually will be able to accurately predict the risk of future onset of many genetic diseases as well as the likely current and future health status of relatives of the patient who share genetic material. Physicians will face a dilemma when a patient chooses not to disclose information that could be significant to genetic relatives. Berry summarizes issues that will need to be reviewed by legislative and judicial lawmakers to clarify under what circumstances may or must a physician disclose genetic information to interested third parties, and under what circumstances may or must the physician, instead, keep such information confidential.[8]

14. I'm confused—can you give me some practical pointers regarding confidentiality and privilege?

The concepts of confidentiality and privilege often are confusing due to overlapping principles and the many exceptions, which have been briefly summarized. Confidentiality is an important element in developing a therapeutic alliance with patients. A breach of confidentiality can result in legal liability, ethical complaints, adverse actions pertinent to a physician's license to practice medicine, and criminal prosecution in certain circumstances.

Practical Pointers Concerning Confidentiality and Privilege

---

1. Follow the general principle to honor a patient's confidences unless a legally cognizable exception applies.

2. Have your own written "Authorization for Release of Medical/Mental Health Information" form that can be tailored to specific circumstances. If requested to release AIDS/HIV information, check with legal counsel or your state's Department of Health to ensure that the authorization you obtain is specific enough to meet legal requirements.

3. When in doubt about the validity of consent to release information, call your patient to discuss information and to verify consent.

4. When performing an evaluation (e.g., worker's compensation), clarify limits of confidentiality at the outset. Explain who will/will not receive a copy of the report.

5. Obtain competent advice before releasing information to anyone after a patient's death.

6. Apprise group therapy members about parameters of confidentiality.

7. When subpoenaed to testify/release records, seek advice from legal counsel. Generally, you will wish to ensure that the patient executes written, informed consent or that a court order is obtained.

8. Do not automatically assume that a managed care company has obtained patient consent to have information released to them. Try to discuss such authorization with the patient at the outset of treatment. Obtain written consent.

9. If using a collection agency or small claims court to collect an unpaid bill, make sure that you send the patient appropriate advance notice in writing and reveal the least amount of information necessary (Caveat: collections often lead to malpractice counterclaims.)

From Macbeth JE, et al: Confidentiality and privilege. In Legal and Risk Management Issues in the Practice of Psychiatry. Washington, D.C., Psychiatrist's Purchasing Group, Inc., 1994; with permission.

BIBLIOGRAPHY

1. American Academy of Child and Adolescent Psychiatry: Code of Ethics. Washington, D.C., AACAP, 1980.
2. American Academy of Psychiatry and the Law: Ethical Guidelines for the Practice of Forensic Psychiatry. Bloomfield, Connecticut, AAPL, 1998.
3. American Psychiatric Association Committee on Confidentiality and Council on Psychiatry and Law: Preserving patient confidentiality in the year of information technology. J Am Acad Psychiatry Law 25:551–559, 1997.
4. American Psychiatric Association Committee on Confidentiality and Council on Psychiatry and Law: American Psychiatric Association resource document on computerized records: A guide to security. J Am Acad Psychiatry Law 25:561–564, 1997.
5. American Psychiatric Association Ethics Committee: The Principles of Medical Ethics With Annotations Especially Applicable to Psychiatry. Washington, D.C., APA, 1998, pp 1–19.

6. Applebaum PS: A "health information infrastructure" and a threat to confidentiality of health records. Psychiatric Services 49:27–33, 1998.
7. Benedek EP: Ethical Issues in Practice. In Schetky DH, Benedek EP (eds): Clinical Handbook of Psychiatry and the Law. Baltimore, Williams & Wilkins, 1993, pp 75–88.
8. Berry RM: The genetic revolution and the physician's duty of confidentiality. J Legal Med 18:401–441, 1997.
9. Council on Ethical and Judicial Affairs: Code of Medical Ethics: Current Opinions with Annotations (1998–1999 ed.) Chicago, American Medical Association, 1998.
10. Gostin L: Health care information and the protection of personal privacy: Ethical and legal considerations. Ann Intern Med 127:683–690, 1997.
11. Macbeth JE: Legal issues in the psychiatric treatment of minors. In Schetky DH, Benedek EP (eds): Clinical Handbook of Child Psychiatry and the Law. Baltimore, Williams & Wilkins, 1992, pp 53–74.
12. Macbeth JE, Wheeler AM, Sither JW, Onek JN: Confidentiality and privilege. In Legal and Risk Management Issues in the Practice of Psychiatry. Washington, D.C., Psychiatrists' Purchasing Group, Inc., 1994.
13. Metzner JL, Dentino AN, Godard SL, et al: Impairment in driving and psychiatric illness. J Neuropsychiatry 5:211–220, 1993.
14. Weintrob A: Confidentiality and its dilemmas in child and adolescent psychiatry. In Rosner R (ed): Principles and Practice of Forensic Psychiatry. New York, Chapman & Hall, 1994, pp 323–330.

81. LEGAL RESPONSIBILITIES WITH CHILD ABUSE AND DOMESTIC VIOLENCE

Ronald Schouten, J.D., M.D.

Discussion of physicians' legal responsibilities in any area of medicine can cause considerable anxiety. This poses a significant problem, because legal issues arise in all aspects of medical practice. Physicians need not have an intricate knowledge of the law, however, any more than lawyers who encounter medical problems need to study medicine. Instead, a general knowledge of legal issues and a sensitivity to situations in which such issues arise are sufficient.

The key to handling medicolegal questions is a willingness to seek consultation from attorneys and colleagues familiar with medicolegal issues. All physicians have access to legal advice through their malpractice insurers, hospital, medical society, or private attorneys familiar with healthcare matters. The reluctance of physicians to ask for help may be the largest obstacle to anxiety reduction and successful resolution of medicolegal issues. For that reason, the response to each of the questions below includes the general advice to ask for help from legal advisors. Such a step provides the maximum protection, the greatest relief from anxiety, and the widest freedom to practice good clincal medicine.

Child abuse and domestic violence are significant social problems. Physicians are in a position to detect and prevent such acts of violence as well as to treat the victims. Society has realized the role that physicians can play in dealing with these problems and has placed obligations on physicians to respond.

CHILD ABUSE

1. What obligations does a physician have when child abuse is suspected?

Every state in the United States has passed legislation that makes physicians and other professionals mandatory reporters of child abuse and neglect. The obligation usually arises at a low level, e.g., when the healthcare professional believes or has a reasonable basis to believe that a child under 18 is a victim of abuse or neglect. Statutes vary with regard to the types of abuse to be reported and whether or not the child must have been seen as a patient by the reporter. The report is made to the state social social service agency responsible for child welfare. Hospital social service offices and attorneys have the name of this agency and should be able to advise the physician on when and how the report is to be made. The penalties for failure to report vary from state to state, but usually they involve a substantial fine and may include criminal penalties. Failure to report also may become the subject of disciplinary actions by the state agency responsible for physician registration.

2. What malpractice risks arise in the area of child abuse?

A physician who fails to diagnose or report child abuse may be held liable for injury or wrongful death of a child as the result of subsequent abuse. Such suits may allege failure to diagnose, failure to report, or failure to conduct a proper investigation. When the child is removed from the home because of suspected child abuse, malpractice suits may arise from negligent selection of placement for the child or failure to monitor the placement. Suits also may arise from alleged wrongful removal of the child from the home, although such suits are unsuccessful when the removal was carried out in good faith.

3. What is child abuse?

Child abuse is broadly defined, although state statutes may have different specific definitions. The Child Abuse Prevention and Treatment Act of 1973 defines child abuse and neglect as:

> … the physical treatment and mental injuring, sexual abuse, negligent treatment, or maltreatment of a child under the age of 18 by a person who is responsible for the child's welfare under circumstances which indicate that the child's health and welfare is harmed or threatened thereby.

Physical abuse may be defined as any injury to a child that is not accidental. Physical neglect refers to a failure to provide for a child's emotional or physical needs. Neglect may include failure to obtain needed medical treatment, even when the failure is consistent with the parents' religious beliefs. Physical neglect is the most common form of physical abuse.

Sexual abuse includes *any* sexual activity (nonconsensual and consensual) between an adult and a child. It includes exhibitionism, oral-genital contact, and fondling as well as intercourse.

4. What are the indicators that a child may be suffering from physical abuse or neglect?

There is no single profile of the abused child or the abusive adult. Child abuse should be included as part of the differential diagnosis of all childhood injuries and unexplained illness.

Elements of the History That May Indicate an Injury Was Inflicted Rather than Accidental

---

- Unexplained delay in bringing the child for treatment after an injury.
- The supervising adult offers an explanation which is implausible or contradictory.
- The explanation of the injury is incompatible with the physical findings.
- The child has had a series of similar or otherwise suspicious injuries, e.g., repeated burns from "touching a hot stove."
- The injury is blamed on a sibling or is attributed to self-injury, e.g., "He keeps throwing himself down the stairs."
- The child has a history of treatment for injuries at various hospitals.
- When interviewed, the child accuses the supervising adult of causing the injury.
- The parents seem to have unrealistic and premature expectations of the child, e.g., "She (a 1-year-old) should know that crying in the middle of the night really upsets me."
- The supervising adult minimizes the injury or seems unconcerned about it.
- The supervising adult has a prior history of having been abused as a child.

Adapted from Green AH: Forensic evaluation of physically and sexually abused children. In Rosner R (ed): Principles and Practice of Forensic Psychiatry. New York, Chapman & Hall, 1994.

Findings on physical exam that may indicate physical abuse include bruises on the buttocks and genitals, burns to the perineum, cigarette burns, abdominal trauma, head injury, multiple fractures of different ages, spiral fractures of long bones, eye injuries, and ear injuries.

The signs of physical neglect may be more subtle but are best summarized by children who present with malnutrition or poor hygiene or merit a diagnosis of failure to thrive. Children who do not meet psychological or physical developmental milestones may be suffering from physical neglect.

5. What is Münchausen's by proxy syndrome?

Münchausen's syndrome is a disorder in which an individual feigns or induces physical illness for the apparent purpose of becoming a patient. Such individuals often are willing to undergo invasive, painful, and debilitating medical procedures, including amputation, as part of the patient role. Indeed, undergoing such procedures may be a motivating force for their behavior. The goal of the behavior is psychological gratification, perhaps by getting attention from physicians, rather than the pursuit of disability claims or monetary reward. When confronted with their behavior, such individuals generally sign out of the hospital against medical advice or drop out of treatment with the confronting physician.

In Münchausen's by proxy syndrome, a parent simulates illness, exaggerates actual illness, or induces illness in a child. The reasons for such behavior are unclear, but they most commonly arise from a desire to get attention from members of the medical profession. The behavior of such parents can range from benign and deceptive to fatal. For example, some parents put cranberry juice in a child's diaper to simulate vaginal bleeding. Others put drops of blood into the child's urine sample to simulate hemorrhagic cystitis. At the other hand of the spectrum are parents who have smothered their children to simulate apnea or injected fecal material subcutaneously to cause fever. Such behavior is a form of child abuse and is reportable to the appropriate agency.

Failure to identify a child who is the victim of Münchausen's by proxy may lead to a malpractice action against the treating physicians. Conversely, negligent assessment that leads to a misdiagnosis of Münchausen's by proxy syndrome also can lead to allegations of malpractice.

Signs and Symptoms of Münchausen's by Proxy

- Medical illnesses that are unusual and for which there is inconsistent explanation.
- Repeated episodes of medical illness in a child with no apparent underlying medical problems, e.g., repeated urinary tract infections in children with normal anatomy.
- Treatment of the child by a number of different physicians at different institutions.
- Treatment of the child in different parts of the country.
- Parental response of resistance or refusal when information is needed from previous treating physicians.
- Parental history of odd, unexplained injuries or illnesses.
- Sibling history of odd, unexplained injuries or illnesses.

Adapted from Schreier HA, Libow J: Hurting for Love: Münchausen's by Proxy Syndrome. New York, Guilford Press, 1993.

6. What resources are available for parents who have difficulty controlling their temper or other problems with parenting skills?

Many state social service agencies and private child welfare programs offer parenting classes, support groups, and day care. In addition, many states have toll-free telephone numbers for parents who feel that they are at risk of physically abusing their children.

7. How do I recognize sexual abuse of a child?

Signs and Symptoms of Child Sexual Abuse

- The child reports a pattern of repetitive, escalating behavior, beginning with exposure of genitals and extending from mutual touching to intercourse or attempted intercourse.
- The child identifies someone well known to him or her as the abuser who told them that the act was "our secret."
- Physical injuries to the perineum and genitalia.
- Occurrence of sexually transmitted diseases or repeated genitourinary infections.
- Anxiety disorders, including symptoms of post-traumatic stress disorder

Table continued on following page

Signs and Symptoms of Child Sexual Abuse (Cont.)

• Increased aggression and impulsivity, including sexually oriented aggression against other children.

• Precocious sexual behavior, compulsive masturbation, and promiscuity may occur. Conversely, adolescents and adults who have been sexually abused may avoid all heterosexually oriented activities.

Adapted from Quinn KM, White S: Interviewing children for suspected child abuse. In Schetky DH, Benedek EP (eds): Clinical Handbook of Child Psychiatry and the Law. Baltimore, Williams & Wilkins, 1992.

8. If a patient confides that he or she has abused a child in the past, is the physician required to report this information?

In most jurisdictions, confidentiality requires that information about past misdeeds, including criminal acts, not be disclosed. Some states require that distant as well as recents acts of abuse be reported. In any jurisdiction, however, if the physician has a reasonable basis to believe that the patient is about to repeat the abuse, there may be an obligation to intervene. Clinical intervention, before a repeat offense occurs, is most helpful. This may include a voluntary request for services from a child welfare agency or entering into structured psychiatric treatment for the individual and family.

9. If an adult patient reports that he or she was sexually abused in the past, does the physician have an obligation to report such information to public authorities?

States generally require that such information be reported only if minor children are in the home and the physician has reason to believe that they also may be at risk of abuse. However, some jurisdictions do require the reporting of child abuse even if it occurred in the distant past.

Allegations of past sexual abuse have become the subject of civil litigation. Law suits against alleged perpetrators of sexual abuse, brought by individuals who report recent recovery of repressed memories, have generated a great deal of controversy. Zealous clinicians have been sued successfully on the basis that they convinced the patient of such "memories" of sexual abuse. Good patient care and informed risk management dictate that the physician receiving such information be supportive of the patient's statements, while at the same time remaining neutral about their accuracy. Documentation of the reports should not comment on the veracity of the claim of abuse. They physician should avoid the use of words such as "alleged" and "claimed," using instead words such as "said" and "reports." The clinician has no way of knowing whether or not the abuse occurred, short of an admission by the accused perpetrator. Hypnosis and narcotherapy (such as amytal interviews) may be helpful therapeutically, but are not valid methods of establishing a historically accurate account of abuse.

10. Can a physician be sued successfully for breach of confidentiality if suspected child abuse is reported?

Threats to sue clinicians who report suspected abuse are to be expected. The child abuse-reporting statutes protect reports from liability by providing an exception to the confidentiality requirements. The exceptions apply when the decision to report is reasonable and made in good faith.

DOMESTIC VIOLENCE

11. What obligations does a physician have when domestic violence is suspected?

In contrast to situations involving child abuse, the physician's legal obligations with regard to domestic violence are unclear. Society has tended to view domestic violence as a private matter into which the state should not intrude. As a result, legislators have begun to address this issue only recently.

Case law arising from situations in which a patient poses a risk of harm to others may be defining. Physicians treating patients with infectious diseases have been found liable for failure to warn nonpatients of the risk of infection. Psychiatrists and other mental health professionals have been found to have a duty to protect third parties against the violent acts of their patients in certain situations. This duty often is called the **Tarasoff duty**, after the California case that first laid out such obligations. The steps taken to protect the third party need not include breach of the patient's confidentiality.

In some jurisdictions, a history of violence and indications that the patient presents a clear risk of violence against an identifiable person in the near future is enough to give rise to the Tarasoff duty. Possibly this obligation could be extended to nonpsychiatrists. Physicians should check with local authorities to determine obligations in their state.

Even when the threat is not explicit, psychiatrists may have an affirmative duty to commit involuntarily a patient who poses a reasonable risk of violence as a result of mental illness. Finally, a physician potentially could be sued for **negligence** when he or she knows, or should know, that a patient is victim of domestic violence but takes no steps to intervene.

12. Give examples of how some states regulate reporting of domestic abuse.

Most states do not specifically require physicians or others to report suspected domestic abuse. There is a growing trend, however, toward enactment of broad-based prevention statutes that impose a requirement to report suspected domestic abuse in a range of cases. For example, the **Kentucky** Adult Protection Act requires that

> Any person, including but not limited to, physician, law enforcement officer, nurse, social worker, department personnel, coroner, medical examiner…, having reasonable cause to suspect that an adult has suffered abuse, neglect, or exploitation, shall report or cause reports to be made in accordance with the provisions of this chapter.

The reports are to be made to the Department of Adult Services. The reporting requirements are not specific to situations of domestic violence; they cover all types of abuse, neglect, or exploitation. failure to report is considered a criminal misdemeanor.

In 1994 **California** passed a new mandatory reporting statute that imposes broad reporting requirements on "any physician or surgeon who has under his or her charge or care any person" whom he or she knows, or reasonably should know, has suffered a wound or other physical injury "where the injury is the result of assaultive or abusive conduct." The statute also recommends documentation of comments about past domestic violence, mapping of injuries, and referrals to local domestic violence services for victims. Failure to report is a misdemeanor "punishable by imprisonment in a county jail for not exceeding six months or by a fine not exceeding one thousand dollars ($1000) or by both that fine and imprisonment."

California's reporting statute is unusual in specifically mentioning domestic violence. Physicians in most states have a legal obligation to report gunshot wounds, suspicious puncture wounds, and unexplained deaths. Thus, the physician who fails to report such events in the context of a domestic dispute may face legal repercussions. State requirements for the reporting of child abuse, elder abuse, or abuse of people with mental or physical disabilities also may come into play.

Colorado, **Connecticut**, and **Hawaii** also require reporting of domestic violence. **Illinois** makes such reporting voluntary, but protects the reporter against law suits.

Although few states specifically mandate the *reporting* of domestic violence, many have been aggressive in enacting and enforcing *laws against* domestic violence. In addition to criminal penalties, the states provide for restraining orders that prohibit the perpetrator from approaching the victim and either threatening or committing violent acts.

13. Is domestic violence a "private matter"?

No. This attitude is one of the biggest barriers in the fight against domestic violence. The belief that assault and battery within the home is somehow permissible as a "private matter" between individuals has led perpetrators to believe that their behavior is acceptable. It has led victims to believe that no one will help them and that reporting such violence is useless. Paradoxically, when victims finally speak out, their complaints often are minimized by those who assume that the delay is indicative of a benign situation.

14. How common is the problem of domestic violence?

Estimates of the incidence and prevalence of domestic violence vary, but they are all dramatic. Between two and four million women per year are believed to be victims of partner violence, including 1 in 7 women seen in general office practices for medical care, 1 in 3 women presenting for care in emergency rooms, 1 in 4 women who commit suicide, and 1 in 4 women who are pregnant. An estimated 50% of the mothers of abused children are victims of domestic violence. *Domestic violence is believed to be the most common single cause of traumatic injury to women.*

15. What constitutes domestic violence?

Domestic or partner violence involves actual or threatened physical injury, sexual assault, psychological abuse, economic control, and progressive social isolation. States differ as to what relationships qualify as "domestic." Massachusetts, for example, takes a broad view. Its domestic violence statue covers current or previous relationships between parties of any combination of genders who are or were married, related by blood, or shared a residence, or are or were involved in "a substantial dating relationship." "Substantial" has been interpreted as a single episode of sexual activity. Other states are more restrictive in defining the relationship.

16. True or false: The routine screening history should address domestic violence.

True. As with other medical conditions, the simplest way to determine whether a patient has been a victim of domestic violence is to ask. Just as we ask simple, nonjudgmental questions about sexual activity, physicians should include a question about domestic violence in the history. This inquiry must be conducted privately, away from the partner or other family members.

A question such as "Has a partner ever hit, kicked, or ortherwise hurt or frightened you?" is a good starting point. If the answer is positive, more details should be elicited in a nonjudgmental, confidential fashion. The Massachusetts Medical Society suggests these questions:

- How were you hurt?
- Has this happened before?
- When did it first happen?
- How badly have you been hurt in the past?
- Have you needed to go to an emergency room for treatment?
- Have you ever been threatened with a weapon, or has a weapon ever been used on you?
- Have the children ever seen you threatened or hurt?
- Have the children ever been threatened or hurt by your partner?

Adapted from Aleprt EJ, Freund KM, et al: partner Violence: How to Recognize and Treat Victims of Abuse. Waltham, MA, Massachusetts Medical Society, 1992.

17. What are important points to remember when interviewing potential victims of partner violence?

Avoid using terms such as "domestic violence," "abused," or "battered," which can be seen as judgmental. In addition, many individuals who are victims of violence do not see themselves as belonging in such categories. Questions about what the patient did to provoke the violence, why she has not left the batterer, or why she returned to the relationship after leaving should be avoided. If the answer to the intial question is negative, the physician should still look for physical indications of violence.

18. How can domestic violence be detected on physical exam?

Physical Signs and Symptoms of Domestic Abuse

- Contusions, abrasions, minor lacerations, fractures, and sprains.
- Neck, head, chest, breast, and abdominal injuries.
- Injuries during pregnancy, especially to the breasts and abdomen.
- Numerous injuries at multiple sites without adequate explanation.

Table continued on following page

Physical Signs and Symptoms of Domestic Abuse (Cont.)

• Chronic pain, psychogenic pain, or pain due to diffuse trauma without visible evidence.
• Physical symptoms related to chronic posttraumatic stress disorder, anxiety disorders, major depression, or stress.
• Gynecologic problems, including frequent genitourinary infections, pelvic pain, and dyspareunia.
• Evidence of rape or other sexual assault.
• Delay between time of injury and arrival at the hospital.
• Previous use of emergency services for trauma.

Adapted from Alpert EJ, Freund KM, et al: Partner Violence: How to Recognize and Treat Victims of Abuse. Waltham, MA, Massachusetts Medical Society, 1992.

Observations suggesting partner violence should be documented carefully in the medical record. Photographs are excellent for documenting injuries and are particulary useful if the pateint or state prosecutor pursues legal action against the batterer.

19. What should the physician do when domestic violence is suspected?

Victims of domestic violence often are reluctant to reveal the causes of their injuries. Reasons for this reluctance include fear of the batterer, lack of alternatives to the violent living arrangement, lack of economic resources, and failure of previous attempts to get help from physicians, law enforcement, and courts.

The physician may take a first step toward overcoming such obstacles by indicating to the patient, "I am concerned for your safety." This expression of concern, along with a clear indication that the violence is unacceptable, against the law, and deserving of action, may be the first support that the patient has received.

Refer the patient for treatment of injuries and for support and counseling. Battered women's programs often have lists of mental health professionals who provide treatment. In addition, such progams may provide shelters for victims and children. Discuss contraception and safe sex practices with the victim. If possible, do *not* give the victim sedating medication. Such medication may limit the patient's ability to escape in the event of further violence; it also may be used to question the patient's credibility in the event of legal proceedings. Consider whether there is a need to report the suspected violence to the appropriate public agency. Finally, put the patient in contact with an advocate for victims of domestic violence so that all alternatives can be explored.

BIBLIOGRAPHY

1. Alpert EJ, Freund KM, et al: Partner Violence: How to Recognize and Treat Victims of Abuse. Waltham, MA, Massachusetts Medical Society, 1992.
2. American Professional Society on the Abuse of Children: Guidelines for psychosocial evaluation of suspected sexual abuse in children. American Professional Society on the Abuse of Children, Chicago, 1997.
3. Appelbaum PA, Gutheil TG: Clinical Handbook of Psychiatry and the Law. Baltimore, Williams & Wilkins, 1991.
4. Barnum R: A suggested framework for forensic consultation in cases of child abuse and neglect. Bull Am Acad Psychiatry Law 25:581–593, 1997.
5. Bulkley JA, Feller JN, Stern P, et al: Child abuse and neglect law and legal proceedings. In Briere J (ed): The APSAC Handbook on Child Maltreatment. Thousand Oaks, CA, 1996.
6. California Penal Code Sec. 11160-1153.2; Amended by ABX1.74, Chapter 19.
7. DeAngelis C: Clinical indicators of child abuse. In Schetky DH, Benedek EP (eds): Clinical Handbook of Child Psychiatry and the Law. Baltimore, Williams & Wilkins, 1992.
8. Flitcraft A, Hadley S, et al: American Medical Association Diagnostic and Treatment Guidelines on Domestic Violence. Chicago, American Medical Association, 1992.
9. Green AH: Forensic evaluation of physically and sexually abused children. In Rosner R (ed): Principles and Practice of Forensic Psychiatry. New York, Chapman & Hall, 1994.
10. Jones JTR: Kentucky tort liability for failure to report family violence. 26 Northern Kentucky Law Review 43 (1999).
11. Kentucky Adult Protection Act, Kentucky Revised Statutes, Chapter 209.
12. Moskowitz S: Saving Granny from the wolf: Elder abuse and neglect—the legal framework. 31 Conn. Law Review 77 (1998).

13. Ohio State Medical Association: Trust Talk: Ohio Physicians' Domestic Violence Project. Columbus, OH, Ohio State Medical Association, 1992.
14. Ostow A: Child abuse. In Hyman SE, Tesar GE (eds): Manual of Psychiatric Emergencies, 3rd ed. Boston, Little, Brown, 1994.
15. Quinn KM, White S: Interviewing children for suspected child abuse. In Schetky DH, Benedek EP (eds): Clinical Handbook of Child Psychiatry and the Law. Baltimore, Williams & Wilkins, 1992.
16. Rand DC, Feldman MD: Misdiagnosis of Muchausen syndrome by proxy: A literature review and four new cases. Harvard Rev Psychiatry 7:94–101, 1999.
17. Reade J: Domestic violence. In Hyman SE, Tesar GE (eds): Manual of Psychiatric Emergencies, 3rd ed. Boston, Little, Brown, 1994.
18. Schouten R: Allegations of sexual abuse: A new area of liability risk. Harv Rev Psychiatry 1:350–352, 1994.
19. Schreier HA, Libow J: Hurting for Love: Münchausen's by Proxy Syndrome. New York, Guilford Press, 1993.
20. Skabronski JC: Elder abuse: Washington's response to a growing epidemic. 31 Gonzaga Law Review 627 (1995/1996).
21. Wardinsky TD: Genetic and congenital defect conditions that mimic child abuse. J Fam Practice 41:377–383, 1995.
22. Yoshimura RM: Empowering battered women: Changes in domestic violence laws in Hawaii. 17 Hawaii Law Review 17:575, 1995.

82. INVOLUNTARY TREATMENT: HOSPITALIZATION AND MEDICATIONS

John A. Menninger, M.D.

1. Why is involuntary hospitalization necessary?

Although the number of involuntary hospitalizations relative to total psychiatric admissions has decreased considerably in the United States from 90% in 1949 to 55% in 1980,[4] civil commitment of the mentally ill remains a frequent route for inpatient treatment. A majority of persons suffering from severe mental illness show **limited insight** into their illness. Schizophrenic patients, in particular, may show no recognition that they have a mental illness or need treatment. Depressed patients who are unable to envision hope or recall a better time may be suicidal and unwilling to seek treatment. Manic individuals who have become markedly grandiose and deny that they have any kind of problem or illness that needs treatment may display behaviors that put themselves or others in danger. Other patients may recognize their symptoms as part of an illness, but disagree with and refuse recommended treatment.

Untreated depression, mania, and psychosis can have devastating effects on both the affected individual and those around him or her: suicide, assaults on others, inadvertent tragedies stemming from delusional thinking, financial and social ruin, and inability to adequately care for one's own needs. Because insight often is lacking, civil commitment may be initiated by others who witness or are the brunt of concerning behavior, whether they be family members, police, or mental health providers.

2. What is the legal basis for involuntary commitment?

The state's authority to commit individuals stems from two legal theories; *parens patriae* and the police power of the state.

Parens patriae, which literally means "parent of the country," provides the sovereign power with authority to protect citizens who, for reasons of mental or physical disability or because they are unsupervised minors, cannot adequately protect or care for themselves. Intervention by the state is indicated for individuals who are deemed unable to make rational decisions for themselves, including the mentally ill who are "gravely disabled" or suicidal. The state also is obligated to make the decision that is in the best interest of the individual and most clearly reflects the choice that the individual would have made if he or she were competent to do so.

The legal theory **police power** provides the state with the authority to act for the protection of society and the general welfare of its citizens. In the process of such protection, isolation and confinement of dangerous individuals may be necessary. Not only the criminal element and persons with highly contagious diseases may be detained, but also the mentally ill who are a risk to others. Whereas *parens patriae* provides for the protection of the individual, police power generally is invoked on behalf of society against the individual.

3. Who can be involuntarily hospitalized?

The legal standards specifying the criteria for civil commitment vary widely from state to state, and may have changed in some states since the publication of this book. The clinician must be aware of the specific criteria for his or her own state. The presence of a **mental illness** is a prerequisite for civil commitment. Other criteria frequently include **dangerous behavior** toward self or others, **grave disability**, and the **need for treatment**. Over the past three decades there has been a general shift among most states from standards based on the individual's need for treatment to standards that require the person to be considered dangerous to self or others. However, some states have recently modified their statutes to allow for involuntary hospitalization of persons who are in need of treatment but are not imminently dangerous to themselves or others.

Less common criteria used by some states include: the responsiveness of the mental illness to treatment and the availability of appropriate treatment at the facility to which the patient will be committed; refusal of voluntary admission; lack of a capacity to consent to or refuse psychiatric treatment or hospitalization; future danger to property; and involuntary hospitalization as the least restrictive alternative.

4. What disorders does the term mentally ill include?

The legal definition of the term mental health, as spelled out in each state's statutes, varies considerably. Except for Utah, the statutes do not include specific psychiatric diagnoses, but instead define mental illness in terms of its effects on the individual's thinking or behavior. Some definitions are rather vague; for example, in the District of Columbia mental illness means "a psychosis or other disease which substantially impairs the mental health of a person." Most definitions include some deleterious effect of the illness. For example, in Georgia mentally ill "shall mean having a disorder of thought or mood which significantly impairs the judgment, behavior, capacity to recognize reality, or ability to cope with the ordinary demands of life." Some definitions are qualified by a reference to the need for treatment. Hawaii's statute specifies that a mentally ill person has "psychiatric disorder or other disease which substantially impairs the person's mental health and necessitates treatment or supervision." Many definitions include aspects of dangerousness. Oregon's statute declares that a mentally ill person is "a person who, because of a mental disorder, is either (a) dangerous to himself or others; or (b) unable to provide for his basic personal needs and is not receiving such care as is necessary for his health or safety."

5. Is someone with a developmental disability considered mentally ill?

Although developmental disability (mental retardation) is described in the Diagnostic and Statistical Manual of Mental Disorders, 4th ed. (DSM-IV), it typically is not considered a mental illness for the purposes of civil commitment. Many statutes completely exclude mental retardation from their definition of mentally ill, whereas others note that such a disorder may not constitute mental illness but does not preclude a comorbid mental illness. A few statutes specifically include mental retardation per se.

6. Are other diagnoses excluded in the definition of mentally ill?

In a few state statutes, the definition of mentally ill specifically excludes other disorders, most commonly alcoholism, drug addiction, and epilepsy. Some exclude "simple intoxication" with either alcohol or drugs. A small number exclude sociopathy, severe personality disorders in general, senility, and organic brain syndrome. Some statutes specifically *include* alcoholism and drug addiction. Maine's statute includes "persons suffering from the effects of the use of drugs, narcotics, hallucinogens or intoxicants, including alcohol, but not including mentally retarded or sociopathic persons."

7. What is grave disability?

The exact definition of grave disability varies from state to state. In general, the term refers to an inability to care adequately for one's own needs. In some states, a person is gravely disabled if he or she cannot care for basic needs without the assistance of others, even if family or friend are currently providing such care. In other states, the person must be without basic needs of food, clothing, shelter, or essential medical care.

8. What are the differences between emergency detention, observational institutionalization, and extended commitment?

Each has a specific purpose, although there often is considerable overlap. All states provide for some form of *emergency detention*, in which the intent is immediate psychiatric intervention to treat what is currently, or soon to become, an emergency situation. Emergency detention allows for an initial psychiatric assessment and at least temporary treatment for an individual who, for example, has presented a danger to self. Some states include statutes that provide for *observational institutionalization*. A person satisfying the appropriate criteria may be hospitalized so that the treatment staff and psychiatrist may further observe him or her to determine the diagnosis and to provide limited treatment. Formal procedures for *extended commitment* can be found in nearly every state. Such commitment allows for continued psychiatric treatment of individuals who meet one or more of the state's specific criteria (usually dangerousness to self or others or grave disability; less common criteria are discussed above) but would otherwise refuse treatment.

9. Who can initiate involuntary hospitalization?

The specifics of which professionals or persons may initiate civil commitment vary among states, and usually within a state depending on the type of commitment sought (e.g., emergency detention or extended commitment). In general, the application for emergency detention is less formal and extended commitment more formal; observational commitment (where available) is somewhere between.

Emergency detention generally may be initiated by another adult, usually a family member or friend who has witnessed the person's deterioration and dangerous behavior. The police also frequently initiate the process, although some states require judicial approval before the person can be detained. A number of states provide for medical certification; that is, an evaluation from a physician stating that the person meets the statutory criterion is adequate to proceed with hospitalization.

Application for **observational commitment** often may be made by any citizen with good reason, although some states limit the application to physicians or hospital personnel. Most states require court approval.

The procedure to request **extended commitment** is the most formal and usually more detailed than the applications for other forms of commitment. In general, one or more of a specific group of people may complete the appropriate forms to request involuntary treatment. Although this group may include spouses, relatives, friends, guardians, and public officials, it typically is limited to physicians, hospital superintendents, and other mental health professionals, such as certain licensed social workers and nurses. Even in states that allow for other persons to initiate commitment, generally only a physician can extend commitment beyond the initial period. Often the application must be accompanied by a certificate or affidavit from a physician in which the person's psychiatric presentation, pertinent history, recent behavior warranting commitment, initial diagnosis, and recommendations for treatment are described in detail. Some states require statements from two physicians or an additional statement from a psychologist, mental health board or similar designee. In virtually all states extended commitment is a judicial process. A hearing is scheduled, and either a judge or a jury decides whether to uphold the request.

10. How long does involuntary hospitalization last?

• Emergency detention is designed to provide for an assessment of a dangerous situation. It is generally limited to a brief period, usually 3–5 days; the period ranges from only 24 hours in a few states to 20 days in New Jersey.

• The length of an observational commitment, in states that allow it, varies from 48 hours in Alaska to 6 months in West Virginia. Before the expiration of the emergency or observational commitment, the patient must either agree to voluntary hospitalization or be discharged; otherwise, civil commitment proceedings must be initiated.

• Extended commitment also is limited; 6 months is a typical period. If at the end of that period the treating psychiatrist recommends continued involuntary treatment, application for further extension of civil commitment may be made. Again the length of time is finite, often $1\frac{1}{2}$–2 times longer than the initial commitment. The possibility for renewal at the end of each period continues as long as it is requested and the patient continues to meet the statutory criteria.

11. Is mental commitment possible on an outpatient basis?

Yes. Many states explicitly provide for outpatient commitment, whereas others simply do not prohibit the extension of civil commitment to outpatient programs. In states with statutes that specifically address outpatient commitment, the length of commitment generally is limited but somewhat longer than for inpatient commitment. The specific criteria and procedures are similar to those for inpatient commitment and likewise vary from state to state. The goal of outpatient commitment may be continued involuntary treatment in a less restrictive setting than the inpatient unit, or an attempt to avoid inpatient treatment for a patient whose condition is deteriorating. If the patient fails to comply with the conditions of treatment, rehospitalization is indicated.

12. Which patients are appropriate for outpatient commitment?

Patients appropriate for outpatient commitment include those who have shown a good response to psychiatric medications in the past, but are **noncompliant** with medications and other aspects of treatment without continued coercion. Involuntary outpatient treatment also is indicated for patients who require considerable **structure** to their lives and support from others to maintain adequate functioning outside the hospital. For outpatient commitment to be realistically tenable, the facility, often a mental health center, should be capable of adequate outreach. Also needed is a high degree of co-operation and communication between the courts authorizing commitment and the outpatient programs, as well as between the outpatient and inpatient facilities.

13. What are the rights of patients who have been involuntarily hospitalized?

Persons involuntarily hospitalized maintain a number of rights, some of which are specifically related to the commitment proceedings and come under the rubric of due process. Such rights usually include notice of commitment, objection to confinement, representation by an attorney, presence at the commitment hearing, trial by jury, independent psychiatric examination, and change to voluntary status. Additional civil rights of the mentally ill, regardless of their legal status, generally include humane care and treatment; treatment in the least restrictive setting; free and open communication with the outside world via telephone or mail; meetings with visitors, particularly their attorney, physician, or clergy; confidentiality of records; possession of their own clothing and money; payment for any work done in the hospital; absentee ballot voting; and being informed of such rights. Many of these rights may be temporarily restricted by the staff if deemed necessary (e.g., while the patient is in restraints or seclusion).

14. Can an involuntary patient be treated?

Treatment cannot be forced. However, involuntary admission does not preclude treatment either. Many patients, despite being hospitalized on a civil commitment, are both amenable and receptive to treatment. They may disagree that they need to be in a hospital, but ironically they do not disagree that they need treatment. It is important to continue to educate patients who deny the need for treatment about their condition, psychiatric diagnosis, and treatment options. The refusal for voluntary hospitalization and voluntary treatment should be sought, explored, and discussed to foster a therapeutic alliance.

Simple education or addressing concerns of the patient may allow him or her to decide to sign into the hospital volitionally and/or to agree to treatment. Severe psychosis, mania, or depression, of course, may result in an impasse that requires the court or judge to decide. However, many patients who are initially brought into the hospital involuntarily may later be willing to sign themselves into the hospital and actively participate in their treatment.

Note that the same therapeutic approaches that help to foster a therapeutic relationship with voluntary patients also help to engage involuntary patients in treatment.

15. May involuntarily hospitalized patients refuse to take medications?

Generally, yes. A majority of states consider all patients, even mentally ill patients hospitalized involuntarily, competent to make personal decisions, including whether to take psychotropic medications, unless they are specifically found legally incompetent by a court of law. Most states provide that an involuntary patient's refusal of medications may be overridden only by court hearing. Many states allow a legally appointed guardian to consent for the patient. A small number of states specifically recognize the right of voluntary patients to refuse medications.

Although a patient's refusal to take medications may stem from delusional thinking or a denial that anything is wrong, the reasons also may be based in reality. The patient may have previously had an intolerable side effect to the medication in question. It is essential to explain the recommended pharmacologic treatments, including expected benefits and possible adverse effects, and to explore fully the reasons behind the patient's refusal. Negotiation and compromise, such as using an alternate medication of the same class or initiating the medication at a lower dose, may be helpful and allow for treatment to proceed.

16. What is the difference between involuntary medications and emergency medications?

Emergency medications are ordered acutely by the treating psychiatrist or physician for a patient who is considered imminently dangerous to self or others, either physically or psychologically, and refuses to take the medications freely. Examples of such situations include the dehydrated and delirious manic patient who is already in restraints but continues to thrash about and bang his or her head against the bed frame. Emergency medications should work acutely (e.g., neuroleptics and benzodiazepines as opposed to antidepressants and mood stabilizers) and must target the serious presenting symptoms. The clinical need for emergency medications must be reassessed frequently, from every several hours to every 24 hours. Often a second opinion about the appropriateness of the emergency medications must be obtained from another physician. Emergency medications usually are limited to a few days.

Involuntary medications are granted by a court in nonemergent situations. Mentally ill persons who require chronic administration of medication and yet have minimal insight into their need may warrant involuntary medications. The treating psychiatrist or physician generally applies for the administration of involuntary medications with an accompanying affidavit supporting the opinion that the patient is mentally ill and incompetent to participate in treatment decisions, and that the medications are clinically indicated. The statement also may need to review the patient's prior noncompliance with medication and expected benefit and potential side effects.

Some states direct that involuntary medications can be requested only for patients who are currently under a civil commitment. The criteria for involuntary medications vary from state to state, but commonly include such aspects as incompetence to participate in decisions about treatment and expected clinical deterioration or dangerous behavior to self or others without the medications.

Court-ordered involuntary medications are time-limited, often lasting only as long as the patient's civil commitment or for a period set by the judge. Extension beyond that time requires a reappraisal of the patient's condition, response to treatment, and likelihood of future compliance.

17. Can electroconvulsive therapy be given involuntarily?

Many states have provisions in their statutes that specifically allow for refusal of electroconvulsive therapy (ECT). If the person is considered incompetent, then a court order or a guardian's consent is required. If the situation is viewed as a life-threatening emergency, some states allow for ECT to be administered without consent of either the patient or a guardian; however, such consent or a court order should be obtained as soon as possible. Often a second opinion about the appropriateness of treatment and the person's competency to consent also must be obtained. Some states limit the use of ECT to certain psychiatric disorders or age groups; some also limit the number of treatments that can be administered to a patient each year.

18. What are the proper indications for seclusion or restraints?

Both seclusion and restraints generally are viewed as appropriate and sometimes necessary parts of inpatient psychiatric treatment, given the proper indications. Restraints are defined as the physical incapacitation of the person, either in total or in part, by tying him or her securely to a bed or chair, frequently with leather straps. Seclusion refers to the placement of an individual in isolated confinement. A seclusion room typically is small, securely built, and unfurnished or minimally furnished, with a lockable door. The door usually has a small window for viewing the patient or a mounted camera for close monitoring.

The most common clinical indications for the use of such external constraints are (1) **prevention of serious injury to self or others** when other treatment techniques are unsuccessful or inappropriate and (2) **prevention of serious physical damage to the inpatient unit or marked disruption of the ward**. Other less common reasons include their use as part of a specific behavior therapy program, or at the patient's own request.

19. What are the legal constraints on the use of seclusion and restraints?

Most states have either specific statutes or administrative rules that regulate the use of restraints. About one-half of states have similar regulations for the use of locked seclusion. In general, the use of restraints and seclusion requires a physician's written order; is limited in duration (often to 24 hours); and must be accompanied by frequent monitoring of the patient's condition, usually by the nursing staff, with documentation of the assessment and reasons for continued seclusion or restraints. If seclusion or restraints are necessary beyond the initial period, a physician must conduct a direct examination, sign another written order, document the behaviors that necessitate continued external constraints, and establish that such measures are the least restrictive intervention. When restraints or seclusion have been used for several consecutive days, a mandatory review by the medical director or superintendent is common.

20. Which is the most restrictive intervention: seclusion, restraints, or involuntary medication?

There is no clearly established hierarchy of intrusiveness. The choice of the most appropriate treatment of a violent psychotic patient varies with the situation, and different clinicians may give opposing views.

21. Who can authorize psychiatric admission of children?

Statutes detailing the psychiatric admission procedures for children often are convoluted and vary widely. In general, children (i.e., legal minors) are considered legally incompetent. This includes incompetence to make a decision about psychiatric hospitalization. The past two decades have seen a number of changes with increased recognition by many states of certain rights of due process for minors. Most states continue to allow a child's parent or guardian to approve admission to a psychiatric hospital regardless of the child's wishes. They also often provide that a child may not be discharged from a mental hospital without authorization from the parents. A number of states have statutes that provide for parentally authorized admission for younger children (up to the age of 13 or 14 years), but older minors have the rights of due process, including a hearing and counsel, either automatically or if they protest their hospitalization.

Once hospitalized, the minor's continued need for inpatient treatment must be reviewed periodically, from every 10 days (in Arizona) to every 60 days in other states. Most states now permit older children to admit themselves voluntarily into a psychiatric hospital. The minimal age ranges from 12 years in Georgia to 17 years in Florida. When a child refuses admission for psychiatric hospitalization and the state does not allow for parental consent, emergency commitment proceedings must be initiated.

22. Do the criteria for civil commitment of children differ from those for adults?

The clinical indications for the commitment of minors may differ from those for adults in particular states. In general, if a child is suicidal or homicidal or has a severe mental illness, he or she may satisfy criteria for involuntary hospitalization. Some state statutes include "being in need of treatment," which allows admission of children who do not respond adequately to intensive outpatient intervention. As with the statutes for adults, the specific criteria and procedures vary markedly among states.

Usually a psychiatrist must conduct an examination to determine the appropriate services for the child. The assessment must include an interview with the child alone and a thorough review of the child's history. The evaluation should use as many possible sources of information as possible, such as parents, school, and social agencies.

23. Can a child's parents authorize involuntary psychotropic medication?

Many states consider a parent's consent for psychiatric treatment adequate to overrule a minor's refusal to take medication. However, if the treatment is considered unusual or hazardous, such as electroconvulsive therapy or high doses of medications, parental consent may be inadequate; in such cases, the clinician should obtain authorization from a court.

24. May a patient who was admitted voluntarily and then wishes to leave be converted to an involuntary patient?

Yes. When a person who has admitted him- or herself voluntarily wishes to be discharged against the recommendation of the physician and treatment team, the staff are provided time to assess whether the patient meets criteria for civil commitment. If such criteria are met, the process of emergency detention must be initiated at once.

25. What is the difference between incompetence and civil commitment?

Competence is divided into legal competence and clinical competence. *Legal competence* refers to a declaration by a court of law that the person is unable to manage adequately his or her assets or to make decisions about personal care and welfare. All adults, including those with severe mental illness, are presumed legally competent until found otherwise. *Clinical competence*, also called decision-making capacity, refers to the ability to comprehend a situation and the consequences of decisions and to communicate such comprehension to others. It refers to a particular question and depends on the patient's understanding and the risks of the proposed intervention. A person may be considered incompetent in one sphere but not another; e.g., the person may be competent to concur with psychiatric hospitalization, but incompetent to consent to ECT.

Patients may be subject to *civil commitment* because they fulfill the particular criteria in that state; e.g., they have a mental illness that renders them markedly delusional with paranoia and suicidal thoughts. However, if they fully understand the risks and benefits of a particular treatment or procedure, whether it is receiving medications, having their teeth pulled, or having surgery for gallstones, they remain competent to accept or refuse, regardless of the decision they make. Conversely, an individual with dementia or mental retardation may not have a major psychiatric illness requiring hospitalization but still be clinically incompetent to make a particular decision.

26. Can mentally ill patients who appear to be incapable of understanding their legal rights with regard to hospitalization be admitted voluntarily?

For the most part, unless someone has already been declared legally incompetent, he or she is presumed to be legally competent to make decisions about personal welfare, including psychiatric admission. Some states, however, specify that a patient's decision for voluntary admission must be competent. In such states, the patient would require civil commitment.

27. Can alcoholics and addicts be involuntarily treated?

It depends upon the state in question. Less than two-thirds of the states have laws allowing for involuntary treatment of alcoholics, and fewer have provisions for drug addicts. Definitions of alcoholism and drug addiction generally include loss of control of intake and imminent risk for self-harm as criteria for civil commitment.

28. Is the person who initiated involuntary hospitalization liable for false imprisonment?

A patient claiming to have been negligently hospitalized may seek malpractice litigation for false imprisonment. Such litigation is rare because of the legal protections that ensure due process. **Important guidelines for clinicians** involved in civil commitments include the following: they should **(1)** be familiar with both the commitment statutes of their state and the appropriate administrative policies for their facility; **(2)** act in good faith; **(3)** conduct a comprehensive psychiatric examination of the person in question; **(4)** complete all aspects of the necessary commitment forms; **(5)** describe the specific behaviors and symptoms that support the presence of mental illness and the need for treatment, including behaviors fulfilling commitment criteria such as dangerousness; **(6)** outline the recommended treatment for the person's condition with consideration for the least restrictive setting; and **(7)** obtain consultation for equivocal cases.

29. Will managed care cost-containment change civil commitment laws?

The potential conflict between the focus on cost reduction by managed care companies and the focus on control of dangerous patients by the courts is currently being played out in many states and likely will result in civil commitment law modification in the future.

BIBLIOGRAPHY

Civil commitment in general
 1. Appelbaum PS: Almost a Revolution: Mental Health Law and the Limits of Change. New York, Oxford University Press, 1994.
 2. Appelbaum PS, Gutheil TG: Clinical Handbook of Psychiatry and the Law, 2nd ed. Baltimore, Williams & Wilkins, 1991.
 3. Bittman BJ, Convit A: Competency, civil commitment, and the dangerousness of the mentally ill. J Forensic Sci 38:1460–1466, 1993.
 4. Brakel SJ, Parry J, Weiner BA: The Mentally Disabled and the Law, 3rd ed. Chicago, American Bar Foundation, 1985.
 5. Hiday VA: Coercion in civil commitment: Process, preferences, and outcome. Int J Law Psychiatry 15:359–377, 1992.
 6. Miller RD: Need-for-treatment criteria for involuntary civil commitment: Impact in practice. Am J Psychiatry 149:1380–1384, 1992.
 7. Munetz MR, Geller JL: The least restrictive alternative in the post institutional era. Hosp Community Psychiatry 44:967–973, 1993.
 8. Weiner BA, Wettstein RM: Legal Issues in Mental Health Care. New York, Plenum Press, 1993.
Involuntary medications
 9. Appelbaum PS: The right to refuse treatment with antipsychotic medications: Retrospect and prospect. Am J Psychiatry 145:413–419, 1988.
 10. Cournos F, McKinnon K, Stanley B: Outcome of involuntary medication in a state hospital system. Am J Psychiatry 148:489–494, 1991.
 11. Schwartz HI, Vingiano W, Beziganian Perez C: Autonomy and the right to refuse treatment: Patient's attitudes after involuntary medications. Hosp Community Psychiatry 39:1049–1054, 1988.
Involuntary ECT
 12. Mahler H, Co BT, Dinwiddle S: Studies in involuntary civil commitment and involuntary electroconvulsive therapy. J Nerv Mental Disorders 174:97–106, 1986.
Outpatient commitment
 13. Geller JL: Clinical guidelines for the use of involuntary outpatient treatment. Hosp Community Psychiatry 41:749–755, 1990.
 14. Miller RD: An update on involuntary civil commitment to outpatient treatment. Hosp Community Psychiatry 43:79–81, 1992.
 15. Mulvey EP, Geller JL, Roth LH: The promise and peril of involuntary outpatient commitment. Am Psychol 42:571–584, 1987.
Restraint and seclusion
 16. Fisher WA: Restraint and seclusion: A review of the literature. Am J Psychiatry 151:1584–1591, 1994.
Insight into mental illness
 17. Amador XF, Strauss DH, Yale SA, Gorman JM: Awareness of illness in schizophrenia. Schizophr Bull 17:113–132, 1991.
Psychiatric diagnoses
 18. American Psychiatric Association: Diagnostic and Statistical Manual of Mental Disorders, 4th ed. Washington, DC, American Psychiatric Association, 1994.

83. COMPETENCE AND INSANITY

Harold J. Bursztajn, M.D., and Archie Brodsky, B.A.

1. Are competence and insanity purely medical concepts?

No. In common usage they are considered legal concepts, because they represent specific judgments made by the courts. However, they also can be regarded as distinct medicolegal concepts. Although clinical data contribute to the determination of both competence and insanity, the determination also requires a knowledge of relevant statutes as well as a comprehensive analysis of both subjective and objective data. Such a deep level of analysis is not normally a part of clinical evaluation. Indeed, the standards for determining competence or insanity are multidimensional and somewhat case-specific. Relevant factors include:

- Applicable laws in the governing jurisdiction (e.g., "insanity" involves judgment of lack of criminal responsibility based on particular standard specified by statute)
- The act or decision for which a person is to be judged competent or incompetent, sane or insane
- Contextual factors defining the meaning of the act for that person at a particular place and time.

Basic Terminology Used in Determinations of Competence or Insanity

Burden of proof: The obligation in court of the moving party to demonstrate the existence of certain facts or to suffer loss of the proceeding.

Competence: The legal recognition of an individual's ability to perform a task. The concept is not applied globally. Rather, it is directed at a specific category of demands.

Deposition: A form of legal discovery in civil proceedings in which the litigants may question potential witnesses under oath to discover the testimony that they are likely to present at trial.

Diminished capacity: The response of a criminal defendant requesting to be partially excused from misconduct on the basis of mental condition.

Expert witness: An individual permitted to present opinion in court on matters of fact that are beyond the expertise of ordinary citizens.

Imperfect self-defense: The response of a criminal defendant requesting to be excused for misconduct on the basis of a mental state of self-defense which is itself substantially influenced by a mental disorder or defect.

Informed consent: Authorization by a person who is free from coercion or undue influence, who has been given adequate information on the decision to be made, and who has the capacity to understand the information disclosed.

Insanity defense: The response of a criminal defendant requesting to be [entirely] excused for misconduct on the basis of mental condition.

Jurisdiction: The scope of a specific court's authority. A court's decision in a particular case sets precedent for all similar cases arising within the court's geographic boundaries.

Standard of proof: The degree of probability to which factual assertions must be proven to allow a moving party to prevail in litigation.

Adapted from Group for the Advancement of Psychiatry, Committee on Psychiatry and Law: The Mental Health Professional and the Legal System (Report No. 131). New York, Brunner/Mazel, 1991, pp 181–186, with permission.

2. Do clinicians make determinations of competence and insanity?

No. Determinations of competence and insanity are made by the courts with the help of assessments by qualified professionals. Ordinarily, such assessments should not be made by a clinician who is treating the person to be evaluated.

3. What professional guidelines apply to combining the roles of treater and evaluator?

The following excerpts from the ethical guidelines of the American Academy of Psychiatry and the Law (AAPL) make clear that an attempt to combine the roles of treater and evaluator involves the clinician in both a **clash of perspectives** and a **conflict of interest**.

> ... the psychiatrist should inform the evaluee that although he is a psychiatrist, he is not the evaluee's "doctor"... There is a continuing obligation to be sensitive to the fact that although a warning has been given, there may be slippage and a treatment relationship may develop in the mind of the examinee.

> A treating psychiatrist should generally avoid agreeing to be an expert witness or to perform an evaluation of his patient for legal purposes because a forensic evaluation usually requires that other people be interviewed and testimony may adversely affect the therapeutic relationship.

4. Discuss the rationale behind the AAPL guidelines.

The reasons for avoiding duality of roles are evident. On the one hand, the empathic, subjective stance that the clinician takes to relieve the patient's suffering and to promote growth is largely incompatible with objective evaluation. On the other hand, the distancing required to perform an objective evaluation, not to mention the loss of confidentiality, tends to undermine the therapeutic alliance. Therefore, when the treating clinician is asked to perform an evaluation for the court, the appropriate response is to refer the patient for a forensic psychiatric evaluation. Likewise, when a forensic evaluation lapses into a treatment relationship despite one's best efforts to the contrary, the wisest response is to refer the patient for further forensic evaluation, especially if the plan is to continue treatment.

5. What is competence—or more accurately, what are competencies?

In **general application**, competence is understood to be the mental soundness necessary to carry out certain legally defined acts. A person is presumed competent unless it is shown that a mental disease or defect impairs his or her ability to understand the nature or consequences of the act in question. Competence is a matter of degree, but for most legal purposes it is the minimal rather than maximal standard of competence that must be met.

Moving beyond general descriptions of the elements of competence (e.g., "understanding of available choices, capacity to make those choices, and freedom from undue influence") to specific **medicolegal applications**, the term has no single definition. Competence is selective and compartmentalized and must be assessed in relation to the decision or act in question: "Competent to do what, and in what context?" Thus, rather than focusing on a single, global competence, ask: "Which are the relevant competencies?" This specification is especially important in assessing the responsibility of organizations for negligent referral and treatment (*Klein v. Solomon and Brown University*, Supreme Court of Rhode Island, 1998) and is pertinent to the increasing trend for the courts to hold managed-care organizations responsible for such deviations.

6. Is the medicolegal application of competence complex?

Yes. Given the many factors that affect competence, the evaluator who goes beyond global assessments often finds that some capacities are impaired, but others are not. The evaluator must be alert for subtle, fluctuating signs of incompetence.

7. Distinguish between determination of competence and assessment of criminal responsibility.

Determination of competence in civil law means the individual is able to give (or withhold) informed consent to medical treatment and make contracts and wills. In criminal law, psychiatrists are asked to assess a defendant's competence to stand trial, confess, waive Miranda rights, or act as his or her own attorney. Psychiatrists also may act as consultants to probation officers or the courts for presentencing and in preparation of probation reports. A psychiatrist is asked to evaluate other areas of competence only on rare occasions: for example, an often neglected question is the defendant's competence to accept a plea bargain. A psychiatrist performing a competence evaluation must ask the attorney to specify which area of competence is in question.

Assessment of criminal responsibility (which may hinge on a determination of sanity or insanity) is different in kind from what is normally referred to as assessment of competence. When a question of diminished capacity arises in relation to criminal responsibility, it refers to a distinct set of faculties such as formation of the intent to commit a particular act, appreciation of moral or legal wrongfulness, or ability to conform one's behavior to the requirements of law.

Questions of competence and criminal responsibility are treated separately in this chapter, as they are in everyday usage. However, the deep connection between the two (i.e., that lack of criminal responsibility by reason of insanity presupposes a generally or specifically disabled and, in some particular sense, incompetent mental state) must be understood.

8. How has the definition of competence evolved?

Classically, competence was defined mainly in terms of **cognitive awareness**. In 1960, in *Dusky v. U.S.*, the U.S. Supreme Court took this conception to its limit, and perhaps beyond, when it defined competence as "not only a factual but a rational understanding."

As understanding of human psychology deepened, psychiatrists also took into account an **affective dimension**. That is, various impairments characterized by overwhelming affect, while not leading to psychosis, may restrict a person's sense of choice or hope for the future. Such conditions include full-fledged post-traumatic stress disorder as well as more subtle but nonetheless real syndromes of trauma response (e.g., pathologic grief and survivor guilt; see Question 12).

9. Distinguish between intrapsychic and interpersonal dimensions of competence.

The intrapsychic dimensions often are addressed first. Thus a forensic evaluation includes a mental status examination (both formal and informal) to look at the person's biologic and intrapsychic integrity, searching for disorders of cognition (e.g., delusions), affect (e.g., hopelessness), or volition (e.g., impulse disinhibition) that may constrain the relevant judgment or behavior. However, a person's competence to consent to treatment cannot be fully assessed without also considering his or her functioning in the interpersonal realm of relationships with the caregivers involved (see Questions 10–14). In the case of testamentary capacity (the competence required to make a last will and testament), interpersonal relationships are even more central to the assessment (see Question 17). Likewise, a person's state of mind at the time of committing a criminal act is often contingent on the interpersonal context, including the perpetrator's perception of self, the victim, and their relationship, as well as the *actual* relationship.

10. What is competence to give informed consent to treatment?

Competent, informed consent consists of three elements: **decision-making capacity**, **requisite information**, and **voluntariness**. Although all three elements usually are viewed as individual assessments, they are also a function of the patient-clinician relationship. The fact that information has been given does not mean that it has been received or retained. For example, information may be conveyed in an overbearing way or may be incomprehensible to a patient who is more visually than verbally oriented. Voluntariness may be compromised by coercive pressures, whether from clinicians who believe that they know what is best for the patient or from an institutional culture that promotes cost-containment. Such deficits in information or voluntariness may overwhelm the patient's decision-making capacity.

Informed consent, therefore, is not a pro forma response to a checklist; rather, it is a **process of mutual engagement in decision making**. Thus, the competence to give informed consent includes the capacity to engage in a dialogue about benefits and risks and to apply the discussion meaningfully to one's present situation. This capacity may be either enhanced or diminished by the manner in which clinicians carry out their side of the dialogue (*Meador v. Stahler and Gheridian*, Mass., 1993).

11. When is a psychiatrist likely to be consulted about a patient's competence to give informed consent?

Consultations on competent, informed consent are requested in several types of situations. Two common ones are: when a general healthcare professional has a patient who refuses medical treatment, and when a mental health professional has a patient who refuses further psychiatric treatment.

12. Describe common pitfalls in the assessment of a patient's competence to give informed consent.

A common bias of clinicians is to obtain a consultation only when the patient refuses treatment, not when the patient agrees to treatment. Note that in terms of risk management as well as the patient's best interest, incompetent consent can be as much an issue as incompetent refusal. When a question of competent consent arises, a forensic psychiatric consultation is helpful.

It is also a mistake to try to assess competence to consent to treatment globally rather than in relation to the specific circumstances of treatment. Competence to consent to treatment, like competence in general, is not an indivisible concept. A patient may be competent to consent to treatment in most circumstances, but not to a particular kind of treatment or to treatment offered by a particular clinician.

For example, a man in severe congestive heart failure secondary to a surgically correctable cardiac condition refused surgery—despite his ability to recite the risks and benefits of the recommended operation. The patient revealed to the consulting psychiatrist that his wife had died 15 years earlier after what had been considered a minor, low-risk operation. The psychiatric consultation gave the patient an opportunity to work through the unresolved grief that impaired his competence to consent. Subsequently he consented and after surgery was grateful that his treating team did not "quit" on him, despite his initial refusal. He described the effect of the psychiatric consultation as "lifting a dark veil."

13. Is assessment of competence affected by the examiner-examinee relationship and the circumstances of the examination?

Yes. Assessment of a patient's capacity to give informed consent may be biased by unrecognized fluctuations in competence resulting from the setting, time of day, variable medication, side effects, rapid changes in pathophysiology, or other factors. The examination may be performed when the patient is at his or her worst or best. Furthermore, a person may be found falsely competent due to overidentification by the examiner, or falsely incompetent due to projection of the examiner's own despair. A breakdown in communication also can occur: for example, a patient who is frightened and not fluent in the examiner's language may respond with greater understanding to a visual model of the heart than to a strictly verbal description of a coronary bypass graft.

14. What other factors can affect assessment of competence?

Medication side effects should not be overlooked as potentially treatable causes of impaired competence. For example, benzodiazepines have a negative effect on memory and can tip even non-Alzheimer's patients into a state of dementia that impairs competence.

Likewise, a patient who reasonably feels he or she has no choice but to accept managed health care's determination of benefits is being coerced and therefore is not giving informed consent. Even in the absence of overt coercion, an atmosphere of pessimism among hospital staff (exacerbated as it may be by managed-care restrictions) may subtly constrain patients' and families' sense of the range of alternatives they are able or even willing to consider. That is, people may disavow what they might actually want if they are conditioned to believe they cannot have it or should not ask for it. Elderly, chronically ill patients and patients of any age with socially stigmatized, chronic illnesses (e.g., AIDS, alcoholism, schizophrenia) are especially vulnerable to such demoralizing influences.

Thus, competence should be assessed in subjective as well as objective terms, in affective as well as cognitive terms, and as a function of the interpersonal and institutional environment as well as individual characteristics.

15. How are questions of patient competence raised in cases of alleged patient-clinician sexual contact?

It is now rare to hear the argument that a patient has given informed consent to sexual contact with a clinician as part of treatment. Not so unusual is the argument that the patient has consented independently to treatment and to concurrent or subsequent sexual contact. The issue, then, is whether the patient is competent to consent to what may be self-destructive physical intimacy with the treating clinician outside of treatment.

Note that when the patient does not have the option of seeing a different doctor or obtaining treatment from another organization, because of managed-care referral, the helplessness and horror the patient experiences and the resulting impairment of competence are magnified.

Questions of consent and of competence to consent often enter implicitly into civil litigation. The degree of damage, as suffered by the plaintiff or as perceived by a jury, often hinges on how competent and active the plaintiff was in initiating and maintaining the alleged sexual relationship. In addressing such questions, a thorough forensic evaluation of the plaintiff must recognize the complex interactions between character defenses and trauma in remembering and communicating.

16. What part does competence play in assessing the risk of suicide or violence?

Clinicians are asked to make decisions involving dangerousness to self or others in various contexts, including involuntary commitment and restriction of freedom during hospitalization. In such decisions, competence is an implicit if not explicit consideration. It becomes explicit in states where the criteria for involuntary commitment (in the presence of mental illness) include the ability to care for oneself as well as dangerousness to self or others.The decision-making process that leads to commitment is thus analogous to the seeking of guardianship on the basis of incompetence to give or withhold informed consent to treatment.

An often neglected and yet essential aspect of the assessment of potential violence is the assessment of the patient's competence to engage in a dialogue with the clinician concerning potential harm to self or others and measures to prevent it. Dangerousness in itself is so salient to clinicians that the equally important question of the patient's capacity to participate responsibly in monitoring his or her dangerousness tends to pale by comparison. The model of dangerousness presented below, in which competence appears as one dimension, illustrates a mindset useful in many areas of clinical decision making, such as addressing the multidimensional complexity of competence itself.

In cases where violence is both foreseeable and preventable, the problem generally is not one of insufficient legal authority to commit, but of inadequate training, poor professional judgement, or limited resources to carry out such a complex assessment.

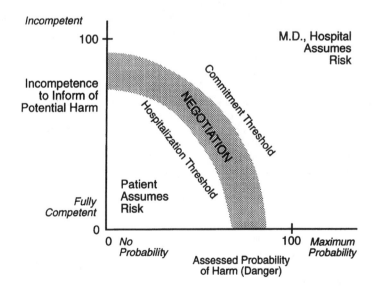

Multidimensional assessment of dangerousness in relation to competence to inform. (From Gutheil TG, Bursztajn HJ, Brodsky A: The multidimensional assessment of dangerousness: Competence assessment in patient care and liability prevention. Bull Am Acad Psychiatry Law 14:123–129, 1986; with permission.)

17. Describe testamentary capacity.

Testamentary capacity is customarily considered the lowest level of competence. Even someone who has a guardian of person may have testamentary capacity, despite a rebuttable presumption that she does not. Making a will is considered to require a lesser degree of competence than entering into a contract, for example, in which case an adverse party seeks an advantageous position. However, clinicians who work with family dynamics may well find an adversarial relationship between the testator and another party or between two parties contending for the inheritance (in which case the testator must act as judge).

18. How do the principles of competence assessment apply to evaluating a last will and testament for testamentary capacity?

Familiarity with state statues and case law is essential for framing the questions to be answered in the forensic psychiatric evaluation of testamentary capacity. Such questions emphasize functional as opposed to diagnostic considerations. For example, the Supreme Judicial Court of Massachusetts, in *Goddard v. Dupree* (1948), defined testamentary capacity as follows:

> *Testamentary capacity requires ability on the part of the testator to understand and carry in mind, in a general way, the nature and situation of his property and his relations to those persons who would naturally have some claim to his remembrance. It requires freedom from delusion which is the effect of disease or weakness and which might influence the disposition of his property. And it requires ability at the time of execution of the alleged will to comprehend the nature of the act of making a will.*

Thus, contrary to the all-too-common stigmatization of the mentally ill, a person with schizophrenia cannot be assumed to lack testamentary capacity unless at least one of these specified functions is impaired. In this as in other areas, diagnosis does not by itself determine competence. At the same time, the evaluator must consider numerous possible sources of functional impairment. Often overlooked are impairments resulting from chronic, partially concealed alcohol use, early-onset organic brain syndromes, or drugs, especially pain-relieving drugs such as morphine, that may have subtle but real euphoric and/or dysphoric effects that alter judgment in relatively low dosages (by *Physician's Desk Reference* standards).

19. What kind of confusion may arise for the clinician addressing testamentary capacity?

With respect to testamentary capacity, as with other forms of competence, the treating clinician should refer the patient to someone in a position to make an objective evaluation. Especially when deathbed revisions of a will are at issue, the treating clinician's proper concern with relieving the patient's suffering precludes such objectivity. The clinician may confuse competence to consent to treatment with competence to dispose of property, each of which must be assessed independently. A treating clinician may either overestimate or underestimate the deceased person's testamentary capacity. Overestimation may occur if the clinician feels threatened by virtue of having already honored the person's acceptance or refusal of treatment, whereas underestimation may occur if the clinician's most salient memories are of the person in a confused rather than coherent state.

20. Is competence to stand trial equivalent to criminal responsibility?

No. The two assessments have different tests, different time contexts, and different purposes. A person is considered competent to stand trial if he or she understands the nature of the charges and is able to cooperate with counsel. The assessment of competence to stand trial is a **present-state** examination, whereas determination of criminal responsibility is **retrospective** and pertains to the person's culpability at the time of the alleged act. Although the criteria for culpability (see Question 26) represent a kind of competence at a deep-structural level, the two determinations are entirely separate matters in everyday practice.

Competence to stand trial usually is considered (subject to jurisdictional variations) the lowest level of competence in the criminal realm, because it is seen to require only a minimum of psychological functioning. However, notwithstanding the understandable desire to have defendants stand trial in a speedy, cost-effective way, the question of whether severely impaired clients have the capacity to assist counsel must be assessed on a case-by-case basis.

21. Should a clinician be trained in forensic psychiatry to determine competence to stand trial?

Yes. When clinicians untrained in forensic psychiatry become involved in competence determinations, essential distinctions may be lost. For example, in a prominent murder case (*New Hampshire v. Colbert*, 1992), the suspect was taken to a hospital emergency department. The clinician's finding that the alleged perpetrator was competent to consent to medical treatment was later equated in the courtroom with the suspect's state of mind at the time of the killings. Such extrapolations are clearly unfounded and unreliable. Moreover, when made by the treating clinician in courtroom testimony, they may be both unethical, because they involve a betrayal of the treatment relationship, and prejudicial, insofar as they unduly influence the jury by creating the impression that the accused must be guilty if the treating clinician is willing to testify against his or her own patient.

Of course, the clinician also should be trained to recognize medical conditions that can affect competence.

22. What other issues surround clinician testimony?

Offering testimony over an imprisoned ex-patient's objection may be considered a violation of professional ethics codes—from that of the American Medical Association to the Hippocratic Oath and the Nuremberg Code—governing duties toward captive patients.

Of course, the clinician whose testimony is compelled by court order must conform to the requirements of the law, but the clinician should clarify (through prior notification) the limits of his or her testimony. The treating clinician can testify only to fact: the primary focus on alleviating the patient's suffering precludes an objective, expert opinion. A referral to colleagues qualified to render an objective opinion may be helpful. Given such prior notification, the court usually is satisfied simply to receive the medical records in lieu of testimony.

23. Why should a person's competence to confess be assessed?

Competence to confess may be vitiated by mental disabilities produced by disorders such as psychotic depression, post-traumatic stress disorder, schizotypal personality, obsessive-compulsive disorder, and organic brain syndromes. After hours of hostile questioning, a person who is cognitively competent but made vulnerable by a major mental illness (e.g., schizophrenia, major depression) may come to "remember" committing a crime that he or she did not, in fact, commit. In Florida, for example, a schizophrenic man spent 9 years in prison for a double murder to which he had falsely confessed. False confessions typically are elicited by coercion and subsequent fear, combined with a conscious or unconscious need to be punished. False confessions also may result from false memory syndrome.

24. Define false memory syndrome.

False memory syndrome often is engendered by overzealous clinicians who cross the boundary between clinical assessment and forensic evaluation—for example, in allegations of child sexual abuse during custody proceedings. Patients who suffer from immature defenses such as hypochondriasis, conversion hysteria (somatization), splitting (dividing people into saints and sinners), and projection (misattributing to others all personal feelings that are unacceptable to oneself) are especially vulnerable to suggestion by the treating clinician. Such patients often attempt to figure out and then conform to the working hypothesis used by the treating clinician to guide treatment.

Memories—whether reported to a therapist, an attorney, or a courtroom—cannot be accepted as accurate without a careful forensic evaluation of their reliability. People in a state of emotional distress readily remember events that did not occur or forget events that did occur. The pressure to repress traumatic memories or to re-establish control by filling in the gaps in memory is too great for reported memories to be taken at face value. Reported memories may be accurate in general outline but inaccurate in detail or vice versa. They may be further distorted by suggestion and even coaching (by therapists, family members, attorneys, or law enforcement personnel) as well as by a need to maintain a close personal attachment by confirming the other person's construction of past events.

25. What other factors may affect memory?

The possibility of deliberate falsification of memory must be considered. The malingering offender who has not been treated is usually more transparent than the one who has had a chance to practice his or her act during treatment. For example, the forensic psychiatric examiner's finding of multiple personality disorder in an untreated examinee may be prima facie more valid than the same finding in a treated examinee. In addition to possible faking, malingering, or exaggerating, the examiner must consider impairments of memory resulting from displacement (to maintain psychic equilibrium), projection (to maintain self-esteem), or the effects of organic conditions, drugs, or personality disorders.

26. What is criminal responsibility in relation to the insanity defense?

State statutes may apply some variation of the following historical standards to establish criminal responsibility:

• The *M'Naghten* **rule** excuses a defendant who, by virtue of a defect of reason or disease of the mind, does not know the nature and quality of the act or that the act is wrong.

• The *Durham* **rule** excuses a defendant whose conduct is the product of mental disease or defect.

• The **American Law Institute test** excuses a defendant who, because of a mental disease or defect, lacks substantial capacity to appreciate the criminality (wrongfulness) of his or her conduct or to conform his or her conduct to the requirements of the law.

• The **Federal Insanity Defense Reform Act** of 1984 excuses a defendant who, "as a result of a severe mental disease or defect, was unable to appreciate the nature and quality or the wrongfulness of his acts."

Of these tests, the *Durham* rule is broadest in application, the *M'Naghten* rule narrowest. The permissive *Durham* rule, although important historically, is now used only in New Hampshire and the Virgin Islands and is generally referred to as the "product of mental illness" test. The American Law Institute test represents an effort to find a middle ground by adding the element of volition to the cognitive standard established by the *M'Naghten* rule. The Federal Insanity Defense Reform Act, by removing the volitional element, essentially reverts to the *M'Naghten* standard. However, although specifying that the mental illness must be "severe," it retains the ALI's term "appreciate," thus allowing the primarily cognitive test to be interpreted as including an affective component.

27. How valid is the public concern that the insanity defense lets dangerous criminals go free?

Especially in the highly publicized cases like that of presidential assailant John Hinckley, the insanity defense is used by its critics as a symbol of the failings of the criminal justice system. However, it is not a cause of such failings. In an eight-state review, the insanity defense was used in only 1% of felony cases and was successful in only 25% of those cases. Indeed, from the point of view of public safety, it may be more effective to treat perpetrators in secure psychiatric facilities than to put them in prison, where they do not have the benefit of treatment and tend to return to the street sooner. In addition, they may become victims of predatory career criminals and/or (because they often are easily impressionable) imitate them. The high rates of recidivism among previously incarcerated offenders offer little comfort to critics who would abolish the insanity defense.

The reality is that, partly because of the widespread fear (promoted by sensationalistic journalism) of letting vicious criminals go free, the insanity defense is rarely successful in contested cases. Emotionally evocative characteristics of both victims and perpetrators reduce the likelihood that an insanity defense will be considered nonprejudicially. The Hinckley verdict was the exception, not the rule.

28. What other factors contribute to the difficulty in persuading juries to accept the insanity defense?

Insanity pleas are more frequently agreed upon by the prosecution and defense than contested. Largely out of public view, a stipulated "not guilty by reason of insanity" (NGRI) verdict is reached in many cases (more than 80% in one Oregon study) in which the question of sanity is raised. In other cases experts from the two sides agree that the defendant does not meet the jurisdiction's standard of insanity. In the small proportion of cases that actually go to trial—relatively well-publicized cases in which the experts disagree—the popular **stereotype of psychiatry as unscientific** is reinforced. Ironically, the fact that most cases do *not* go to trial (because of the high interrelater reliability with which most psychiatric diagnoses are made) leaves juries with the impression that psychiatrists always disagree. With this impression as a baseline and with two experts in front of them who disagree, jurors naturally tend to disbelieve the field as a whole and deliver a guilty verdict.

Besides having to overcome popular **stereotypes of mental illness** as either fiction or the paradigm of the incoherent "madman," the defense expert faces other difficulties. Prosecution experts characterize complex acts such as concealment as evidence of rational behavior, even when a deeper analysis reveals that such concealment is regressive behavior driven by psychosis. Moreover, defense experts often are hampered by **limited funds**, which make it difficult to budget both a comprehensive forensic evaluation and the time needed for preparation of testimony to rebut a prosecution expert's negative findings. Finally, **gender- and relationship-specific stereotypes**, which predispose juries to deliver NGRI verdicts for women who kill their children or for children who kill their parents, result in guilty verdicts for men who kill.

29. What is diminished capacity?

There are two kinds of diminished capacity:

1. An element of the charged crime is negated by showing that the defendant lacked the requisite mental state to be found guilty of the crime as charged. This defense, when successful, usually results in a conviction on a lesser charge rather than outright acquittal. For example, a person found to have lacked the mental state necessary to commit first-degree murder (i.e., premeditation) may be convicted of second-degree murder. For a person found to have lacked the intent to kill, the charge may be reduced to involuntary manslaughter.

2. A partial insanity defense that is not concerned with whether the defendant entertained a particular mental state is mounted. It addresses why and how the defendant was in a state of mind that precluded full responsibility for his or her actions. Again, reduction of charges is more likely than dismissal. This variant of diminished capacity resembles the insanity defense in that it provides a basis for extenuation (albeit a controversial one), even if all the elements of the charged crime have been proved. It often centers on impaired decision making resulting from post-traumatic stress disorder and its numerous offshoots, such as battered woman syndrome. It raises the question of both intrapsychic and interpersonal capacity. Typically, a person in an oppressive relationship believes options are limited. For example, a battered woman who kills her abusive partner may argue that sustained abuse left her feeling that "she had no other choice."

30. How is the claim of diminished capacity used?

In the current climate, the claim of diminished capacity is more likely to lead to just dispute resolution than the insanity defense. Given the limited applicability of the insanity defense and the odds against it prevailing in court, diminished capacity is used with increasing frequency as a flexible (if partial) alternative, filling the need for some assessment of a defendant's mental state as a factor in criminal responsibility.

Diminished capacity also is taken into account in the application of the new federal sentencing guidelines, which, after guilt has been determined, allow departure from otherwise mandated sentences if diminished capacity can be shown. Some states—for example, New Jersey—also have adopted this approach to sentencing.

31. Do considerations of diminished capacity form the basis for a claim of imperfect self-defense?

Imperfect self-defense is a prime example of the second variant of diminished capacity. To support a claim of imperfect self-defense, data about the defendant's state of mind at the time of the alleged crime must include the perception that the act was an act of self-defense. For example, a Vietnam war veteran who hears a truck backfire while he is arguing with another driver after a traffic accident may react as if he were under fire. Such a "false-alarm syndrome" may constitute the basis of an imperfect self-defense claim.

32. Are conditions such as battered-woman syndrome, rape trauma syndrome, child sexual abuse accommodation syndrome, and patient-therapist sex syndrome now recognized as legitimate bases for a defense of diminished capacity?

Expert testimony about battered-woman syndrome is admitted with increasing frequency in criminal cases. The courts also are grappling with the admissibility of other such syndromes. Descriptively, all of these labels have some basis in experience. Women are at serious risk of domestic violence, for example, and such abuse (like rape or sexual exploitation in therapy) has traumatic effects.

Nevertheless, reliance on putative abuse and trauma syndromes presents serious pitfalls both for the treating psychiatrist and for the expert psychiatric witness. Such diagnoses are not recognized in the Diagnostic and Statistical Manual–IV (DSM–IV) and do not take the place of other diagnoses. They raise questions of unreliability of evidence (including false memories), stereotyping, and stigmatization. Labeling people as victims does not allow for the enormous range of reactions to adversity of which people are capable. It is necessary, therefore, to evaluate each case individually rather than to assume an a priori syndrome.

For example, patient-therapist sex syndrome is merely a hypothetical, schematic construction. A victim of such abuse in fact may suffer from any or all of the claimed symptoms, but each individual case requires careful examination to determine which, if any, of the symptoms are present. Moreover, the presence of such symptoms is not by itself proof that the specifically alleged trauma in fact took place.

33. What other mental disorders affect criminal responsibility?

Psychosis, by whatever diagnosis or etiology, is the mental disorder that most commonly serves as a basis for an insanity defense. In addition, people with **organic brain syndromes** may fail to make the connection between actions and consequences. **Multiple-personality disorder** also needs to be ruled out.

Court decisions in different jurisdictions have been inconsistent about voluntary **intoxication** as an extenuating factor. In general, mental impairment resulting from either acute voluntary intoxication or chronic substance abuse may result in some degree of diminished capacity, but not in acquittal by reason of insanity. An insanity defense, on the other hand, may be successful in cases of involuntary intoxication, delirium tremens, idiosyncratic intoxication, unpredictable variations in tolerance, or permanent psychosis (such as Korsakoff's psychosis) due to chronic alcohol use.

34. List the steps to follow in conducting a forensic psychiatric assessment.

There is no simple formula for conducting a forensic psychiatric assessment; the method of examination must be tailored to the person being examined and to the factual and legal questions at issue. Although a forensic psychiatrist may be asked to assess a person's *current* functioning (as in a disability evaluation), usually the request entails reconstruction of a *prior* mental state. Such an examination is akin to filling in a crossword puzzle; data from the events in question are merged with data from the present examination.

35. Are there general guidelines for performing a forensic psychiatric assessment?

The examiner must maintain objectivity, conducting the examination with an openness to evidence and an attitude of informed skepticism. A proper assessment is always an in-depth process and often an extended one. Typically, it includes multiple interviews of the examinee, interviews with others involved in the case, and review of other relevant data such as depositions, police and medical reports, and audiotape and videotape; when appropriate, site visits are made. If needed, the examiner may request additional specialized medical consultations and testing, such as a sleep/awake electroencephalograph, which may reveal an underlying seizure disorder. Such data are analyzed with a view toward internal coherence, subtle verbal and nonverbal cues, and corroboration of the examinee's story by other evidence.

As noted in the AAPL ethical guidelines, "An evaluation for forensic purposes begins with notice to the evaluee of any limitation on confidentiality." This so-called Lamb warning serves not only to set the stage for proceeding ethically with a forensic evaluation, but also to prepare the evaluee for hearing a report of the results, as in the context of distressing courtroom testimony.

36. Can hypnosis serve as a useful check on the unreliability of an examinee's memories of key events?

Given the heightened suggestibility of hypnotized subjects, *under no circumstances* should memories uncovered during hypnosis be considered reliable, especially in criminal cases. Hypnosis decreases the examinee's autonomy; instead, strive to enhance autonomy—for example, by allowing a portion of the interview to be unstructured and associational. Confrontation has a place, but not to the extent that the examinee will say anything to decrease the anxiety induced by the interview. Advanced training in modes of forensic examination—including the recognition of countertransference, avoidance of accidentally conveying subtle cues and suggestions, creation of an atmosphere conducive to open communication, and use of unstructured interview techniques—helps to build expertise in data gathering and evaluation of memories.

37. How useful is psychological testing in the forensic psychiatric assessment?

In selected cases, psychological testing provides useful corroborative evidence, but only if it is used appropriately as an adjunct to—not a substitute for—forensic psychiatric examination. Because testing may disrupt the working alliance needed for the forensic examination, it should occur (when indicated) after, rather than before, the examination. Tests must be carefully administered by the examiner to minimize invalid results driven by anxiety, fatigue, reading difficulty, or misunderstanding. Moreover, test results require careful interpretation because: (1) a person's state of mind at the time of testing is not necessarily the same as the person's state of mind at the time of the events in question; (2) the results obtained in the forensic context may be invalidated by anxiety and confusion or by attempted manipulation.

38. Can dreams provide reliable data for medicolegal purposes?

Asking the examinee to communicate dreams (as well as memories, thoughts, and feelings) may yield useful data, but only in the context of a comprehensive forensic psychiatric examination by a psychoanalytically informed examiner with sufficient training and experience. By listening skeptically but carefully to everything communicated by the examinee, including dreams, the forensic psychiatrist gains the required entry into an examinee's internal reality. Dreams cannot be taken as a representation of literal truth; nor can the dream as communicated be assumed to be the dream as dreamt. Rather, one must listen to the dream as one would to any other communication: At what point in the examination was it communicated? Was it communicated spontaneously or at the examiner's inquiry? What associations preceded and followed it? What was the accompanying affect?

39. How might dreams be indicative of an examinee's credibility?

Dream communications may contribute to overall assessment of an examinee's credibility, because dreams are hard to fake. People are much more practiced at lying and exaggerating about waking events than about dreams. Specifically, after a genuine trauma (but not a fabricated one), dreams tend to progress from direct representations of the experience to more and more disguised versions. Likewise, the natural progression of emotional reactions in the wake of trauma typically runs from anxiety to depression, whereas a person who is embellishing may emphasize one reaction but not the other.

40. Does the presence or absence of dreams have meaning?

In DSM-IV, "recurrent distressing dreams" are listed as a possible diagnostic indicator of posttraumatic stress disorder (PTSD). Although vivid dream imagery is sometimes evidence of trauma, as in PTSD, it also may be a manifestation of an underlying hysterical personality disorder or simply a personal characteristic with no diagnostic significance. At the other extreme, the absence of dreams may be significant. For example, a man who had been in an airplane crash reported vivid dreams until the night preceding the anniversary of the crash, at which time he said that he simply felt terrified but had no dreams. Such a detail enables the examiner to explore further the impact of a major life event.

41. In what other ways are dreams helpful?

Even when dreams are not reported, it may be worthwhile to inquire about them, especially in the case of people who are not psychologically minded and, at the extreme, alexythymic. Both characteristics may occur as a result of trauma. When a person has difficulty with expressing feelings, whether for reasons of personality, trauma, or the public nature of the forensic examination, dreams may be a useful vehicle for exploring the examinee's psychic functioning.

42. How does countertransference affect the assessment?

An awareness of how your own reactions color assessment of another person is essential, regardless of your subspecialty (e.g., psychopharmacology) or mode or school of treatment. In psychoanalytic terms, this dynamic process is called countertransference. It operates primarily through the mechanisms of projection and identification. You may project your own competence or incompetence, either in general or in a particular relationship, onto the person being examined. Such projection, as well as overidentification, may affect the assessment of competence in any area discussed in this chapter.

43. What is positive countertransference?

Positive countertransference occurs when you assess an examinee uncritically—especially an examinee with whom you overidentify on the basis of similar demographic or personal characteristics—because you wish to see the examinee as healthy and self-sufficient. A desire to protect the examinee from distress may lead you to avoid exploring emotionally charged areas in which the examinee may be found incompetent. Likewise, a justifiable concern to avoid stigmatization may divert attention from areas of real incompetence.

44. What is negative countertransference?

Negative countertransference occurs when you find a person competent out of a desire to maintain control and to protect yourself and society from the person's dissembling—so that the defendant, for example, will not "get away with" the crime. On the other hand, you may inaccurately assess someone as incompetent because of failure to establish a communicative alliance for the purposes of the assessment. In this case, the denial of your helplessness to establish such an alliance may result in projecting the incompetence of the alliance onto the examinee.

45. What specific countertransference dangers should be watched for by the examiner?

The examiner who is retained by one party in a legal action may be susceptible to any of several typical countertransference reactions. It is relatively easy to recognize identification with the attorney (plaintiff, prosecution, or defense) who has retained your services. More subtle is the reaction-formation by which you identify with the opposing side. A most insidious (yet common) tendency, especially in response to an anxiety-provoking examinee, is to remove yourself to the safe ground of being the judge. Such detachment may take the form of false certainty in the face of confusing and ambiguous data.

46. What other factors may affect the assessment of criminal responsibility?

The assessment may be biased by "false sanity" resulting from the use of psychotropic drugs or from the setting in which the examination takes place. It is difficult to recognize psychotic states in examinees who have recompensated through medication, psychotherapy, tincture of time, removal from the stressful setting of the events in question, or placement in a structured medical or correctional setting. Conducting an examination in a jail or prison may either mask or induce psychosis, depending on whether the examinee experiences the facility as supportive or stressful. Other factors that may bias the assessment include a restricted emphasis on the appearance of the criminal act (e.g., planning, flagrancy, concealment, flight) without due regard to the psychological facts (e.g., people who are in the midst of a paranoid psychosis often flee or conceal without the requisite intent to obstruct justice).

47. Do special issues arise in the assessment of competence and criminal responsibility in children?

Yes. Common areas of competence assessment in children include consent to medical care, such as abortion, and emancipation of minors. In a clearcut instance of the interpersonal dimension of competence, the family must be included in assessments that involve a child or adolescent.

Age also is taken into account in the assessment of criminal responsibility. Age may be an absolute legal barrier to criminal responsibility, as in a state in which children under a certain age are considered incapable of forming the intent to kill. Age also may be a relative barrier in terms of a particular child's capacity to think and make decisions independently.

48. Does competence assessment play a part in product liability suits?

Yes. The forensic psychiatrist may be asked to review package inserts and warning labels or signs with an understanding of how people make choices about potentially dangerous products. Questions of cognitive awareness and affective maturity arise in assessing a person's capacity to assume the risk of using such a product. In the case of children, such questions commonly arise with respect to toys and playground equipment.

49. Do indigent defendants have a right to a court-appointed forensic psychiatric expert in cases in which mental status may be a factor in determining guilt?

According to the U.S. Supreme Court in the landmark case *Ake v. Oklahoma* (1985), indigent defendants have this right. There is no substitute for a forensic psychiatric evaluation in gathering and interpreting the data needed to determine criminal responsibility. Therefore, recourse to such expertise is essential to a fair trial in cases in which mental status may be relevant.

In practice, however, access to court-appointed psychiatric expertise often is restricted in ways that compromise both the expert's independence and the defendant's right to due process. It has been proposed, therefore, that any indigent defendant who shows a reasonable need for forensic expertise be provided with a private psychiatrist of his or her own choosing who is paid for, but not controlled by, the state. At present, this entitlement must be advocated for, both in individual cases and at the policy level.

Note that the forensic psychiatrist must be aware of the dangers of performing an incomplete evaluation because of limited funds. If such a limited evaluation is unavoidable, it should be acknowledged in the psychiatrist's report and/or testimony.

50. How important is an understanding of ethical issues in the practice of forensic psychiatry?

Such an understanding is essential. The AAPL Ethical Guidelines for the Practice of Forensic Psychiatry consider much of what has been discussed in this chapter from an explicitly ethical perspective, with a view toward distinguishing between the methods of forensic and clinical assessment. In forensic psychiatric practice, issues of competence, consent, and responsibility frequently are intertwined with the ethical and epistemologic issues surrounding agency, autonomy, authenticity, and moral choice. Therefore, it often is useful to seek not only collegial ethical consultation with practicing forensic psychiatrists but also consultation with a trained ethicist for a transdisciplinary perspective.

51. What recent and forthcoming Supreme Court decisions are likely to affect general and forensic psychiatric practice with respect to the determination of competence?

Recent Supreme Court decisions in areas ranging from the Americans with Disabilities Act (ADA) to sexual harassment have emphasized the competence of both the plaintiff and the defendants in judging whether a plaintiff's claim or a defendant's accommodation response is "reasonable" (*Olmstead vs. L.C*, 1999).*

• For plaintiffs, whether a claim is reasonable under the ADA is considered in terms of how competence-impairing a given disorder is with respect to social and work function. For defendants, the determination of whether an accommodation for a worker's disability is reasonable may involve raising as a defense the question of whether competent medical and mental-health care has been provided. The latter may have far-reaching implications for managed-care organizations.

• In cases of sexual harassment (*Oncale v. Sundowner Offshore Services, Inc., et al.*, 1998), the determination of whether an employee's perception was reasonable may rest in part on factors impairing the employee's competence to perceive reasonably. A company's competent preventive measures (e.g., in hiring, training, and supervision) and responses to harassment claims are available affirmative defenses.

• The importance of competence as a factor in health law is highlighted by a recent Supreme Court decision bearing upon the standards for emergency care and transfer, which underscored the need for engaging in an informed-consent process with patients in cases where economic factors play a major role in influencing care (*Roberts v. Galen of Virginia, Inc.*, 1999).

• Finally, given the Supreme Court's reaffirmation of a "reliable and relevant" standard for all expert testimony (*Daubert v. Merrell Dow Pharmacetuicals, Inc.*, 1993; *Kumho Tire Co. v. Carmichael*, 1999), it is likely that general psychiatrists wishing to subspecialize in forensic psychiatry will find it helpful to reinforce their training and experience with relevant psychodynamically informed perspectives (gleaned from the literature, colleagues, and so forth) regarding the varieties of "competencies," as applied to both the individual and the organizational environment.

---

* For further information on the cases cited here, including links to complete case texts, please see Dr. Bursztajn's website (http://www.forensic-psych.com).

ACKNOWLEDGMENTS

Phillip J. Resnick and Robert I. Simon contributed highly detailed comments on this chapter, some of which were incorporated essentially verbatim into the text. James C. Beck, Thomas G. Gutheil, Mark J. Mills, Herbert C. Modlin, Jonas R. Rappeport, and Larry H. Strasburger also contributed close readings that much improved the final draft. Alan A. Stone's thought-provoking lectures on the aftermath of the Hinckley verdict and, more recently, Alan M. Dershowitz's exposition of the imperfect self-defense have been most useful. Patricia M. L. Illingworth provided an invaluable perspective on an ethical framework for psychiatric and legal issues. Buz Scherr illuminated with helpful clarity the distinction between "simple intent" and "specific intent" crimes. None of these generous advisers, however, should be held responsible for anything with which readers may disagree.

BIBLIOGRAPHY

1. Bursztajn HJ, Brodsky A: Captive patients, captive doctors: Clinical dilemmas and interventions in caring for patients in managed health care. Gen Hosp Psychiatry 21:239–248, 1999.
2. Bursztajn HJ, Brodsky A: Ethical and legal dimensions of benzodiazepine prescription: A commentary. Psychiatr Annals 28:121–128, 1998.
3. Bursztajn HJ, Brodsky A: A new resource for managing malpractice risks in managed care. Arch Intern Med 156:2057–2063, 1996.
4. Bursztajn HJ, Harding HP, Gutheil TG, Brodsky A: Beyond cognition: The role of disordered affective states in impairing competence to consent to treatment. Bull Am Acad Psychiatry Law 19:383–388, 1991.
5. Bursztajn HJ, Scherr AE, Brodsky A: The rebirth of forensic psychiatry in light of recent historical trends in criminal responsibility. Psychiatr Clin North Am 17:611–635, 1994.
6. Forensic Psychiatry & Medicine website: http://www.forensic-psych.com
7. Grisso T, Appelbaum PS: Assessing Competence to Consent to Treatment: A Guide for Physicians and Other Health Professionals. New York, Oxford University Press, 1998.
8. Group for the Advancement of Psychiatry, Committee on Psychiatry and Law: The Mental Health Professional and the Legal System (Report No. 131). New York, Brunner/Mazel, 1991.
9. Parry J (ed): State Justice Institute Benchbook on Psychiatric and Psychological Evidence. Chicago, American Bar Association, 1998.
10. Perlin ML: Mental Disability Law: Civil and Criminal. Charlottesville, VA, Michie, 1989–1993.
11. Rosner R (ed): Principles and Practice of Forensic Psychiatry. New York, Chapman & Hall, 1994.
12. Stone AA: Law, Psychiatry, and Morality. Washington, DC, American Psychiatric Press, 1984.

84. ETHICS AND THE DOCTOR–PATIENT RELATIONSHIP

Claire Zilber, M.D.

The regimen I adopt shall be for the benefit of my patients according to my ability and judgment, and not for their hurt or any wrong. . . . Whatsoever house I enter, there will I go for the benefit of the sick, refraining from all wrongdoing or corruption, and especially from any act of seduction, male or female.

Oath of Hippocrates

1. What is a fiduciary relationship?

The Hippocratic oath expresses the essence of the fiduciary relationship between a physician and each of his patients. The physician has a duty to act in the patient's best interest and to refrain from exploiting the patient. Respecting the fiduciary relationship and the trust of the patient is a cornerstone of the ethical physician's practice.

2. What is a boundary violation?

In the context of the physician–patient relationship, a boundary violation refers to any behavior on the part of a physician that transgresses the limits of the professional relationship. Boundary violations have the potential to exploit or harm patients. Boundary *violations* differ from boundary *crossings,* which occur whenever the patient–physician interaction goes beyond the usual therapeutic framework but is not necessarily harmful to a patient. For example, if a therapist happens to encounter a patient in a social setting, that is a boundary crossing—but it is neither harmful nor unethical as long as the therapist does not violate confidentiality. However, if the therapist plans to meet the patient for dinner, it is a boundary violation.

The potential areas of exploitation include personal or social boundary violations, business relationships, and sexual activity. Examples of personal or social boundary violations include seeing patients in unorthodox settings for the convenience of the physician, loaning a patient money, or burdening the patient with personal information. Business ventures with a patient or taking advantage of insider information revealed by the patient are examples of unethical business relationships. Any form of sexual activity with a patient is a clear boundary violation.

3. A patient is looking for financial investors in a project that promises to be lucrative, and he invites the physician to invest in the project. May the physician ethically participate? The same patient gives a hot stock tip. Is it ethical to act on it?

The ethical physician will not take advantage of either of these scenarios. In the first scenario, participation in a business relationship with the patient may harm the patient's treatment. If the business fails, feelings of anger, guilt, or resentment may emerge between the physician and the patient. The physician may lose the objectivity necessary to provide competent and compassionate treatment if he or she resents having lost money as a result of the business venture. The patient may have similar negative feelings that make it difficult to seek help from the physician for medical problems. Even if the business succeeds, the physician is no longer an impartial and objective person for the patient. In the case of psychiatric treatment, the psychiatrist's relative neutrality and abstinence, central to the healing nature of the therapeutic relationship, cannot be preserved if a business relationship exists between the patient and psychiatrist.

In the second scenario, the physician would be "exploiting information furnished by the patient."[10] In addition, by acting on insider information, the physician may be breaking the law, which in itself is unethical behavior.[10] This applies equally to psychiatrists and other physicians.

4. Why is sexual activity with a consenting adult patient considered unethical?

Transference and countertransference are psychiatric concepts that help to explain why sexual activity, even with a consenting patient or former patient, is unethical. **Transference** is a phenomenon of unconscious displacement of earlier relationship experiences and expectations onto the physician and may cause a wide range of feelings in the patient, from rage to love and sexual attraction. **Countertransference** is the corresponding unconscious emotional reaction of the physician to the patient. Transference and countertransference may continue even after the termination of treatment; for this reason, psychiatrists may not ethically enter into a sexual relationship with a former patient, no matter how long ago the treatment ended. Many consider the same dynamics applicable to other medical specialists and would extend the prohibition to all physicians. At present, the proscription against sexual activity with a former patient is unique to psychiatry, but sexual activity with a current patient is generally considered unethical in all fields of medicine.

Sexual activity with a patient damages the healing capacity of psychiatric treatment. One survey of psychiatrists found that 65% of those who had been sexually involved with patients felt that they were in love with the patient, and 92% believed that the patient was in love with them.[4] In fact, such feelings may have had their origins in transference and countertransference; by acting on the feelings rather than working in therapy to understand them, the psychiatrist harms the treatment and the fiduciary relationship. Freud observed that it is deleterious to the patient if countertransference is acted out: "If the patient's advances were returned, it would be a great triumph for her, but a complete defeat of the treatment. . . . The love relationship, in fact, destroys the patient's susceptibility to influence from analytic treatment."[3]

5. Are feelings of sexual attraction toward a patient unethical?

No. Sexual feelings toward a patient are quite common. In one survey, 87% of psychotherapists (95% of men and 76% of women) acknowledged having been sexually attracted to one or more of their patients.[9] It is important not to act on such feelings. It may be helpful to seek supervision in the treatment of these patients to ensure that the sexual countertransference does not impede the treatment.

6. As you discuss a case with a colleague, she tells you that she has been trying a new approach with an emotionally "needy" patient. She has extended the session time beyond the customary 45 minutes, seeing him at the end of the day for $1\frac{1}{2}$ hours. She also begins and ends each session with a hug, which she feels is necessary to assure the patient of her care and concern. Is this behavior ethical?

This psychiatrist is sliding down the slippery slope of boundary crossings, but she probably has not yet behaved in an unethical manner. Sexual transgressions frequently are preceded by such boundary crossings. Although some may say that no sexual activity has occurred, others may see the hugs as sexual. It is difficult to know whether the patient experiences the hugs as sexual. Even without the hugs, the circumstances under which the physician is seeing the patient are unorthodox and may harm the treatment. The psychiatrist is also at risk for a formal ethical complaint and a lawsuit. Fifteen percent of lawsuits against psychiatrists involve sexual boundary violations.[11]

7. A patient has just informed the physician of a plan to kill someone. The physician wants to ensure the other person's safety, but also is concerned about confidentiality. What may the physician ethically do?

The Principles of Medical Ethics direct physicians to "safeguard patient confidence within the constraints of the law."[10] The law requires the physician to warn the person at risk or to intervene so that no harm may be done. The ethical physician discloses only the information that is necessary and relevant to the situation. Fantasy material, sexual orientation, or other sensitive information usually does not need to be disclosed. The welfare and privacy of the patient should still be protected as much as possible.

Whenever possible, it is preferable to involve the patient in the ethical dilemma that the physician faces. For example, by working with the homicidal patient, the physician may be able to obtain a release of information from the patient to warn the person at risk or to persuade the patient to accept hospitalization until the homicidal ideation subsides. If the homicidal patient will not cooperate with the physician's efforts to ensure the safety of all involved, the physician is legally obligated to warn the person at risk.

8. A patient has been repeatedly resistant to treatment. He has missed numerous appointments, has not been following treatment recommendations, and is abrasive when the physician raises concerns about such behavior. Frustrated, the physician suggests that the patient seek treatment with someone else. He retorts, "I hired you to be my doctor. I can fire you, but you can't fire me!" Is he right?

No. A physician may choose not to treat a patient provided that it is not an emergency and that the physician has provided suitable notice and referrals. Generally, the ethical physician works with the patient to achieve as smooth a transition as possible. *The Principles of Medical Ethics* states, "A physician shall, in the provision of appropriate care, except in emergencies, be free to choose whom to serve, with whom to associate, and the environment in which to provide medical services.[10] If a physician has strong and persistent negative feelings toward a patient, he or she will have difficulty providing objective treatment. Likewise, if a physician feels obligated to treat someone regardless of the circumstances, problems with treatment may arise. As an old maxim advises, *you can't treat someone who you can't not treat.*

9. A physician suspects that a colleague has been abusing alcohol. One morning, while on hospital rounds, the physician smells alcohol on the colleague's breath. Is the physician obligated to take action?

The physician is not obligated, but is strongly encouraged to report impairment in colleagues. According to *The Principles of Medical Ethics*, "Special consideration should be given to those psychiatrists who, because of mental illness, jeopardize the welfare of their patients and their own reputations and practices. It is ethical, even encouraged, for another psychiatrist to intercede in such situations."[10] This ethical principle is easily extended to physicians and other specialties. Furthermore, in some states physicians are mandated to report impaired colleagues to the medical licensing board. The bylaws of most hospitals and health maintenance organizations also require reporting of suspected or proved impairments.

Once reported, impaired physicians are strongly encouraged to enter into treatment. Every effort is made to assist the physician to get help so that he or she may retain medical license and practice. Physicians are often reluctant to report their impaired colleagues because they do not want to be responsible for jeopardizing another doctor's professional practice; in fact, reporting is an excellent way to help impaired colleagues and to facilitate their entry into treatment.

10. A 35-year-old man in the final stages of acquired immunodeficiency syndrome (AIDS) asks for the physician's help. He is in constant pain and homebound, with no appreciable quality of life. He would like to overdose on medications to stop his suffering, but does not have enough of a stockpile to ensure a lethal overdose. He informs the physician of his plan and asks the physician, who sympathizes with his plight, to write a prescription for a lethal dose of narcotics. What may an ethical physician do in this situation?

The Principles of Medical Ethics explicitly states, "A physician shall respect the law and also recognize a responsibility to seek changes in those requirements which are contrary to the best interests of patients. . . . It is conceivable that an individual could violate a law without being guilty of unethical behavior."[10] At present it is illegal to assist in a suicide, although a few states have introduced legislation that would allow physician-assisted suicide. In the above case, the physician may not legally prescribe a lethal dose of narcotics. Many physicians feel strongly that their role is to treat illness and to save lives, not to assist in taking a life. They also raise concerns about the limits of physician-assisted suicide: for whom is it appropriate, who decides it is appropriate, and how is it regulated? The possibility of abuse of the law raises many concerns for physicians who otherwise may have no moral objections to physician-assisted suicide.

Some physicians may disagree with the prohibition against physician-assisted suicide. Such individuals may ethically organize to change the law. *The Principles of Medical Ethics* allows for the possibility that a physician who assists a suicide may be acting ethically, even though the action is illegal.

In fact, many doctors have quietly hastened death in some of their patients with terminal illness, acting on their belief that relieving hopeless suffering is consistent with their role as a physician.

Regardless of a particular physician's stance on the issue of assisted suicide, he or she should do everything else in his or her power to treat the patient's pain and to improve the patient's quality of life. In many instances ameliorable conditions, such as chronic cancer pain, lead patients to seek death. When the pain is treated and the patient feels comforted, suicidal wishes may be alleviated.

ACKNOWLEDGMENT

The author is grateful to David Wahl, M.D., and Michael Weissberg, M.D., for reviewing this chapter.

BIBLIOGRAPHY

1. Appelbaum PS: Statutes regulating patient-therapist sex. Hosp Community Psychiatry 41:15–16, 1990.
2. Carr M, Robinson GE: Fatal attraction: The ethical and clinical dilemma of patient-therapist sex. Can J Psychiatry 35:122–127, 1990.
3. Freud S: Observations on Transference Love (1914), in The Standard Edition of the Complete Psychological Works of Sigmund Freud, Vol. 12. Translated and edited by J. Strachey, London, Hogarth Press, 1958, pp 157–171.
4. Gartrell N, Herman J, Olarte S, et al: Psychiatrist-patient sexual contact: Results of a national survey: I. Prevalence. Am J Psych 143:1126–1131, 1986.
5. Gutheil TG, Gabbard GO: The concept of boundaries in clinical practice: Theoretical and risk-management dimensions. Am J Psychiatry 150:188–196, 1993.
6. Lazarus JA: Sex with former patients almost always unethical. Am J Psychiatry 149:855–857, 1992.
7. Menninger WW, Gabbard GO (eds): Sexual boundary violations. Psychol Am 21:644–680, 1991.
8. Menninger WW: Inappropriate Doctor-patient Relationships. Presented at the Menninger Winter Psychiatry Conference, Park City, Utah, 1993.
9. Pope KS, Keith-Spiegel P, Tabachnick BG: Sexual attraction to clients: The human therapist and the (sometimes) inhuman training system. Am Psychol 41:147–158, 1986.
10. The Principles of Medical Ethics with Annotations Especially Applicable to Psychiatry. Washington, DC, American Psychiatric Association, 1998.
11. Simon R: Clinical Psychiatry and the Law. Washington, DC, American Psychiatric Press, 1987.

INDEX

Page numbers in **boldface type** indicate complete chapters.

503